A Life Course Approach to Women's Health

A Life Course Approach to Adult Health Series

A Life Course Approach to Chronic Disease Epidemiology, Second Edition
Edited by Diana Kuh and Yoav Ben Shlomo
9780198578154

A Life Course Approach to Women's Health
Edited by Diana Kuh and Rebecca Hardy
9780192632890

Epidemiological Methods in Life Course Research
Edited by Andrew Pickles, Barbara Maughan, and Michael Wadsworth
9780198528487

Designing, Analysing and Understanding Family Based Studies in Life Course Epidemiology
Edited by Deborah A Lawlor and Gita D Mishra
9780199231034

A Life Course Approach to Mental Disorders
Edited by Karestan C Koenen, Sasha Rudenstine, Ezra Susser, and Sandro Galea
9780199657018

A Life Course Approach to Healthy Ageing
Edited by Diana Kuh, Rachel Cooper, Rebecca Hardy, Marcus Richards, and Yoav Ben-Shlomo
9780199656516

A Life Course Approach to Women's Health

Second Edition

Editors

Gita D Mishra

Director, Australian Women and Girl's Health Research Centre, Professor of Life Course Epidemiology, School of Public Health, The University of Queensland, Brisbane, Australia

Rebecca Hardy

Professor of Epidemiology and Medical Statistics, School of Sport, Exercise and Health Sciences, Loughborough University, Loughborough, UK

Diana Kuh

Emeritus Professor of Life Course Epidemiology, MRC unit for Lifelong Health and Ageing, University College London, London, UK

Consultant Editor

Anna Murray

Professor of Human Genetics, Department of Clinical and Biomedical Sciences, University of Exeter, Exeter, UK

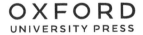

OXFORD
UNIVERSITY PRESS

OXFORD
UNIVERSITY PRESS

Great Clarendon Street, Oxford, OX2 6DP,
United Kingdom

Oxford University Press is a department of the University of Oxford.
It furthers the University's objective of excellence in research, scholarship,
and education by publishing worldwide. Oxford is a registered trade mark of
Oxford University Press in the UK and in certain other countries

First Edition published in 2002
Second Edition published in 2023

Published in the United States of America by Oxford University Press
198 Madison Avenue, New York, NY 10016, United States of America

British Library Cataloguing in Publication Data

Data available

Library of Congress Control Number: 2022951899

ISBN 978–0–19–286464–2

DOI: 10.1093/oso/9780192864642.001.0001

Printed and bound in the UK by
TJ Books Limited

For Gita's late babu and ma,
for Rebecca's daughter Abby,
and for Diana's granddaughter Martha

Preface

Gita D. Mishra, Rebecca Hardy, and Diana Kuh

Two decades have passed since publication of the first edition of *A Life Course Approach to Women's Health* in 2002, the second text in this ground-breaking Life Course Epidemiology Series. That book addressed core questions on the extent to which life course models provide explanations for disease outcomes across life, and their relevance in understanding the future health of women. It highlighted the epidemiologic evidence on the long-term importance of fetal and childhood experience in the development of common chronic diseases and disorders that pose the main threats to physical and mental health in midlife and beyond. Reviewers both recognised the text as a major contribution to the field and recommended it as essential reading for anyone with an interest in women's health. Since then, and particularly over the last decade, we have seen extraordinary gains in the evidence on women's health across the life course and advances in methodology and analytical techniques. In some cases, this has opened up new fields of research, such as in the emerging area of integrative omics, that would barely have been conceivable at the time of original publication. So, this second edition not only has a wealth of new material and novel topics to cover, but also much to live up to in the process. That being the case, its aim remains essentially the same: to provide an up-to-date and comprehensive review of scientific evidence and methodological developments in life course epidemiology as applied to women's health.

The editors share a long-term interest in childhood influences on adult health that intersected in the early 2000s with our collaborative work on the Medical Research Council National Survey of Health and Development (NSHD), also known as the 1946 British Birth Cohort. This is a prospective longitudinal study of over 5000 women and men who have been followed up since their birth in England, Scotland, and Wales in March 1946. Our interest in women's health in midlife was stimulated by the information we collected from the women in this cohort about their health and social experiences during the menopause transition. Since then, NSHD and other cohort studies have matured to the extent that it allows research, increasingly using big data from across these cohorts on many of the chronic conditions of older age, including cardiovascular disease, chronic obstructive pulmonary disease (COPD), and dementia. One of the constant sources of interest is how the health and well-being of women relate in all kinds of expected and novel ways to their life history, in particular the arc of women's reproductive characteristics from menarche to menopause. It is with this shared perspective that we invited 50 researchers working on women's health and well-being from diverse fields to contribute to this new edition.

This text includes a range of topics not covered previously that reflect the focus of recent research, advances in technology, and the evolving nature of the field with its application in practice and policy. We have included new chapters on endometriosis, lung function, cognition, gynaecological cancer, integrative omics, structural sexism, violence, health service use, and Knowledge Translation. Even for topics covered in the original edition, the update and review reveal the substantial progress in women's health research. As previously, each chapter reflects the views of individual authors, within a common life course framework to provide a consistent approach across the book. This conceptual framework is summarised in the introductory chapter, with an outline of each topic covered. Key findings, common themes, and theoretical and methodological challenges are highlighted in the concluding chapter.

For us as the editors, this book has been an exciting and tremendous challenge, particularly considering the COVID-19 pandemic which spread just as our contributors began to engage in writing their first draft. We, therefore, have immense gratitude for our contributors and all their hard work despite the difficulties. In the end, it has been a privilege to edit the text, and we have all gained an enormous amount from doing so. We acknowledge the contribution of our consultant editor, Professor Anna Murray, for her crucial expertise in genetics and related fields. We are also grateful to Dr Hsiu-Wen Chan, who has provided invaluable and meticulous assistance in the final stages of assembling the chapters as a coherent body of work. Finally, special thanks are extended to our families, friends, and colleagues who have been so supportive of our involvement in this project.

Acknowledgements

The authors would like to thank the following for permission to reproduce published material:

Figure 8.1 reproduced from Bui DS, Lodge, CJ, Burgess JA, et al. Childhood predictors of lung function trajectories and future COPD risk: a prospective cohort study from the first to the sixth decade of life. *Lancet Respir Med.* 2018;6(7):535–44, by permission from Elsevier. Figure 8.2 reproduced from Jenkins CR, Chapman KR, Donohue JF, et al. Improving the management of COPD in women. *Chest.* 2017;151:686–96, by permission from Elsevier. Figure 15.2 reproduced from Mishra GD, Ben-Shlomo Y, and Kuh D. 2010. A life course approach to health behaviors: theory and methods. In: Steptoe A, ed. *Handbook of behavioral medicine.* New York: Springer. pp. 525–39, by permission from Springer Nature. Figure 16.1 reproduced from NCD Risk Factor Collaboration (NCD-RisC), 2016. Trends in adult body-mass index in 200 countries from 1975 to 2014: a pooled analysis of 1698 population-based measurement studies with 19·2 million participants. *Lancet.* 387(10026):1377–1396, by Elsevier; Figure 16.2 reproduced from Johnson W, Li L, Kuh D, Hardy R. How has the age-related process of overweight or obesity development changed over time? Co-ordinated analyses of individual participant data from five United Kingdom birth cohorts. *PLoS Medicine.* 2015;12(5):e1001828, with permission from PLoS. Figure 20.2 reproduced from Heise LL. What works to *prevent partner violence? an evidence overview,* published December 2011 with permission from Lori Heise. Figure 20.4 reproduced from World Health Organization. 2018. *Violence against women prevalence estimates, 2018: global, regional and national prevalence estimates for intimate partner violence against women and global and regional prevalence estimates for non-partner sexual violence against women.* Geneva, WHO; published 9 March 2021 with permission from the World Health Organization. Figures 21.1 and 21.3 were reproduced from Stephenson J, Kuh D, Shawe J, et al. *Why should we consider a life-course approach to women's health care?* Scientific Impact Paper No. 27. Royal College of Obstetrics & Gynaecology 2011, with permission from Judith Stephenson.

The authors would also like to thank the following researchers for their contribution: Ms Shamta Warang for her literature review on oral contraception use and type 2 diabetes in Chapter 6; Dr Katrina Moss from the Australian Women and Girls' Health Research Centre at the University of Queensland for contributions on prenatal and early life exposures and assistance with editing and referencing for Chapter 9; and Dr Raisa Cassim at the University of Melbourne for creating Figure 8.3.

Contents

Contributors   xiii

PART I **Introduction**

1 A Life Course Approach to Women's Health   3
   Gita D. Mishra, Diana Kuh, and Rebecca Hardy

PART II **Reproductive health**

2 A Life Course Approach to Women's Reproductive Health   19
   Maria C. Magnus and Abigail Fraser

3 A Life Course Approach to Endometriosis   33
   Gita D. Mishra, Ingrid J. Rowlands, Hsiu-Wen Chan, and Grant W. Montgomery

4 Menopause and Hysterectomy: A Life Course Perspective   49
   Gita D. Mishra, Hsin-Fang Chung, Martha Hickey, Diana Kuh, and Rebecca Hardy

PART III **Health, ageing, and disease**

5 A Life Course Approach to Cardiovascular Disease   73
   Jane A.H. Masoli and Rebecca Hardy

6 A Life Course Approach to Diabetes   93
   Emily Papadimos, Jedidiah Morton, Jessica Harding, and Elizabeth Barr

7 A Life Course Approach to Musculoskeletal Ageing   115
   Rachel Cooper, Kate A. Ward, and Avan Aihie Sayer

8 A Life Course Approach to Lung Function Impairment and COPD   135
   Dinh S. Bui and Shyamali C. Dharmage

9 Depression and Psychological Distress   153
   Barbara Maughan

10 Cognition Function and Dementia: A Life Course Perspective   169
   Erin E. Sundermann, Sarah J. Banks, and Carlos Araujo Menendez

11 The Life Course Epidemiology of Breast Cancer   189
   Lauren C. Houghton, Nancy Potischman, and Rebecca Troisi

12 Gynaecological Cancers: A Life Course Perspective   203
   Susan J. Jordan and Penelope M. Webb

PART IV **Biological and behavioural pathways**

13   Integrative Omics for Women's Health   221
Anna Murray and Katherine S. Ruth

14   Endocrine Pathways Across the Life Course   237
*Marta Bianchini, Alfonsina Chiefari, Rosa Lauretta, Marilda Mormando,
Giulia Puliani, and Marialuisa Appetecchia*

15   A Life Course Perspective on Women's Health Behaviours   257
Hsin-Fang Chung and Gita D. Mishra

16   A Life Course Approach to Body Weight   273
Rebecca Hardy and Laura D. Howe

PART V **Social issues impacting women's health**

17   Life Course Socioeconomic Trajectories and Health   295
Rebecca Hardy

18   Women's Social Relationships and Links with Health and
Well-being over the Life Course   313
Anne McMunn

19   Structural Sexism Across the Life Course: How Social Inequality
Shapes Women's Later-Life Health   327
Jessica A. Kelley and Marissa Gilbert

20   The Influence of Gender-Based Violence Across the Life Course   343
Elizabeth McLindon, Minerva Kyei-Onanjiri, and Kelsey Hegarty

PART VI **From evidence to practice**

21   A Life Course Approach to Women's Health Care   359
Judith Stephenson, Jennifer Hall, and Louise F. Wilson

22   Translating Women's Health Research into Policy and Practice   371
Helen Brown, Stephanie Best, and Trina Hinkley

PART VII **Conclusion**

23   A Life Course Approach to Women's Health: Linking the Past, Present,
and Future   385
Rebecca Hardy, Diana Kuh, and Gita D. Mishra

Index   407

Contributors

Marialuisa Appetecchia
Director, Oncological Endocrinology Unit
IRCCS Regina Elena National Cancer Institute,
Rome, Italy
Email: marialuisa.appetecchia@ifo.it

Sarah J. Banks
Associate Professor and Neuropsychologist,
Department of Neuroscience and Department of
Psychiatry
University of California, San Diego,
California, USA
Email: sbanks@ucsd.edu

Elizabeth Barr
Senior Research Fellow, Division of Wellbeing
and Preventable Chronic Disease
Menzies School of Health Research, Darwin,
Australia
Email: Elizabeth.Barr@menzies.edu.au

Stephanie Best
Associate Professor and Senior Research Lead,
Department of Health Services Research
Peter MacCallum Cancer Centre, Melbourne,
Australia
Email: Stephanie.Best@pctcrmac.org

Marta Bianchini
Medical Doctor, Endocrinologist, Oncological
Endocrinology Unit
IRCCS Regina Elena National Cancer Institute,
Rome, Italy
Email: marta.bianchini@ifo.it

Helen Brown
Senior Lecturer, School of Exercise and Nutrition
Sciences
Deakin University, Melbourne, Australia
Email: h.brown@deakin.edu.au

Dinh S. Bui
Research Fellow, Melbourne School of
Population of Global Health
The University of Melbourne, Melbourne,
Australia
Email: dinh.bui@unimelb.edu.au

Hsiu-Wen Chan
Senior Research Assistant, School of
Public Health
The University of Queensland, Brisbane,
Australia
Email: h.chan4@uq.edu.au

Alfonsina Chiefari
Diabetes Unit
ASL Viterbo, Italy
Email: alfonsinachiefari@gmail.com

Hsin-Fang Chung
Research Fellow, School of Public Health
The University of Queensland, Brisbane,
Australia
Email: h.chung1@uq.edu.au

Rachel Cooper
Professor of Translational Epidemiology, AGE
Research Group, Faculty of Medical Sciences
Newcastle University, Newcastle upon Tyne, UK
Email: rachel.cooper@newcastle.ac.uk

Shyamali C. Dharmage
Professor of Life Course Epidemiology of
Allergies and Chronic Respiratory Diseases
Melbourne School of Population and
Global Health
The University of Melbourne, Melbourne,
Australia
Email: s.dharmage@unimelb.edu.au

Abigail Fraser
Professor of Epidemiology, Population Health
Science, Bristol Medical School
MRC Integrative Epidemiology Unit at the
University of Bristol, Bristol, UK
Email: Abigail.Fraser@bristol.ac.uk

Marissa Gilbert
Doctoral student, Department of Sociology
Case Western Reserve University, Cleveland,
Ohio, USA
Email: mxg557@case.edu

Jennifer Hall
Clinical Associate Professor, Institute for
Women's Health
University College London, London, UK
Email: jennifer.hall@ucl.ac.uk

Jessica Harding
Assistant Professor, Division of Transplantation
Department of Surgery, Emory University School
of Medicine, Atlanta, Georgia, USA
Email: jessica.harding@emory.edu

Rebecca Hardy
Professor of Epidemiology and Medical Statistics,
School of Sport, Exercise and Health Sciences
Loughborough University, Loughborough, UK
Emil: R.J.Hardy@lboro.ac.uk

Kelsey Hegarty
Professor of Family Violence Prevention,
Department of General Practice and Primary
Health Care
The University of Melbourne, Melbourne,
Australia
Centre for Family Violence Prevention, Royal
Women's Hospital, Melbourne Australia
Email: k.hegarty@unimelb.edu.au

Martha Hickey
Professor of Obstetrics and Gynaecology, The
University of Melbourne, Melbourne
Director of the Gynaecology Research Centre,
Royal Women's Hospital, Victoria, Australia
Email: hickeym@unimelb.edu.au

Trina Hinkley
Honorary Fellow, School of Exercise and
Nutrition Sciences
Deakin University, Geelong, Australia
Email: think.research@outlook.com

Lauren C. Houghton
Assistant Professor of Epidemiology, Mailman
School of Public Health
Columbia University, New York, New York, USA
Email: lh2746@columbia.edu

Laura D. Howe
Professor of Epidemiology and Medical Statistics
Bristol Population Health Science Institute,
Bristol Medical School
MRC Integrative Epidemiology Unit, University
of Bristol, Bristol, UK
Email: Laura.Howe@bristol.ac.uk

Susan J. Jordan
Associate Professor of Epidemiology, School of
Public Health
The University of Queensland, Brisbane,
Australia
Email: s.jordan@uq.edu.au

Jessica Kelley
Professor of Sociology, Department of Sociology
Case Western Reserve University, Cleveland,
Ohio, USA
Email: jak119@case.edu

Diana Kuh
Emeritus Professor of Life Course Epidemiology,
MRC Lifelong Health and Ageing
University College London, London, UK
Email: d.kuh@ucl.ac.uk

Minerva Kyei-Onanjiri
Research Fellow, Department of General Practice
and Primary Health Care
The University of Melbourne, Melbourne,
Australia
Email: minerva.kyeionanjiri@unimelb.edu.au

Rosa Lauretta
Medical Doctor, Endocrinologist, Oncological
Endocrinology Unit
IRCCS Regina Elena National Cancer Institute,
Rome, Italy
Email: rosa.lauretta@ifo.it

Maria C. Magnus
Senior Research Associate, Centre for Fertility
and Health
Norwegian Institute of Public Health,
Oslo, Norway
Email: mariachristine.magnus@fhi.no

Jane A.H. Masoli
Consultant in Geriatric Medicine, National
Institute for Health and Care Research Senior
Clinical Research Fellow in Ageing
Faculty of Health and Life Sciences, University of
Exeter, Exeter
Email: J.Masoli@exeter.ac.uk

Barbara Maughan
Professor of Developmental Epidemiology,
Social, Genetic and Developmental
Psychiatry Centre
Kings College London, London, UK
Email: barbara.maughan@kcl.ac.uk

Elizabeth McLindon
Research Fellow, Department of General Practice
and Primary Health Care
The University of Melbourne, Melbourne,
Australia
Centre for Family Violence Prevention, Royal
Women's Hospital, Melbourne Australia
Email: elizabeth.mclindon@unimelb.edu.au

Anne McMunn
Professor of Social Epidemiology, Institute of
Epidemiology & Health Care
University College London, London, UK
Email: a.mcmunn@ucl.ac.uk

Carlos Araujo Menendez
Research Associate, Department of Psychiatry
University of California, San Diego,
California, USA
Email: cearaujo@ucsd.edu

Gita D. Mishra
Director, Australian Longitudinal Study on
Women's Health
Professor of Life Course Epidemiology, School of
Public Health
The University of Queensland, Brisbane,
Australia
Email: g.mishra@uq.edu.au

Grant W. Montgomery
NHMRC Leadership Fellow, Institute for
Molecular Biosciences
The University of Queensland, Brisbane Australia
Email: g.montgomery1@uq.edu.au

Marilda Mormando
Medical Doctor, Endocrinologist, Oncological
Endocrinology Unit
IRCCS Regina Elena National Cancer Institute,
Rome, Italy
Email: marilda.mormando@ifo.it

Jedidiah Morton
PhD candidate, Baker Heart & Diabetes Institute,
Melbourne, Australia
School of Public Health and Preventive Medicine,
Monash University, Clayton, Australia
Email: jedidiah.morton@baker.edu.au

Anna Murray
Professor of Human Genetics, Department of
Clinical and Biomedical Sciences, University of
Exeter, Exeter, UK
Email: A.Murray@exeter.ac.uk

Emily Papadimos
Paediatric Endocrinologist and PhD candidate
Menzies School of Health Research, Darwin,
Australia
Email: emily.papadimos@menzies.edu.au

Nancy Potischman
Nutritional Epidemiologist
Director, Population Studies Program, Office of
Dietary Supplements, Rockville, Maryland, USA
Email: potischn@mail.nih.gov

Giulia Puliani
Medical Doctor, Emdocrinologist, PhD,
Oncological Endocrinology Unit
IRCCS Regina Elena National Cancer Institute,
Rome, Italy
Email: giulia.puliani@ifo.it

Ingrid J. Rowlands
Research Fellow, School of Public Health
The University of Queensland, Brisbane,
Australia
Email: i.rowlands@uq.edu.au

Katherine S. Ruth
Research Fellow, Department of Clinical and
Biomedical Sciences, University of Exeter,
Exeter, UK
Email: K.S.Ruth@exeter.ac.uk

Avan Aihie Sayer
William Leech Professor of Geriatric Medicine,
AGE Research Group, Faculty of Medical
Sciences
Newcastle University, Newcastle upon Tyne, UK
Email: avan.sayer@newcastle.ac.uk

Judith Stephenson
Margaret Pyke Professor of Sexual &
Reproductive Health
University College London, London, UK
Email: judith.stephenson@ucl.ac.uk

Erin E. Sundermann
Assistant Professor of Psychiatry, Department of
Psychiatry
University of California, San Diego, USA
Email: esundermann@ucsd.edu

Rebecca Troisi
Professor and Epidemiologist, Division of Cancer
Epidemiology and Genetics, National Cancer
Institute
National Institutes of Health, Department
of Health and Human Services, Bethesda,
Maryland, USA
Email: Ttroisir@mail.nih.gov

Kate A. Ward
Professor of Global Musculoskeletal Health,
MRC Lifecourse Epidemiology, Centre, Human
Development and Health
University of Southampton, Southampton, UK
Email: kw@mrc.soton.ac.uk

Penelope M. Webb
Professor and Program Director of
Population Health
QIMR Berghofer Medical Research Institute,
Australia
Email: penny.webb@qimrberghofer.edu.au

Louise F. Wilson
Postdoctoral Research Fellow, School of
Public Health
The University of Queensland, Brisbane,
Australia
Email: l.wilson8@uq.edu.au

PART I
INTRODUCTION

1

A Life Course Approach to Women's Health

Gita D. Mishra, Diana Kuh, and Rebecca Hardy

1.1 Introduction and Preview

This second edition of *A Life Course Approach to Women's Health* is part of the Life Course Epidemiology Series from Oxford University Press. The first edition, published in 2002, addressed whether a life course perspective can provide explanations for women's health and disease outcomes across life. The term 'life course epidemiology' was coined in 1997 in the first book in the series, *A Life Course Approach to Chronic Disease Epidemiology*.[1,2] The editors of that founding text, Kuh and Ben-Shlomo, defined *life course epidemiology* as:

> … the study of long-term biological, behavioural and psychosocial processes that link adult health and disease risk to physical or social exposures acting during gestation, childhood, adolescence, earlier or adult life, or across generations.

This definition has stood the test of time and has led to the other texts in the series on methodology,[3] family-based designs,[4] and healthy ageing,[5] and a second edition of the original text.[6] Yet as these books and the growing corpus of scientific papers in the field demonstrate life course epidemiology has continued to evolve. This includes new conceptual developments, methodological innovations, a broadening of health outcomes under investigation, and increased understanding of the biological mechanisms and social pathways linking earlier life risk and protective factors to later life health outcomes.[7]

Women's health, with its fundamental axis of reproductive health and ageing across life, has played a substantial role in the evolution of life course epidemiology over the last two decades. So, the central aim of this new edition is to update and review the scientific evidence and methodological developments in life course epidemiology as applied to women's health. This second edition reviews the new and considerably strengthened body of evidence on the biological and social factors at each stage of life that are linked with major age-related noncommunicable diseases. New chapters address a series of health outcomes not included previously and which have become feasible for investigation as cohort studies have matured to cover older age groups, including dementia and chronic obstructive pulmonary disease (COPD). There is also a new chapter on endometriosis—a complex and debilitating condition that has recently gained research attention. Another covers the emerging field of omics (i.e. the study of the entire complement of genes, proteins, and metabolites) that describes the rapid technological advances in genome sequencing and the proliferation of studies investigating the role of genetic and epigenetic factors influencing women's health. Two new chapters address how emerging scientific knowledge is interpreted and translated to inform

Gita D. Mishra, Diana Kuh, and Rebecca Hardy, *A Life Course Approach to Women's Health* In: *A Life Course Approach to Women's Health*. Second Edition. Edited by: Gita D Mishra, Rebecca Hardy, and Diana Kuh, Oxford University Press. © Oxford University Press 2023.
DOI: 10.1093/oso/9780192864642.003.0001

policy development and preventive health interventions, and how these are codeveloped with specific groups of women.

The European Institute for Gender Equality[8] defines *sex* as referring to:

> Biological and physiological characteristics that define humans as female or male. These sets of biological characteristics are not mutually exclusive, as there are individuals who possess both, but these characteristics tend to differentiate humans as females or males.

They refer to *gender* as 'the social attributes and opportunities associated with being female and male', including 'the relationships between women and men and girls and boys, as well as to the relations between women and those between men'. Their key point is that gender is a social construct that is 'context- and time-specific, and changeable'. In this context, they define *woman* in both biological and gender terms as referring to 'a person assigned as female sex at birth, or a person who defines herself as a woman'.

This book is concerned with both the biological aspects and the implications of societal constructs on women's health. The terms *woman* and *women* are mainly used with the findings typically contrasted with those for men. This binary gender construct reflects the way much of the evidence has been disaggregated to date; for example, survey data collected over decades from cohort studies generally refers to biological sex, rather than self-identified gender. The findings, however, also may be relevant to people from nonbinary and gender-diverse groups who may experience menstrual cycles, pregnancy, endometriosis, and the menopause. These groups also require access to women's health and reproductive services, and this is clearly an area that needs further research to build the evidence base. The evidence presented here on women's health should inform policy and preventive health initiatives that are respectful and responsive to individual needs and are inclusive of those from nonbinary and gender-diverse groups.

1.2 An Introduction to Life Course Epidemiology

A life course approach offers an interdisciplinary framework or orientation for guiding and structuring research on health, human development, and ageing. Epidemiologists were relatively late to adopt this approach compared with researchers from other scientific disciplines, including psychology, sociology, demography, anthropology, and biology (as discussed in Kuh and Davey Smith;[9] Kuh, et al.;[10] and Alwin[11]). Further, many of the initial concepts and ideas in life course epidemiology were borrowed from these other scientific disciplines.

Two areas of public health research led to a revival of interest in a life course epidemiological perspective and its central premise that biological and social factors throughout life independently, cumulatively, and interactively influence health and disease. The first was the seminal work of David Barker and colleagues in the 1980s and 1990s on the fetal origins of adult disease hypothesis which posited that environmental insults, such as undernutrition during critical periods of growth and development in early life, have long-term effects on the risk of cardiovascular and other chronic adult diseases by 'programming' the structure or function of organs, tissues, or body systems.[12] The second was the research from maturing birth cohort studies that revealed long-term effects of early social conditions on adult health that were independent of adult conditions.[13-17] Life course epidemiology extended both these research areas, investigating the long-term effects of growth and development during childhood and adolescence on adult health and disease risk, the drivers and consequences of functional change, and the impact of continuity and change in lifetime lifestyles and social conditions.[7] Over time, there has been a convergence of research interests; for example, the field of developmental origins of health and disease (DOHaD) emerged after 2003, with an increasing focus on evolutionary concepts and the multiple pathways linking developmental factors to later health and resilience.[18] Life course epidemiology has increasingly emphasised the importance of understanding age-related patterns of change in functional capability and biological function, which complement the study of disease outcomes. It is interested in understanding developmental trajectories to provide clues to the early life exposures influencing development of peak function, as well as the influences on the age-related decline.

1.2.1 Life Course Models

The theoretical framework for the focus of life course epidemiology—identifying causal pathways for the observed associations—is based on a series of models. The critical period described above can be thought of as a special case of the more general *sensitive period model*, where the impact of an exposure during a time window, such as adolescence, may have a greater effect than outside that time window. This, in turn, may be seen as a variation on the *accumulation model*, where the effect of each time period of exposure is cumulative; for instance, the time spent in a disadvantaged socioeconomic position or the number of years smoking. While accumulation models have generally been applied to repeated measures of the same exposure over the life course, they were initially conceptualised to consider the accumulation of different exposures and exposures that clustered together. Another type of model is the *chain of risk model*, where a series of linked exposures across each time period led to the outcome being more likely, but where the elimination of one risk factor breaks the chain of risk and the causal mechanism, and the risk is mitigated. Study design or data limitations may mean it is appropriate to assume or hypothesise a specific life course model a priori, though this should be acknowledged and justified by supporting evidence on plausible causal pathways. While these original life course models were represented using simplified causal diagrams, the development of directed acyclic graphs within the causal inference literature has been applied to life course concepts.[19] It can be an analytically challenging process to select the best life course model to provide more rigorous insights. Although the technical details are beyond the scope of this text, the last decade or so has seen the development of innovative statistical methods to identify the life course model that best fits the overall association identified, including mediation analysis, counterfactual frameworks, and Bayesian approaches.[20-24]

More broadly, life course epidemiology investigates the contribution of early life factors jointly with later life risk factors to identify risk and protective pathways across the life course. We need to investigate whether childhood risk factors operate mainly through their effects on conventional adult risk factors, or whether they add independent risk or act interactively with later life factors to affect adult disease. Identification of pathways across the life course may have important policy implications, by highlighting the type and timing of interventions for maximum impact on health. When interpreting such evidence for current policy, however, it is important to consider the extent that the characteristics of the cohort being studied (such as childhood environmental exposures, dietary patterns, and cultural norms) may have changed over time, which can impact the relevance to current generations. Similarly, a major event, such as disruption during wartime, national disasters, or a pandemic (e.g. COVID-19), can have very particular impacts on a cohort. These may be revealing from the perspective of research on the consequences of such exposures but render the evidence of limited direct applicability to current cohorts. These are known as cohort and period effects, respectively.

1.2.2 Women's Health and the Life Course Approach

When the first edition of this book was published, life course epidemiology had studied women less than men, and it is an indicator of how much has changed that this is now arguably no longer the case. Partly the focus on men reflected the original interest in the developmental origins of cardiovascular disease, where little attention was paid to the condition in women. The early postwar cohorts that were set up to investigate the role of proximal risk factors (such as hypertension or diabetes) and aspects of adult lifestyle on cardiovascular disease were generally limited to white middle-aged men.[25] Many cohorts were based on occupation, so in an era when gender disparities in the workplace were even greater than they are today, if women were included in the studies their numbers were often small and they were not representative of the general population. As often happens in research, many of the same cohorts were used for studies in other areas, such as effects of social inequality and social mobility on disease risk,[26-29] and even the childhood origins of adult chronic disease.[14,15,30,31] Historical cohorts that have been used to investigate the fetal origins of adult chronic diseases also have fewer women than men and sometimes none, partly because of the increased administrative burden to trace women who change their names on marriage.

Thus far, the case has been made for a life course approach, but not specifically a life course approach to women's health. We consider a life course approach to women's health as the study of all health outcomes of importance to women, but particularly noncommunicable diseases (NCDs), sometimes also referred to as *chronic conditions*, and biological function. This is distinct from the often-implicit assumption that women's health is limited to reproductive and maternal health. Rather, the reproductive events and characteristics of women's lives, from menarche to menopause and beyond, form a reproductive axis that is fundamental to their lives and to the life course approach. For example, oestrogen exposure varies across life, including timing of menarche, childbearing and breastfeeding, exogenous hormone use (oral contraceptives and menopausal hormone therapy), and type and timing of menopause. Alongside the gender-based social structures, it is a key reason for a distinct approach to NCDs in women. These sex and gender differences are evident in four main ways:

- The prevalence of common diseases differs between men and women (e.g. women are about twice as likely to experience depression[32] and three-to-four times as likely to have osteoporosis than men,[33,34] and have diseases that are unique to women, such as gynaecological cancers);
- Some risk factors are more common in women than men (e.g. sexual abuse[35]), and associations between risks and NCDs may be different for women (e.g. diabetes increases the risk of heart disease fourfold in women, but doubles the risk for men);[36,37]

- As women generally live longer than men, they comprise a higher proportion of the older age groups that suffer from age-related NCDs (e.g. dementia and Alzheimer disease)[38–40] and spend more time in poor health;[39,41]
- The characteristics of a woman's reproductive axis are linked with risk of many NCDs.[42,43]

It is also the case that women's reproductive axis characterises much of their health services use from adolescence to midlife, and so represents a sex-specific public health platform for tailored preventive strategies and monitoring.

1.3 Overview of Chapters

The core of this book has five main parts, commencing in Part II on Reproductive Health and its drivers. Chapter 2 describes the separate and joint effects of factors in early and adult life that may affect reproductive health across this life stage, from the timing of menarche, through to fertility and pregnancy complications (e.g. fetal loss, preeclampsia, gestational diabetes, and preterm birth), to the experience of the menopausal transition (e.g. early menopause and vasomotor symptoms). Chapter 3 is a new chapter examining endometriosis, specifically the risk factors for and consequences of this condition. After considerable neglect, this condition has received increased attention in research and public health policy in recent years. Chapter 4 reviews the evidence for biological and social factors across the life course that affect the timing of menopause, and the factors leading to decision-making about hysterectomy. It also covers vasomotor symptoms over the menopausal transition and the current guidelines on use of menopausal hormone therapy.

Part III, Health, Ageing, and Disease, focuses on the main NCDs or chronic conditions experienced by women. Cardiovascular disease (CVD) (Chapter 5) remains a leading cause of morbidity and mortality among women. While many of the classic risk factors (e.g. smoking and obesity) are similar for women as for men, the chapter highlights the female-specific risk factors, including adverse pregnancy outcomes and early menopause. Diabetes is the focus of Chapter 6, where evidence not only highlights the role of in utero exposures but also maternal risk factors during pregnancy. As with CVD, women who experience pregnancy complications (e.g. gestational diabetes) or early age at menopause are more likely to have type 2 diabetes in later life.

Musculoskeletal conditions (which covers osteoporosis, sarcopenia, and osteoarthritis) described in Chapter 7 are far more prevalent in women than men. Sex hormones are of interest as there are plausible mechanisms whereby changes in endogenous hormone levels that women experience, such as during menopause, can impact bone, muscle, and joints. Body weight and health behaviours across life are also important factors and show some gender differences.[44] Across life, females tend to have smaller lungs and airways, and their lung function levels are lower than in males.[45] The implication of these and other factors are part of the evidence review in Chapter 8 of COPD in women, which is characterised by a gender-specific pattern of risk factors, disease pathogenesis, presentation, and prognosis as well as disparity in diagnosis and treatment of women across the life course.

Mental health is a particularly important topic for women (Chapter 9), as from early adolescence onwards, women are about twice as likely to experience depression as men, and forms of depression-related conditions are specific to women, including premenstrual dysphoric disorder, postpartum depression, and postmenopausal depression and anxiety. This chapter also provides an overview of recent evidence on genetic factors, exposure to adverse perinatal and childhood experiences, and more proximate stressors that may be involved in the development of depression and psychological distress.

As populations age, women comprise a higher proportion of older age groups with implications for diseases, such as dementia and Alzheimer disease (AD). Chapter 10 discusses the contributing factors in women's lives to their higher rates of AD, greater pathology burden of AD, and a steeper decline prior to AD dementia diagnosis, but more favourable clinical profile in prodromal AD than men. The chapter includes an evidence review of how life-long sex differences in cognition, brain function, and reproductive ageing may contribute to gender differences.

Diseases of particular concern to women are addressed in Chapter 11 (breast cancer) and Chapter 12 (gynaecological cancer). From a life course perspective, breast cancer development is particularly illustrative, with risk factors spanning pubertal and adolescent development, pregnancy, and menopause. For example, earlier age at menarche is a well-established risk factor for breast cancer,[46-49] while physical activity in childhood and adolescence appears protective. Chapter 12 focuses on the three most common gynaecological cancers: endometrial, ovarian, and cervical. Similar to breast cancer, it is likely that ovulatory/hormonal exposures across the life course have a role in the risk, as illustrated by associations of longer duration of breastfeeding with reduced risk[50,51] and older age at natural menopause with increased risk[52,53] of endometrial and ovarian cancer. Higher levels of physical activity are linked with lower risk of endometrial cancer independent of obesity, while women who reported being inactive or sedentary prior to diagnosis were at increased risk of ovarian cancer.[54,55]

In Part IV, Biological and Behavioural Pathways, we shift from specific disease outcomes to how different types of factors or exposures operate across the life course. Chapter 13 presents the new topic of omics, which refers to the shift in the last 20 years from studies of individual genes, proteins, and molecules and their function to considering the total complement in a single experiment. Omics approaches support hypothesis-free studies that have had considerable success in identifying novel biological pathways. Although the heritability for timing of menarche and menopause are estimated at around 50% (i.e. genetic influences account for 50% of the variation), these are multifactorial traits where the genetic predisposition is due to many individual variants, each having small effects. Chapter 14 reviews current evidence on the development and ageing of the endocrine system in women. The authors describe how the hormonal pathways across the life course play a key role in the maintenance of health. The final chapters in Part III take a life course perspective to health behaviours (Chapter 15) and body weight (Chapter 16). The extent that these disease risk factors have their origins earlier in life may help to explain the links between the childhood environment and adult health. Adult health behaviours and obesity are strongly related to lifetime socioeconomic circumstances, while the changing environment and changes in cultural norms over time have impacted trends in these factors that have resulted in cohort differences in life course exposure.

Part V, Social Issues Impacting Women's Health, addresses the social dimensions of a life course approach to women health. The chapter on socioeconomic trajectories (Chapter 17) compares life course social mobility trends in women and men and the effects on later health outcomes of experience of disadvantaged socioeconomic position in childhood, and the potential cumulative impact of exposure to disadvantage through adolescence into adulthood. The chapter also discusses the variety of potential pathways which may be involved, including socially patterned health risk behaviours and exposure to adverse childhood experiences. Chapter 18 addresses how women's changing social relationships across the life course influence their health outcomes, including a discussion of how early life circumstances and life course transitions influence social relationships. The different aspects of such relationships, including the network size or composition, emotional or instrumental support, and engagement with organisations or communities may play a different role at each life stage.

Chapter 19 is a new chapter to this volume, and it examines women's health through the lens of structural sexism and how this impacts women's health across the life course. This goes beyond the interactional level of social life (i.e. discrimination, bias, and roles) to the more fundamental gendered forces that operate at all levels to shape women's lives. The extent to which these forces shape gender differences and explain women's health and well-being, and their relative importance compared with biological differences such as the role of sex hormones, remains both a contentious and evolving debate. The societal context and gender disparities are a key theme of Chapter 20 in a new chapter on gender-based violence against women and its impact across the life course, from early life through adolescence and adulthood, including during pregnancy, to elder abuse. This chapter highlights the Ecological Framework for violence against women[56]—a multidisciplinary perspective that highlights a key aspect of the life course approach.

Last, Part VI addresses a new topic of understanding how best the life course approach can be applied in policy and practice. Chapter 21 looks specifically at the relevance of a life course approach to women's health care. As the authors illustrate, the consultation rates for women are around twice those of men through midlife from 15 to 60 years of age. This is most clearly seen during women's reproductive life stage, but the consultation rates are still markedly higher than men even without including reproductive events. From the life course perspective, this extended use of reproductive health services may represent an opportunistic platform both to improve maternal and child health and well-being, and to reduce NCDs in later life. Chapter 22 addresses the new topic of knowledge translation (KT) that has emerged to enable evidence to be effectively adopted into practice. The chapter outlines some methodologies or KT frameworks, such as the Knowledge to Action (K2A) cycle,[57] that is now adopted by the World Health Organization (WHO). These typically follow three steps or stages: understanding the need, selecting and trialling appropriate mechanisms for change, and evaluating effectiveness. KT frameworks highlight the importance of understating barriers and enabling factors to bring about effective and sustained change, as well as engaging with key participants, including disadvantaged women from the community and health professionals working in practice, in the codesign of new tools, protocols, and resources.

1.4 The Life Course Approach in Women's Health Policy

The new chapters on applying evidence and translating knowledge in practice are timely as there are growing indications that the life course perspective is gaining traction in development of policy on women's health at international and national levels. Both the WHO and UNICEF have adopted a life course framework to inform recommendations for mainstreaming NCD prevention across childhood, adolescence, and reproductive life.[58–61] Some earlier signs of the life course approach influencing policy have been developed on specific topics (e.g. the 2011 call to action on obesity in England)[62] or on women's health but applied within a limited jurisdiction (e.g. 2010 NSW Women's Health Framework in Australia).[63] More recently, however, there are indications of a sustained policy shift in some countries. In late 2019, the Royal College of Obstetricians and Gynaecologists in the UK published its proposal for a national women's health strategy, entitled *Better for women: Improving the Health and Wellbeing of Girls and Women*,[64] with the first chapter devoted to a life course approach. The following year the UK government set out its response to a public call for evidence with *Our Vision for the Women's Health Strategy for England*,[65] that declared a life course approach as its central focus for the development of the strategy itself. The *Strategy*, published in July 2022, has a 10-year aim to boost the health outcomes of all women and girls and radically improved the way in which the health care system engages and listens to them.[66] The strategy specifically states that it will achieve its aims by, among other things, taking a life course approach.

There have been two national women's health policy announcements that give the life course perspective a central role in their comprehensive and detailed guidance. First, in early 2019, the Australian government published its *National Women's Health Strategy:2020–2030*[67] that specified a life course approach, alongside gender equity, health equity, and prevention, as one of its core principles. Specifically, this refers to the development of 'health initiatives that focus on improving health and target risk factors and critical intervention points for women across the life course'. They categorise the burden of disease, health focus, the key intervention points in terms of four main life stages: girls (split into birth to 5 years and 5–14 years), adolescents (15–24 years), adult women (25–44 years and 45–64 years), and older women (64–74 years and 75 years and older). The approach is followed through into the priority areas, such as chronic conditions and preventive health, where the first two specific actions are to: increase awareness and primary prevention of chronic conditions and associated risk factors for women and girls and embed a life course approach in policy and practice, and invest in targeted prevention, timely detection, and intervention of chronic conditions affecting women and girls. These are followed by more specific details and a series of suggested measures for success.

In 2021, Scotland's *Women's Health Plan*[68] similarly integrated the life course approach within objectives to address inequalities (e.g. health and vulnerable groups), gender equality and intersectionality, and respectful and inclusive services. It, then, outlined key issues and health needs across using a simplified three stages of life: girls and young women, middle years, and later years. The plan identifies a series of actions that cut across all priorities, where the leading long-term action is to 'adopt a life course approach in all services to improve women's health holistically'. Since CVD remains the leading cause of death for women in Scotland, *heart health* is defined as a key priority, with the first action listed as: 'In all heart health consultations, opportunities should be taken to provide individualised advice and care to women, and in all pregnancy and pre-pregnancy discussions and interactions opportunities should be taken to optimise women's heart health to optimise women's holistic health as part of the life course approach.'

The first point to note is that we are unaware of similar types of women's health policy documents being adopted in other locations, such as in the countries of Europe, North America, or Asia. This may reflect where life course epidemiological research is less well-established and influential. In low- and middle-income countries (LMICs) and even in high-income countries (HICs), such as some European nations, there may be a tendency to follow international agencies; for instance, it was the WHO Regional Office for Europe that funded the 2019 report on measuring implementation of the life course approach, and this may eventually lead to its explicit adoption in these countries. The second point is that we have yet to gain a clear sense of how a life course approach is specifically being implemented in clinical practice, or on progress to date, such as in new monitoring protocols for pregnant women at risk of cardiometabolic diseases. In Australia, we can point to the National Action Plan for Endometriosis[69] and accompanying longer term funding, which might have in part arisen out of the National Women's Health Strategy, even though it was published earlier. It is also fair to say that attention was diverted from this national strategy by the COVID-19 pandemic, which occurred just subsequent to its publication.

1.4.1 The COVID-19 Pandemic and Noncommunicable Disease

The contributing authors have written much of this second edition in the shadow of the COVID-19 pandemic, with some including sections in their chapter to outline its implications for women's health at different life stages, including those due to the stay-at-home policy responses. There were initial concerns that the overwhelming policy focus on COVID-19 would obscure the less-visible epidemic of NCDs.[70] These have been justified fears. For example, considerable harm has been done in disrupting public health strategies, such as breast and cervical cancer screening, and the existing management and treatment healthcare plans of cancer patients.[71,72] Inevitably, this is likely to result in an increase in fatalities, as it appears will be the case for breast cancer.[73] We also know the policy for people to stay at home and the associated socioeconomic stress led to a marked increase in the incidence of domestic violence,[74,75] with longer term consequences for women's mental health, health risk behaviours, and subsequent adverse NCD outcomes. Time will tell whether the pandemic has derailed women's health policy initiatives, with their focus on gender disparities, NCD prevention, and access to health services. The impact of the COVID-19 pandemic on women is discussed in many chapters in this book, and the challenges and implications for life course epidemiology are discussed further in the concluding chapter.

1.5 Conclusion

Life course epidemiology is the study of the contribution of biological and social factors acting independently, interactively, and cumulatively during gestation, childhood, adolescence, and adult life on health outcomes in later life. The purpose is to identify long-term risk and protective processes that explain variation in individual disease risk and healthy ageing, and in changing patterns of risk and protective factors and diseases over time or across populations. In so doing, the life course approach can inform the development of women's health policy and tailored and timely preventive health strategies to improve health and well-being. The contributors in this book provide an up-to-date review of the current evidence available across an array of topics, including new areas that have emerged and developed in importance since the first edition. This includes considering the wider issues of implementing and evaluating a life course approach to women's health in policy and practice. By bringing together these different strands, this book makes a unique contribution to interdisciplinary research, offers important new insights into the causes of women's health, and provides challenges for future life course research.

References

1. Kuh D, Ben-Shlomo Y, ed. *A life course approach to chronic disease epidemiology*. Oxford: Oxford University Press; 1997.
2. Kuh D, Hardy R, ed. *A life course approach to women's health*. Oxford: Oxford University Press; 2002.
3. Pickles A, Maughan B, Wadsworth M, ed. *Epidemiological methods in life course research*. Oxford: Oxford University Press; 2007.
4. Lawlor DA, Mishra GD, ed. *Family matters: designing, analysing and understanding family-based studies in life course epidemiology* Oxford: Oxford University Press; 2009.
5. Kuh D, Cooper R, Hardy R, Ben-Shlomo Y, ed. *A life course approach to healthy ageing*. Oxford: Oxford University Press; 2013.
6. Kuh D, Ben Shlomo Y, ed. *A life course approach to chronic disease epidemiology*. Oxford: Oxford University Press; 2004.
7. Ben-Shlomo Y, Cooper R, Kuh D. The last two decades of life course epidemiology, and its relevance for research on ageing. *International Journal of Epidemiology*. 2016;45(4):973–88.
8. European Institute for Gender Equality. A–Z index. EIGE; 2022 [updated on unknown date; cited 31 Aug. 2022]. Available from: https://eige.europa.eu/thesaurus/.
9. Kuh D, Davey Smith G. When is mortality risk determined? Historical insights into a current debate. *Social History of Medicine*. 1993;6(1):101–23.
10. Kuh D, Ben-Shlomo Y, Lynch J, Hallqvist J, Power C. Life course epidemiology. *Journal of Epidemiology and Community Health*. 2003;57(10):778–83.
11. Alwin DF. Commentary: it takes more than one to tango. Life course epidemiology and related approaches. *International Journal of Epidemiology*. 2016;45(4):988–93.
12. Lucas A. Programming by early nutrition in man. In: Bock GR, Whelan J, eds. *The childhood environment and adult disease*. Chichester: John Wiley and Sons; 1991. pp. 38–55.
13. Kuh DJ, Wadsworth ME. Physical health status at 36 years in a British national birth cohort. *Social Science & Medicine*. 1993;37(7):905–16.
14. Blane D, Hart CL, Smith GD, Gillis CR, Hole DJ, Hawthorne VM. Association of cardiovascular disease risk factors with socioeconomic position during childhood and during adulthood. *BMJ*. 1996;313(7070):1434–8.
15. Heslop P, Davey Smith G, Macleod J, Hart C. The socioeconomic position of employed women, risk factors and mortality. *Social Science & Medicine*. 2001;53(4):477–85.
16. Krieger N, Chen JT, Selby JV. Class inequalities in women's health: combined impact of childhood and adult social class—a study of 630 US women. *Public Health*. 2001;115(3):175–85.
17. Kuh D, Power C, Blane D, Bartley M. Social pathways between childhood and adult health. In: Kuh D, Ben-Shlomo Y, eds. *A life course approach to chronic disease epidemiology: tracing the origins of ill-health from early to adult life*. Oxford: Oxford University Press; 1997. pp. 169–200.
18. Hanson M, Gluckman P. Commentary: developing the future. Life course epidemiology, DOHaD and evolutionary medicine. *International Journal of Epidemiology*. 2016;45(4):993–6.
19. De Stavola BL, Daniel RM. Commentary: incorporating concepts and methods from causal inference into life course epidemiology. *International Journal of Epidemiology*. 2016;45(4):1006–10.
20. Howe LD, Smith AD, Macdonald-Wallis C, Anderson EL, Galobardes B, Lawlor DA, et al. Relationship between mediation analysis and the structured life course approach. *International Journal of Epidemiology*. 2016;45(4):1280–94.

21. Smith AD, Hardy R, Heron J, Joinson CJ, Lawlor DA, Macdonald-Wallis C, et al. A structured approach to hypotheses involving continuous exposures over the life course. *International Journal of Epidemiology*. 2016;45(4):1271–9.
22. Mishra G, Nitsch D, Black S, De Stavola B, Kuh D, Hardy R. A structured approach to modelling the effects of binary exposure variables over the life course. *International Journal of Epidemiology*. 2008;38(2):528–37.
23. Chumbley J, Xu W, Potente C, Harris KM, Shanahan M. A Bayesian approach to comparing common models of life-course epidemiology. *International Journal of Epidemiology*. 2021;50(5):1660–70.
24. Madathil S, Joseph L, Hardy R, Rousseau M-C, Nicolau B. A Bayesian approach to investigate life course hypotheses involving continuous exposures. *International Journal of Epidemiology*. 2018;47(5):1623–35.
25. Kuh D, Davey Smith G. The life course and adult chronic disease: an historical perspective with particular reference to coronary heart disease. In: Kuh D, Ben-Shlomo Y, eds. *A life course approach to chronic disease epidemiology: tracing the origins of ill-health from early to adult life*. Oxford: Oxford University Press; 1997. pp. 15–44.
26. Rose G, Marmot MG. Social class and coronary heart disease. *British Heart Journal*. 1981;45(1):13–19.
27. Marmot MG, Shipley MJ, Rose G. Inequalities in death—specific explanations of a general pattern? *Lancet*. 1984;323(8384):1003–6.
28. Baker IA, Sweetnam PM, Yarnell JWG, Bainton D, Elwood PC. Haemostatic and other risk factors for ischaemic heart disease and social class: evidence from the Caerphilly and Speedwell studies. *International Journal of Epidemiology*. 1988;17(4):759–65.
29. Smith GD, Shipley MJ, Rose G. Magnitude and causes of socioeconomic differentials in mortality: further evidence from the Whitehall study. *Journal of Epidemiology and Community Health*. 1990;44(4):265–70.
30. Kaplan GA, Salonen JT. Socioeconomic conditions in childhood and ischaemic heart disease during middle age. *BMJ*. 1990;301(6761):1121–3.
31. Lynch JW, Kaplan GA, Cohen RD, Wilson TW, Smith NL, Kauhanen J, et al. Childhood and adult socioeconomic status as predictors of mortality in Finland. *Lancet*. 1994;343(8896):524–7.
32. Kuehner C. Why is depression more common among women than among men? *Lancet Psychiatry*. 2017;4(2):146–58.
33. Alswat KA. Gender disparities in osteoporosis. *Journal of Clinical Medical Research*. 2017;9(5):382–7.
34. Australian Institute of Health and Welfare. Osteoporosis. Canberra: AIHW; 2020 [updated 20 August 2020; cited 17 August 2022]. Available from: https://www.aihw.gov.au/reports/chronic-musculoskeletal-conditions/osteoporosis/contents/what-is-osteoporosis.
35. Stoltenborgh M, van IJzendoorn MH, Euser EM, Bakermans-Kranenburg MJ. A global perspective on child sexual abuse: meta-analysis of prevalence around the world. *Child Maltreatment*. 2011;16(2):79–101.
36. Huxley R, Barzi F, Woodward M. Excess risk of fatal coronary heart disease associated with diabetes in men and women: meta-analysis of 37 prospective cohort studies. *BMJ*. 2006;332(7533):73–8.
37. Ding EL, Song Y, Malik VS, Liu S. Sex differences of endogenous sex hormones and risk of type 2 diabetes: a systematic review and meta-analysis. *JAMA*. 2006;295(11):1288–99.
38. Cao Q, Tan C-C, Xu W, Hu H, Cao X-P, Dong Q, et al. The prevalence of dementia: a systematic review and meta-analysis. *Journal of Alzheimer's Disease*. 2020;73:1157–66.
39. Niu H, Álvarez-Álvarez I, Guillén-Grima F, Aguinaga-Ontoso I. Prevalence and incidence of Alzheimer's disease in Europe: a meta-analysis. *Neurología (English Edition)*. 2017;32(8):523–32.
40. Nichols E, Szoeke CEI, Vollset SE, Abbasi N, Abd-Allah F, Abdela J, et al. Global, regional, and national burden of Alzheimer's disease and other dementias, 1990–2016: a systematic analysis for the global burden of disease study 2016. *Lancet Neurology*. 2019;18(1):88–106.
41. Freedman VA, Wolf DA, Spillman BC. Disability-free life expectancy over 30 years: a growing female disadvantage in the US population. *American Journal of Public Health*. 2016;106(6):1079–85.

42. Zhu D, Chung H-F, Dobson AJ, Pandeya N, Giles GG, Bruinsma F, et al. Age at natural menopause and risk of incident cardiovascular disease: a pooled analysis of individual patient data. *Lancet Public Health*. 2019;4(11):e553–e564.

43. Grandi SM, Filion KB, Yoon S, Ayele HT, Doyle CM, Hutcheon JA, et al. Cardiovascular disease-related morbidity and mortality in women with a history of pregnancy complications. *Circulation*. 2019;139(8):1069–79.

44. Holliday KL, McWilliams DF, Maciewicz RA, Muir KR, Zhang W, Doherty M. Lifetime body mass index, other anthropometric measures of obesity and risk of knee or hip osteoarthritis in the GOAL case-control study. *Osteoarthritis and Cartilage*. 2011;19(1):37–43.

45. LoMauro A, Aliverti A. Sex differences in respiratory function. *Breathe (Sheff)*. 2018;14(2):131–40.

46. Barnard ME, Boeke CE, Tamimi RM. Established breast cancer risk factors and risk of intrinsic tumor subtypes. *Biochimica et Biophysica Acta (BBA)—Reviews on Cancer*. 2015;1856(1):73–85.

47. Anderson KN, Schwab RB, Martinez ME. Reproductive risk factors and breast cancer subtypes: a review of the literature. *Breast Cancer Research and Treatment*. 2014;144(1):1–10.

48. Yang XR, Sherman ME, Rimm DL, Lissowska J, Brinton LA, Peplonska B, et al. Differences in risk factors for breast cancer molecular subtypes in a population-based study. *Cancer Epidemiology, Biomarkers & Prevention*. 2007;16(3):439–43.

49. Fuhrman BJ, Moore SC, Byrne C, Makhoul I, Kitahara CM, Berrington de González A, et al. Association of the age at menarche with site-specific cancer risks in pooled data from nine cohorts. *Cancer Research*. 2021;81(8):2246–55.

50. Babic A, Sasamoto N, Rosner BA, Tworoger SS, Jordan SJ, Risch HA, et al. Association between breastfeeding and ovarian cancer risk. *JAMA Oncology*. 2020;6(6):e200421.

51. Jordan SJ, Na R, Johnatty SE, Wise LA, Adami HO, Brinton LA, et al. Breastfeeding and endometrial cancer risk: an analysis from the Epidemiology of Endometrial Cancer Consortium. *Obstetrics & Gynecology*. 2017;129(6):1059–67.

52. Wentzensen N, Poole EM, Trabert B, White E, Arslan AA, Patel AV, et al. Ovarian cancer risk factors by histologic subtype: an analysis from the Ovarian Cancer Cohort Consortium. *Journal of Clinical Oncology*. 2016;34(24):2888–98.

53. Dossus L, Allen N, Kaaks R, Bakken K, Lund E, Tjonneland A, et al. Reproductive risk factors and endometrial cancer: the European prospective investigation into cancer and nutrition. *International Journal of Cancer*. 2010;127(2):442–51.

54. Cannioto R, LaMonte MJ, Risch HA, Hong C-C, Sucheston-Campbell LE, Eng KH, et al. Chronic recreational physical inactivity and epithelial ovarian cancer risk: evidence from the Ovarian Cancer Association Consortium. *Cancer Epidemiology, Biomarkers & Prevention*. 2016;25(7):1114–24.

55. Biller VS, Leitzmann MF, Sedlmeier AM, Berger FF, Ortmann O, Jochem C. Sedentary behaviour in relation to ovarian cancer risk: a systematic review and meta-analysis. *European Journal of Epidemiology*. 2021;36(8):769–80.

56. Sánchez OR, Vale DB, Rodrigues L, Surita FG. Violence against women during the COVID-19 pandemic: an integrative review. *International Journal of Gynecology & Obstetrics*. 2020;151(2):180–7.

57. Straus SE, Tetroe J, Graham I. Defining knowledge translation. *Canadian Medical Association Journal*. 2009;181(3–4):165–8.

58. Mikkelsen B, Williams J, Rakovac I, Wickramasinghe K, Hennis A, Shin H-R, et al. Life course approach to prevention and control of non-communicable diseases. *BMJ*. 2019;364:l257.

59. Azenha GS, Parsons-Perez C, Goltz S, Bhadelia A, Durstine A, Knaul F, et al. Recommendations towards an integrated, life-course approach to women's health in the post-2015 agenda. *Bulletin of the World Health Organization*. 2013;91(9):704–6.

60. UNICEF. *Programme guidance for early life prevention of non-communicable diseases*. New York: UNICEF; 2019.

61. Jacob CM, Cooper C, Baird J, Hanson M. *What quantitative and qualitative methods have been developed to measure the implementation of a life-course approach in public health policies at the national level?* Copenhagen: WHO Regional Office for Europe; Health Evidence Network (HEN) Synthesis Report 63; 2019.

62. UK Department of Health. *Healthy lives, healthy people: a call to action for obesity in England*. London: UK Department of Health; 2011.

63. NSW Ministry of Health. *NSW women's health framework 2019*. St Leonards: NSW Ministry of Health; 2019.
64. Royal College of Obstetricians & Gynaecologists. *Better for women: improving the health of wellbeing of girls and women*. London: Royal College of Obstetricians & Gynaecologists; 2019.
65. UK Department of Health and Social Care. *Our vision for the women's health strategy for England*. London: UK Department of Health and Social Care; 2021.
66. UK Department of Health & Social Care. *Women's health strategy for England*. London: UK Department of Health & Social Care; 2022.
67. Australian Department of Health and Aged Care. *National women's health strategy 2020–2030*. Canberra: Australian Department of Health and Aged Care; 2018.
68. The Scottish Government. *Women's health plan: a plan for 2021–2024*. Edinburgh: The Scottish Government; 2021.
69. Australian Department of Health and Aged Care. *National action plan for endometriosis*. London: Australian Department of Health and Aged Care; 2018.
70. Allen LN, Feigl AB. Reframing non-communicable diseases as socially transmitted conditions. *Lancet Global Health*. 2017;5(7):e644–e646.
71. Alkatout I, Biebl M, Momenimovahed Z, Giovannucci E, Hadavandsiri F, Salehiniya H, et al. Has COVID-19 affected cancer screening programs? A systematic review. *Frontiers in Oncology*. 2021;11:675038.
72. Riera R, Bagattini ÂM, Pacheco RL, Pachito DV, Roitberg F, Ilbawi A. Delays and disruptions in cancer health care due to COVID-19 pandemic: systematic review. *JCO Global Oncology*. 2021;7:311–23.
73. Maringe C, Spicer J, Morris M, Purushotham A, Nolte E, Sullivan R, et al. The impact of the COVID-19 pandemic on cancer deaths due to delays in diagnosis in England, UK: a national, population-based, modelling study. *Lancet Oncology*. 2020;21(8):1023–34.
74. Piquero AR, Jennings WG, Jemison E, Kaukinen C, Knaul FM. Domestic violence during the COVID-19 pandemic—evidence from a systematic review and meta-analysis. *Journal of Criminal Justice*. 2021;74:101806.
75. Arenas-Arroyo E, Fernandez-Kranz D, Nollenberger N. Intimate partner violence under forced cohabitation and economic stress: evidence from the COVID-19 pandemic. *Journal of Public Economics*. 2021;194:104350.

PART II

REPRODUCTIVE HEALTH

2

A Life Course Approach to Women's Reproductive Health

Maria C. Magnus and Abigail Fraser

2.1 Introduction

The World Health Organization defines reproductive health as:

> ... a state of complete physical, mental and social well-being and not merely the absence of disease or infirmity, in all matters relating to the reproductive system and to its functions and processes. Reproductive health implies that people are able to have a satisfying and safe sex life and that they have the capability to reproduce and the freedom to decide if, when and how often to do so.[1]

It is clear from this definition that women's reproductive health is multifaceted. It encompasses physical and mental health, individual choices about reproductive health-related behaviours, and the sociolegal environment that enables or limits women's ability and freedom to make these choices. We cannot do justice to all these facets of reproductive health here; we, therefore, devote most of this chapter to the different stages of the female reproductive lifespan: puberty, the reproductive years characterised by (in)fertility and pregnancy, and the transition through the menopause. We describe secular trends for age at puberty and natural menopause, related symptoms, and life course determinants of reproductive health. We focus on body mass index (BMI) and smoking as examples of how exposures may affect reproductive health throughout the lifespan. In addition to being important health outcomes, women's reproductive characteristics are associated with noncommunicable diseases in later life; we give several examples in the latter part of this chapter and address underlying mechanisms.

2.2 Stages of Women's Reproductive Lifespan and Reproductive Health Indicators

2.2.1 Puberty and Menarche

Age at menarche, or the onset of menses, indicates the start of the female reproductive lifespan. It occurs during the latter stages of the pubertal transition, preceded by breast (thelarche) and pubic hair (pubarche) development.[2] Age at pubertal onset has declined over

Maria C. Magnus and Abigail Fraser, *A Life Course Approach to Women's Reproductive Health* In: *A Life Course Approach to Women's Health*. Second Edition. Edited by: Gita D Mishra, Rebecca Hardy, and Diana Kuh, Oxford University Press. © Oxford University Press 2023. DOI: 10.1093/oso/9780192864642.003.0002 time. A systematic review of 30 studies in which thelarche was assessed in a physical or clinical examination by a trained paediatrician using Tanner staging found that between 1977 and 2013, age at thelarche (Tanner breast stage 2) declined by just under three months per decade.[3] Similarly, an evaluation of 218 reports including 220,037 European women born between 1795 and 1981 found that age at menarche—the more commonly used indicator of pubertal timing—decreased about two to three months per decade.[4] A decrease in age at menarche has also been observed in more recent years, suggesting that this trend may not yet have plateaued in Western countries, as indicated by some studies.[5,6] A British study including 94,170 women found a decline from a mean age of 13.5 years among women born between 1908 and 1919 to 12.6 years among women born in 1945–49 and 12.3 years among women born in 1990–93.[7] Evidence of a decrease in age at menarche was also reported from Asian and South American countries.[8,9] For example, a Japanese study found a mean age at menarche of 13.8 years among women born in the 1930s compared with 12.2 years among women born in the 1980s.[10] This overall trend for a decline in age at menarche, therefore, appears to be seen across geographical regions and ethnic backgrounds.

Women of reproductive age, between the ages of 15 and 49 years,[1] make up ~25% of the world's population. Menstrual characteristics such as cycle length, regularity, premenstrual symptoms, and pain are therefore important and still understudied health traits that affect a large proportion of the population. Menstruation and its symptoms can adversely impact quality of life as well as productivity[11] and school attendance.[12] Hormonal imbalances that characterise conditions such as polycystic ovary syndrome (PCOS) affect cycle length and regularity and are associated with chronic disease risk (see Section 2.4) and mortality.[13,14]

2.2.2 Fertility and Pregnancy

Fertility can be indicated by how long it takes a woman to conceive or be characterised based on sex hormone levels and ovarian reserve.[15] Notably, findings from the global burden of disease project indicated that, on average, the global fertility rate decreased from 4.7 live births in 1950 to 2.4 live births in 2017,[16] and this decrease is projected to continue in the coming decades.[17] This is likely explained in large parts by the secular trend of delayed childbearing and has resulted in an increased number of couples struggling to conceive and using assisted reproductive technologies.[18,19] It is estimated that between 10% and 15% of couples are affected by subfertility, defined as trying to conceive for more than 12 months, and that female fertility problems are the main or contributing cause in about half of these cases.[20,21]

It is during these reproductive years that women experience pregnancy and its related complications such as fetal death (miscarriage or stillbirth), hypertensive disorders of pregnancy, gestational diabetes, preterm birth, and fetal growth restriction.[22,23] It is estimated that one in five pregnancies ends in miscarriage, and a third of pregnancies are affected by other complications.[24]

2.2.3 Menopause

Female reproductive ageing is characterised by the gradual decrease in oocyte quantity and quality. A women's fertility potential is virtually nonexistent in the 10 years prior to natural menopause,[25] which is defined as the absence of menstruation over a period of 12 months when not caused by medical treatment or surgery and marks the end of a woman's reproductive lifespan (see Chapter 4). Findings from 15 cohorts in the InterLACE consortium, including more than 300,000 women, indicated that the mean age of natural menopause is 50 years, 4.7% had early menopause (at 40–44 years of age) and 1.2% had premature menopause (< 40 years of age).[26] A large systematic review which included 46 studies from 24 countries found that the age at menopause was lowest among women in Africa, Asia, and Middle Eastern countries, and highest in Europe and Australia, followed by the United States.[27] It is unclear whether the age at natural menopause has changed over time. While some evidence indicates that age at natural menopause might have increased from the beginning of the 1900s until the 1950s,[28,29] few studies have investigated the trend in age at menopause in women born after 1950.[30,31] Findings from the InterLACE consortium that include women with different ethnic backgrounds did not support a change in age at menopause over time. Other large studies of European women reported an increase in age at natural menopause between women born in 1920 and 1932 and women born in 1925 and 1944, and a decrease after this time.[30,31]

Evidence suggests that 50%–80% of women in high-income settings report experiencing vasomotor symptoms, such as night sweats and hot flushes, at some point during the menopausal transition,[32,33] and that a third of women experienced vaginal dryness in the postmenopausal years.[30] It has also been suggested that menopause—independently of age—may adversely affect women's continence, mental health,[30] and physical[34] and cognitive functioning.[35] But evidence is inconclusive, and the biosocial mechanisms that may explain any causal effects remain to be clarified.

2.2.4 Relationships Between Indicators of Women's Reproductive Health

As observable indicators of women's reproductive health are likely to reflect a woman's underlying hormonal milieu, associations between indicators are plausible. However, these indicators span the life course, from puberty to menopause, and are affected by multiple exposures across the different stages of life (as discussed in Sections 2.3.2–2.3.5), including broader societal conditions. Indeed, studies investigating the relationship between age at menarche, age at menopause, and duration of women's reproductive lifespan have yielded conflicting results.[36,37] In the large UK Biobank, age at menarche and age at menopause are not correlated (r = 0.007). The InterLACE consortium found that the combination of early menarche and nulliparity was associated with over a fivefold greater risk for premature menopause (< 40 years) and a doubling of the risk of early menopause (40–44 years) compared with women who experienced menarche at age 12 or above and who had two or more children,[38] providing some evidence in support of a continuity of the reproductive axis across the life course. Other studies reported associations between pairs of reproductive health indicators such as earlier age at menarche and pregnancy complications,[39,40] and parity and age at menopause,[41] but the evidence base is often limited and inconsistent.[42] Moreover, the mechanisms underlying these associations are yet to be determined, with adiposity, subclinical cardiovascular health, shared genetic architecture, and direct causal effects all thought to play a role. The increasing availability of genome-wide data on large sample sizes has enabled researchers to investigate the extent of shared genetic architecture across indicators of women's reproductive health and to use Mendelian randomization (MR) approaches to investigate whether relationships are likely to be causal or not. This body of work is discussed in the following section (Section 2.3.1; see also Chapter 13).

2.3 Determinants of Female Reproductive Health Indicators

2.3.1 Genetic Determinants

Genetics has a clear role in women's reproductive health. Several genome-wide association studies (GWAS) have identified genetic markers linked to multiple female reproductive health indicators. The most recent GWAS reported 389 independent single nucleoid polymorphisms (SNPs), which predicted age at menarche and explained 7% of the total variation.[43] An investigation of genetic predictors of reproductive behaviour found 12 SNPs associated with total number of offspring or age at first birth, out of which 10 predicted age at first birth and 2 predicted the total number of offspring.[44] With regard to pregnancy outcomes, 12 maternal SNPs located in 10 genes have been linked to offspring birthweight, and these explain only 1.4% of the offspring birthweight variation,[45] while 6 maternal SNPs in 4 genes are robustly associated with offspring gestational age.[46] More recent studies have attempted to disentangle the respective roles of maternal and fetal genotypes in these pregnancy outcomes, supporting the notion that the risk of pregnancy complications is likely influenced by a complex interplay between maternal and offspring genetic composition.[47,48] Only two SNPs were found to predict preeclampsia in a meta-analysis from a large international consortium.[49] For age at natural menopause, a total of 54 independently predictive SNPs have been identified, and these were found to explain 6% of the variation in age at natural menopause.[50] Notably, the genetic correlation between age at natural menopause and age at menarche is fairly low (only 0.14).[50] The genetic drivers of early menarche and menopause, therefore, appear to be largely independent.

MR uses genetic variants that are robustly associated with an exposure of interest as instrumental variables, under the assumption that they are randomly allocated at conception and are, therefore, unrelated to potential confounding factors. Multiple MR studies have investigated the relationships between indicators of women's reproductive health.[51–54] The most comprehensive report examined the genetic correlations and causal relationships between eight indicators of female reproductive health in UK Biobank and found positive effects of age at menarche, age at first sexual intercourse, and age at first birth, for example, on age at last birth and age at menopause.[54]

2.3.2 Prenatal Environment

Women are born with a finite number of oocytes.[55] It is, therefore, plausible that the intra-uterine environment to which they are exposed might affect their development and women's later reproductive health. Birthweight is often used as a general marker of the quality of the intra-uterine environment, as it is an easily attainable measure. Systematic reviews of the available evidence indicate that low birthweight is associated with a younger age at menarche, but preterm birth is not.[56,57] This may simply reflect the inverse association between birthweight and childhood BMI.[58] Alternatively, in utero growth or determinants of growth may causally affect pubertal timing. Studies also indicate that other factors which may influence the intra-uterine environment, such as maternal prepregnancy BMI, smoking, and alcohol intake, might influence daughters' age at menarche.[59-62] The intra-uterine environment may also affect women's future fertility, with some—but not all studies[63-65]—reporting that women born small-for-gestational-age or preterm have a reduced fertility potential and a higher likelihood of being diagnosed with infertility. Own low birthweight appears to be associated with an increase in the risks of having a pregnancy affected by preeclampsia and gestational diabetes.[66-68] Women who are low birthweight or small-for-gestational-age at birth are also reported to have a younger age at natural menopause and to be at increased risk of premature ovarian failure (natural menopause before 40 years of age).[69,70] Whilst it is unclear what the underlying mechanisms are and, indeed, if associations reflect causal effects (as opposed to confounding—by shared genetic and/or environmental risk factors), available evidence does not negate the notion that the intra-uterine environment may contribute to shaping women's reproductive health throughout the lifespan.

2.3.3 Childhood and Adolescent Environment

Whilst the number of oocytes a woman has is determined in utero, oocytes continue to mature across childhood and adolescence; the postnatal environmental might, therefore, influence this process with potential consequences for reproductive health later in life.[55] The most robust relationship currently established is a clear inverse relationship between childhood weight gain and BMI with age at menarche, as summarised in a systematic review, although the magnitude of this association varies greatly across studies.[57] This finding has been further substantiated by evidence from MR analysis.[71] This is important because triangulating evidence from analyses with different potential sources of bias boosts confidence in 'convergent' results.[72]

Second-hand smoke exposure during childhood is also reported to be associated with a younger age at menarche.[73,74] Other childhood environmental exposures hypothesised to contribute to a younger age at menarche are endocrine-disrupting chemicals, although the existing evidence is inconsistent, which can reflect regional and socioeconomic differences in the likelihood of exposure to these chemicals and the age at which the exposure to the chemicals was measured.[75-77] Childhood obesity is also linked to adult fertility problems and some studies indicate that there might be a nonlinear relationship, where both underweight and overweight during childhood are associated with a higher risk of adult infertility.[78,79] This is also highlighted by an increased risk of PCOS among women with a history of childhood obesity.[80,81] Inconsistent evidence links environmental tobacco smoke exposure during childhood with adult fertility in divergent directions, indicating that this relationship is yet to be clarified.[82-84] Women who were obese as children, or who experienced a greater change in their BMI from childhood to early adulthood have a higher risk of pregnancy complications, including gestational diabetes and hypertensive disorders of pregnancy.[85-87] In contrast,

BMI during childhood does not appear to influence age at natural menopause, although the number of studies that have investigated this relationship is limited.[88] Notably, because of the strong tracking of BMI across the life course, it is difficult to disentangle the role of BMI during specific periods of life. Overall, there appears to be a role for the childhood environment in female puberty timing, fertility, and some pregnancy complications, however its role in the timing of menopause is less clear.

2.3.4 Adult Environment

Health-related behaviours in adulthood are linked to fertility, risk of pregnancy loss and complications, and age at natural menopause (see Chapter 4 for indications for surgical menopause). Being overweight or obese and smoking influences the fertility potential as measured by reproductive hormone levels and the ovarian reserve (anti-Müllerian hormone levels) among women of reproductive age[89] and are linked to poorer rates of success among women undergoing fertility treatment.[90,91] These factors also influence the risk of most adverse pregnancy outcomes. Notably, while smoking increases the risk of preterm birth, low birthweight, and small-for-gestational-age,[92] it is also consistently associated with a lower risk of preeclampsia.[93]

BMI appears to have a nonlinear relationship with pregnancy complications, with an increased risk of preeclampsia, preterm birth, small-for-gestational-age, and gestational diabetes observed among both underweight and overweight or obese women.[94,95] Higher intensity of smoking, longer duration, higher cumulative dose, earlier age at start smoking, and shorter time since quitting smoking are all associated with a higher risk of premature and early menopause.[96] Women who are underweight are at a higher risk of early menopause (< 45 years), while women with overweight or obesity are more likely to have late menopause (≥56 years).[97]

2.3.5 Socioeconomic Determinants of Female Reproductive Health Throughout the Lifespan

Socioeconomic factors influence a woman's environment and health throughout the life course. Findings from the National Health Examination and Nutrition Survey point to substantial socioeconomic differences in age at menarche.[98] A large cross-cohort analysis including women across different countries and regions supported the notion that women with higher education levels had fewer children, were older when they had their first birth, and experienced later menopause than women with lower education levels.[30] It is likely that an older age at first birth and lower total number of children among women with higher education reflects the fact that women are inclined to postpone having children until after they have completed their education. Socially disadvantaged women also appear to have a higher risk of various pregnancy complications.[99–101] A greater risk of early natural menopause among women with lower educational levels has also been identified in MR analyses.[102] Lower socioeconomic position translates into a continuous exposure to more adverse health circumstances, as well as cumulative psychosocial stress, resulting in accelerated ageing which might also be reflected in earlier menopause.[27]

2.4 Indicators of Reproductive Health and Noncommunicable Disease Risk

It has long been recognised that indicators of women's reproductive health reflect general health, providing clues relatively early on in the life course about future noncommunicable disease risk.[103] Some associations between reproductive health indicators and disease are likely to reflect a causal effect, with mechanisms relatively well established. For example, earlier age at menarche, later age at menopause, and shorter breastfeeding duration are associated with increased breast cancer risk (discussed in more detail in Chapter 11).[52,104,105] MR studies confirm these findings, in particular with oestrogen receptor-positive cancer,[106] as well as the postulated mechanism; greater lifetime exposure to reproductive hormones increased breast cancer risk.[50,107] Another such example is the known effects of reproductive hormones on bone density and subsequent fracture risk. Primary ovarian insufficiency, pregnancy, lactation, and menopause are all associated with a decline in or low bone density,[108] and MR studies suggest modest causal effects of later puberty and earlier menopause on fracture risk.[109]

In comparison, the mechanism underlying well-documented associations between indicators of reproductive health, such as earlier age at menarche, PCOS, parity, pregnancy complications, and cardiovascular disease (CVD) risk, are less clear and remain very active areas of research (see Chapter 5).[110] Accumulating evidence from both MR studies[52,71] and a study using repeat measures of adiposity across childhood and adulthood,[111] suggest that childhood BMI (which tracks into adulthood) is a major driver of the association between younger age at menarche and increased CVD risk. Multiple studies report a positive association between parity and CVD risk in parous women; in some but not all studies, the risk is elevated in nulliparous women. This association could reflect confounding, by socioeconomic position for example, or causal adverse effects of pregnancy, and/or child rearing on CVD risk. Studies that have compared the parity-CVD relationships in men and women in an attempt to determine whether confounding—which would affect associations in both sexes—is the main mechanism, have yielded inconclusive results.[112] Interestingly, pregnancy has a lasting lowering effect on blood pressure. The Norwegian HUNT study that includes measures of cardiovascular risk factors both pre- and postpregnancy shows that blood pressure drops after each pregnancy.[113] Another study used sex of first offspring as an instrument for number of offspring, exploiting the preference for sons in an Indian population.[114] This study found that women—but not men—with a first-born daughter (a proxy for having an additional child) had lower blood pressure, suggesting that either pregnancy or a female-specific child rearing effect (which is less likely), causally reduces blood pressure. Blood pressure is an important CVD risk factor, but it is possible the positive association of parity with CVD is mediated by pathways other than blood pressure (e.g. via lipids)[115] and that these 'cancel out' the protective effect of pregnancy on blood pressure. The identification of genetic variants robustly associated with parity, in combination with large scale datasets such as UK Biobank and the Chinese Kadoorie Biobank, means that MR studies may provide further insight into the mechanisms driving the parity-CVD association.

Women who experience pregnancy complications have a twofold risk of CVD compared to those who do not.[24] Results from HUNT suggest that this association may be driven by women's prepregnancy cardiometabolic health as opposed to a direct causal effect.[116]

Regardless, pregnancy complications identify women at increased CVD risk, and, therefore, several studies have investigated whether they have predictive value above and beyond established CVD risk factors and have found that the added value is negligible.[117] This does not mean that the 'unmasking' of women at increased CVD risk is not valuable. Pregnancy and its complications affect young women who may benefit from knowing about their risk and from support to reduce it. Moreover, as women are in contact with medical providers around pregnancy, this is an opportunity to intervene to reduce CVD relatively early in the life course.

2.5 Conclusions

Women's reproductive health spans at least three decades of the life course. It, therefore, includes multiple health 'events', choices, and behaviours and should be seen in terms of its implications for health across the life course. Although further research is needed, reproductive health has the potential to be leveraged as an opportunity for early risk assessment and prevention of adverse health conditions as women engage with health providers around contraception and pregnancy. The increasing visibility and open public discourse about women's reproductive health, including menstruation, miscarriage, and menopause, will hopefully bring about greater investment in this area, including in research, that will benefit women—their reproductive and overall health, and their well-being in later life.

Key messages and implications

- Women's reproductive health is multifaceted and encompasses the physical, mental, and social well-being aspects related to the reproductive system.
- The reproductive years span over three decades. The onset of menses marks the beginning of the reproductive years, while (in)fertility, pregnancy, and pregnancy complications play major roles in women's lives during early adulthood. Menopause, the cessation of menses, is another major transition and occurs in middle age.
- The prenatal, childhood, and adult environment influence women's reproductive health, as is illustrated by the effects of prenatal exposure to maternal smoking and obesity, own smoking, and obesity during childhood and adulthood on several reproductive health indicators.
- Female reproductive health indicators predict the risk of various chronic diseases in later life, such as CVD, osteoporosis, and breast cancer, and may, therefore, be used to identify high-risk women and intervene to reduce that risk early on in the life course.

References

1. World Health Organization. *Reproductive health indicators: guidelines for their generation, interpretation and analysis for global monitoring.* World Health Organization; 2006.

2. Angold A, Worthman CW. Puberty onset of gender differences in rates of depression: a developmental, epidemiologic and neuroendocrine perspective. *Journal of Affective Disorders*. 1993;29(2):145–58.

3. Eckert-Lind C, Busch AS, Petersen JH, Biro FM, Butler G, Bräuner EV, et al. Worldwide secular trends in age at pubertal onset assessed by breast development among girls: a systematic review and meta-analysis. *JAMA Pediatrics*. 2020;174(4):e195881.

4. Wyshak G, Frisch RE. Evidence for a secular trend in age of menarche. *New England Journal of Medicine*. 1982;306(17):1033–5.

5. Finer LB, Philbin JM. Trends in ages at key reproductive transitions in the United States, 1951–2010. *Women's Health Issues: Official Publication of the Jacobs Institute of Women's Health*. 2014;24(3):e271–e279.

6. Gentry-Maharaj A, Glazer C, Burnell M, Ryan A, Berry H, Kalsi J, et al. Changing trends in reproductive/lifestyle factors in UK women: descriptive study within the UK Collaborative Trial of Ovarian Cancer Screening (UKCTOCS). *BMJ Open*. 2017;7(3):e011822.

7. Morris DH, Jones ME, Schoemaker MJ, Ashworth A, Swerdlow AJ. Secular trends in age at menarche in women in the UK born 1908–93: results from the Breakthrough Generations Study. *Paediatric and Perinatal Epidemiology*. 2011;25(4):394–400.

8. Deng Y, Liang J, Zong Y, Yu P, Xie R, Guo Y, et al. Timing of spermarche and menarche among urban students in Guangzhou, China: trends from 2005 to 2012 and association with Obesity. *Scientific Reports*. 2018;8(1):263.

9. Petersohn I, Zarate-Ortiz AG, Cepeda-Lopez AC, Melse-Boonstra A. Time trends in age at menarche and related non-communicable disease risk during the 20th century in Mexico. *Nutrients*. 2019;11(2):394.

10. Hosokawa M, Imazeki S, Mizunuma H, Kubota T, Hayashi K. Secular trends in age at menarche and time to establish regular menstrual cycling in Japanese women born between 1930 and 1985. *BMC Women's Health*. 2012;12:19.

11. Schoep ME, Adang EMM, Maas JWM, De Bie B, Aarts JWM, Nieboer TE. Productivity loss due to menstruation-related symptoms: a nationwide cross-sectional survey among 32 748 women. *BMJ Open*. 2019;9(6):c026186.

12. Hennegan J, Shannon AK, Rubli J, Schwab KJ, Melendez-Torres GJ. Women's and girls' experiences of menstruation in low- and middle-income countries: a systematic review and qualitative metasynthesis. *PLoS Medicine*. 2019;16(5):e1002803.

13. Wang YX, Arvizu M, Rich-Edwards JW, Stuart JJ, Manson JE, Missmer SA, et al. Menstrual cycle regularity and length across the reproductive lifespan and risk of premature mortality: prospective cohort study. *BMJ*. 2020;371:m3464.

14. ACOG Committee opinion, no. 651. Menstruation in girls and adolescents: using the menstrual cycle as a vital sign. *Obstetrics and Gynecology*. 2015;126(6):e143–e146.

15. ACOG Committee opinion, no. 781. Infertility workup for the women's health specialist: *Obstetrics and Gynecology*. 2019;133(6):e377–e384.

16. GBD 2017 Population and Fertility Collaborators. Population and fertility by age and sex for 195 countries and territories, 1950–2017: a systematic analysis for the global burden of disease study 2017. *Lancet (London, England)*. 2018;392(10159):1995–2051.

17. Vollset SE, Goren E, Yuan CW, Cao J, Smith AE, Hsiao T, et al. Fertility, mortality, migration, and population scenarios for 195 countries and territories from 2017 to 2100: a forecasting analysis for the Global Burden of Disease Study. *Lancet (London, England)*. 2020;396(10258):1285–306.

18. Eurostat. *Women in the EU are having their first child later [Internet]*. 24 Feb. 2021 [cited 19 Nov. 2021]. Available from: https://ec.europa.eu/eurostat/web/products-eurostat-news/-/ddn-20210224-1.

19. Human Reproduction and Embryology (ESHRE), Wyns C, De Geyter C, Calhaz-Jorge C, Kupka MS, Motrenko T, Smeenk J, Bergh C, et al. Assisted reproductive technology in Europe, 2017: results generated from European registries by ESHRE. *Human Reproduction Open*. 2021;3:hoab026.

20. Smith S, Pfeifer SM, Collins JA. Diagnosis and management of female infertility. *JAMA*. 2003;290(13):1767–70.

21. Deshpande PS, Gupta AS. Causes and prevalence of factors causing infertility in a public health facility. *Journal of Human Reproductive Science*. 2019;12(4):287–93.

22. McIntyre HD, Catalano P, Zhang C, Desoye G, Mathiesen ER, Damm P. Gestational diabetes mellitus. *Nature Reviews Disease Primers*. 2019;5(1):47.

23. Vest AR, Cho LS. Hypertension in pregnancy. *Cardiology Clinics*. 2012;30(3):407–23.

24. Rich-Edwards JW, Fraser A, Lawlor DA, Catov JM. Pregnancy characteristics and women's future cardiovascular health: an underused opportunity to improve women's health? *Epidemiologic Reviews*. 2014;36(1):57–70.

25. Kumari M, Head J, Marmot M. Prospective study of social and other risk factors for incidence of type 2 diabetes in the Whitehall II Study. *Archives of Internal Medicine*. 2004;164(17):1873–80.

26. Zhu D, Chung HF, Dobson AJ, Pandeya N, Giles GG, Bruinsma F, et al. Age at natural menopause and risk of incident cardiovascular disease: a pooled analysis of individual patient data. *Lancet Public Health*. 2019;4(11):e553–e564.

27. Schoenaker DA, Jackson CA, Rowlands JV, Mishra GD. Socioeconomic position, lifestyle factors and age at natural menopause: a systematic review and meta-analyses of studies across six continents. *International Journal of Epidemiology*. 2014;43(5):1542–62.

28. Lewington S, Li L, Murugasen S, Hong LS, Yang L, Guo Y, et al. Temporal trends of main reproductive characteristics in ten urban and rural regions of China: the China Kadoorie biobank study of 300 000 women. *International Journal of Epidemiology*. 2014;43(4):1252–62.

29. Park CY, Lim JY, Park HY. Age at natural menopause in Koreans: secular trends and influences thereon. *Menopause*. 2018;25(4):423–9.

30. El Khoudary SR, Greendale G, Crawford SL, Avis NE, Brooks MM, Thurston RC, et al. The menopause transition and women's health at midlife: a progress report from the Study of Women's Health Across the Nation (SWAN). *Menopause*. 2019;26(10):1213–27.

31. Gottschalk MS, Eskild A, Hofvind S, Gran JM, Bjelland EK. Temporal trends in age at menarche and age at menopause: a population study of 312 656 women in Norway. *Human Reproduction*. 2020;35(2):464–71.

32. Gold EB, Colvin A, Avis N, Bromberger J, Greendale GA, Powell L, et al. Longitudinal analysis of the association between vasomotor symptoms and race/ethnicity across the menopausal transition: study of women's health across the nation. *American Journal of Public Health*. 2006;96(7):1226–35.

33. Chung H-F, Zhu D, Dobson A, Kuh D, Gold E, Crawford S, et al. Age at menarche and risk of vasomotor menopausal symptoms: a pooled analysis of six studies. *BJOG*. 2021;128(3):603–13.

34. Cooper R, Mishra G, Clennell S, Guralnik J, Kuh D. Menopausal status and physical performance in midlife: findings from a British birth cohort study. *Menopause*. 2008;15(6):1079–85.

35. Kilpi F, Soares ALG, Fraser A, Nelson SM, Sattar N, Fallon SJ, et al. Changes in six domains of cognitive function with reproductive and chronological ageing and sex hormones: a longitudinal study in 2411 UK mid-life women. *BMC Women's Health*. 2020;20(1):177.

36. Forman MR, Mangini LD, Thelus-Jean R, Hayward MD. Life-course origins of the ages at menarche and menopause. *Adolescent Health, Medicine and Therapeutics*. 2013;4:1–21.

37. Bjelland EK, Hofvind S, Byberg L, Eskild A. The relation of age at menarche with age at natural menopause: a population study of 336 788 women in Norway. *Human Reproduction*. 2018;33(6):1149–57.

38. Mishra GD, Pandeya N, Dobson AJ, Chung H-F, Anderson D, Kuh D, et al. Early menarche, nulliparity and the risk for premature and early natural menopause. *Human Reproduction (Oxford, England)*. 2017;32(3):679–86.

39. Wang L, Yan B, Shi X, Song H, Su W, Huang B, et al. Age at menarche and risk of gestational diabetes mellitus: a population-based study in Xiamen, China. *BMC Pregnancy and Childbirth*. 2019;19(1):138.

40. Li H, Song L, Shen L, Liu B, Zheng X, Zhang L, et al. Age at menarche and prevalence of preterm birth: results from the healthy baby cohort study. *Scientific Reports*. 2017;7(1):12594.

41. Roman Lay AA, do Nascimento CF, Horta BL, Dias Porto Chiavegatto Filho A. Reproductive factors and age at natural menopause: a systematic review and meta-analysis. *Maturitas*. 2020;131:57–64.

42. Gold EB. The timing of the age at which natural menopause occurs. *Obstetrics and Gynecology Clinincs of North America*. 2011;38(3):425–40.
43. Day FR, Thompson DJ, Helgason H, Chasman DI, Finucane H, Sulem P, et al. Genomic analyses identify hundreds of variants associated with age at menarche and support a role for puberty timing in cancer risk. *Nature Genetics*. 2017;49(6):834–41.
44. Barban N, Jansen R, de Vlaming R, Vaez A, Mandemakers JJ, Tropf FC, et al. Genome-wide analysis identifies 12 loci influencing human reproductive behavior. *Nature Genetics*. 2016;48(12):1462–72.
45. Beaumont RN, Warrington NM, Cavadino A, Tyrrell J, Nodzenski M, Horikoshi M, et al. Genome-wide association study of offspring birth weight in 86 577 women identifies five novel loci and highlights maternal genetic effects that are independent of fetal genetics. *Human Molecular Genetics*. 2018;27(4):742–56.
46. Zhang G, Feenstra B, Bacelis J, Liu X, Muglia LM, Juodakis J, et al. Genetic associations with gestational duration and spontaneous preterm birth. *New England Journal of Medicine*. 2017;377(12):1156–67.
47. Tiensuu H, Haapalainen AM, Karjalainen MK, Pasanen A, Huusko JM, Marttila R, et al. Risk of spontaneous preterm birth and fetal growth associates with fetal SLIT2. *PLoS Genetics*. 2019;15(6):e1008107.
48. Liu X, Helenius D, Skotte L, Beaumont RN, Wielscher M, Geller F, et al. Variants in the fetal genome near pro-inflammatory cytokine genes on 2q13 associate with gestational duration. *Nature Communications*. 2019;10(1):3927.
49. Steinthorsdottir V, McGinnis R, Williams NO, Stefansdottir L, Thorleifsson G, Shooter S, et al. Genetic predisposition to hypertension is associated with preeclampsia in European and Central Asian women. *Nature Communications*. 2020;11(1):5976.
50. Day FR, Ruth KS, Thompson DJ, Lunetta KL, Pervjakova N, Chasman DI, et al. Large-scale genomic analyses link reproductive aging to hypothalamic signaling, breast cancer susceptibility and BRCA1-mediated DNA repair. *Nature Genetics*. 2015;47(11):1294–303.
51. Lawn RB, Sallis HM, Wootton RE, Taylor AE, Demange P, Fraser A, et al. The effects of age at menarche and first sexual intercourse on reproductive and behavioural outcomes: a Mendelian randomization study. *PLoS One*. 2020;15(6):e0234488.
52. Magnus MC, Guyatt AL, Lawn RB, Wyss AB, Trajanoska K, Küpers LK, et al. Identifying potential causal effects of age at menarche: a Mendelian randomization phenome-wide association study. *BMC Medicine*. 2020;18(1):71.
53. Ruth KS, Beaumont RN, Tyrrell J, Jones SE, Tuke MA, Yaghootkar H, et al. Genetic evidence that lower circulating FSH levels lengthen menstrual cycle, increase age at menopause and impact female reproductive health. *Human Reproduction*. 2016;31(2):473–81.
54. Prince C, Sharp GC, Howe LD, Fraser A, Richmond RC. The relationships between women's reproductive factors: a Mendelian randomization analysis. *MC Medicine*. 2021 20(1):103.
55. Woodruff TK. Making eggs: is it now or later? *Nature Medicine*. 2008;14(11):1190–1.
56. James E, Wood CL, Nair H, Williams TC. Preterm birth and the timing of puberty: a systematic review. *BMC Pediatrics*. 2018;18(1):3.
57. Juul F, Chang VW, Brar P, Parekh N. Birth weight, early life weight gain and age at menarche: a systematic review of longitudinal studies. *Obesity Reviews*. 2017;18(11):1272–88.
58. Barker DJ. The developmental origins of chronic adult disease. *Acta Paediatrica (Oslo, Norway: 1992) Supplement*. 2004;93(446):26–33.
59. Brix N, Ernst A, Lauridsen LLB, Parner ET, Arah OA, Olsen J, et al. Maternal pre-pregnancy body mass index, smoking in pregnancy, and alcohol intake in pregnancy in relation to pubertal timing in the children. *BMC Pediatrics*. 2019;19(1):338.
60. Lawn RB, Lawlor DA, Fraser A. Associations between maternal prepregnancy body mass index and gestational weight gain and daughter's age at menarche: the Avon Longitudinal Study of Parents and Children. *American Journal of Epidemiology*. 2018;187(4):677–86.
61. Brix N, Ernst A, Lauridsen LLB, Arah OA, Nohr EA, Olsen J, et al. Maternal pre-pregnancy obesity and timing of puberty in sons and daughters: a population-based cohort study. *International Journal of Epidemiology*. 2019;48(5):1684–94.

62. Brix N, Ernst A, Lauridsen LLB, Parner ET, Olsen J, Henriksen TB, et al. Maternal smoking during pregnancy and timing of puberty in sons and daughters: a population-based cohort study. *American Journal of Epidemiology*. 2019;188(1):47–56.

63. deKeyser N, Josefsson A, Bladh M, Carstensen J, Finnström O, Sydsjö G. Premature birth and low birthweight are associated with a lower rate of reproduction in adulthood: a Swedish population-based registry study. *Human Reproduction*. 2012;27(4):1170–8.

64. Thorsted A, Lauridsen J, Høyer B, Arendt LH, Bech B, Toft G, et al. Birth Weight for Gestational Age and the risk of infertility: a Danish cohort study. *Human Reproduction*. 2020;35(1):195–202.

65. Vikström J, Hammar M, Josefsson A, Bladh M, Sydsjö G. Birth characteristics in a clinical sample of women seeking infertility treatment: a case-control study. *BMJ Open*. 2014;4(3):e004197.

66. Dempsey JC, Williams MA, Luthy DA, Emanuel I, Shy K. Weight at birth and subsequent risk of preeclampsia as an adult. *American Journal of Obstetrics and Gynecology*. 2003;189(2):494–500.

67. Innes KE, Byers TE, Marshall JA, Barón A, Orleans M, Hamman RF. Association of a woman's own birth weight with subsequent risk for gestational diabetes. *JAMA*. 2002;287(19):2534–41.

68. Andraweera PH, Dekker G, Leemaqz S, McCowan L, Myers J, Kenny L, et al. Effect of birth weight and early pregnancy BMI on risk for pregnancy complications. *Obesity (Silver Spring)*. 2019;27(2):237–44.

69. Bjelland EK, Gran JM, Hofvind S, Eskild A. The association of birthweight with age at natural menopause: a population study of women in Norway. *International Journal of Epidemiology*. 2020;49(2):528–36.

70. Ruth KS, Perry JR, Henley WE, Melzer D, Weedon MN, Murray A. Events in early life are associated with female reproductive ageing: a UK Biobank study. *Scientific Reports*. 2016;6:24710.

71. Bell JA, Carslake D, Wade KH, Richmond RC, Langdon RJ, Vincent EE, et al. Influence of puberty timing on adiposity and cardiometabolic traits: a Mendelian randomisation study. *PLoS Medicine*. 2018;15(8):e1002641.

72. Lawlor DA, Tilling K, Davey Smith G. Triangulation in aetiological epidemiology. *International Journal of Epidemiology*. 2016;45(6):1866–86.

73. Reynolds P, Hurley SE, Hoggatt K, Anton-Culver H, Bernstein L, Deapen D, et al. Correlates of active and passive smoking in the California teachers study cohort. *Journal of Women's Health (Larchmt)*. 2004;13(7):778–90.

74. Windham GC, Lum R, Voss R, Wolff M, Pinney SM, Teteilbaum SL, et al. Age at pubertal onset in girls and tobacco smoke exposure during pre- and postnatal susceptibility windows. *Epidemiology*. 2017;28(5):719–27.

75. Watkins DJ, Téllez-Rojo MM, Ferguson KK, Lee JM, Solano-Gonzalez M, Blank-Goldenberg C, et al. In utero and peripubertal exposure to phthalates and BPA in relation to female sexual maturation. *Environmental Research*. 2014;134:233–41.

76. Wolff MS, Pajak A, Pinney SM, Windham GC, Galvez M, Rybak M, et al. Associations of urinary phthalate and phenol biomarkers with menarche in a multiethnic cohort of young girls. *Reproductive Toxicology*. 2017;67:56–64.

77. Zhang Y, Cao Y, Shi H, Jiang X, Zhao Y, Fang X, et al. Could exposure to phthalates speed up or delay pubertal onset and development? A 1.5-year follow-up of a school-based population. *Environment International*. 2015;83:41–9.

78. He Y, Tian J, Oddy WH, Dwyer T, Venn AJ. Association of childhood obesity with female infertility in adulthood: a 25-year follow-up study. *Fertility and Sterility*. 2018;110(4):596–604.e1.

79. Jacobs MB, Bazzano LA, Pridjian G, Harville EW. Childhood adiposity and fertility difficulties: the Bogalusa Heart Study. *Pediatric Obesity*. 2017;12(6):477–84.

80. He Y, Tian J, Blizzard L, Oddy WH, Dwyer T, Bazzano LA, et al. Associations of childhood adiposity with menstrual irregularity and polycystic ovary syndrome in adulthood: the childhood determinants of adult health study and the Bogalusa heart study. *Human Reproduction*. 2020;35(5):1185–98.

81. Laitinen J, Taponen S, Martikainen H, Pouta A, Millwood I, Hartikainen AL, et al. Body size from birth to adulthood as a predictor of self-reported polycystic ovary syndrome symptoms. *International Journal of Obesity and Related Metabolic Disorders*. 2003;27(6):710–5.

82. Jensen TK, Joffe M, Scheike T, Skytthe A, Gaist D, Petersen I, et al. Early exposure to smoking and future fecundity among Danish twins. *International Journal of Andrology*. 2006;29(6):603–13.

83. Peppone LJ, Piazza KM, Mahoney MC, Morrow GR, Mustian KM, Palesh OG, et al. Associations between adult and childhood second-hand smoke exposures and fecundity and fetal loss among women who visited a cancer hospital. *Tobaco Control*. 2009;18(2):115–20.

84. Wilcox AJ, Baird DD, Weinberg CR. Do women with childhood exposure to cigarette smoking have increased fecundability? *American Journal of Epidemiology*. 1989;129(5):1079–83.

85. Pedersen DC, Bjerregaard LG, Nohr EA, Rasmussen KM, Baker JL. Associations of childhood BMI and change in BMI from childhood to adulthood with risks of hypertensive disorders in pregnancy. *American Journal of Clinical Nutrition*. 2020;112(5);1180–7.

86. Leeners B, Rath W, Kuse S, Irawan C, Neumaier-Wagner P. The significance of under- or over-weight during childhood as a risk factor for hypertensive diseases in pregnancy. *Early Human Development*. 2006;82(10):663–8.

87. Wallace M, Bazzano L, Chen W, Harville E. Maternal childhood cardiometabolic risk factors and pregnancy complications. *Annals of Epidemiology*. 2017;27(7):429–34.

88. Hardy R, Mishra GD, Kuh D. Body mass index trajectories and age at menopause in a British birth cohort. *Maturitas*. 2008;59(4):304–14.

89. Moslehi N, Shab-Bidar S, Ramezani Tehrani F, Mirmiran P, Azizi F. Is ovarian reserve associated with body mass index and obesity in reproductive aged women? A meta-analysis. *Menopause*. 2018;25(9):1046–55.

90. Sermondade N, Huberlant S, Bourhis-Lefebvre V, Arbo E, Gallot V, Colombani M, et al. Female obesity is negatively associated with live birth rate following IVF: a systematic review and meta-analysis. *Human Reproduction Update*. 2019;25(4):439–51.

91. Budani MC, Fensore S, Di Marzio M, Tiboni GM. Cigarette smoking impairs clinical outcomes of assisted reproductive technologies: a meta-analysis of the literature. *Reproductive Toxicology*. 2018;80:49–59.

92. Philips EM, Santos S, Trasande L, Aurrekoetxea JJ, Barros H, von Berg A, et al. Changes in parental smoking during pregnancy and risks of adverse birth outcomes and childhood overweight in Europe and North America: an individual participant data meta-analysis of 229,000 singleton births. *PLoS Medicine*. 2020;17(8):e1003182.

93. Wei J, Liu CX, Gong TT, Wu QJ, Wu L. Cigarette smoking during pregnancy and pree-clampsia risk: a systematic review and meta-analysis of prospective studies. *Oncotarget*. 2015;6(41):43667–78.

94. Santos S, Voerman E, Amiano P, Barros H, Beilin LJ, Bergström A, et al. Impact of maternal body mass index and gestational weight gain on pregnancy complications: an individual participant data meta-analysis of European, North American and Australian cohorts. *BJOG*. 2019;126(8):984–95.

95. Goto E. Dose-response association between maternal body mass index and small for gestational age: a meta-analysis. *Journal of Maternal Fetal and Neonatal Medicine*. 2017;30(2):213–8.

96. Zhu D, Chung HF, Pandeya N, Dobson AJ, Cade JE, Greenwood DC, et al. Relationships between intensity, duration, cumulative dose, and timing of smoking with age at menopause: a pooled analysis of individual data from 17 observational studies. *PLoS Medicine*. 2018;15(11):e1002704.

97. Zhu D, Chung HF, Pandeya N, Dobson AJ, Kuh D, Crawford SL, et al. Body mass index and age at natural menopause: an international pooled analysis of 11 prospective studies. *European Journal of Epidemiology*. 2018;33(8):699–710.

98. Krieger N, Kiang MV, Kosheleva A, Waterman PD, Chen JT, Beckfield J. Age at menarche: 50-year socioeconomic trends among US-born black and white women. *American Journal of Public Health*. 2015;105(2):388–97.

99. Bo S, Menato G, Bardelli C, Lezo A, Signorile A, Repetti E, et al. Low socioeconomic status as a risk factor for gestational diabetes. *Diabetes & Metabolism*. 2002;28(2):139–40.

100. Peacock JL, Bland JM, Anderson HR. Preterm delivery: effects of socioeconomic factors, psychological stress, smoking, alcohol, and caffeine. *BMJ*. 1995;311(7004):531–5.

101. Silva LM, Coolman M, Steegers EA, Jaddoe VW, Moll HA, Hofman A, et al. Low socioeconomic status is a risk factor for preeclampsia: the generation R study. *Journal of Hypertension*. 2008;26(6):1200–8.

102. Ding X, Tang R, Zhu J, He M, Huang H, Lin Z, et al. An appraisal of the role of previously reported risk factors in the age at menopause using mendelian randomization. *Frontiers in Genetics*. 2020;11:507.

103. Rich-Edwards JW. Reproductive health as a sentinel of chronic disease in women. *Women's Health (London, England)*. 2009;5(2):101–5.

104. Menarche, menopause, and breast cancer risk: individual participant meta-analysis, including 118 964 women with breast cancer from 117 epidemiological studies. *Lancet Oncology*. 2012;13(11):1141–51.

105. Burgess S, Thompson DJ, Rees JMB, Day FR, Perry JR, Ong KK. Dissecting causal pathways using Mendelian randomization with summarized genetic data: application to age at menarche and risk of breast cancer. *Genetics*. 2017;207(2):481–7.

106. Day FR, Thompson DJ, Helgason H, Chasman DI, Finucane H, Sulem P, et al. Genomic analyses identify hundreds of variants associated with age at menarche and support a role for puberty timing in cancer risk. *Nature Genetics*. 2017;49(6):834–41.

107. Ruth KS, Day FR, Hussain J, Martínez-Marchal A, Aiken CE, Azad A, et al. Genetic insights into biological mechanisms governing human ovarian ageing. *Nature*. 2021;596(7872):393–7.

108. Mills EG, Yang L, Nielsen MF, Kassem M, Dhillo WS, Comninos AN. The relationship between bone and reproductive hormones beyond estrogens and androgens. *Endocrine Reviews*. 2021;42(6):691–719.

109. Trajanoska K, Morris JA, Oei L, Zheng HF, Evans DM, Kiel DP, et al. Assessment of the genetic and clinical determinants of fracture risk: genome wide association and mendelian randomisation study. *BMJ*. 2018;362:k3225.

110. Thangaratinam S, Thomas GN, Nirantharakumar K, Adderley NJ. Association between the reproductive health of young women and cardiovascular disease in later life: umbrella review. *BMJ (Clinical Research Ed.)*. 2020;371:m3502.

111. O'Keeffe LM, Frysz M, Bell JA, Howe LD, Fraser A. Puberty timing and adiposity change across childhood and adolescence: disentangling cause and consequence. *Human Reproduction*. 2020;35(12):2784–92.

112. Magnus MC, Iliodromiti S, Lawlor DA, Catov JM, Nelson SM, Fraser A. Number of offspring and cardiovascular disease risk in men and women: the role of shared lifestyle characteristics. *Epidemiology*. 2017;28(6):880–8.

113. Haug EB, Horn J, Markovitz AR, Fraser A, Macdonald-Wallis C, Tilling K, et al. The impact of parity on life course blood pressure trajectories: the HUNT study in Norway. *European Journal of Epidemiology*. 2018;33(8):751–61.

114. Teufel F, Geldsetzer P, Sudharsanan N, Subramanyam M, Yapa HM, De Neve J-W, et al. The effect of bearing and rearing a child on blood pressure: a nationally representative instrumental variable analysis of 444 611 mothers in India. *International Journal of Epidemiology*. 2021;50(5):1671–83.

115. Markovitz AR, Haug EB, Horn J, Fraser A, Macdonald-Wallis C, Tilling K, et al. Does pregnancy alter life-course lipid trajectories? Evidence from the HUNT Study in Norway. *Journal of Lipid Research*. 2018;59(12):2403–12.

116. Haug EB, Horn J, Markovitz AR, Fraser A, Vatten LJ, Macdonald-Wallis C, et al. Life course trajectories of cardiovascular risk factors in women with and without hypertensive disorders in first pregnancy: the HUNT study in Norway. *Journal of the American Heart Association*. 2018;7(15):e009250.

117. Markovitz AR, Stuart JJ, Horn J, Williams PL, Rimm EB, Missmer SA, et al. Does pregnancy complication history improve cardiovascular disease risk prediction? Findings from the HUNT study in Norway. *European Heart Journal*. 2019;40(14):1113–20.

3

A Life Course Approach to Endometriosis

Gita D. Mishra, Ingrid J. Rowlands, Hsiu-Wen Chan, and Grant W. Montgomery

3.1 Introduction

Endometriosis is one of the most common, yet under-appreciated, chronic gynaecological disorders. However, increasing political and clinical focus on the disease in HICs may be generating change.[1,2] In broad terms, endometriosis is characterised by growth or lesions of endometrial-like tissue outside the uterus, usually in the pelvic area such as on the ovaries, fallopian tubes, the peritoneum, and the outside of the uterus. The resultant inflammation and scarring, including adhesions, can lead to a range of symptoms, including chronic pelvic pain, back pain, headaches or migraines, dysmenorrhoea (painful menstruation with heavy bleeding), and dyspareunia (painful intercourse), as well as accompanying tiredness or weakness.[3,4] At the time of diagnosis, the total number of symptoms experienced by women with suspected endometriosis is higher than for women with surgically confirmed endometriosis, which may reflect poor control from nonsurgical methods of treatment or no intervention. Limited life course research into endometriosis may mean that the full spectrum of symptoms experienced is more extensive or variable. Around a third of women with confirmed endometriosis experience infertility.[5]

Currently, there is no cure for endometriosis, and surgical management is appropriate only when symptoms reach a level of severity to justify the risk, with one study finding progressions of lesions postsurgery in 29% of patients.[6] Pharmacological treatment focuses on management of the condition, such as with analgesics and suppression of oestrogen with the aim of inhibiting tissue proliferation and inflammation. For dysmenorrhoea or chronic pelvic pain, prescribing an oral contraceptive (OC) represents part of the first-line treatment.

The life course approach provides an ideal framework for investigating outcomes with long latency and diseases that arise from a complex set of processes, as exemplified by endometriosis. The approach focuses on the timing and duration of exposures during critical or sensitive windows during development, especially from early life through to adolescence, during which many known or potential risk factors for this condition have been identified (see Figure 3.1). Similarly, throughout adulthood, existing and new exposures and the manifestation of the condition may have an impact on health and well-being, including disruption to education, career, relationships, and family planning. In this way, the life course approach can not only help provide early identification of groups of women at most risk, but the optimal time for preventive health strategies and/or monitoring.

Gita D. Mishra, Ingrid J. Rowlands, Hsiu-Wen Chan, and Grant W. Montgomery, *A Life Course Approach to Endometriosis* In: *A Life Course Approach to Women's Health*. Second Edition. Edited by: Gita D Mishra, Rebecca Hardy, and Diana Kuh, Oxford University Press.
© Oxford University Press 2023. DOI: 10.1093/oso/9780192864642.003.0003

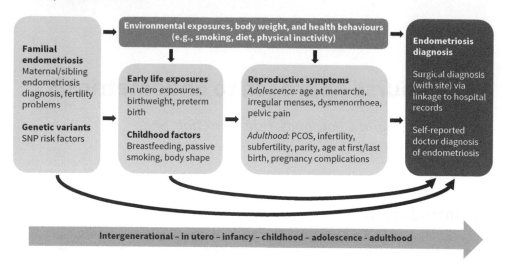

Figure 3.1 Life course conceptual framework for potential risk factors and consequences of endometriosis.

3.2 Prevalence and Burden

Estimates for women with asymptomatic endometriosis range from 2% to 11%.[7–9] Similarly, large community-based studies on endometriosis in the United States and Australia have reported a prevalence of 11% to 11.5%.[7,10] In symptomatic adolescents, 65% of girls undergoing laparoscopic investigation were diagnosed with endometriosis, rising to a rate of 75% for those with pain that did not respond to conventional medical therapy.[11] Accurate population level statistics are problematic, however, because of the current requirement for surgical visualisation for confirmation. Differences across studies in diagnostic criteria, the data collection method (self-report vs medical record linkage), and the sample population used also contribute to variations in prevalence estimates.

Historically, endometriosis was described as more common among white, career-driven women from socially advantaged backgrounds.[12] Much of this rhetoric was based on small, hospital-based studies that over-represented women from higher socioeconomic groups.[13] The social patterning of endometriosis is a likely outcome of the sociocultural and medical challenges associated with diagnosis. The accessibility, affordability, and acceptability of health care among individuals within a population plays an important role. In Australia, national hospital data recorded more hospitalisations for endometriosis among women living in higher socioeconomic areas than lower socioeconomic areas.[14] Further, Australian women with surgically confirmed endometriosis were more likely to have private health insurance than those without endometriosis.[4] Timely and equitable diagnosis of endometriosis remains a priority.

3.2.1 Variations in Prevalence by Ethnicity

The prevalence of endometriosis varies by race/ethnicity. Black and Hispanic women are about half as likely to be diagnosed with endometriosis than white women, whereas Asian women were around 60% more likely to have a diagnosis of endometriosis.[15] In Australia, there are fewer hospital admissions for endometriosis among indigenous Australians than nonindigenous Australians.[14] Although variation across race/ethnicity may indicate a genetic predisposition to the condition, another explanation is that racial/ethnic minorities experience greater socioeconomic and cultural barriers to obtaining a confirmed diagnosis of endometriosis.

3.2.2 Incidence Rates

The Australian Longitudinal Study on Women's Health revealed that endometriosis diagnosis rises rapidly in women in their 20s to a peak in the early 30s.[10] As this peak corresponds with the typical childbearing years of women in Australia, it may indicate that increased diagnosis for endometriosis is occurring as part of reproductive or prepregnancy related health services use, such as with fertility treatments.[16] It should be noted that women may have been living with or managing the condition with (or without) symptoms for many years prior to receiving a clinical diagnosis of endometriosis.

A cross-study comparison, including studies from the UK, United States, and Sweden, showed similar trends where the incidence of endometriosis peaked in the later 20s to early 30s.[17] In China, the risk of endometriosis was greatest for women born in 1938–42 and steadily declined amongst women who were born thereafter.[18] Although more studies are needed to confirm this finding, the cohort effect could be due to a reduction in risk factors for endometriosis over time (e.g. a decline in the prevalence of smoking during pregnancy[19,20] and the withdrawal of endocrine-disrupting agents for medical treatment).[21]

3.2.3 Challenges in the Diagnosis of Endometriosis

A key issue with this disease is that the standard for reliable clinical diagnosis still requires surgical visualisation, typically laparoscopy, supported by histologic confirmation. The risks associated with surgical intervention mean that there is a growing international trend towards a clinical diagnosis that combines symptoms with noninvasive approaches, including ultrasound and magnetic resonance imaging. Timely diagnosis, however, remains a problematic, with reports indicating that women will typically need to consult seven health professionals before diagnosis,[22,23] spend 6–10 years awaiting diagnosis,[24-26] with chronic pelvic pain first occurring in most women during adolescence.[23]

Wide variation exists in how the condition manifests, in terms of the location and form of the lesions, cysts, or nodules. However, three apparently distinct phenotypes of endometriosis with increasing severity are recognised: superficial (or peritoneal) endometriosis (SUP), ovarian endometrioma (OMA), and deep infiltrating endometriosis (DIE).[27] In addition, a detailed classification system used for the different stages and severity of endometrioses has been set out by the American Society of Reproductive Medicine.[27] Some have questioned, the value of such classification systems as a diagnostic tool in practice, where, for women with severe endometriosis, they appear not to correlate with the symptoms, treatment response, or prognosis.[9,28]

3.2.4 What Is the Economic and Broader Burden of the Condition?

For many women, endometriosis can also lead to psychological, physical, and social difficulties,[29,30] and subsequent economic burden from both direct (e.g. hospitalisation) and indirect (e.g. workplace absenteeism) costs.[31] A large international study has estimated the total annual cost per woman with endometriosis in Europe, the UK, and the United States to be almost €10,000 (or US$11,000), with over 60% of this due to absence from work in 2017–18.[31] In Australia, the estimated annual costs of endometriosis per woman (and averaged across all age groups) were almost twice that of US figures (US$21,000 equivalent), with over 80% of the total attributable to lost productivity.[32] The total direct health costs were estimated to have exceeded AU$506 million in 2017–18 in Australia.[33] Although these figures carry considerable uncertainty, the scale of economic burden attributable to endometriosis appears on a par, or higher than, other chronic diseases, including heart disease and diabetes. This should not be surprising as the timing and duration of the impact of endometriosis occurs not just during the reproductive life stage but also the most economically productive phase of women's lives. The impact of endometriosis often commences from adolescence and persists into later life.[34]

3.2.5 Impact on Quality of Life

Endometriosis has been described as a 'biographical disruption' that renders many women unable to lead the anticipated lives they had envisioned, requiring significant readjustment and reappraisal of the future.[35,36] The physical and psychosocial effects of endometriosis can emerge in adolescence and young adulthood,[37] but long diagnostic delays mean that many women cope for up to 10 years without adequate treatment and support.[38] Women's attempts to manage the physical symptoms of the disease for years without professional guidance can disrupt their self-concept, intimate relationships, family planning, and broader social lives including educational attainment and participation in work.[35,36,39,40]

A holistic approach to supporting women after a diagnosis of endometriosis is also essential. Adjusting to a diagnosis of endometriosis can be an ongoing process that negatively affects women's life trajectories. The fluctuating, unpredictable symptoms that women can experience over time may require a combination of medical, surgical, and infertility treatments.[9] The chronic and recurrent nature of the disease means that frequent medical review and treatment changes are often required.[41] The need for intervention may intensify as the disease progresses, severely affecting quality of life. The potential for early menopause and increased chronic disease risk means that women with endometriosis need ongoing support and monitoring as they learn to adapt and live with the disease across the life course. Furthermore, onset of menopausal symptoms (triggered by the dramatic reduction in oestrogen levels) is commonly treated with menopausal hormone therapy (MHT). As oestrogen-stimulated growth of endometrial lesions is one pathophysiological characteristics of endometriosis, it is possible that MHT may reactivate or exacerbate growth of endometrial deposits, as evidenced in an animal study.[42] Therefore, clinicians need to consider the risk and benefits of prescribing MHT to women with endometriosis.

3.3 Aetiology of Endometriosis

The aetiology of endometriosis, both its pathogenesis and development, is poorly under-stood as reflected by the range of postulated causal pathways. While endometriosis is a dis-ease that is most often clinically detected among women in their early 30s,[43] symptoms often emerge during adolescence following menarche.[34] Very little research on endometriosis in childhood exists, but the disease could result from endometrial cells shed during neonatal uterine bleeding[44,45] and may be triggered by early life exposures that contribute to the pro-gression of the disease in adulthood. Sampson's theory of retrograde menstruation[46] is gen-erally regarded as a likely part of the explanation for the pathogenesis of the condition. This refers to backward flow of menstrual debris, including viable endometrial cells through the fallopian tubes, and these then 'seed' inside peritoneal cavity. Although a number of studies support this theory,[47,48] retrograde menstruation is commonplace among women and most do not develop endometriosis.[34] Other theories for the source of the condition include stem cells,[49] coelomic metaplasia (the abnormal transformation of extrauterine cells into endo-metrial cells),[50] the spread of cells via the lymphatic and vascular system,[51] as well as the role of potential genetic or epigenetic factors.[52] Further details on the theories of endometriosis pathogenesis are beyond the scope of this chapter and are described elsewhere.[9,53] While this remains an active area of research, it is likely that multiple factors and mechanisms will be needed to explain full spectrum of how endometriosis manifests in women.

3.4 Risk Factors for Endometriosis Across the Life Course

Before summarising the evidence on risk factors across the life course, it is worth highlighting that considerable caution is needed in interpreting the evidence, which is typically based on laparoscopically confirmed endometriosis (that usually occurs long after disease onset). Comparison of the research is hindered by the various methodological limitations and design differences between studies, including retrospective data collection, inconsistent methods for identifying endometriosis cases, and inappropriate control groups used for comparison. Additionally, because of the lengthy time to diagnosis, a bidirectional relationship is possible such as between the symptoms of endometriosis and physical inactivity. Here, we review some of the risk factors that have been identified for endometriosis.

3.4.1 Heritability and Genetic Factors

The overall heritability of endometriosis based on twin studies is estimated at 47%–51%; thus, genetic variation accounts for around half of the disease risk.[54,55] It has been known for some decades that a family history of endometriosis appears to predispose women to the condi-tion. An early case-control study of women with confirmed endometriosis reported a preva-lence of 6.9% among first-degree relatives, compared with just 1% for the control group.[56] More recently, a large Swedish study reported that women whose mother had endometriosis were more than twice as likely to be diagnosed with endometriosis than other women.

In terms of genetic factors, large population-based genome-wide association studies (GWAS) have found that common genetic variations account for around 26% of the risk of endometriosis.[57] The most recent meta-analysis of 10 GWAS of European and Japanese women identified 18 significant loci associated with endometriosis, with 9 robustly replicated.[58-60] A key objective of this genetic research is to identify how specific genetic variants contribute to the pathogenesis of the condition. Potential insights from the research on causal pathways can enable better predictions about who is most at risk of endometriosis. Improved risk predictions can generate new methods to support the earlier diagnosis of endometriosis and provide targets for therapeutics to slow or stop the development of the disease.

3.4.2 In Utero Exposures

3.4.2.1 Maternal Smoking During Pregnancy

A Swedish study found that maternal smoking in early pregnancy was clearly linked with an increased risk of endometriosis in their daughters, including a dose response from moderate to heavy maternal smoking, after adjusting for maternal endometriosis and sociodemographic factors.[29] It is still not clear if mothers ceased smoking in response to the advice they received or if they continued to smoke through the rest of the pregnancy and beyond. The limited information on the duration of maternal smoking means we cannot disentangle the negative effects of in utero exposure to smoking from any passive smoking during infancy on the daughter's endometriosis risk. Similarly, maternal smoking is an established risk factor for low birthweight (see Section 3.4.3), which is also associated with endometriosis. In this study, more than a quarter of the total associations between maternal smoking and the daughter's endometriosis risk was mediated via birthweight.[29]

3.4.2.2 Other in Utero Exposures

A range of hormonal exposures during gestation could present a risk for endometriosis.[61] For instance, diethylstilbestrol (DES) is a synthetic form of oestrogen previously used to prevent miscarriages and pregnancy complications that has been linked with reproductive tract structural abnormalities and altered oestrogen receptor expression.[62] A US cohort study reported that women who had in utero exposure to maternal DES are 80% more likely to develop endometriosis,[63] suggesting this an area worthy of further research. More broadly, Benagiano and Brosens (2014) discussed a range of potential sources of hormonal exposures (pharmaceutical or environmental), such as dioxins and other endocrine-disrupting chemicals, which have been previously associated with adverse fetal developmental outcomes;[64] evidence of a link with endometriosis from small studies or animal models, however, were inconclusive.

3.4.2.3 Birth Characteristics

Recent findings from the Swedish registry study reported that women with a low birthweight were 16% more likely to have an endometriosis diagnosis, even after accounting for maternal endometriosis and gestational age.[29] In addition, the study found a clear linear relationship of increased risk for endometriosis with lower birthweight categories. However, the presence of an association after adjusting for maternal endometriosis has raised doubts given the high degree of heritability for the condition.[63,65] The evidence for links with gestational age is far more limited, with a recent review reporting that only one out of five studies detected an association for preterm birth.

3.4.2.4 Childhood and Adolescence

Some evidence points to links between growth rates in childhood and endometriosis risk. A 2012 review identified five studies, including three prospective cohort studies, that together showed body size in childhood had a consistent inverse relationship for subsequent endometriosis diagnosis, even after adjusting for factors such as age, birthweight, age at menarche, parity, and OC use.[66] In 2017, a major French study also reported a reduced risk of endometriosis for women who recalled having a large versus lean body shape at age 8 years and at menarche.[67] However, low body weight as a risk factor for endometriosis may be a product of methodological issues, or a sign of systemic problems in the diagnosis of endometriosis, including difficulties for girls and women who are overweight or obese to access appropriate care in clinical practice.

Women with an early age at menarche consistently have a higher risk of endometriosis,[68–70] More recent research delved further into this relationship but was unable to detect any variation in age at menarche across the three endometriosis phenotypes (SUP, OMA, and DIE).[71] Regarding menstrual characteristics, a US cohort study found that late adolescent women (aged 18–22 years) with shorter cycles had a higher prevalence of endometriosis,[68] an association that was also evident in adult women.[70]

Another aspect of the condition among adolescents (and adults) is the high prevalence of multiple comorbidities, including pain disorders that may reflect a general hypersensitivity to pain, referred to as central sensitisation.[72] The Women's Health Study reported that adolescents (aged 21 years or less) with endometriosis were over four times more likely to experience migraines than those without endometriosis; the strength of the association increased with the severity of the migraines.[73] The Women's Health Study also found that adolescents with both endometriosis and migraines were more likely to experience dysmenorrhoea than those without migraines. A case study of 138 adolescents (diagnosed by age 21) identified a high prevalence of comorbid pain syndromes (56%), mood conditions (48%), and asthma (26%).[74] Similarly, another small case study of adolescents with endometriosis found that more than half had genitourinary or gastrointestinal symptoms.[75] A recent meta-analysis reported patients with endometriosis were three times more likely to have irritable bowel syndrome.[76] Further evidence is needed, however, from large community-based cohort studies to gain a more comprehensive understanding of these comorbidities as a whole.

3.4.5 Adult Factors

3.4.5.1 Reproductive Characteristics

Much of the evidence available on endometriosis is from studies with adult women since the 1980s, and this has served to produce a somewhat clearer picture on adult risk factors and potential causal pathways. In general, the pattern of associations seen in adolescence is strengthened in adulthood but is often limited by small case studies. In terms of menstrual characteristics, worsening or persistent dysmenorrhoea is recognised as a one of the primary symptoms for health professionals to investigate an endometriosis diagnosis.[77] Additionally, and as with adolescents, there is consistent evidence that adult women with shorter cycle lengths have an increased risk of the disease; however, the evidence appears mixed or limited on associations with the length and heaviness of flow, irregularity, and other menstrual characteristics.[8] The use of combined OCs substantially reduces the volume of flow and regulates the cycle length to 28 days. The progestins in OCs have anti-inflammatory properties,[78] and prescribing OCs is part of standard treatment for pelvic pain and endometriosis. A meta-analysis of 18 studies reported a 37% lower relative risk of diagnosed endometriosis for current OC users, but around a 20% increased risk for past or ever users of OCs.[79] Despite the methodological drawbacks of some contributing studies, the evidence suggests a protective effect of current OC use. A higher risk of endometriosis after OC use ceases may reflect delayed diagnosis; further high-quality studies are needed to confirm these findings.

Infertility is an established risk factor for and/or consequence of endometriosis. Women with incident infertility had twice the risk of endometriosis; yet over 83% of these women with endometriosis had successfully given birth by the age of 40. An early diagnosis of endometriosis appears to offer advantages to women wanting to become pregnant.[16] A population-based Australian study reported that women who received a diagnosis of endometriosis before starting assisted reproductive treatment (ART) were more likely to give birth and have fewer cycles of ART than women who were diagnosed with endometriosis after starting ART.[16] There is currently limited evidence examining the reproductive outcomes for women with endometriosis.

As with pregnancy, breastfeeding affects hormone levels, yet there is very little evidence on breastfeeding and endometriosis. A US cohort study reported that exclusive breastfeeding (6 months) was associated with lower risk of endometriosis, and there was an inverse linear relationship with the duration of breastfeeding.[68] Maternal breastfeeding also appears to provide a protective effect for endometriosis in the daughter.[80]

3.4.5.2   Health Behaviours and Body Size

Body weight across the life course has most consistently been associated with endometriosis. Lower adult BMI[67,81] and lower weight gain in adulthood is associated with endometriosis[82] Similarly, women with a smaller waist-to-hip ratio had three times the risk of endometriosis than women with a larger waist-to-hip ratio.[67,81] The waist-to-hip ratio has implications for hormone levels, including the ratio of oestrogens to androgens. However, because oestrogen and chronic inflammation are thought to play a role in the aetiology of endometriosis, the absence of an association between obesity and endometriosis is somewhat perplexing. An Australian cohort study reported that women diagnosed with suspected endometriosis were more likely to be overweight and obese.[82] Social and health care challenges for women who are overweight or obese to access timely and appropriate investigations for endometriosis may mean they are never surgically diagnosed, creating a diagnostic bias in the research.[82]

For alcohol consumption, a meta-analysis of 15 studies found that women with any alcohol intake had a 24% increased risk of endometriosis compared with women who did not consume alcohol.[83]

Regarding dermatologic characteristics, cohort studies from France[84] and more recently Scotland[85] have both identified an increased risk of melanoma among women with endometriosis relative to age-matched women without the disease.[84] Skin and pigmentary characteristics common to people who develop melanoma are also more likely among women with endometriosis including sun sensitivity, a greater number of freckles and moles on the body[86,87] and, to a lesser extent, red hair.[8] Genetics, oestrogen dominance, and chronic inflammation may be shared mechanisms that contribute to the development of both endometriosis and skin changes. However, the lack of ethnic diversity in the research related to endometriosis means that links between dermatologic characteristics and endometriosis should be further examined.

There is a growing body of research examining the role of synthetically produced environmental chemicals or endocrine-disrupting chemicals (EDC) in the diagnosis of endometriosis.[88] Previous reviews of the literature reported inconclusive findings regarding EDC and endometriosis, possibly arising from small sample sizes.[8,89] Methodological shortcomings, particularly around the timing and measurement of chemical exposures and the timing of endometriosis diagnosis, have made it difficult to identify convincing links between environmental chemical exposures and endometriosis.[90]

Although a review of the literature reported associations between pesticides and endometriosis, effect sizes were small and there was a considerable risk of bias in the research overall.[91] Another recent review of the literature reported associations between phthalates, bisphenol A, and persistent organic pollutants (i.e. dioxins, pesticides, and polychlorinated biphenyls) and endometriosis.[90] The authors acknowledged that the extent to which these chemicals, alone or together, might influence endometriosis could not be determined because of methodological differences between the studies assessed.[90]

3.5 Endometriosis and Chronic Disease Risk

Although much of the current evidence from epidemiologic studies varies considerably in terms of quality and quantity, there are indications that women with endometriosis face increased risk for other chronic conditions.[8] One of the methodological challenges is accounting for treatments related to the management of endometriosis, and other interventions related to reproductive health, that can directly or indirectly affect hormone levels. For example, apart from being prescribed OCs to address pelvic pain, women with endometriosis are more likely to have a hysterectomy and/or oophorectomy, which if done early relative to the menopausal transition, are linked with increased risk of cardiovascular disease[92] and other conditions in later life. Common causes may also be an issue. The symptoms of endometriosis may lead to poor health behaviours that are mediating factors for a range of chronic conditions and adverse health outcomes. Any associations between endometriosis and other chronic diseases need to be interpreted in a way that recognises the potential role of other shared or mediating factors, as well as reverse causation.

3.5.1 Ovarian Cancer

Studies have shown a clear link between endometriosis and ovarian cancer.[93] Further, the Ovarian Cancer Association Consortium found that women who reported a history of endometriosis were one and a half times more likely to develop invasive ovarian cancer, three times as likely to have the clear-cell subtype, and twice as likely to have low-grade serous or endometrial invasive subtypes of ovarian cancer than the control group.[94] As no links were identified with high-grade serous or mucinous subtypes of ovarian cancer, this suggests there are specific mechanisms involved in the relationship between endometriosis and some types of ovarian cancer.

3.5.2 Other Cancers

Few studies have investigated the relationship between endometriosis and other reproductive cancers, with mixed and inconclusive findings on links with breast and endometrial cancer.[93] Some evidence points to an inverse relationship with cervical cancer, though these studies had limited statistical power.[93] Similarly, there is mixed or insufficient evidence available on the relationship between endometriosis and a range of nongynaecological cancers, including cutaneous melanoma, non-Hodgkin's lymphoma, brain cancer, and endocrine or thyroid cancers.[93]

3.5.3 Autoimmune Diseases, Allergies, and Asthma

Female hormones may contribute to the higher prevalence of autoimmune diseases among women, such as rheumatoid arthritis and multiple sclerosis. Endometriosis is associated with abnormalities in the immune system at the cellular level and a heightened humoral (or antibody-mediated) immune response, which mirror those seen in women with autoimmune diseases.[95] A large Danish retrospective cohort study found that women with endometriosis had an increased risk for a range of autoimmune and related diseases.[96,97] Most links between autoimmune disease and endometriosis were attenuated when the analysis was restricted to those with surgically confirmed diagnosis; however, associations were strengthened for multiple sclerosis, ulcerative colitis, and Crohn's disease.[97] Additionally, a Swedish cohort study found women with endometriosis were at increased risk of celiac disease.[98] And patients with surgically diagnosed endometriosis were twice as likely to have asthma and four times more likely to have allergies than controls.[99]

3.5.4 Cardiovascular Diseases

Endometriosis is linked to local and systemic chronic inflammation, markers of oxidative stress, and an adverse atherogenic lipid profile, which are associated with coronary heart disease (CHD).[93] Whilst most studies are under-powered to detect associations, the US Nurses' Health Study found an increased risk of myocardial infarction, angina, or coronary-related procedures (artery bypass surgery or stent) among women with endometriosis. There was also a 62% increased risk of these CHD outcomes combined among women with endometriosis compared to women without endometriosis.[100] More recently, a UK population-based cohort study also reported a higher risk of cardiovascular disease (CVD, including ischaemic heart disease, cerebrovascular disease, arrhythmia, and hypertension) among women with endometriosis compared to women without endometriosis.[101] The risk of CVD in both studies was attenuated when accounting for those women who had hysterectomy or oophorectomy, highlighting the potential role of endometriosis treatments on the causal pathway to chronic disease outcomes.

3.6 Conclusions

The diagnosis of endometriosis has historically been difficult and remains a current public health challenge. Noninvasive methods of endometriosis will significantly change the diagnostic landscape for endometriosis, and new methods are key to reduce diagnostic delay. However, robust diagnostic methods that are cost-effective and can be easily implemented at the population level are not widely available. In addition, our understanding of the factors that drive the disease remains largely theoretical. Continued research into the aetiology of endometriosis, therefore, remains central to identifying new methods of diagnosis.

Few risk factors for endometriosis have been identified. Much of the work on the aetiology of endometriosis has focused on adulthood and the emergence of symptoms during this period. Research focusing on early life periods—including childhood and adolescence—is limited but needed to understand whether there are ways we can intervene earlier and change the origins and course of the disease. The exception is low body weight, which appears to be influential to endometriosis across the life course.

At the broader level, social, medical, and political influences are central to improving the diagnosis of endometriosis. The clinical focus on surgery to confirm diagnosis, coupled with the limited social and clinical awareness of the disease,[102,103] are major barriers to early diagnosis. The normalisation of women's menstrual pain in social and medical contexts,[36] reinforced by the social stigma related to menstruation, have also discouraged women from seeking adequate social and professional support for endometriosis.[104] Advocates for endometriosis have called for widespread change to how we diagnose, treat, and talk to women. There has been some success, with political recognition of endometriosis as a public health issue in Australia, UK, United States, and, more recently, France. Both Australia and France have implemented national strategies for endometriosis that are aimed at increasing public awareness and education, improving treatment, and investing in research. Such strategies reinforce the need for a multilevel approach that targets individual, social, health care, and political barriers to the diagnosis of endometriosis.

Key messages and implications

- There is a clear need for large community-based, longitudinal studies with prospective data to undertake epidemiologic research into endometriosis.
- Longitudinal endometriosis-focused studies are crucial to disentangling the timing of the endometriosis diagnosis in relation to key risk factors.
- Understanding how key risk factors might mediate the endometriosis diagnosis and future chronic disease outcomes will build a more integrated picture.

References

1. Armour M, Sinclair J, Ng CHM, Hyman MS, Lawson K, Smith CA, et al. Endometriosis and chronic pelvic pain have similar impact on women, but time to diagnosis is decreasing: an Australian survey. *Scientific Reports.* 2020;10(1):16253.

2. Soliman AM, Fuldeore M, Snabes MC. Factors associated with time to endometriosis diagnosis in the United States. *Journal of Women's Health.* 2017;26(7):788–97.

3. Becker K, Heinemann K, Imthurn B, Marions L, Moehner S, Gerlinger C, et al. Real world data on symptomology and diagnostic approaches of 27,840 women living with endometriosis. *Scientific Reports.* 2021;11(1):20404.

4. Rowlands I, Hockey R, Abbott J, Montgomery G, Mishra G. Longitudinal changes in employment following a diagnosis of endometriosis: findings from an Australian cohort study. *Annals of Epidemiology.* 2022;69:1–8.

5. Prescott J, Farland LV, Tobias DK, Gaskins AJ, Spiegelman D, Chavarro JE, et al. A prospective cohort study of endometriosis and subsequent risk of infertility. *Human Reproduction.* 2016;31(7):1475–82.

6. Evers JLH. Is adolescent endometriosis a progressive disease that needs to be diagnosed and treated? *Human Reproduction.* 2013;28(8):2023.

7. Olšarová K, Mishra GD. Early life factors for endometriosis: a systematic review. *Human Reproduction Update.* 2020;26(3):412–22.

8. Shafrir AL, Farland LV, Shah DK, Harris HR, Kvaskoff M, Zondervan K, et al. Risk for and consequences of endometriosis: a critical epidemiologic review. *Best Practice & Research. Clinical Obstetrics and Gynaecology.* 2018;51:1–15.

9. Zondervan KT, Becker CM, Missmer SA. Endometriosis. *New England Journal of Medicine.* 2020;382(13):1244–56.

10. Rowlands IJ, Abbott JA, Montgomery GW, Hockey R, Rogers P, Mishra GD. Prevalence and incidence of endometriosis in Australian women: a data linkage cohort study. *BJOG: An International Journal of Obstetrics and Gynaecology.* 2020;128(4):657–65.

11. Janssen EB, Rijkers AC, Hoppenbrouwers K, Meuleman C, D'Hooghe TM. Prevalence of endometriosis diagnosed by laparoscopy in adolescents with dysmenorrhea or chronic pelvic pain: a systematic review. *Human Reproduction Update.* 2013;19(5):570–82.

12. Farland L, Horne A. Disparity in endometriosis diagnoses between racial/ethnic groups. *BJOG: An International Journal of Obstetrics & Gynaecology.* 2019;126(9):1115–6.

13. Mangtani P, Booth M. Epidemiology of endometriosis. *Journal of Epidemiology and Community Health.* 1993;47(2):84.

14. Australian Institute of Health and Welfare. *Endometriosis in Australia: prevalence and hospitalisations.* Canberra: Australian Institute of Health and Welfare; 2019. Report no. PHE 247.

15. Bougie O, Yap MI, Sikora L, Flaxman T, Singh S. Influence of race/ethnicity on prevalence and presentation of endometriosis: a systematic review and meta-analysis. *BJOG: An International Journal of Obstetrics and Gynaecology.* 2019;126(9):1104–15.

16. Moss KM, Doust J, Homer H, Rowlands IJ, Hockey R, Mishra GD. Delayed diagnosis of endometriosis disadvantages women in ART: a retrospective population linked data study. *Human Reproduction.* 2021;36(12):3074–82.

17. Rowlands IJ, Mishra GD, Abbott JA. Global epidemiological data on endometriosis. In: Oral E, ed. *Endometriosis and adenomyosis: global perspectives across the lifespan.* Cham: Springer International Publishing; 2022. pp. 15–28.

18. Feng J, Zhang S, Chen J, Yang J, Zhu J. Long-term trends in the incidence of endometriosis in China from 1990 to 2019: a join point and age–period–cohort analysis. *Gynecological Endocrinology.* 2021;37(11):1041–5.

19. Havard A, Tran DT, Kemp-Casey A, Einarsdóttir K, Preen DB, Jorm LR. Tobacco policy reform and population-wide antismoking activities in Australia: the impact on smoking during pregnancy. *Tobacco Control.* 2018;27(5):552–9.

20. Azagba S, Manzione L, Shan L, King J. Trends in smoking during pregnancy by socioeconomic characteristics in the United States, 2010–2017. *BMC Pregnancy and Childbirth.* 2020;20(1):52.

21. Zamora-Leon P. Are the effects of DES over? A tragic lesson from the past. *International Journal of Environmental Research and Public Health.* 2021;18(19):10309.

22. Ballard K, Lowton K, Wright JJF. What's the delay? A qualitative study of women's experiences of reaching a diagnosis of endometriosis. *Fertility Sterility.* 2006;86(5):1296–301.

23. Nnoaham KE, Hummelshoj L, Webster P, d'Hooghe T, de Cicco Nardone F, de Cicco Nardone C, et al. Impact of endometriosis on quality of life and work productivity: a multicenter study across ten countries. *Fertility Sterility*. 2011;96(2):366–73e8.

24. Dreyer NA, Tunis SR, Berger M, Ollendorf D, Mattox P, Gliklich R. Why observational studies should be among the tools used in comparative effectiveness research. *Health Affairs*. 2010;29(10):1818–25.

25. Bernuit D, Ebert AD, Halis G, Strothmann A, Gerlinger C, Geppert K, et al. Female perspectives on endometriosis: findings from the uterine bleeding and pain women's research study. *Journal of Endometriosis*. 2011;3(2):73–85.

26. Staal AHJ, van der Zanden M, Nap AW. Diagnostic delay of endometriosis in the Netherlands. *Gynecologic and Obstetric Investigation*. 2016;81(4):321–4.

27. Vermeulen N, Abrao MS, Einarsson JI, Horne AW, Johnson NP, Lee TTM, et al. Endometriosis classification, staging and reporting systems: a review on the road to a universally accepted endometriosis classification. *Human Reproduction Open*. 2021;2021(4):hoab025.

28. Schliep KC, Mumford SL, Peterson CM, Chen Z, Johnstone EB, Sharp HT, et al. Pain typology and incident endometriosis. *Human Reproduction*. 2015;30(10):2427–38.

29. Gao M, Scott K, Koupil I. Associations of perinatal characteristics with endometriosis: a nationwide birth cohort study. *International Journal of Epidemiology*. 2020;49(2):537–47.

30. Ferreira ALL, Bessa MMM, Drezett J, de Abreu LC. Quality of life of the woman carrier of endometriosis: systematized review. *Reprodução & Climatério*. 2016;31(1):48–54.

31. Simoens S, Dunselman G, Dirksen C, Hummelshoj L, Bokor A, Brandes I, et al. The burden of endometriosis: costs and quality of life of women with endometriosis and treated in referral centres. *Human Reproduction*. 2012;27(5):1292–9.

32. Armour M, Lawson K, Wood A, Smith CA, Abbott J. The cost of illness and economic burden of endometriosis and chronic pelvic pain in Australia: a national online survey. *PLoS One*. 2019;14(10):e0223316.

33. Ernst & Young. *The cost of endometriosis in Australia*. Sydney: Ernst & Young; 2019.

34. Shim JY, Laufer MR. Adolescent endometriosis: an update. *Journal of Pediatric and Adolescent Gynecology*. 2020;33(2):112–19.

35. Hudson N, Culley L, Law C, Mitchell H, Denny E, Raine-Fenning N. 'We needed to change the mission statement of the marriage': biographical disruptions, appraisals and revisions among couples living with endometriosis. *Sociology of Health & Illness*. 2016;38(5):721–35.

36. Manderson L, Warren N, Markovic M. Circuit breaking: pathways of treatment seeking for women with endometriosis in Australia. *Qualitative Health Research*. 2008;18(4):522–34.

37. Rowlands IJ, Teede H, Lucke J, Dobson AJ, Mishra GD. Young women's psychological distress after a diagnosis of polycystic ovary syndrome or endometriosis. *Human Reproduction*. 2016;31(9):2072–81.

38. Ballard KD, Seaman HE, de Vries CS, Wright JT. Can symptomatology help in the diagnosis of endometriosis? Findings from a national case-control study—Part 1. *BJOG: An International Journal of Obstetrics and Gynaecology*. 2008;115(11):1382–91.

39. Culley L, Law C, Hudson N, Denny E, Mitchell H, Baumgarten M, et al. The social and psychological impact of endometriosis on women's lives: a critical narrative review. *Human Reproduction Update*. 2013;19(6):625–39.

40. Young K, Fisher J, Kirkman M. Women's experiences of endometriosis: a systematic review and synthesis of qualitative research. *The Journal of Family Planning and Reproductive Health Care*. 2015;41(3):225–34.

41. Rowe HJ, Hammarberg K, Dwyer S, Camilleri R, Fisher JR. Improving clinical care for women with endometriosis: qualitative analysis of women's and health professionals' views. *Journal of Psychosomatic Obstetrics and Gynaecology*. 2021;42(3):174–80.

42. Wang C-T, Wang D-B, Liu K-R, Li Y, Sun C-X, Guo C-S, et al. Inducing malignant transformation of endometriosis in rats by long-term sustaining hyperestrogenemia and type II diabetes. *Cancer Science*. 2015;106(1):43–50.

43. Rowlands I, Abbott J, Montgomery G, Hockey R, Rogers P, Mishra G. Prevalence and incidence of endometriosis in Australian women: a data linkage cohort study. *BJOG: An International Journal of Obstetrics and Gynaecology*. 2021;128(4):657–65.

44. Gargett CE, Schwab KE, Brosens JJ, Puttemans P, Benagiano G, Brosens I. Potential role of endo-metrial stem/progenitor cells in the pathogenesis of early-onset endometriosis. *Molecular Human Reproduction.* 2014;20(7):591–8.

45. Brosens I, Gargett CE, Guo S-W, Puttemans P, Gordts S, Brosens JJ, et al. Origins and progression of adolescent endometriosis. *Reproductive Sciences.* 2016;23(10):1282–8.

46. Sampson JA. Metastatic or embolic endometriosis, due to the menstrual dissemination of endo-metrial tissue into the venous circulation. *American Journal of Pathology.* 1927;3(2):93–110 43.

47. Harirchian P, Gashaw I, Lipskind ST, Braundmeier AG, Hastings JM, Olson MR, et al. Lesion kin-etics in a non-human primate model of endometriosis. *Human Reproduction.* 2012;27(8):2341–51.

48. Burney RO, Giudice LC. Pathogenesis and pathophysiology of endometriosis. *Fertility and Sterility.* 2012;98(3):511–19.

49. Figueira PG, Abrao MS, Krikun G, Taylor HS. Stem cells in endometrium and their role in the pathogenesis of endometriosis. *Annals of the New York Academy of Sciences.* 2011;1221:10–17.

50. Matsuura K, Ohtake H, Katabuchi H, Okamura H. Coelomic metaplasia theory of endometri-osis: evidence from in vivo studies and an in vitro experimental model. *Gynecologic and Obstetric Investigation.* 1999;47(Suppl 1):18–20; discussion 2.

51. Sampson JA. Metastatic or embolic endometriosis, due to the menstrual dissemination of endo-metrial tissue into the venous circulation. *American Journal of Pathology.* 1927;3:109.

52. Koninckx PR, Ussia A, Adamyan L, Wattiez A, Gomel V, Martin DC. Pathogenesis of endometri-osis: the genetic/epigenetic theory. *Fertility and Sterility.* 2019;111(2):327–40.

53. Chapron C, Marcellin L, Borghese B, Santulli P. Rethinking mechanisms, diagnosis and manage-ment of endometriosis. *Nature Reviews Endocrinology.* 2019;15(11):666–82.

54. Saha R, Pettersson HJ, Svedberg P, Olovsson M, Bergqvist A, Marions L, et al. Heritability of endo-metriosis. *Fertility and Sterility.* 2015;104(4):947–52.

55. Treloar SA, O'Connor DT, O'Connor VM, Martin NG. Genetic influences on endometriosis in an Australian twin sample. *Fertility and Sterility.* 1999;71(4):701–10.

56. Simpson JL, Elias S, Malinak LR, Buttram VC, Jr. Heritable aspects of endometriosis. I. Genetic studies. *American Journal of Obstetrics and Gynecology.* 1980;137(3):327–31.

57. Lee SH, Harold D, Nyholt DR, ANZGene Consortium, International Endogene Consortium, Genetic and Environmental Risk for Alzheimer's disease Consortium, et al. Estimation and partitioning of polygenic variation captured by common SNPs for Alzheimer's disease, multiple sclerosis and endometriosis. *Human Molecular Genetics.* 2013;22(4):832–41.

58. Sapkota Y, Steinthorsdottir V, Morris AP, Fassbender A, Rahmioglu N, De Vivo I, et al. Meta-analysis identifies five novel loci associated with endometriosis highlighting key genes involved in hormone metabolism. *Nature Communications.* 2017;8(1):15539.

59. Nyholt DR, Low SK, Anderson CA, Painter JN, Uno S, Morris AP, et al. Genome-wide association meta-analysis identifies new endometriosis risk loci. *Nature Genetics.* 2012;44(12):1355–9.

60. Rahmioglu N, Nyholt DR, Morris AP, Missmer SA, Montgomery GW, Zondervan KT. Genetic variants underlying risk of endometriosis: insights from meta-analysis of eight genome-wide asso-ciation and replication datasets. *Human Reproduction Update.* 2014;20(5):702–16.

61. Louis GMB. Early origins of endometriosis: role of endocrine disrupting chemicals. In: Giudice L, Evers JLH, Healy D, eds. *Endometriosis: science and practice.* Oxford: Wiley-Blackwell Publishers; 2012. pp. 153–63.

62. Newbold R. Cellular and molecular effects of developmental exposure to diethylstilbestrol: im-plications for other environmental estrogens. *Environmental Health Perspectives.* 1995;103(Suppl 7):83–7.

63. Missmer SA, Hankinson SE, Spiegelman D, Barbieri RL, Michels KB, Hunter DJ. In utero exposures and the incidence of endometriosis. *Fertility and Sterility.* 2004;82(6):1501–8.

64. Benagiano G, Brosens I. In utero exposure and endometriosis. *Journal of Maternal-Fetal & Neonatal Medicine.* 2014;27(3):303–8.

65. Wolff EF, Sun L, Hediger ML, Sundaram R, Peterson CM, Chen Z, et al. In utero exposures and endometriosis: the endometriosis, natural history, disease, outcome (ENDO) study. *Fertility and Sterility.* 2013;99(3):790–5.

66. Vigano P, Somigliana E, Panina P, Rabellotti E, Vercellini P, Candiani M. Principles of phenomics in endometriosis. *Human Reproduction Update*. 2012;18(3):248–59.

67. Farland LV, Missmer SA, Bijon A, Gusto G, Gelot A, Clavel-Chapelon F, et al. Associations among body size across the life course, adult height and endometriosis. *Human Reproduction*. 2017;32(8):1732–42.

68. Missmer SA, Hankinson SE, Spiegelman D, Barbieri RL, Malspeis S, Willett WC, et al. Reproductive history and endometriosis among premenopausal women. *Obstetrics and Gynecology*. 2004;104(5 Pt 1):965–74.

69. Nnoaham KE, Webster P, Kumbang J, Kennedy SH, Zondervan KT. Is early age at menarche a risk factor for endometriosis? A systematic review and meta-analysis of case-control studies. *Fertility and Sterility*. 2012;98(3):702–12.e6.

70. Matalliotakis IM CH, Fragouli YG, Goumenou AG, Mahutte NG, Arici A. Epidemiological characteristics in women with and without endometriosis in the Yale series. *Archives of Gynecology and Obstetrics*. 2008;277(5):389–93.

71. Marcellin L, Santulli P, Pinzauti S, Bourdon M, Lamau MC, Borghese B, et al. Age at menarche does not correlate with the endometriosis phenotype. *PLoS One*. 2019;14(7):e0219497.

72. Stratton P, Khachikyan I, Sinaii N, Ortiz R, Shah J. Association of chronic pelvic pain and endometriosis with signs of sensitization and myofascial pain. *Obstetrics and Gynecology*. 2015;125(3):719–28.

73. Miller JA, Missmer SA, Vitonis AF, Sarda V, Laufer MR, DiVasta AD. Prevalence of migraines in adolescents with endometriosis. *Fertility and Sterility*. 2018;109(4):685–90.

74. Smorgick N, Marsh CA, As-Sanie S, Smith YR, Quint EH. Prevalence of pain syndromes, mood conditions, and asthma in adolescents and young women with endometriosis. *Journal of Pediatric and Adolescent Gynecology*. 2013;26(3):171–5.

75. Dun EC, Kho KA, Kearney S, Nezhat CH. Endometriosis in adolescents: referrals, diagnosis, treatment, and outcomes. *Journal of Minimally Invasive Gynecology*. 2015;22(6 S):S176.

76. Nabi MY, Nauhria S, Reel M, Londono S, Vasireddi A, Elmiry M, et al. Endometriosis and irritable bowel syndrome: a systematic review and meta-analyses. *Frontiers in Medicine*. 2022;9:914356.

77. Giudice LC. Clinical practice: endometriosis. *New England Journal of Medicine*. 2010;362(25):2389–98.

78. Vercellini P, Fedele L, Pietropaolo G, Frontino G, Somigliana E, Crosignani PG. Progestogens for endometriosis: forward to the past. *Human Reproduction Update*. 2003;9(4):387–96.

79. Vercellini P, Eskenazi B, Consonni D, Somigliana E, Parazzini F, Abbiati A, et al. Oral contraceptives and risk of endometriosis: a systematic review and meta-analysis. *Human Reproduction Update*. 2011;17(2):159–70.

80. Sasamoto N, Farland LV, Vitonis AF, Harris HR, DiVasta AD, Laufer MR, et al. In utero and early life exposures in relation to endometriosis in adolescents and young adults. *European Journal of Obstetrics & Gynecology and Reproductive Biology*. 2020;252:393–8.

81. Shah DK, Correia KF, Vitonis AF, Missmer SA. Body size and endometriosis: results from 20 years of follow-up within the nurses' health study II prospective cohort. *Human Reproduction*. 2013;28(7):1783–92.

82. Rowlands IJ, Hockey R, Abbott JA, Montgomery GW, Mishra GD. Body mass index and the diagnosis of endometriosis: findings from a national data linkage cohort study. *Obesity Research & Clinical Practice*. 2022;16(3):235–41.

83. Parazzini F, Cipriani S, Bravi F, Pelucchi C, Chiaffarino F, Ricci E, et al. A meta-analysis on alcohol consumption and risk of endometriosis. *American Journal of Obstetrics and Gynecology*. 2013;209(2):106e1–10.

84. Farland LV, Lorrain S, Missmer SA, Dartois L, Cervenka I, Savoye I, et al. Endometriosis and the risk of skin cancer: a prospective cohort study. *Cancer Causes and Control*. 2017;28(10):1011–19.

85. Saraswat L, Ayansina D, Cooper KG, Bhattacharya S. Risk of melanoma in women with endometriosis: a Scottish national cohort study. *European Journal of Obstetrics & Gynecology and Reproductive Biology*. 2021;257:144–8.

86. Kvaskoff M, Mesrine S, Clavel-Chapelon F, Boutron-Ruault M-C. Endometriosis risk in relation to naevi, freckles and skin sensitivity to sun exposure: the French E3N cohort. *International Journal of Epidemiology*. 2009;38(4):1143–53.

87. Kvaskoff M, Han J, Qureshi AA, Missmer SA. Pigmentary traits, family history of melanoma and the risk of endometriosis: a cohort study of US women. *International Journal of Epidemiology*. 2013;43(1):255–63.

88. García-Peñarrubia P, Ruiz-Alcaraz AJ, Martínez-Esparza M, Marín P, Machado-Linde F. Hypothetical roadmap towards endometriosis: prenatal endocrine-disrupting chemical pollutant exposure, anogenital distance, gut-genital microbiota and subclinical infections. *Human Reproduction Update*. 2020;26(2):214–46.

89. Smarr MM, Kannan K, Buck Louis GM. Endocrine disrupting chemicals and endometriosis. *Fertility and Sterility*. 2016;106(4):959–66.

90. Sirohi D, Al Ramadhani R, Knibbs LD. Environmental exposures to endocrine disrupting chemicals (EDCs) and their role in endometriosis: a systematic literature review. *Reviews on Environmental Health*. 2021;36(1):101–15.

91. Matta K, Koual M, Ploteau S, Coumoul X, Audouze K, Le Bizec B, et al. Associations between exposure to organochlorine chemicals and endometriosis: a systematic review of experimental studies and integration of epidemiological evidence. *Environmental Health Perspectives*. 2021;129(7):76003.

92. Zhu D, Chung HF, Dobson AJ, Pandeya N, Brunner EJ, Kuh D, et al. Type of menopause, age of menopause and variations in the risk of incident cardiovascular disease: pooled analysis of individual data from 10 international studies. *Human Reproduction*. 2020;35(8):1933–43.

93. Kvaskoff M, Mu F, Terry KL, Harris HR, Poole EM, Farland L, et al. Endometriosis: a high-risk population for major chronic diseases? *Human Reproduction Update*. 2015;21(4):500–16.

94. Pearce CL, Templeman C, Rossing MA, Lee A, Near AM, Webb PM, et al. Association between endometriosis and risk of histological subtypes of ovarian cancer: a pooled analysis of case-control studies. *Lancet Oncology*. 2012;13(4):385–94.

95. Eisenberg VH, Zolti M, Soriano D. Is there an association between autoimmunity and endometriosis? *Autoimmunity Reviews*. 2012;11(11):806–14.

96. Nielsen NM, Jorgensen KT, Pedersen BV, Rostgaard K, Frisch M. The co-occurrence of endometriosis with multiple sclerosis, systemic lupus erythematosus and Sjogren syndrome. *Human Reproduction*. 2011;26(6):1555–9.

97. Jess T, Frisch M, Jorgensen KT, Pedersen BV, Nielsen NM. Increased risk of inflammatory bowel disease in women with endometriosis: a nationwide Danish cohort study. *Gut*. 2012;61(9):1279–83.

98. Stephansson O, Falconer H, Ludvigsson JF. Risk of endometriosis in 11,000 women with celiac disease. *Human Reproduction*. 2011;26(10):2896–901.

99. Matalliotakis I, Cakmak H, Matalliotakis M, Kappou D, Arici A. High rate of allergies among women with endometriosis. *Journal of Obstetrics and Gynaecology*. 2012;32(3):291–3.

100. Mu F, Rich-Edwards J, Rimm EB, Spiegelman D, Missmer SA. Endometriosis and risk of coronary heart disease. *Circulation. Cardiovascular Quality and Outcomes*. 2016;9(3):257–64.

101. Okoth K, Wang J, Zemedikun D, Thomas G, Nirantharakumar K, Adderley N. Risk of cardiovascular outcomes among women with endometriosis in the United Kingdom: a retrospective matched cohort study. *BJOG: An International Journal of Obstetrics & Gynaecology*. 2021;128(10):1598–609.

102. Young K, Fisher J, Kirkman M. Clinicians' perceptions of women's experiences of endometriosis and of psychosocial care for endometriosis. *The Australian & New Zealand Journal of Obstetrics & Gynaecology*. 2017;57(1):87–92.

103. Agarwal SK, Chapron C, Giudice LC, Laufer MR, Leyland N, Missmer SA, et al. Clinical diagnosis of endometriosis: a call to action. *American Journal of Obstetrics and Gynecology*. 2019;220(4):354e1–e12.

104. Seear K. The etiquette of endometriosis: stigmatisation, menstrual concealment and the diagnostic delay. *Social Science & Medicine*. 2009;69(8):1220–7.

4

Menopause and Hysterectomy

A Life Course Perspective

Gita D. Mishra, Hsin-Fang Chung, Martha Hickey,
Diana Kuh, and Rebecca Hardy

4.1 Introduction

Menopause is the end of menstruation following the cessation of ovulation.[1] It may be spontaneous (natural menopause; defined by 12 months of amenorrhea) or iatrogenic, such as the removal of both ovaries (bilateral oophorectomy; defined as *surgical menopause*), or secondary to chemotherapy or radiation treatment.[1] Menopause marks the end of a woman's reproductive life, where the permanently lowered oestrogen exposure has significant biological and social implications.[2] The timing of menopause is recognised as a sentinel for chronic disease risk in later life,[2] while symptoms related to the menopause (especially physiological symptoms) impact the quality of life, work productivity, and employment rate.[3,4] Systematic reviews and meta-analyses have concluded that earlier menopause is associated with an increased risk of all-cause mortality,[5] cardiovascular disease,[5] type 2 diabetes,[6] osteoporosis,[7] fracture,[8] and depression,[9] while later menopause is associated with an increased risk of breast, endometrial, and ovarian cancer.[10,11]

Age at natural menopause varies across different countries, regions, and ethnic groups. Recent epidemiological estimates give a median age at natural menopause of 50–52 years among women from HICs,[2,12,13] while the median age is around 48 years or younger in African, Latin American, Middle East, and some Asian countries.[2] This may be due to genetic variations, but may also reflect differences in sociodemographic and behavioural factors.[2] A secular increase in the age at menopause has been reported in most countries.[14-18] In China, the age at menopause rose steadily from 47.9 to 49.3 years among women born between 1930 and 1950.[18] Across all birth cohorts, Chinese women living in urban areas experienced menopause on average 7 months later than women living in rural areas.[18] In the United States, the mean age at menopause increased by 1.5 years (from 48.4 to 49.9 years) over the past 6 decades.[17] However, the prevalence of spontaneous premature (< 40 years) and early menopause (40–44 years) has not declined over time.[19,20] This may be because some risk factors for premature and early menopause (discussed in Section 4.2.2) are increasing.[13,21] With the increasing number of childhood and young cancer survivors (e.g. breast cancer), the prevalence of premature and early menopause that results from chemotherapy and radiotherapy treatment may have increased, especially in HICs, but there are no data available regarding the secular trend.

Gita D. Mishra, Hsin-Fang Chung, Martha Hickey, Diana Kuh, and Rebecca Hardy, *Menopause and Hysterectomy* In: *A Life Course Approach to Women's Health*. Second Edition. Edited by: Gita D Mishra, Rebecca Hardy, and Diana Kuh, Oxford University Press.
© Oxford University Press 2023. DOI: 10.1093/oso/9780192864642.003.0004

Some women do not experience natural menopause but instead undergo bilateral oophorectomy (surgical menopause), usually as an additional procedure to hysterectomy (removal of the uterus). Hysterectomy is the second most common gynaecological procedure performed worldwide after caesarean section. In HICs, between 20% and 45% of women will have had a hysterectomy by age 60–70 years,[22–24] and of these, 30%–50% had a concomitant bilateral oophorectomy.[23,25] Hysterectomy rates vary by geographical location, even across regions within a country, and over time. The rates peaked in the 1980s[26,27] and then substantially declined over the last decade, largely driven by a decline in rates of hysterectomy for benign conditions.[27–32] This decline may be predominantly explained by the development of alternative, less invasive procedures and pharmacological treatments for uterine fibroids and dysfunctional uterine bleeding.[29,30] For example, the National Institute for Health and Care Excellence (NICE) guidelines on heavy menstrual bleeding direct clinicians first to consider levonorgestrel-releasing intrauterine system (Mirena) and pharmacological therapies rather than surgical options.[33] An increase in mean age at hysterectomy has been reported in some countries, such as Denmark (from 46 years in 1977–81 to 50 years in 2006–11)[34] and Sweden (from 47.3 years in 1987–90 to 52.2 years in 2002–03),[32] indicating that conservative treatment does not completely avert hysterectomy but may defer it until later ages. The indications for hysterectomy in older postmenopausal women are more likely to be cancer and prolapse.

As birth cohort studies have matured over recent decades with participants reaching older ages, there has been increasing interest in the developmental life course perspective for reproductive ageing research, and in women's health experiences and treatment choices during the menopausal transition.[35] This chapter reviews the factors across different life stages that affect the timing of natural menopause (see Section 2.2), the indications to undergo an oophorectomy and hysterectomy (see Sections 2.3 & 2.4), the level of symptoms experienced during the menopausal transition, and the decision to take menopausal hormone therapy (MHT) (see Section 1.5). We then conclude with a brief outline of implications for health policy and future research (see Section 1.6).

4.2 Natural Menopause

Menopause is a natural stage of reproductive ageing that usually occurs between 45 and 55 years of age. Cessation of menstruation before the age of 40 years is commonly referred to as premature menopause, but *premature ovarian insufficiency* (POI) is currently considered the most apposite term to denote spontaneous loss of ovarian activities before age 40 years.[36] The cause of POI is usually unknown but may be related to genetic or autoimmune factors.[36] Menopause that occurs between 40 and 45 years is termed *early menopause*.[36] In the general population of HICs, the prevalence of POI is 2% (range 1%–3%) and of early menopause is 7.6% (range 5%–10%), suggesting that almost one in ten women experience menopause before age 45.[21] A meta-analysis showed the prevalence of POI is higher in medium (4.9%) and low (4.3%) Human Development Index countries;[2] the Human Development Index is a summary measure of life expectancy, education, and income indicators developed by the United Nations Development Programme. The prevalence of POI (nonsurgical) in survivors of paediatric and young adult cancer is generally higher than in the general population but varies immensely depending on patient characteristics, cancer diagnosis, and treatment exposures, ranging from 2.1% to 82.2%.[37]

4.2.1 Biology of Menopause

Women are born with their entire lifetime supply of primordial follicles, which may potentially develop into mature oocytes. While most follicles are lost during prenatal life, normal female ovaries contain about 1–2 million follicles at birth (from a peak of 5–7 million follicles at the fifth month of gestation).[38] By the time of puberty, only around 25% of this total remains (approximately 400,000). Thereafter, there is a steady loss of follicles throughout a woman's reproductive life through recruitment and ovulation.[38] The rate of follicle loss accelerates from the mid-30s, and menopause occurs when the number of follicles has been depleted to approximately 1000.[12,38] The menopausal transition includes gradual biological and endocrinological changes, with an associated decline in fertility in the late 30s. Traditionally, it has been thought that circulating concentrations of oestradiol (E2) decline towards the end of reproductive life, but recent studies suggest that elevated E2 levels can occur throughout early menopausal transition.[39] Elevations in E2 are largely confined to the menstrual and luteal phases of ovulatory cycles during the menopausal transition. Progesterone declines towards menopause as it is produced only if ovulation occurs.[40] As circulating levels of oestrogen increase and progesterone decline, the menopausal transition is often characterised by irregular, heavier, and prolonged menstrual cycles, and the occurrence of menopausal symptoms (mainly hot flushes, night sweats, and vaginal dryness).

4.2.2 Risk Factors for Earlier Age at Menopause

Age at menopause has strong genetic components, and cigarette smoking is a marked behavioural risk factor for early menopause. Little is known about the early life factors that affect the primordial follicle pool and why the majority of these follicles undergo atresia before birth.[35] Much of the evidence described here is from observational studies that report on associations for risk factors with the timing of menopause. These observational associations may not necessarily indicate a causal relationship, but some Mendelian randomisation studies have provided evidence to support the causality.[11–43]

4.2.2.1 Genetic Factors

Heritability estimates of age at menopause provide support for genetic factors contributing to the timing of menopause. The Framingham Heart Study found that around 50% of the interindividual variability in age at menopause can be explained by genetic factors, with similar estimates of heritability for mother-daughter (42%) and sister-sister pairs (44%).[44] Twin studies have shown heritability to range from 31% to 72%.[45–47] Strong genetic predictors of premature and early menopause include a family history of premature and early menopause, being a child of a multiple pregnancy (e.g. twins), and genetic causes (e.g. chromosomal abnormalities, Fragile X syndrome, and autosomal gene mutations).[48,49] Women with a family history of early menopause (≤ 45 years) in a mother, sister, aunt or grandmother had a sixfold increased odds (95% CI 3.9–9.4) of early menopause.[50] The odds of early menopause was greatest for family history in a sister or multiple relatives (9- to 12-fold increased odds).[50] Twins and other multiple pregnancy offspring have a higher prevalence of POI and early menopause than the general population,[51,52] and ages at menopause were more concordant among identical than among non-identical twins.[51] If one twin experienced POI, her identical sister was almost seven times as likely to experience menopause at the same age, indicating a strong heritability effect.[51] The mechanisms linking multiple pregnancy and POI are still unclear. Poor intrauterine growth, manifested as lower birthweight, has been hypothesised to cause a decreased peak number of primordial follicles, which in turn may lead to earlier menopause.[53] However, twin studies found no association between differences in birthweight and differences in age at menopause in twin pairs;[51,53] instead, there were some indications that twins with POI had a heavier birthweight than twins with normal or later menopause.[53]

Recent meta-analyses of genome-wide association studies have identified over 50 loci associated with variations in age at menopause[54,55] and some variants associated with early menopause.[56] Although genetic factors explain a substantial proportion of the variation in age at menopause, there remains scope for the influence of early life, reproductive, and social environmental factors.

4.2.2.2 Fetal Development and Adverse Childhood Experiences

The number of follicles retained at birth may determine age at menopause.[38,57] Intrauterine and childhood adverse conditions may also influence the timing of menopause through the regulation of the primordial follicle pool (ovarian reserve).[57] Given that the primordial follicle pool is formed during prenatal life, it is biologically plausible that restricted prenatal growth could influence the number of ovarian follicles and potentially lead to earlier menopause. However, a systematic review of eleven studies found that nine studies reported no association between low birthweight and age at menopause,[58] while two studies reported an association of higher birthweight and greater adiposity with earlier menopause.[59,60] Larger size at birth is associated with higher maternal concentrations of oestrogen. It is possible that higher birthweight may indicate changes to the development of the ovary related to exposure to elevated hormonal levels in utero, as reflected by higher maternal concentrations.[60] Previous studies found that women prenatally exposed to cigarette smoke were more likely to be postmenopausal but only among those who had never smoked in adult life.[61] Recent large cohort studies, including the Nurses' Health Study II, did not find an association between in utero smoking exposure and early age at menopause.[62-64]

There is accumulating evidence that adverse socioeconomic circumstances in childhood have a greater impact on the timing of menopause than adverse circumstances experienced in adulthood,[65-67] partly mediated by poor early life nutrition and poor childhood growth.[67] Earlier age at menopause is associated with prenatal and childhood famine (particularly for severe famine experienced between ages 2–6 years),[68,69] low childhood weight (at age 1 or 2 years),[59,65,70] and not having been breastfed.[65,70] Cognitive function and emotional stress could also underlie this social gradient.[66] Two British birth cohort studies found that poor cognitive function across the life course was associated with earlier age at menopause, and the effect was strongest in childhood.[71,72] Early life experience of abuse and household dysfunction (e.g. parental divorce, parental absence, violence) may affect ovarian function and reproductive ageing via dysregulation of the body's stress responses, particularly the hypothalamic-pituitary-adrenal (HPA) axis.[73,74] There is evidence that childhood abuse may lead to neuroendocrine disruption, thereby affecting ovarian hormones during the menopausal transition.[73] Women who experienced childhood sexual abuse[75] and parental divorce before the age of 5 years[66,76] tended to have earlier age at menopause, suggesting that early life stressors may be a contributing factor.

4.2.2.3 Age at Menarche and Reproductive Factors Across the Life Course

It is hypothesised that fewer ovulatory cycles will tend to result in later menopause.[12] Late menarche indicates the delayed onset of ovulatory cycles; long and irregular menstrual cycles lead to fewer ovulatory cycles; while pregnancy and breastfeeding contribute to periods of anovulation, all of which would be expected to delay menopause. Using pooled data from the International Collaboration for a Life Course Approach to Reproductive Health and Chronic Disease Events (InterLACE), early menarche (≤ 11 vs 13 years) was associated with an increased risk of premature and early menopause among women from western HICs.[21] The China Kadoorie Biobank also showed that women with early menarche (≤ 12 vs 15 years) were at higher risk of premature and early menopause.[77] Recent Mendelian randomisation analyses support the causal association between age at menarche and age at menopause.[41–43]

Nulliparity and lower parity have been associated with earlier onset of menopause, while higher parity, particularly among women of advantaged socioeconomic position (SEP), has been related to later age at menopause,[21,77–81] consistent with the theory that fewer ovulatory cycles result in later menopause.[12] Nulliparity strengthens the association between early menarche and the risk of premature and early menopause.[21] Women who had early menarche (≤ 11 years) and nulliparity had a much higher risk of premature and early menopause, compared with women with menarche at ≥12 years and with two or more children.[21] The Nurses' Health Study found that among parous women, a longer total duration of breastfeeding was associated with a lower risk of early menopause (< 45 years) even after accounting for parity.[81] However, there is a possibility of the reverse relationship that greater ovarian reserve may lead to higher parity and also later menopause.

There is some evidence that short menstrual cycles (< 25 vs 26–31 days) and very regular cycles (± 3 days vs always irregular/no periods) at age 18–22 years are associated with a higher risk of early menopause (< 45 years).[82] Women with shorter and very regular cycles tend to have lower levels of anti-Müllerian hormone (AMH), which is a biomarker of ovarian reserve.[82] It is possible that the size of the primordial follicle pool (ovarian reserve) may influence a woman's whole reproductive life, influencing menstrual characteristics, fertility, as well as the timing of menopause.[35]

4.2.2.4 Adult Social and Behavioural Factors

The pattern of regional differences in age at menopause supports the role of SEP and lifestyle factors. A meta-analysis of studies across six continents found that women living in LMICs tended to have an earlier age at menopause than those living in HICs, and across countries, those with lower levels of education and manual occupations had an earlier onset of menopause in a dose-response manner.[2] It has been speculated that adverse socioeconomic conditions across the life course may be related to an early decline in ovarian function through exposures, such as lifestyle factors, that influence the rate of oocyte depletion.[2]

Of all the behavioural factors investigated, current cigarette smoking is the most consistently associated with an earlier age at menopause of approximately one year.[2] Smoking is linked with hormonal production and metabolism, including decreased oestrogen levels and increased production of adrenal androgens,[83,84] contributing towards an antioestrogen effect leading to earlier menopause. However, smoking may influence ovarian sex steroid production in a way that is reversible upon smoking cessation. Pooled data from the InterLACE consortium showed that compared with never smokers, former smokers still had around 10%–15% higher risk of premature and early menopause, but the risk was much lower than that of current smokers (twice the risk).[85] Smokers who had quit for more than 10 years had a similar risk to never smokers, highlighting the clear benefits of early cessation of smoking (preferably before the age of 30 years) to lower excess risk of early menopause.[85] Smoking could also be a factor mediating adverse experiences and age at menopause. A longitudinal study found that the effect of intimate partner violence on early menopause was largely explained by cigarette smoking.[86] However, Mendelian randomisation analyses failed to confirm a causal association between current smoking habit and earlier age at menopause.[41]

Both body size and fat distribution have been related to the timing of menopause.[87] A pooled analysis from the InterLACE supports earlier evidence that women who are overweight or obese in midlife have a 50% higher risk of experiencing late menopause (≥ 56 years) compared with those who are normal weight, while those who are underweight have over twice the risk of early menopause (< 45 years).[88] It is hypothesised that the higher peripheral production of oestrogen in the adipose tissue leads to later onset of menopause.[87] In contrast, being underweight may trigger early menopause as a result of malnutrition, over-exercising, and weight reduction diets,[89-91] as less adipose tissue is linked to lower levels of leptin and hence oestrogen leading to early menopause.[92] For the association of diet and physical activity with age at menopause, the current evidence is inconclusive because of the wide range of measurements used across different studies.[2]

4.3 Surgical Menopause

Surgical menopause refers to the removal of both ovaries (bilateral oophorectomy) before natural menopause. This results in an abrupt reduction in ovarian steroids (oestrogen, progesterone, and testosterone). Bilateral oophorectomy is commonly performed at the time of hysterectomy for benign conditions or to prevent ovarian cancer in those at high inherited risk.[93] The 2005 US National Inpatient Sample found that among women who underwent hysterectomy for a benign condition, 46% had a concomitant bilateral oophorectomy, and 11% had unilateral oophorectomy.[25] In 2005, the prevailing practice was to avoid oophorectomy for women under age 40,[94] except for women at high inherited risk of ovarian and breast cancer (carrying pathogenic gene mutations such as BRCA1 or BRCA2)[95] and women with a strong family history of ovarian cancer.[93] A recent US study showed that both unilateral and bilateral oophorectomy declined after 2005, which was most pronounced for women who underwent oophorectomy concurrently with hysterectomy or did not have any ovarian indication.[96]

Women with endometriosis, pelvic infection, pelvic pain, or ovarian cyst were significantly more likely to undergo bilateral oophorectomy, while women with fibroids, abnormal bleeding, or prolapse were more likely to have hysterectomy alone.[25] Older age (over 40 years), lack of health insurance (in the United States), low income, and low education attainment were significant predictors of bilateral oophorectomy.[25,97] Case-control studies found that women who experienced childhood abuse[98] and who had a history of mood, anxiety, and somatoform disorders[99] were at higher risk of undergoing bilateral oophorectomy for a benign condition.

4.4 Hysterectomy

Hysterectomy, a surgical procedure that removes the uterus, is one of the most common gynaecological procedures performed worldwide.[100] Hysterectomy may lead to changes in blood supply to the ovaries, which may induce menopause occurring on average 2–4 years earlier than average.[101,102] In HICs, the median age at hysterectomy is around 47 years for women undergoing a hysterectomy for benign conditions,[23,25,29] with an older median age for women having a hysterectomy because of malignant diseases (61 years in Denmark).[29] In contrast, the median age of Indian women at hysterectomy was lower at 42 years,[103] while another population-based study conducted in Gujarat, India, found the mean age of hysterectomy among women with low income to be 36 years old.[104]

4.4.1 Indications for Hysterectomy

For women, the decision to undergo a hysterectomy for benign disease is part of a social context related to education, childbearing plans, and health care use, all of which may be shaped by earlier life experiences.[35] In clinical practice, the majority of hysterectomies are performed for benign conditions, most commonly for uterine fibroids (accounting for approximately 30% of hysterectomies)[105,106] and dysfunctional uterine bleeding (17%).[106] Endometriosis is another common gynaecological disorder treated by hysterectomy (accounting for 12%)[106] and is discussed separately in Chapter 3. Uterine fibroids are noncancerous growths in the wall of the uterus associated with heavy menstrual bleeding and pelvic pain.[107] The incidence rates of fibroids increase with age, reaching a peak at around 50 years, before declining after menopause.[107–109] There is a large variation in the prevalence of fibroids. An international internet-based survey found the prevalence of self-reported fibroids ranged from 4.5% (UK) to 9.8% (Italy).[110] A review of registry, single-centre, and other observational studies found a higher prevalence (mostly between 10% and 40%), depending on study populations and diagnostic methods (e.g. ultrasound).[107]

4.4.2 Risk Factors for Hysterectomy and Fibroids

4.4.2.1 Genetic Factors
Twin studies found that genetic influences on liability to hysterectomy and fibroid hospitalisation were substantial.[45,111,112] Hysterectomy showed a considerable heritability (59%), as a result of its two main indications: fibroids (69%) and heavy menstrual bleeding (55%).[45] Familial aggregation of fibroids indicates that genetic factors may underlie fibroid development.[107–109] African American women have also been consistently reported to have a higher incidence of fibroids across all ages, by two- to threefold compared with white women and after adjustment for known risk factors.[107–109] They tend to be diagnosed earlier, have multiple and larger fibroids, and have symptoms that are more severe compared to other ethnic groups.[108,109] They also have a 2.4-fold increased risk of undergoing hysterectomy and a 6.8-fold increased risk of myomectomy (a surgical procedure to remove uterine fibroids) compared with white women.[113] The higher incidence rates of fibroids, hysterectomy, and

myomectomy in African American women do not seem to be attributable to differences in the types and severity of symptoms, use of health care, or prevalence of other putative risk factors, suggesting a genetic basis for the difference.[107–109]

4.4.2.2 Age at Menarche and Menstrual and Reproductive Characteristics

Menstrual characteristics that increase the levels of oestrogen may promote the growth of fibroids. Circulating oestradiol concentrations are high in those who experience early menarche, while both early menarche and late menopause indicates a longer oestrogen exposure. Pregnancy, accompanied by sharp elevations and declines in the production of oestrogen and progesterone in the early gestation and postpartum period, can have a dramatic effect on fibroid growth.[108] Systematic reviews and meta-analyses have concluded that earlier age at menarche is associated with an increased risk of fibroids,[108,109] as well as hysterectomy.[100] No studies so far have specifically investigated the association between late menopause and the risk of fibroids, but the incidence declines for postmenopausal women (over 70% of fibroids are diagnosed at age 40–54),[114,115] suggesting that later age at menopause is associated with a greater risk of developing fibroids. Higher parity has been consistently associated with a lower risk of fibroids; however, the protective effect is considered to be overestimated because the presence of fibroids can lead to infertility or subfertility.[107–109] A recent meta-analysis of eight studies did not show an association between parity and risk of hysterectomy,[100] but women who were sterilised (tubal ligation) were more likely to undergo hysterectomy than those who were not sterilised.[103,104,116] There is evidence to suggest that earlier age at first birth (≤ 25 years) and longer time since last birth (≥5 years) were associated with increased risk of fibroids in both African American and white women in the United States.[114,117,118] Meanwhile, the relationship between menstrual cycle patterns and fibroids is less clear.[109] In the Nurses' Health Study II, longer menstrual cycles were associated with a reduced risk of fibroids,[118] but no such link was found in other studies.[109] The association between the use of oral contraceptive pills (OCPs) and fibroids has been studied extensively, but no consistent findings have emerged.[109] Two studies reported an increased risk of fibroids only among women who initiated the use of OCPs at younger ages (before 17 years),[117,119] suggesting that early sexual activity and exposure to sexually transmitted infections may play a role in aetiology.[109]

4.4.2.3 Socioeconomic Position

Hysterectomy is the result of a range of factors, including biological, cultural, and social factors. Hysterectomy for benign disease is more common at a younger age than hysterectomy for cancer.[120] More disadvantaged SEP, particularly lower levels of education, has been associated with increased risk of hysterectomy, but the effect size varies by ethnicity, geographic location, and across birth cohorts.[121–123] A meta-analysis of 10 studies in HICs showed a dose-response relationship with a 17% higher risk of hysterectomy with each lower level of education.[100] A similar situation was found in LMICs, such as India, where women with no or primary school education were more likely to undergo hysterectomy than women who had education levels of matriculation and above.[103] However, women from wealthy households with health insurance were more likely to have a hysterectomy than women from poor households without health insurance.[103] Findings of another study in India showed that women with lower income, with at least two or more children, and living in rural areas, underwent hysterectomy at higher rates than other women.[104] It is possible that women experiencing more disadvantaged SEP are more likely to have children early, and hysterectomy rates are higher for women who have completed their family, with a young age of sterilisation at 27.5 years among low-income Indian women.[104]

4.4.2.4 Body Weight and Health-Related Behaviours

Higher BMI has generally been associated with a modestly increased risk of developing fibroids. Most studies found a nonlinear association, with the risk increasing up through the overweight groups and then decreasing slightly among the heaviest or obese groups. though this decline may reflect difficulties in ascertaining a diagnosis.[109] Weight gain during adulthood has also been consistently associated with a higher risk of fibroids,[114,124,125] but no association was found with body size in childhood and adolescence.[125] This relationship may be explained through hormonal and inflammatory mechanisms. An increase in body weight and fat tissue is correlated with an increase in the peripheral conversion of androgen to oestrogen and reduced production of sex-hormone-binding globulin, resulting in more unbound active oestrogens in overweight and obese women.[109] Visceral fat, but not subcutaneous fat, is associated with the presence of fibroids.[126] Further, visceral fat is a hormonally active tissue and excess visceral fat has been shown to increase the production of proinflammatory mediators.[126]

The associations between cigarette smoking and the risk of fibroids have been mixed. A recent meta-analysis showed a small reduced risk of fibroids for current and former smokers, with consistent results in the cohort studies.[127] Although earlier studies suggested that smoking seemed to reduce the risk of fibroids,[128–130] subsequent studies showed an increased risk[131,132] or no association.[133,134] Smoking has been shown to decrease levels of circulating oestrogen; conversely, it may also exert adverse oestrogen-related effects on the uterus that could promote cell proliferation.[135,136] Alcohol consumption also seems to affect the development of fibroids. A meta-analysis study showed that ever and current use of alcohol was associated with increased risk of fibroids in cohort studies, but this was not consistent with findings from case-control studies.[137] Alcohol can decrease oestrogen metabolism, thereby increasing levels of endogenous oestrogen and bioavailable oestrogen.[138,139] High consumption of red and processed meats was also associated with an increased risk of fibroids, while exercise and higher intakes of vegetables and fruit may be protective against fibroids.[108,109] Physical activity and a plant-based diet may decrease fibroid risk by reducing the bioavailability of circulating oestrogen.[108,109] Early studies suggested that soy intake may reduce fibroid risk because soy exhibits antioestrogenic activity among women with high levels of endogenous oestrogen, but subsequent studies did not find any association between soy intake and fibroids.[140,141] Stress could also have an indirect effect on fibroid risk. Stress has been linked to high BMI, alcohol consumption, physical inactivity, and elevated blood pressure, which may all increase the risk of fibroids.[108] In addition, stress influences the HPA and gonadal axes, thereby affecting the bioavailability of oestrogen[142] and increasing the risk of fibroid development and growth.[108]

4.4.2.5 Health Services Use

Earlier experience of health care use could influence a woman's decision about hysterectomy. Australian studies of middle-aged women have found that having more dilatation and curettage procedures and other nongynaecological operations, the use of prescription medications, having private health insurance, and more visits to general practitioners

(GPs) were associated with hysterectomy.[143,144] Gynaecologists (62%) and GPs (16%) were the most influential sources of information about hysterectomy in Australia.[145] These results indicate that pre-existing gynaecological problems (e.g. heavy menstrual bleeding) and nongynaecological treatment and previous surgery may influence women's decision-making in hysterectomy. It raises the possibility that some women are more prone to surgery or medical interventions than others.[35] A greater number of visits to a health professional may also provide more opportunities to discuss available treatments including a hysterectomy.[35]

4.5 Symptomatology During the Menopausal Transition and Hormone Therapy Use

4.5.1 Continuity and Change in Symptom Reporting and Lifetime Risk Factors

During the menopausal transition, changes in gonadotrophins and sex steroid hormones may lead to a range of symptoms. Vasomotor symptoms (VMS), including hot flushes and night sweats, are often considered the cardinal symptoms of menopause. Cohort data from the UK and Australia found that the experience of VMS through midlife formed distinct groups.[146,147] About 14% of British women in the first national birth cohort study had an 'early severe' profile, with symptoms declining progressively during postmenopause, and one in ten women had a 'late severe' profile with the peak in symptom prevalence occurring 1 to 2 years into postmenopause, while about one in four women followed a similar trajectory but with more moderate symptoms (Figure 4.1).[146] One in two women experienced mild or no symptoms.[146] A range of midlife sociodemographic factors and health behaviours have been

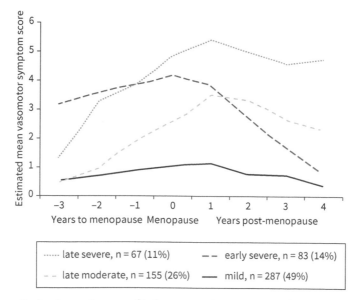

Figure 4.1 Longitudinal symptoms profile for vasomotor menopausal symptoms relative to time at menopause for British women (adapted from Mishra and Kuh (2012)).[146]

Source: Mishra GD, Kuh D. Health symptoms during midlife in relation to menopausal transition: British prospective cohort study. *BMJ* 2012;344:e402. doi:10.1136/bmj.e402

consistently associated with VMS, including being overweight or obese, smoking, disadvantaged SEP, anxiety, depressive symptoms, and perceived stress.[146,148-150] Earlier life reproductive factors may also be associated with VMS. Women with early age at menarche (≤ 11 vs ≥14 years) were more likely to experience frequent VMS, but midlife BMI played a role in modifying the association.[151] In addition, women with a history of premenstrual symptoms were more likely to report VMS.[152]

Psychological symptoms, such as depressed mood, anxiety, and sleep disturbance, are also common during menopause. In the British birth cohort study, one in ten women experienced psychological symptoms that peaked in the first 2 years postmenopause.[146] However, for the majority of women who experienced psychological symptoms during midlife, it is less clear whether these were directly due to menopause. Those symptoms could be the result of concurrent life events since menopause occurs at a life stage when women are also more likely to experience physical and psychological stressors, become a carer for parents, and experience children moving out of home.[35] Risk factors across life may also explain midlife psychological symptoms.[153] Women who experienced a high level of psychological distress in midlife were more likely to come from divorced families (particularly if they also experienced marital breakdown), scored highly on the neuroticism scale or exhibited antisocial behaviour when they were teenagers, and had a prior history of mental and physical health problems or certain social factors (e.g. perceived lack of access to help in a crisis) in adult life.[153] Further, women who experienced VMS were more likely to have concurrent and subsequent depressed mood, but the association was largely explained by sleep difficulties.[150]

Somatic symptoms (e.g. migraine, joint pain, and back pain) and urogynaecological symptoms (e.g. urinary incontinence, urinary tract infection) tend to follow a constant profile through midlife, unrelated to the timing of menopause,[146,147] with around 25% of British women reporting severe or very severe somatic symptoms.[146] Women of manual social class at childhood or adulthood, lower education level, and obese BMI were more likely to have severe somatic symptoms, but no association was found with smoking status and physical level.[146] For sexual discomfort, about 14% of British women reported an increasing prevalence in late perimenopause through to menopause, and 4% had very severe sexual discomfort throughout the menopausal transition.[146] Vaginal dryness was the major risk factor for change in sex life and difficulties with intercourse.[154] Being married, surgical menopause, hysterectomy, and anxiety were associated with vaginal dryness, regardless of sexual activity.[155]

A significant limitation of current studies is the variation in measurement tools used to assess symptoms associated with the menopause across studies and populations, which restricts effective data synthesis, limiting the usefulness of research to inform clinical practice. To address these methodological concerns, an international collaboration (the COMMA initiative: Core Outcome Set in Menopause) was established to achieve consensus on standardised measures used to collect and report menopausal symptoms. This will enhance the availability of comparable data across diverse populations and facilitate research to improve evidence-based patient care.[156,157]

4.5.2 Menopausal Hormone Therapy

For women who seek medical advice for VMS, MHT (previously known as hormone replacement therapy) is usually an effective treatment. MHT use started in the 1960s, with very high use in the 1990s of up to 40% in some HICs.[158] The use of MHT dropped substantially following adverse findings from the Women's Health Initiative (WHI) study published in 2002.[159] The WHI started a large, randomised trial in 1998 to evaluate the effect of MHT (estrogen plus progestin) on the risk of all cause mortality and disability (mainly cardiovascular disease and breast cancer) in postmenopausal women without hysterectomy. After a 5-year follow-up, the results showed an increased risk of coronary heart disease, stroke, and breast cancer among hormone users, suggesting that overall health risks exceeded benefits, and the trial was discontinued.[159] Since publication of the WHI data, there has been ongoing controversy around study design (observational studies and randomised controlled trials) and conclusions, and recommendations from authorities on the usage of MHT have fluctuated.[158] Clinical trials that focused on the effects of MHT for women close to the onset of menopause, testing the so-called *timing hypothesis*, have shown mixed results. One (ELITE) showed less increase in carotid artery-intima thickness (a subclinical measure of atherosclerosis) when MHT was initiated within 6 years of menopause,[160] while another (KEEPs) failed to show a significant effect on biomarkers of cardiovascular disease in younger postmenopausal women.[161] Recent trials of younger women also showed no improved cognition with MHT use.[162,163] A retrospective study from a US insurance database reported that MHT use was associated with a reduced risk of all neurodegenerative diseases, including for Alzheimer's disease and dementia,[164] but there is no clear evidence of benefit for these outcomes from clinical trials yet.[165]

The 2017 Cochrane Review on MHT concluded that the treatment is not indicated for primary or secondary prevention of cardiovascular disease or dementia, nor for the preservation of cognitive function in postmenopausal women.[166] Similarly, a 2022 synthesis report and systematic review for the US Preventive Services Task Force concluded that while MHT (both oestrogen only and combined oestrogen and progestin) was associated with some benefits, it was also linked with increased risk of harms, with some differences between the use of oestrogen only and combined oestrogen and progestin, with insufficient evidence to support the timing hypothesis.[167] This review led the US Preventive Services Task Force to recommend that doctors should only provide MHT for symptom relief and not for the primary prevention of chronic disease.[168]

The 2022 hormone therapy position statement of the North American Menopause Society, however, takes a different stance. It recommends MHT as an effective treatment for VMS, and argues that it prevents bone demineralisation and fracture for the duration of use.[169] The statement acknowledges the risks of MHT differ by type, dose, duration, route of administration, timing of initiation, and the use of and amount of exposure to progestogen. It concludes that for women who are within 10 years of menopause or younger than 60 years of age and have no contraindications, the benefits may outweigh the risk for the treatment of VMS and prevention of bone loss or fracture. However, for women who initiate MHT more than 10 years from menopause onset or are aged 60 years or older, they argue that the opposite is the case because of the greater absolute risks of coronary heart disease, stroke, venous thromboembolism, and dementia.[169] In addition, the statement recommends that women with POI, early menopause, induced menopause, or surgical menopause before the age of 45 (particularly those before aged 40 years) should use MHT until the median age of menopause unless contraindicated (e.g. history of oestrogen-sensitive cancer). Health practitioners are encouraged to consider patient preferences for management of VMS (including alternative treatments and strategies), taking into consideration medical history and life course risk factors for chronic disease.

In term of the factors links with MHT use before the WHI trials, a British cohort study showed that more educated women were more likely to take MHT for long-term prevention of osteoporosis, while less educated women were more likely to take MHT to relieve menopausal symptoms based on their doctor's advice.[170] Hysterectomy, particularly where an oophorectomy had also been performed, was identified as the major factor associated with MHT uptake and longer, more continuous use. Among women without hysterectomy or oophorectomy, previous use of health services for menstrual disorders, previous use of oral contraception, smoking, and disadvantaged social class were associated with early use of MHT.[170] A large Italian study showed that despite the decreasing prevalence of MHT use after the WHI (from 17.6% in 1997–99 to 11.4% in 2002–03), the determinants of MHT uptake remained largely unchanged.[171] Surgical menopause was still the major factor for MHT use, but the MHT prescription appeared to decrease over the study period. A recent narrative review on the determinants of MHT uptake after surgical menopause showed that younger age and higher education were associated with MHT use, but the effect of social class varied across studies.[172] It is possible that the influence of lifetime individual factors for MHT uptake was swamped by ever-changing external factors, such as physician's recommendation, information sources (media, family, and friends), and evidence about the safety of MHT.[172]

4.6 Conclusions

The timing of natural menopause is of clinical and public health interest because it is associated with numerous health outcomes in later life. Although around 50% of the variation in menopause age among women is attributed to genetic components, a growing body of evidence has linked early life, reproductive, social, and behavioural factors to age at menopause. Of these nongenetic factors, cigarette smoking, being underweight, early menarche, and nulliparity or low parity are predictors of premature (< 40 years) and early natural menopause (40–44 years). With early menarche and delayed childbearing becoming more common as countries transition into higher income economies, further population studies are needed to identify temporal trends in premature and early menopause.

Hysterectomy is one of the most common surgical procedures, and fibroids are a common indication for hysterectomy (30%). Current evidence suggests that oestrogen plays an important role in the development of fibroids. It is unclear whether it is cumulative exposure to oestrogen or exposure at a critical/sensitive stage of life (e.g. puberty and pregnancy) that is most important. The pathways to fibroid development are further complicated by factors such as OCP use that affect oestrogen exposures. Almost all health behaviours are confounded by SEP. More research is warranted on the association between childhood adverse experiences and the development of gynaecological disorders. Both the biological indications and social preference for hysterectomy may have their origins earlier in life, which reflects in a woman's gynaecological history and shapes social class, childbearing plan, and health care use. Thus, a life course approach is needed to determine the temporal sequence of reproductive events and the impact of social factors.

Future longitudinal studies should use standardised measurement tools to collect symptoms that are or may be associated with the menopause, in order to be able to pool and/or compare data across studies to strengthen the evidence identifying women at risk of troublesome symptoms. Studies should also investigate the life course characteristics of women who do not experience troublesome menopausal symptoms which could highlight successful strategies for prevention. MHT use over the past decades have shown different patterns of use by birth cohorts, influenced by the changing evidence from observational studies and clinical trials, and changes in public discourse. Discussions about the use of MHT should consider symptom severity; patient's wishes; life course risk factors for chronic disease; other health conditions, including any contraindications to MHT use; and alternative treatments and strategies.

Key messages and implications

- Women with genetic risk factors for premature and early menopause, and those who have had early menarche (especially those with no children), should be encouraged to quit smoking early and maintain optimal weight to reduce the risk and consequences of premature and early menopause.
- Consideration for hysterectomy, especially for benign conditions, should include a discussion of economic, social, and cultural factors.
- For practitioners and women, the decision to use MHT should consider symptom severity; patient's wishes; life course risk factors for chronic disease; other health conditions, including any contraindications to MHT use; and alternative treatments and strategies.

References

1. Davis SR, Lambrinoudaki I, Lumsden M, Mishra GD, Pal L, Rees M, et al. Menopause. *Nature Reviews. Disease Primers.* 2015;1:15004.
2. Schoenaker DA, Jackson CA, Rowlands JV, Mishra GD. Socioeconomic position, lifestyle factors and age at natural menopause: a systematic review and meta-analyses of studies across six continents. *International Journal of Epidemiology.* 2014;43(5):1542–62.
3. Whiteley J, DiBonaventura M, Wagner JS, Alvir J, Shah S. The impact of menopausal symptoms on quality of life, productivity, and economic outcomes. *Journal of Women's Health.* 2013;22(11):983–90.
4. Bryson A, Conti G, Hardy R, Peycheva D, Sullivan A. The consequences of early menopause and menopause symptoms for labour market participation. *Social Science and Medicine.* 2022;293:114676.
5. Muka T, Oliver-Williams C, Kunutsor S, Laven JS, Fauser BC, Chowdhury R, et al. Association of age at onset of Menopause and time since onset of menopause with cardiovascular outcomes, intermediate vascular traits, and all-cause mortality: a systematic review and meta-analysis. *JAMA Cardiology.* 2016;1(7):767–76.
6. Anagnostis P, Christou K, Artzouchaltzi AM, Gkekas NK, Kosmidou N, Siolos P, et al. Early menopause and premature ovarian insufficiency are associated with increased risk of type 2 diabetes: a systematic review and meta-analysis. *European Journal of Endocrinology.* 2019;180(1):41–50.
7. Gallagher JC. Effect of early menopause on bone mineral density and fractures. *Menopause.* 2007;14(3 Pt 2):567–71.
8. Anagnostis P, Siolos P, Gkekas NK, Kosmidou N, Artzouchaltzi AM, Christou K, et al. Association between age at menopause and fracture risk: a systematic review and meta-analysis. *Endocrine.* 2019;63(2):213–24.

9. Georgakis MK, Thomopoulos TP, Diamantaras AA, Kalogirou EI, Skalkidou A, Daskalopoulou SS, et al. Association of age at menopause and duration of reproductive period with depression after menopause: a systematic review and meta-analysis. *JAMA Psychiatry.* 2016;73(2):139–49.

10. Collaborative Group on Hormonal Factors in Breast Cancer. Menarche, menopause, and breast cancer risk: individual participant meta-analysis, including 118 964 women with breast cancer from 117 epidemiological studies. *Lancet Oncology.* 2012;13(11):1141–51.

11. Pike MC, Pearce CL, Wu AH. Prevention of cancers of the breast, endometrium and ovary. *Oncogene.* 2004;23(38):6379–91.

12. Gold EB. The timing of the age at which natural menopause occurs. *Obstetrics and Gynecology Clinics of North America.* 2011;38(3):425–40.

13. InterLACE Study Team. Variations in reproductive events across life: a pooled analysis of data from 505 147 women across 10 countries. *Human Reproduction.* 2019;34(5):881–93.

14. Rodstrom K, Bengtsson C, Milsom I, Lissner L, Sundh V, Bjourkelund C. Evidence for a secular trend in menopausal age: a population study of women in Gothenburg. *Menopause.* 2003;10(6):538–43.

15. Pakarinen M, Raitanen J, Kaaja R, Luoto R. Secular trend in the menopausal age in Finland 1997–2007 and correlation with socioeconomic, reproductive and lifestyle factors. *Maturitas.* 2010;66(4):417–22.

16. Gottschalk MS, Eskild A, Hofvind S, Gran JM, Bjelland EK. Temporal trends in age at menarche and age at menopause: a population study of 312 656 women in Norway. *Human Reproduction.* 2020;35(2):464–71.

17. Appiah D, Nwabuo CC, Ebong IA, Wellons MF, Winters SJ. Trends in age at natural menopause and reproductive life span among US women, 1959–2018. *JAMA.* 2021;325(13):1328–30.

18. Lewington S, Li L, Murugasen S, Hong LS, Yang L, Guo Y, et al. Temporal trends of main reproductive characteristics in ten urban and rural regions of China: the China Kadoorie Biobank study of 300 000 women. *International Journal of Epidemiology.* 2014;43(4):1252–62.

19. Choe SA, Sung J. Trends of premature and early Menopause: a comparative study of the US national health and nutrition examination survey and the Korea national health and nutrition examination survey. *Journal of Korean medical science.* 2020;35(14):e97.

20. Golezar S, Ramezani Tehrani F, Khazaei S, Ebadi A, Keshavarz Z. The global prevalence of primary ovarian insufficiency and early menopause: a meta-analysis. *Climacteric.* 2019;22(4):403–11.

21. Mishra GD, Pandeya N, Dobson AJ, Chung HF, Anderson D, Kuh D, et al. Early menarche, nulliparity and the risk for premature and early natural menopause. *Human Reproduction.* 2017;32(3):679–86.

22. Rositch AF, Nowak RG, Gravitt PE. Increased age and race-specific incidence of cervical cancer after correction for hysterectomy prevalence in the United States from 2000 to 2009. *Cancer.* 2014;120(13):2032–8.

23. Loxton D, Byles J, Tooth L, Barnes I, Byrne E, Cavenagh D, et al. *Reproductive health: contraception, conception and change of life—findings from the Australian longitudinal study on women's health.* Canberra: ALSWH; 2021.

24. Howard BV, Kuller L, Langer R, Manson JE, Allen C, Assaf A, et al. Risk of cardiovascular disease by hysterectomy status, with and without oophorectomy: the women's health initiative observational study. *Circulation.* 2005;111(12):1462–70.

25. Jacoby VL, Vittinghoff E, Nakagawa S, Jackson R, Richter HE, Chan J, et al. Factors associated with undergoing bilateral salpingo-oophorectomy at the time of hysterectomy for benign conditions. *Obstetrics and Gynecology.* 2009;113(6):1259–67.

26. Hammer A, Rositch AF, Kahlert J, Gravitt PE, Blaakaer J, Sogaard M. Global epidemiology of hysterectomy: possible impact on gynecological cancer rates. *American Journal of Obstetrics and Gynecology.* 2015;213(1):23–9.

27. Redburn JC, Murphy MF. Hysterectomy prevalence and adjusted cervical and uterine cancer rates in England and Wales. *BJOG: An International Journal of Obstetrics and Gynaecology.* 2001;108(4):388–95.

28. Chen I, Choudhry AJ, Tulandi T. Hysterectomy trends: a Canadian perspective on the past, present, and future. *Journal of Obstetrics and Gynaecology Canada.* 2019;41(Suppl 2):S340–S342.

29. Lycke KD, Kahlert J, Damgaard R, Mogensen O, Hammer A. Trends in hysterectomy incidence rates during 2000–2015 in Denmark: shifting from abdominal to minimally invasive surgical procedures. *Clinical Epidemiology*. 2021;13:407–16.

30. Wilson LF, Pandeya N, Mishra GD. Hysterectomy trends in Australia, 2000–2001 to 2013–2014: joinpoint regression analysis. *Acta obstetricia et gynecologica Scandinavica*. 2017;96(10):1170–9.

31. Wright JD, Herzog TJ, Tsui J, Ananth CV, Lewin SN, Lu YS, et al. Nationwide trends in the performance of inpatient hysterectomy in the United States. *Obstetrics and Gynecology*. 2013;122(2 Pt 1):233–41.

32. Lundholm C, Forsgren C, Johansson AL, Cnattingius S, Altman D. Hysterectomy on benign indications in Sweden 1987–2003: a nationwide trend analysis. *Acta obstetricia et gynecologica Scandinavica*. 2009;88(1):52–8.

33. National Institute for Health and Care Excellence. *Heavy menstrual bleeding: assessment and management (NG88)*. London: National Institute for Health and Care Excellence; 2018.

34. Lykke R, Blaakaer J, Ottesen B, Gimbel H. Hysterectomy in Denmark 1977–2011: changes in rate, indications, and hospitalization. *European Journal of Obstetrics, Gynecology, and Reproductive Biology*. 2013;171(2):333–8.

35. Hardy R, Kuh D. Menopause and gynaecological disorders: a life course perspective. In: Kuh D, Hardy R, eds. *A life course approach to women's health, 1st edition*. Oxford: Oxford University Press; 2002. pp. 64–85.

36. European Society for Human Reproduction Embryology Guideline Group on POI, Webber L, Davies M, Anderson R, Bartlett J, Braat D, et al. ESHRE Guideline: management of women with premature ovarian insufficiency. *Human Reproduction*. 2016;31(5):926–37.

37. Gargus E, Deans R, Anazodo A, Woodruff TK. Management of primary ovarian insufficiency symptoms in survivors of childhood and adolescent cancer. *Journal of the National Comprehensive Cancer Network*. 2018;16(9):1137–49.

38. Ginsberg J. What determines the age at the menopause? *BMJ*. 1991;302(6788):1288–9.

39. Hale GE, Zhao X, Hughes CL, Burger HG, Robertson DM, Fraser IS. Endocrine features of menstrual cycles in middle and late reproductive age and the menopausal transition classified according to the staging of reproductive aging workshop (STRAW) staging system. *Journal of Clinical Endocrinology and Metabolism*. 2007;92(8):3060–7.

40. O'Connor KA, Ferrell R, Brindle E, Trumble B, Shofer J, Holman DJ, et al. Progesterone and ovulation across stages of the transition to menopause. *Menopause*. 2009;16(6):1178–87.

41. Ding X, Tang R, Zhu J, He M, Huang H, Lin Z, et al. An appraisal of the role of previously reported risk factors in the age at menopause using mendelian randomization. *Frontiers in Genetics*. 2020;11:507.

42. Louwers YV, Visser JA. Shared genetics between age at menopause, early menopause, POI and other traits. *Frontiers in Genetics*. 2021;12:676546.

43. Prince C, Sharp GC, Howe LD, Fraser A, Richmond RC. The relationships between women's reproductive factors: a Mendelian randomisation analysis. *BMC Medicine*. 2022;20(1):103.

44. Murabito JM, Yang Q, Fox C, Wilson PW, Cupples LA. Heritability of age at natural menopause in the Framingham heart study. *Journal of Clinical Endocrinology and Metabolism*. 2005;90(6):3427–30.

45. Snieder H, MacGregor AJ, Spector TD. Genes control the cessation of a woman's reproductive life: a twin study of hysterectomy and age at menopause. *Journal of Clinical Endocrinology and Metabolism*. 1998;83(6):1875–80.

46. de Bruin JP, Bovenhuis H, van Noord PA, Pearson PL, van Arendonk JA, te Velde ER, et al. The role of genetic factors in age at natural menopause. *Human Reproduction*. 2001;16(9):2014–8.

47. Treloar SA, Do KA, Martin NG. Genetic influences on the age at menopause. *Lancet*. 1998;352(9134):1084–5.

48. Mishra GD, Chung HF, Cano A, Chedraui P, Goulis DG, Lopes P, et al. EMAS position statement: predictors of premature and early natural menopause. *Maturitas*. 2019;123:82–8.

49. Qin Y, Jiao X, Simpson JL, Chen ZJ. Genetics of primary ovarian insufficiency: new developments and opportunities. *Human Reproduction Update*. 2015;21(6):787–808.

50. Cramer DW, Xu H, Harlow BL. Family history as a predictor of early menopause. *Fertility and Sterility*. 1995;64(4):740–5.
51. Gosden RG, Treloar SA, Martin NG, Cherkas LF, Spector TD, Faddy MJ, et al. Prevalence of premature ovarian failure in monozygotic and dizygotic twins. *Human Reproduction*. 2007;22(2):610–5.
52. Ruth KS, Perry JR, Henley WE, Melzer D, Weedon MN, Murray A. Events in early life are associated with female reproductive ageing: a UK Biobank study. *Scientific Reports*. 2016;6:24710.
53. Treloar SA, Sadrzadeh S, Do KA, Martin NG, Lambalk CB. Birth weight and age at menopause in Australian female twin pairs: exploration of the fetal origin hypothesis. *Human Reproduction*. 2000;15(1):55–9.
54. Zhang L, Wei XT, Niu JJ, Lin ZX, Xu Q, Ni JJ, et al. Joint genome-wide association analyses identified 49 novel loci for age at natural menopause. *Journal of Clinical Endocrinology and Metabolism*. 2021;106(9):2574–91.
55. Stolk L, Perry JR, Chasman DI, He C, Mangino M, Sulem P, et al. Meta-analyses identify 13 loci associated with age at menopause and highlight DNA repair and immune pathways. *Nature Genetics*. 2012;44(3):260–8.
56. Perry JR, Corre T, Esko T, Chasman DI, Fischer K, Franceschini N, et al. A genome-wide association study of early menopause and the combined impact of identified variants. *Human Molecular Genetics*. 2013;22(7):1465–72.
57. Finch C, Kirkwood T. *Chance, development and ageing*. Oxford: Oxford University Press; 2000.
58. Sadrzadeh S, Verschuuren M, Schoonmade LJ, Lambalk CB, Painter RC. The effect of adverse intrauterine conditions, early childhood growth and famine exposure on age at menopause: a systematic review. *Journal of Developmental Origins of Health and Disease*. 2018;9(2):127–36.
59. Cresswell JL, Egger P, Fall CH, Osmond C, Fraser RB, Barker DJ. Is the age of menopause determined in-utero? *Early Human Development*. 1997;49(2):143–8.
60. Tom SE, Cooper R, Kuh D, Guralnik JM, Hardy R, Power C. Fetal environment and early age at natural menopause in a British birth cohort study. *Human Reproduction*. 2010;25(3):791–8.
61. Strohsnitter WC, Hatch EE, Hyer M, Troisi R, Kaufman RH, Robboy SJ, et al. The association between in utero cigarette smoke exposure and age at menopause. *American Journal of Epidemiology*. 2008;167(6):727–33.
62. Langton CR, Whitcomb BW, Purdue-Smithe AC, Sievert LL, Hankinson SE, Manson JAE, et al. Association of in utero exposures with risk of early natural menopause. *American Journal of Epidemiology*. 2022;191(5):775–86.
63. Honorato TC, Haadsma ML, Land JA, Boezen MH, Hoek A, Groen H, et al. In utero cigarette smoke exposure and the risk of earlier menopause. *Menopause*. 2018;25(1):54–61.
64. Steiner AZ, D'Aloisio AA, DeRoo LA, Sandler DP, Baird DD. Association of intrauterine and early-life exposures with age at menopause in the sister study. *American Journal of Epidemiology*. 2010;172(2):140–8.
65. Hardy R, Kuh D. Does early growth influence timing of the menopause? Evidence from a British birth cohort. *Human Reproduction*. 2002;17(9):2474–9.
66. Hardy R, Kuh D. Social and environmental conditions across the life course and age at menopause in a British birth cohort study. *BJOG: An International Journal of Obstetrics and Gynaecology*. 2005;112(3):346–54.
67. Lawlor DA, Ebrahim S, Smith GD. The association of socio-economic position across the life course and age at menopause: the British women's heart and health study. *BJOG: An International Journal of Obstetrics and Gynaecology*. 2003;110(12):1078–87.
68. Yarde F, Broekmans FJ, van der Pal-de Bruin KM, Schonbeck Y, te Velde ER, Stein AD, et al. Prenatal famine, birthweight, reproductive performance and age at menopause: the Dutch hunger winter families study. *Human Reproduction*. 2013;28(12):3328–36.
69. Elias SG, van Noord PAH, Peeters PHM, Tonkelaar ID, Grobbee DE. Caloric restriction reduces age at menopause: the effect of the 1944–1945 Dutch famine. *Menopause*. 2018;25(11):1232–7.
70. Mishra G, Hardy R, Kuh D. Are the effects of risk factors for timing of menopause modified by age? Results from a British birth cohort study. *Menopause*. 2007;14(4):717–24.
71. Richards M, Kuh D, Hardy R, Wadsworth M. Lifetime cognitive function and timing of the natural menopause. *Neurology*. 1999;53(2):308–14.

72. Kuh D, Butterworth S, Kok H, Richards M, Hardy R, Wadsworth ME, et al. Childhood cognitive ability and age at menopause: evidence from two cohort studies. *Menopause.* 2005;12(4):475–82.

73. Allsworth JE, Zierler S, Krieger N, Harlow BL. Ovarian function in late reproductive years in relation to lifetime experiences of abuse. *Epidemiology.* 2001;12(6):676–81.

74. Allsworth JE, Zierler S, Lapane KL, Krieger N, Hogan JW, Harlow BL. Longitudinal study of the inception of perimenopause in relation to lifetime history of sexual or physical violence. *Journal of Epidemiology and Community Health.* 2004;58(11):938–43.

75. Magnus MC, Anderson EL, Howe LD, Joinson CJ, Penton-Voak IS, Fraser A. Childhood psychosocial adversity and female reproductive timing: a cohort study of the ALSPAC mothers. *Journal of Epidemiology and Community Health.* 2018;72(1):34–40.

76. Mishra GD, Cooper R, Tom SE, Kuh D. Early life circumstances and their impact on menarche and menopause. *Women's Health (London).* 2009;5(2):175–90.

77. Wang M, Gong WW, Hu RY, Wang H, Guo Y, Bian Z, et al. Age at natural menopause and associated factors in adult women: Findings from the China Kadoorie Biobank study in Zhejiang rural area. *PLoS ONE.* 2018;13(4):e0195658.

78. Parazzini F, Progetto Menopausa Italia Study G. Determinants of age at menopause in women attending menopause clinics in Italy. *Maturitas.* 2007;56(3):280–7.

79. Li L, Wu J, Pu D, Zhao Y, Wan C, Sun L, et al. Factors associated with the age of natural menopause and menopausal symptoms in Chinese women. *Maturitas.* 2012;73(4):354–60.

80. Perez-Alcala I, Sievert LL, Obermeyer CM, Reher DS. Cross cultural analysis of factors associated with age at natural menopause among Latin-American immigrants to Madrid and their Spanish neighbors. *American Journal of Human Biology.* 2013;25(6):780–8.

81. Langton CR, Whitcomb BW, Purdue-Smithe AC, Sievert LL, Hankinson SE, Manson JE, et al. Association of parity and breastfeeding with risk of early natural menopause. *JAMA Network Open.* 2020;3(1):e1919615.

82. Whitcomb BW, Purdue-Smithe A, Hankinson SE, Manson JE, Rosner BA, Bertone-Johnson ER. Menstrual cycle characteristics in adolescence and early adulthood are associated with risk of early natural menopause. *Journal of Clinical Endocrinology and Metabolism.* 2018;103(10):3909–18.

83. Baron JA, La Vecchia C, Levi F. The antiestrogenic effect of cigarette smoking in women. *American Journal of Obstetrics and Gynecology.* 1990;162(2):502–14.

84. Khaw KT, Tazuke S, Barrett-Connor E. Cigarette smoking and levels of adrenal androgens in postmenopausal women. *New England Journal of Medicine.* 1988;318(26):1705–9.

85. Zhu D, Chung HF, Pandeya N, Dobson AJ, Cade JE, Greenwood DC, et al. Relationships between intensity, duration, cumulative dose, and timing of smoking with age at menopause: a pooled analysis of individual data from 17 observational studies. *PLoS Medicine.* 2018;15(11):e1002704.

86. Mishra GD, Chung HF, Gelaw YA, Loxton D. The role of smoking in the relationship between intimate partner violence and age at natural menopause: a mediation analysis. *Women's Midlife Health.* 2018;4:1.

87. Tao X, Jiang A, Yin L, Li Y, Tao F, Hu H. Body mass index and age at natural menopause: a meta-analysis. *Menopause.* 2015;22(4):469–74.

88. Zhu D, Chung HF, Pandeya N, Dobson AJ, Kuh D, Crawford SL, et al. Body mass index and age at natural menopause: an international pooled analysis of 11 prospective studies. *European Journal of Epidemiology.* 2018;33(8):699–710.

89. Bromberger JT, Matthews KA, Kuller LH, Wing RR, Meilahn EN, Plantinga P. Prospective study of the determinants of age at menopause. *American Journal of Epidemiology.* 1997;145(2):124–33.

90. Jungari SB, Chauhan BG. Prevalence and determinants of premature menopause among Indian women: issues and challenges ahead. *Health and Social Work.* 2017;42(2):79–86.

91. Master-Hunter T, Heiman DL. Amenorrhea: evaluation and treatment. *American Family Physician.* 2006;73(8):1374–82.

92. Sarac F, Oztekin K, Celebi G. Early menopause association with employment, smoking, divorced marital status and low leptin levels. *Gynecological Endocrinology.* 2011;27(4):273–8.

93. Parker WH, Jacoby V, Shoupe D, Rocca W. Effect of bilateral oophorectomy on women's long-term health. *Women's Health (London).* 2009;5(5):565–76.

94. Olive DL. Dogma, skepsis, and the analytic method: the role of prophylactic oophorectomy at the time of hysterectomy. *Obstetrics and Gynecology.* 2005;106(2):214–5.

95. Rebbeck TR, Kauff ND, Domchek SM. Meta-analysis of risk reduction estimates associated with risk-reducing salpingo-oophorectomy in BRCA1 or BRCA2 mutation carriers. *Journal of the National Cancer Institute.* 2009;101(2):80–7.

96. Erickson Z, Rocca WA, Smith CY, Gazzuola Rocca L, Stewart EA, Laughlin-Tommaso SK, et al. Time trends in unilateral and bilateral oophorectomy in a geographically defined American population. *Obstetrics and Gynecology.* 2022;139(5):724–34.

97. Progetto Menopausa Italia Study G. Determinants of hysterectomy and oophorectomy in women attending menopause clinics in Italy. *Maturitas.* 2000;36(1):19–25.

98. Gazzuola Rocca L, Smith CY, Grossardt BR, Faubion SS, Shuster LT, Stewart EA, et al. Adverse childhood or adult experiences and risk of bilateral oophorectomy: a population-based case-control study. *BMJ Open.* 2017;7(5):e016045.

99. Gazzuola Rocca L, Smith CY, Bobo WV, Grossardt BR, Stewart EA, Laughlin-Tommaso SK, et al. Mental health conditions diagnosed before bilateral oophorectomy: a population-based case-control study. *Menopause.* 2019;26(12):1395–404.

100. Wilson LF, Mishra GD. Age at menarche, level of education, parity and the risk of hysterectomy: a systematic review and meta-analyses of population-based observational studies. *PLoS ONE.* 2016;11(3):e0151398.

101. Farquhar CM, Sadler L, Harvey SA, Stewart AW. The association of hysterectomy and menopause: a prospective cohort study. *BJOG: An International Journal of Obstetrics and Gynaecology.* 2005;112(7):956–62.

102. Moorman PG, Myers ER, Schildkraut JM, Iversen ES, Wang F, Warren N. Effect of hysterectomy with ovarian preservation on ovarian function. *Obstetrics and Gynecology.* 2011;118(6):1271–9.

103. Prusty RK, Choithani C, Gupta SD. Predictors of hysterectomy among married women 15–49 years in India. *Reproductive Health.* 2018;15(1):3.

104. Desai S, Campbell OM, Sinha T, Mahal A, Cousens S. Incidence and determinants of hysterectomy in a low-income setting in Gujarat, India. *Health Policy and Planning.* 2017;32(1):68–78.

105. Weaver F, Hynes D, Goldberg JM, Khuri S, Daley J, Henderson W. Hysterectomy in Veterans Affairs medical centers. *Obstetrics and Gynecology.* 2001;97(6):880–4.

106. Merrill RM. Hysterectomy surveillance in the United States, 1997 through 2005. *Medical Science Monitor.* 2008;14(1):CR24–31.

107. Stewart EA, Cookson CL, Gandolfo RA, Schulze-Rath R. Epidemiology of uterine fibroids: a systematic review. *BJOG: An International Journal of Obstetrics and Gynaecology.* 2017;124(10):1501–12.

108. Pavone D, Clemenza S, Sorbi F, Fambrini M, Petraglia F. Epidemiology and risk factors of uterine fibroids. *Best Practice and Research. Clinical Obstetrics & Gynaecology.* 2018;46:3–11.

109. Wise LA, Laughlin-Tommaso SK. Epidemiology of uterine fibroids: from menarche to menopause. *Clinical Obstetrics & Gynecology.* 2016;59(1):2–24.

110. Zimmermann A, Bernuit D, Gerlinger C, Schaefers M, Geppert K. Prevalence, symptoms and management of uterine fibroids: an international internet-based survey of 21,746 women. *BMC Women's Health.* 2012;12:6.

111. Treloar SA, Martin NG, Dennerstein L, Raphael B, Heath AC. Pathways to hysterectomy: insights from longitudinal twin research. *American Journal of Obstetrics and Gynecology.* 1992;167(1):82–8.

112. Luoto R, Kaprio J, Rutanen EM, Taipale P, Perola M, Koskenvuo M. Heritability and risk factors of uterine fibroids—the Finnish twin cohort study. *Maturitas.* 2000;37(1):15–26.

113. Wechter ME, Stewart EA, Myers ER, Kho RM, Wu JM. Leiomyoma-related hospitalization and surgery: prevalence and predicted growth based on population trends. *American Journal of Obstetrics and Gynecology.* 2011;205(5):492.e1–492.e4925.

114. Templeman C, Marshall SF, Clarke CA, DeLellis Henderson K, Largent J, Neuhausen S, et al. Risk factors for surgically removed fibroids in a large cohort of teachers. *Fertility and Sterility.* 2009;92(4):1436–46.

115. Whiteman MK, Kuklina E, Jamieson DJ, Hillis SD, Marchbanks PA. Inpatient hospitalization for gynecologic disorders in the United States. *American Journal of Obstetrics and Gynecology.* 2010;202(6):541.e1–541.e5416.

116. Hillis SD, Marchbanks PA, Tylor LR, Peterson HB. Higher hysterectomy risk for sterilized than nonsterilized women: findings from the U.S. collaborative review of sterilization. The U.S. Collaborative Review of Sterilization Working Group. *Obstetrics and Gynecology.* 1998;91(2):241–6.

117. Wise LA, Palmer JR, Harlow BL, Spiegelman D, Stewart EA, Adams-Campbell LL, et al. Reproductive factors, hormonal contraception, and risk of uterine leiomyomata in African American women: a prospective study. *American Journal of Epidemiology.* 2004;159(2):113–23.

118. Terry KL, De Vivo I, Hankinson SE, Missmer SA. Reproductive characteristics and risk of uterine leiomyomata. *Fertility and Sterility.* 2010;94(7):2703–7.

119. Marshall LM, Spiegelman D, Goldman MB, Manson JE, Colditz GA, Barbieri RL, et al. A prospective study of reproductive factors and oral contraceptive use in relation to the risk of uterine leiomyomata. *Fertility and Sterility.* 1998;70(3):432–9.

120. Marshall SF, Hardy RJ, Kuh D. Socioeconomic variation in hysterectomy up to age 52: national, population based, prospective cohort study. *BMJ.* 2000;320(7249):1579.

121. Powell LH, Meyer P, Weiss G, Matthews KA, Santoro N, Randolph JF, Jr., et al. Ethnic differences in past hysterectomy for benign conditions. *Women's Health Issues.* 2005;15(4):179–86.

122. Cooper R, Lucke J, Lawlor DA, Mishra G, Chang JH, Ebrahim S, et al. Socioeconomic position and hysterectomy: a cross-cohort comparison of women in Australia and Great Britain. *Journal of Epidemiology and Community Health.* 2008;62(12):1057–63.

123. Hautaniemi SI, Leidy Sievert L. Risk factors for hysterectomy among Mexican American women in the US Southwest. *American Journal of Human Biology.* 2003;15(1):38–47.

124. Wise LA, Palmer JR, Spiegelman D, Harlow BL, Stewart EA, Adams-Campbell LL, et al. Influence of body size and body fat distribution on risk of uterine leiomyomata in U.S. black women. *Epidemiology.* 2005;16(3):346–54.

125. Terry KL, De Vivo I, Hankinson SE, Spiegelman D, Wise LA, Missmer SA. Anthropometric characteristics and risk of uterine leiomyoma. *Epidemiology.* 2007;18(6):758–63.

126. Ciavattini A, Delli Carpini G, Moriconi L, Clemente N, Orici F, Boschi AC, et al. The association between ultrasound-estimated visceral fat deposition and uterine fibroids: an observational study. *Gynecological Endocrinology.* 2017;33(8):634–7.

127. Chiaffarino F, Ricci E, Cipriani S, Chiantera V, Parazzini F. Cigarette smoking and risk of uterine myoma: systematic review and meta-analysis. *European Journal of Obstetrics, Gynecology, and Reproductive Biology.* 2016;197:63–71.

128. Lumbiganon P, Rugpao S, Phandhu-fung S, Laopaiboon M, Vudhikamraksa N, Werawatakul Y. Protective effect of depot-medroxyprogesterone acetate on surgically treated uterine leiomyomas: a multicentre case—control study. *British Journal of Obstetrics and Gynaecology.* 1996;103(9):909–14.

129. Parazzini F, Negri E, La Vecchia C, Rabaiotti M, Luchini L, Villa A, et al. Uterine myomas and smoking. Results from an Italian study. *Journal of Reproductive Medicine.* 1996;41(5):316–20.

130. Ross RK, Pike MC, Vessey MP, Bull D, Yeates D, Casagrande JT. Risk factors for uterine fibroids: reduced risk associated with oral contraceptives. *British Medical Journal (Clinical Research Edition).* 1986;293(6543):359–62.

131. Chen CR, Buck GM, Courey NG, Perez KM, Wactawski-Wende J. Risk factors for uterine fibroids among women undergoing tubal sterilization. *American Journal of Epidemiology.* 2001;153(1):20–6.

132. Dragomir AD, Schroeder JC, Connolly A, Kupper LL, Hill MC, Olshan AF, et al. Potential risk factors associated with subtypes of uterine leiomyomata. *Reproductive Sciences.* 2010;17(11):1029–35.

133. Wise LA, Palmer JR, Harlow BL, Spiegelman D, Stewart EA, Adams-Campbell LL, et al. Risk of uterine leiomyomata in relation to tobacco, alcohol and caffeine consumption in the black women's health study. *Human Reproduction.* 2004;19(8):1746–54.

134. Marshall LM, Spiegelman D, Manson JE, Goldman MB, Barbieri RL, Stampfer MJ, et al. Risk of uterine leiomyomata among premenopausal women in relation to body size and cigarette smoking. *Epidemiology.* 1998;9(5):511–7.

135. Marom-Haham L, Shulman A. Cigarette smoking and hormones. *Current Opinion in Obstetrics and Gynecology.* 2016;28(4):230–5.

136. Ohtake F, Takeyama K, Matsumoto T, Kitagawa H, Yamamoto Y, Nohara K, et al. Modulation of oestrogen receptor signalling by association with the activated dioxin receptor. *Nature*. 2003;423(6939):545–50.

137. Chiaffarino F, Cipriani S, Ricci E, La Vecchia C, Chiantera V, Bulfoni A, et al. Alcohol consumption and risk of uterine myoma: A systematic review and meta-analysis. *PLoS ONE*. 2017;12(11):e0188355.

138. Muti P, Trevisan M, Micheli A, Krogh V, Bolelli G, Sciajno R, et al. Alcohol consumption and total estradiol in premenopausal women. *Cancer Epidemiology, Biomarkers and Prevention*. 1998;7(3):189–93.

139. Reichman ME, Judd JT, Longcope C, Schatzkin A, Clevidence BA, Nair PP, et al. Effects of alcohol consumption on plasma and urinary hormone concentrations in premenopausal women. *Journal of the National Cancer Institute*. 1993;85(9):722–7.

140. Wise LA, Radin RG, Palmer JR, Kumanyika SK, Rosenberg L. A prospective study of dairy intake and risk of uterine leiomyomata. *American Journal of Epidemiology*. 2010;171(2):221–32.

141. Nagata C, Nakamura K, Oba S, Hayashi M, Takeda N, Yasuda K. Association of intakes of fat, dietary fibre, soya isoflavones and alcohol with uterine fibroids in Japanese women. *British Journal of Nutrition*. 2009;101(10):1427–31.

142. Puder JJ, Freda PU, Goland RS, Ferin M, Wardlaw SL. Stimulatory effects of stress on gonadotropin secretion in estrogen-treated women. *Journal of Clinical Endocrinology and Metabolism*. 2000;85(6):2184–8.

143. Dennerstein L, Shelley J, Smith AM, Ryan M. Hysterectomy experience among mid-aged Australian women. *Medical Journal of Australia*. 1994;161(5):311–3.

144. Byles JE, Mishra G, Schofield M. Factors associated with hysterectomy among women in Australia. *Health Place*. 2000;6(4):301–8.

145. Janda M, Armfield NR, Page K, Kerr G, Kurz S, Jackson G, et al. Factors influencing women's decision making in hysterectomy. *Patient Education and Counseling*. 2018;101(3):504–10.

146. Mishra GD, Kuh D. Health symptoms during midlife in relation to menopausal transition: British prospective cohort study. *BMJ*. 2012;344:e402.

147. Mishra GD, Dobson AJ. Using longitudinal profiles to characterize women's symptoms through midlife: results from a large prospective study. *Menopause*. 2012;19(5):549–55.

148. Thurston RC, Joffe H. Vasomotor symptoms and menopause: findings from the study of Women's health across the nation. *Obstetrics and Gynecology Clinics of North America*. 2011;38(3):489–501.

149. Anderson DJ, Chung HF, Seib CA, Dobson AJ, Kuh D, Brunner EJ, et al. Obesity, smoking, and risk of vasomotor menopausal symptoms: a pooled analysis of eight cohort studies. *American Journal of Obstetrics and Gynecology*. 2020;222(5):478 e1–e17.

150. Chung HF, Pandeya N, Dobson AJ, Kuh D, Brunner EJ, Crawford SL, et al. The role of sleep difficulties in the vasomotor menopausal symptoms and depressed mood relationships: an international pooled analysis of eight studies in the InterLACE consortium. *Psychological Medicine*. 2018;48(15):2550–61.

151. Chung HF, Zhu D, Dobson AJ, Kuh D, Gold EB, Crawford SL, et al. Age at menarche and risk of vasomotor menopausal symptoms: a pooled analysis of six studies. *BJOG: An International Journal of Obstetrics and Gynaecology*. 2021;128(3):603–13.

152. Gold EB, Block G, Crawford S, Lachance L, FitzGerald G, Miracle H, et al. Lifestyle and demographic factors in relation to vasomotor symptoms: baseline results from the study of Women's health across the nation. *American Journal of Epidemiology*. 2004;159(12):1189–99.

153. Kuh D, Hardy R, Rodgers B, Wadsworth ME. Lifetime risk factors for women's psychological distress in midlife. *Social Science and Medicine*. 2002;55(11):1957–73.

154. Mishra G, Kuh D. Sexual functioning throughout menopause: the perceptions of women in a British cohort. *Menopause*. 2006;13(6):880–90.

155. Waetjen LE, Crawford SL, Chang PY, Reed BD, Hess R, Avis NE, et al. Factors associated with developing vaginal dryness symptoms in women transitioning through menopause: a longitudinal study. *Menopause*. 2018;25(10):1094–104.

156. The University of Melbourne Department of Obstetrics & Gynaecology. *COMMA: core outcomes in menopause [Internet]*. Melbourne: The University of Melbourne; 2016 [updated on unknown

date; cited 29 July 2021]. Available from: https://medicine.unimelb.edu.au/school-structure/obstetrics-and-gynaecology/research/COMMA.

157. Lensen S, Bell RJ, Carpenter JS, Christmas M, Davis SR, Giblin K, et al. A core outcome set for genitourinary symptoms associated with menopause: the COMMA (core outcomes in menopause) global initiative. *Menopause*. 2021;28(8):859–66.

158. Cagnacci A, Venier M. The controversial history of hormone replacement therapy. *Medicina (Kaunas)*. 2019;55(9):602.

159. Rossouw JE, Anderson GL, Prentice RL, LaCroix AZ, Kooperberg C, Stefanick ML, et al. Risks and benefits of estrogen plus progestin in healthy postmenopausal women: principal results from the Women's Health Initiative randomized controlled trial. *JAMA*. 2002;288(3):321–33.

160. Hodis HN, Mack WJ, Henderson VW, Shoupe D, Budoff MJ, Hwang-Levine J, et al. Vascular effects of early versus late postmenopausal treatment with estradiol. *New England Journal of Medicine*. 2016;374(13):1221–31.

161. Miller VM, Taylor HS, Naftolin F, Manson JE, Gleason CE, Brinton EA, et al. Lessons from KEEPS: the Kronos early estrogen prevention study. *Climacteric*. 2021;24(2):139–45.

162. Henderson VW, St John JA, Hodis HN, McCleary CA, Stanczyk FZ, Shoupe D, et al. Cognitive effects of estradiol after menopause: a randomized trial of the timing hypothesis. *Neurology*. 2016;87(7):699–708.

163. Gleason CE, Dowling NM, Wharton W, Manson JE, Miller VM, Atwood CS, et al. Effects of hormone therapy on cognition and mood in recently postmenopausal women: findings from the randomized, controlled KEEPS-cognitive and affective study. *PLoS Medicine*. 2015;12(6):e1001833; discussion e.

164. Kim YJ, Soto M, Branigan GL, Rodgers K, Brinton RD. Association between menopausal hormone therapy and risk of neurodegenerative diseases: implications for precision hormone therapy. *Alzheimer's and Dementia*. 2021;7(1):e12174.

165. Guo H, Liu M, Zhang L, Wang L, Hou W, Ma Y, et al. The critical period for neuroprotection by estrogen replacement therapy and the potential underlying mechanisms. *Current Neuropharmacology*. 2020;18(6):485–500.

166. Marjoribanks J, Farquhar C, Roberts H, Lethaby A, Lee J. Long-term hormone therapy for perimenopausal and postmenopausal women. *Cochrane Database Systematic Reviews*. 2017;1:CD004143.

167. Schwimmer M, Kahwati L. Hormone therapy for the primary prevention of chronic conditions in postmenopausal persons: updated evidence report and systematic review for the US Preventive Services Task Force. *JAMA*. 2022;328(17):1747–65.

168. US Preventive Services Task Force, Mangione CM, Barry MJ, et al. Hormone therapy for the primary prevention of chronic conditions in postmenopausal persons: US Preventive Services Task Force recommendation statement. *JAMA*. 2022;328(17):1740–6.

169. Faubion SS, Crandall CJ, Davis L, El Khoudary SR, Hodis HN, Lobo RA, Maki PM, Manson JE, Pinkerton JV, Santoro NF, Shifren JL. The 2022 hormone therapy position statement of The North American Menopause Society. *Menopause*. 2022;29(7):767–94.

170. Kuh D, Hardy R, Wadsworth M. Social and behavioural influences on the uptake of hormone replacement therapy among younger women. *BJOG: An International Journal of Obstetrics and Gynaecology*. 2000;107(6):731–9.

171. Parazzini F, Progetto Menopausa Italia Study G. Trends of determinants of hormone therapy use in Italian women attending menopause clinics, 1997–2003. *Menopause*. 2008;15(1):164–70.

172. Siyam T, Carbon J, Ross S, Yuksel N. Determinants of hormone therapy uptake and decision-making after bilateral oophorectomy (BO): a narrative review. *Maturitas*. 2019;120:68–76.

PART III
HEALTH, AGEING, AND DISEASE

5

A Life Course Approach to Cardiovascular Disease

Jane A.H. Masoli and Rebecca Hardy

5.1 Introduction

Cardiovascular disease (CVD) remains the leading cause of mortality and morbidity world-wide.[1] As shown in Figure 5.1, cardiovascular disease prevalence increases across the life course. In 2019, 34.6% of deaths in women were attributed to cardiovascular disease globally, and 47% in Europe.[2,3] Global estimates of deaths from CVD and disability-adjusted life years increased linearly in females between 1990 and 2019.[1] In HICs, cardiovascular mortality plateaued and declined in men between 1990 and 2011, with a subsequent decline in cardiovascular mortality in women lagging behind men by 10 years.[4] However, the higher prevalence of obesity, physical inactivity, and poor diet in younger individuals has seen an increase in the proportion of CVD in those aged < 50.[5] Deceleration in the rate of decline in cardiovascular mortality after 2011 is likely due to a combination of an ageing population and increased prevalence of cardiovascular risk factors at a population level.[6] In European countries, females had a higher overall incidence of CVD than males between 1990 and 2017, but lower median rates after age-standardisation (1006 per 100,000 population compared to 1291 in males).[3] This can be mostly explained by the consistently higher life expectancy of women. Estimates in CVD during and immediately after the COVID-19 pandemic were affected by changes to medical services and delayed presentation of disease. Risk factor optimisation opportunities through measurement and lifestyle advice were reduced,[7] although thought to be equal by sex, which may have a further effect on postpandemic CVD estimates.

There are sex and gender differences that affect risk, pathophysiology, research, clinical presentation, and management of CVD, some of which vary through the life course.[4,9] In this chapter, we will discuss these differences in the context of specific cardiovascular risk factors and outcomes, as well as genetic risk and differences at specific life stages.

5.2 Cardiovascular Outcomes

5.2.1 Coronary Heart Disease

Coronary heart disease (CHD) is the most common form of CVD,[3] and is the leading cause of cardiovascular mortality.[10] Women have a lower incidence of CHD than men across the

Jane A.H. Masoli and Rebecca Hardy, *A Life Course Approach to Cardiovascular Disease* In: *A Life Course Approach to Women's Health*. Second Edition. Edited by: Gita D Mishra, Rebecca Hardy, and Diana Kuh, Oxford University Press. © Oxford University Press 2023.
DOI: 10.1093/oso/9780192864642.003.0005

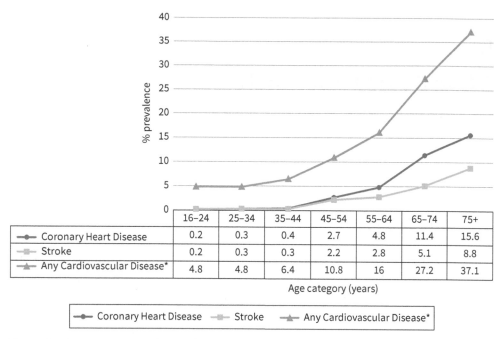

	16–24	25–34	35–44	45–54	55–64	65–74	75+
Coronary Heart Disease	0.2	0.3	0.4	2.7	4.8	11.4	15.6
Stroke	0.2	0.3	0.3	2.2	2.8	5.1	8.8
Any Cardiovascular Disease*	4.8	4.8	6.4	10.8	16	27.2	37.1

Age category (years)

Coronary Heart Disease — Stroke — Any Cardiovascular Disease*

Figure 5.1 Percentage prevalence of cardiovascular disease across the life course in men and women in England (2017). Source: British Heart Foundation Heart and Circulatory Disease Statistics, 2022.[8]

life course. In 2017, the median age-standardised rate of CHD across 54 European countries was estimated at 132 per 100,000 compared to 236 in males.[3] In addition, CHD is associated with a nearly threefold increase in the disability-adjusted life years (combining life years lost through premature death and years lived with CHD) in men compared to women.[3]

5.2.2 Cerebrovascular Disease

Stroke is the major clinical outcome of cerebrovascular disease and 87% of strokes are ischaemic.[11] The association between sex and stroke risk varies over the life course, with a higher lifetime risk in women than men at age 55 to 75 years at one in five in women compared to one in six men,[12] largely because of increased longevity. While men are more likely to experience CHD as the first cardiovascular event, in women the first event is more likely to be stroke.[13] Both sex and gender effects have been found to influence stroke care and research.[13] There is now good evidence that women have higher stroke severity and worse outcomes than men.[14,15] It is uncertain to what degree sex differences in premorbid functional status may account for this,[16] as women are more likely to have strokes in older age with frailty and multimorbidity.[11] An alternative explanation is difference in stroke presentation between men and women.[17,18]

5.3 Cardiovascular Risk Factors

CVD is largely dependent on a combination of genetics and known cardiovascular risk factors driving atherosclerosis. While cardiovascular outcomes predominate in middle to older age, the process of atherosclerosis is influenced over the life course.[19] Smoking, diet, obesity, hypercholesterolaemia, diabetes, physical inactivity, and excess alcohol consumption in younger people contribute to the development of CVD in later life. The National Health and Nutrition Examination Survey in the United States has shown that hypertension, obesity, diabetes and hypercholesterolaemia were more common in older individuals, while smoking and unhealthy diet were more common in younger individuals.[5] Sex differences in the prevalence of obesity, diet, alcohol consumption, and smoking are covered in Chapter 15.

Optimising cardiovascular risk factors is associated with reduced all-cause mortality, cardiovascular mortality, and cardiovascular outcomes.[11] A study estimating the proportion of US adults with 'ideal' cardiovascular health, as defined by American Heart Association metrics on seven risk factors, found that more women than men had high cardiovascular health based on the total score across all risk factors. More women met the ideal criteria for smoking, body mass index (BMI), blood pressure (BP) and glycated haemoglobin (HbA1c), while more men met the criteria for ideal physical activity and cholesterol health.[20] There was a consistent association between higher cardiovascular health scores and lower risk of cardiovascular events, with absolute risk increasing across the life course.[20] Understanding how such cardiovascular risk factors change across life are important for understanding the development of CVD and for disease prevention.

5.3.1 Cholesterol

The Avon Longitudinal Study of Parents and Children measured lipid metabolites at ages 8, 16, 18, and 25 years old, and parents at mean age 50, and found that low-density lipoprotein (LDL) was higher in females at age 8, but higher in males from age 16, with larger differences between the sexes in young adulthood.[19] In adults, total cholesterol values are similar in women and men.[3] Cardiovascular risk increases linearly as cholesterol, specifically LDL cholesterol, blood concentrations increase.[21,22] In pooled analysis of the trajectory for LDL cholesterol across the life course in 36,030 participants, elevated LDL cholesterol as a young adult aged 18 to 39 years was associated with a 64% increased risk of CHD, independent of later life exposures.[23]

5.3.2 Blood Pressure

Analysis from eight longitudinal studies in the UK showed that systolic BP (SBP) increases with age from early life, with slower increases in early adulthood, an acceleration in midlife, and a levelling off or even decline in older age.[24] A greater increase in SBP in boys compared with girls was observed in childhood, and SBP was markedly higher in men compared with women in early adulthood. But a greater midlife increase occurred in women, so that by around 60 years of age, mean SBP was higher in women.[24] The age-related increase in average SBP in this study, however, is likely driven by lifestyle factors typical in HICs. This is backed up by studies which demonstrate little age-related rise in BP in samples from four non-industrialised remote populations, including those followed longitudinally.[25]

Hypertension is the most common chronic disease globally and the leading preventable risk factor for cardiovascular disease and all-cause mortality.[26,27] Hypertension has had a longstanding definition of SBP ≥140 mmHg or diastolic BP ≥90 mmHg.[28] However, there is an evolving definition of hypertension, with several international hypertension guidelines released since 2016 recommending lower treatment targets in specific groups.[29,30] The estimated global age-standardised prevalence of hypertension in adults aged ≥20 years in 2010 was 31.9% in men and 30.1% in women.[31] However, at ages older than 70 years, the global prevalence was estimated at 68.6% in men and 75.8% in women.[31] Hypertension is more strongly associated with CHD in women than in men, with a population-attributable risk of 36% for myocardial infarction (MI).[4]

A systematic review and meta-analysis found a graded, progressive association between higher BP categories at ages 18 to 45 and increased risk of cardiovascular events.[32] The Prospective Studies Collaboration also found that BP was strongly associated with age-specific stroke and CHD mortality.[33]

BP in late adolescence or early adulthood is also related to CHD and stroke mortality in follow-ups of cohorts of university alumni and military conscripts.[34-36] Evidence is accumulating to suggest that the midlife rise in BP has implications for subsequent disease development as it has been associated with coronary artery atherosclerosis[37] and poorer cardiac structure and function.[38,39] The Lifetime Risk Pooling Project found that those who were consistently hypertensive over at least 10 years and those whose BP increased to the level of hypertension had high cumulative lifetime risks of CHD, but those experiencing a decrease in BP to normal levels had risk similar to those with BP consistently normal.[40] In support of a causal association between cumulative SBP and CHD, a Mendelian randomisation (MR) study suggests that single-nucleotide polymorphisms associated with lower SBP were related to a slower age-related rise in SBP and a greater reduction in risk of CHD than has been found in observational studies.[41]

5.4 Sex-Specific Risk Factors

Research has examined the role of risk factors that reflect the unique exposure of women to sex hormones, as it has been widely believed that the narrowing of the CVD gender gap in midlife is down to the cardioprotective effect of oestrogen. Although there is little evidence that postmenopausal levels of endogenous oestrogen are associated with CHD,[42] it may be lifetime levels or accumulation of life course oestrogen exposure which are more important.

Existing studies do not include oestrogen measured repeatedly over the life course. Time from age at menarche to age at menopause has been used to estimate duration of endogenous oestrogen exposure, with some studies accounting for pregnancy and breastfeeding. If oestrogen is cardioprotective, then the risk of CVD would be hypothesised to increase with a later age at menarche and an earlier age at menopause. In a pooled analysis of 307,855 women from 12 studies in the InterLACE consortium, short reproductive life span was indeed associated with an increased risk of CVD events in midlife—a relationship which was largely explained by early menopause rather than late menarche.[43] However, women with both a short reproductive span and particularly early menarche (≤ 11 years) had greatest risk.

5.4.1 Age at Menarche

Contrary to the hypothesis of a cardioprotective effect of oestrogen, a meta-analysis of 12 cohort studies (2,341,769 women) found that a 1-year later age at menarche was related to a small decrease in risk of CVD mortality, CHD mortality, and stroke mortality,[44] although there was considerable heterogeneity between the studies. Similarly, an MR phenome-wide association study (MR-pheWAS) of age at menarche in UK Biobank identified an effect of earlier menarche on greater risk of CHD, ischaemic stroke, angina, and hypertension.[45]

Early menarche has consistently been found to be associated with adult obesity, raising the possibility that BMI is a mediator of the menarche-CVD relationship. However, rapid childhood growth triggers menarche, and, thus, it is difficult to disentangle the effects of age at menarche from life course tracking of overweight from childhood. Observational evidence relating age at menarche to cardiovascular risk factors, such as blood pressure and lipids, have been mixed. MR studies agree with the lack of causal associations,[46,47] supporting confounding by prepubertal obesity as the most likely explanation for any associations in observational studies.

5.4.2 Age at Menopause

While the evidence relating to age at menarche remains equivocal, there is stronger evidence to suggest an effect of age at menopause. An InterLACE paper analysing data from 15 cohorts studies found that women with premature (< 40 years) and early menopause (40–44 years) had an increased risk of a nonfatal CVD before the age of 60 years, but not after age 70 years, compared with women who had menopause at age 50–51.[48] This association is supported by an MR study that showed that genetic variants associated with earlier age at natural menopause were associated with increased CVD risk.[49] Compared with natural menopause, women who had surgical menopause had a 20% higher risk of CVD and in analysis stratified by type of menopause, younger age at period cessation was associated with increased risk.[48] Women who experienced surgical menopause at earlier ages (< 50 years) and who used menopausal hormone therapy (MHT) had lower risk of incident CHD than those who were not users of MHT.

If associations of age at period cessation and CVD events are causal, it is unclear whether changes in conventional cardiovascular risk factors are an important mediating pathway, as longitudinal studies with repeated measures of cardiovascular risk factors across midlife show little impact of menopause. The Study of Women's Health across the Nation (SWAN) found that only total cholesterol, LDL cholesterol, and apolipoprotein B showed increases within the 1-year interval before and after the final menstrual period.[50] There were only small changes in BMI, waist circumference, and HbA1c (and none for BP or lipid levels) in the MRC (Medical Research Council) National Survey of Health and Development.[51] There were also no changes in the expected direction observed with hysterectomy in the SWAN,[52] or in the Coronary Artery Risk Development in Young Adults (CARDIA) study.[53] Larger longitudinal studies are, therefore, required to provide more precise estimates of associations between age at menopause and cardiovascular risk factors, In addition, there may be other possible intermediate phenotypes that require further study, such as carotid atherosclerosis which may vary with age at period cessation.[54]

An alternative to the view that the oestrogen drop during the menopausal transition triggers somatic ageing and increases CVD risk is that ovarian ageing may be a result of underlying ageing or disease processes or their common antecedents. Analysis of the Framingham cohort found higher BP and poorer lipid profile in the premenopausal period was associated with earlier menopause leading the authors to suggest that detrimental changes in cardiovascular risk factors may determine age at menopause.[55] A more recent study pooling multiple studies found that when compared with women without premenopausal CVD events, women who experienced a first CVD event before the age 35 years had double the risk of early menopause.[56]

A few studies have shown that women who suffer from vasomotor symptoms during the menopause transition have an increased risk of subsequent CVD outcomes[57-59] with severity rather than frequency being more important.[60] However, it is not possible to determine whether associations are causal, cardiovascular changes precede vasomotor symptoms, symptoms are a marker of underlying cardiovascular changes, or whether there are common antecedents.

5.4.3 Parity

Although oestrogen rises during pregnancy, it dips afterwards and during breastfeeding, and so it has been hypothesised that pregnancy may 'reset' oestrogen levels. Thus, increasing parity may reflect a lower lifetime exposure. Pregnancy also causes detrimental metabolic changes necessary for fetal growth, although BP drops after each pregnancy (see Chapter 2). The long-term impact of such changes remains unclear. Among parous women, increasing parity has been found to be associated with increased risk of CVD, particularly for those with high numbers of children[61-64] with the suggestion that this reflects a long-term biological effect of more pregnancies. However, studies have not been entirely consistent with others showing no association.[65,66] There are a few studies that compare associations between women and men, which can help to disentangle the pathways (as described in Chapter 15). Although some find evidence of associations in men as well as women, with disease outcomes and cardiovascular risk factors suggestive of a lifestyle explanation, they have not been entirely consistent.[67-69] Further research is needed to distinguish those not having children through choice from those suffering from infertility, as nulliparous women tend to have increased risk of CVD compared with women with one or two children.[64,70] A prolonged time to pregnancy (TTP), suggestive of fertility problems, showed a small increased CVD risk in the Norwegian Mother, Father, and Child Cohort Study for both women (14% for TTP >12 months compared with 0–3 months) and men (7%).[71]

5.4.4 Pregnancy Outcomes

Pregnancy has been described as a 'stress test' that reveals underlying susceptibility to disease as a result of the adverse cardiometabolic changes that occur. In support of this, hypertensive disorders of pregnancy,[72–75] preterm delivery,[76–78] small-for-gestational-age delivery,[79] and pregnancy loss are consistently associated with subsequent CVD. In addition, gestational diabetes is very strongly linked with subsequent type 2 diabetes.[80] Recently, the American Heart Association acknowledged the importance of recognising such adverse pregnancy outcomes when evaluating CVD risk in women, although highlighted that their value in reclassifying risk is not established.[81]

5.4.5 Hormonal Contraception and Menopausal Hormone Therapy

There is considerable evidence that current users of combined oral contraceptives have an increased risk of stroke compared with noncurrent users,[82] with a greater risk for ischaemic than haemorrhagic stroke.[83,84] Risk was also increased among those on higher doses of oestrogen, and in women who were smokers and who had hypertension. The association with the progesterone-only pill is more inconsistent.[85,86]

There has been controversy over the relationship between MHT and CVD. Initial observational studies showed an apparently beneficial of MHT on risk of CVD,[87] but women who took MHT were healthier, more physically active, and thinner than those who did not, and residual confounding remained a problem. Discontinuation of the Women's Health Initiative (WHI) randomised controlled trial (RCT) because of the unexpected increased risks of CVD in the combined MHT treatment arm in 2002, resulted in new guidelines on MHT use (see Chapter 4). However, as those enrolled in WHI were older postmenopausal women, the so-called window-of-opportunity hypothesis was subsequently proposed stating that the timing of initiation of MHT relative to menopause was related to the benefits and harms.[88] A systematic review of 31 RCTs[89] aiming to assess evidence related to this hypothesis found no association with cardiac mortality among women over the age of 60 years (for initiators of MHT versus controls) and a slight decrease in odds among users in the MHT initiator group in younger women. An increased risk of stroke was observed at all ages in the MHT group compared to controls. In another systematic review,[90] a decreased risk of MI in MHT users was seen in the observational studies, but not in the RCTs. Subgroup analysis did find heterogeneity in associations by timing of initiation, but also by underlying disease, regimen type, and route of administration which require further examination.

5.5 Social Risk Factors

5.5.1 Socioeconomic Position Across the Life Course

Social inequalities, according to a range of markers of socioeconomic position (SEP), in CVD have been widely documented across HICs. A systematic review, including over 1 million incident events, found that the social inequality in CHD and CVD was greater in women than men.[91] For example, the age-adjusted ratio of the relative risks comparing men and women for CHD for manual versus non-manual occupation was 1.14. This excess risk may be due to greater inequalities in cardiovascular risk factors, particularly obesity, among women, or greater inequalities in the stress-related response, or in access and use of health care.

Greater disadvantage in childhood, as measured by parental markers of SEP,[92] is also related to increased CVD risk in both sexes. The development of social inequalities in cardiovascular risk factors across the life course is likely key to explaining at least some of the association. A systematic review found little evidence of an association between SEP and BP measured in childhood and adolescence, but a number of studies have found that those from a more disadvantaged childhood SEP have higher BP in adulthood.[93] Disadvantaged childhood SEP has also been associated with adverse lipid and glucose profiles in adulthood. A study attempting to disentangle how life course SEP influenced cardiovascular risk factors found that the accumulation model was predominant in women, whereas childhood appeared to be a sensitive period among men,[94] which is consistent with the greater social inequalities by adult SEP in women.

Although education is often used as a marker of adult SEP, it also captures childhood SEP, and has been suggested as a mediator of the relationship between childhood SEP and CVD. Education, like adult SEP, may be more strongly related to CVD in women than men.[91] The causality of an association was backed up by an MR study where each standard deviation of years of education (3.6 years) was associated with lower odds of CHD,[95] although sex differences were not considered. For both observational and MR analyses, BMI, SBP, and smoking behaviour were demonstrated to mediate a substantial proportion of the education effect.

5.5.2 Social Roles

Being in a partnership represents a direct form of social support and may reduce the risk of unhealthy behaviours, while being single may lead to lower levels of social networks, and increased loneliness. Being unmarried, compared with being married, is associated with greater risk of CVD and CHD mortality for both sexes, although for CVD this appears weaker in women than men.[96] CVD mortality is greater in divorced and separated men than women, but no sex difference in risk was observed among those who were widowed or never married. Job strain and long working hours, markers of work stress have been consistently related to increased risk of incident CHD, including in a review of 27 cohort studies, which also suggested small differences in associations between men and women.[97]

5.6 Genetic Risk

Over the past 20 years, there has been significant progress in genetic profiling, and there is potential utility of genetic risk scores in CVD. Genetic risk is assigned at conception and is largely stable from birth, therefore providing a baseline risk that runs throughout the life course.[98] Polygenic risk scores have been developed for CVD and for individual cardiovascular risk factors. These could be used as an early biomarker for identification of higher risk earlier in the life course. There remains insufficient evidence for clinical utility of polygenic risk scores for CVD prevention at present because of a combination of cost and performance limitations. However, there is scope for incorporation of genetic risk into existing risk scores in the future if performance is proven and costs reduce, or genotyping becomes integrated with the clinical record.

5.7 Early Life

5.7.1 Birth Size

The fetal origins of adult disease hypothesis, subsequently, the developmental origins of adult health and disease, states that an adverse fetal environment leads to developmental adaptations that programme body structure, physiology and metabolism resulting in disease in later life.[99] Low birthweight, considered a proxy marker of adverse intrauterine conditions and reduced growth, has been associated with an increased risk in CHD with a meta-analysis estimating an odds ratio of 0.83 per kilogram of birthweight.[100,101] Some studies also find that those of particularly high birthweight (>4.0kg), may be at increased risk compared with those within a 'normal' birthweight range,[102] which could be due in part to maternal obesity and gestational diabetes.[103] There is less consistent evidence of associations between birthweight and cardiovascular risk factors, such as BP[104–106] or lipid levels.[107,108] Few sex differences have been reported, although one study found an association with total cholesterol to be weaker in women than men[109] and there have been conflicting findings for insulin resistance.[110,111]

As birthweight is only a proxy marker of the intrauterine environment, the mechanisms underlying the observed associations are yet to be fully understood. Although confounding by environmental factors, such as SEP, was originally proposed as an alternative explanation for the associations between birthweight and health, studies which have been able to adjust the relationship have not found this to be the case.[101] There is growing evidence to suggest that relationship between birthweight and cardiometabolic health is, at least in part, the result of shared genetic effects.[112] Novel MR approaches which consider maternal genotypes related offspring birthweight and health risk after conditioning on offspring genotype are being developed, which may further elucidate the mechanisms.[113] One study, which separated the direct fetal, from the indirect maternal, genetic effects and applied MR to assess causal mechanisms, favoured a genetic, rather than intrauterine, explanation for the association of birthweight with blood pressure.[114] Although there appears to be little evidence of sex differences in associations in the offspring, elucidating the causal mechanisms through which birthweight is associated with offspring health is important for mothers. Health messages and interventions during pregnancy are based on such findings, and it has been suggested that the assumption of the prime importance of the intrauterine environment can lead to unnecessary maternal blame and guilt.[115]

While older studies were limited to using birth-size measures as markers of in utero growth, more recent studies have been able to directly measure growth and cardiovascular development in utero. For example, the Generation R study demonstrated associations between length and weight growth from later pregnancy to the age of 2 years with BP at 2 years.[116] In the same study, sex differences in cardiovascular function in fetuses have been observed with males demonstrating increased preload, but reduced afterload, compared to females raising the possibility that differences in cardiovascular function initiate in utero.[117] Further, many historical studies were unable to distinguish birth size from gestational age. With increasing numbers of preterm babies surviving, the health implications are increasingly important. Shorter gestation and preterm birth have been consistently related to increased risk of stroke and higher BP through to midlife[118–120] with one study suggesting a stronger effect in women than men.[121] Despite these associations, there is less consistent evidence relating preterm birth with CHD, possibly a result of short follow-up and/or survivor bias in earlier studies.

A study of over 2 million singletons births in Sweden from 1973–94 found increased rates of CHD at 30–43 years in those born preterm compared to full term, which were stronger in women (93% higher) than men (37% higher).[122] Increased left ventricular mass and remodelling of the hearts of adults who were born preterm has also been observed.[123]

5.7.2   Childhood Growth and Nutrition

Short stature in adulthood has consistently been related to higher risk of CHD in observational and MR studies for both women and men[124,125] and it has been suggested that leg length is more strongly associated with CHD than total or trunk length.[126] Leg growth is determined more by early childhood exposures,[127] suggesting a greater impact of pre-adult exposures on disease risk. A large Danish cohort with repeated measures of BMI found that the positive associations between BMI and CHD were strengthened with the older age of BMI measurement from 7 to 13 years.[128] Rapid increases in BMI in childhood and adolescence in both sexes have been associated with higher risk of CHD and cardiovascular risk factors,[129,130] while longitudinal observational studies find evidence for accumulation of BMI from childhood for CHD[131] and risk factors.[132] Disentangling a potential sensitive period during adolescence from the effect of lifetime accumulation or adult overweight is challenging.[133] MR analyses using genetic risk scores for childhood BMI and adult BMI suggest that the association between childhood body size and CVD risk is likely due to those with a high BMI in childhood having persisting high BMI into adulthood.[134]

An association between breastfeeding and cardiovascular risk factors has been found in multiple studies, but there is less evidence of an association with CHD.[135,136] However, most studies were from HICs where breastfeeding is distributed by SEP and may, thus, be confounded by a whole range of related behavioural characteristics. Evidence from LMICs, where there is no or little SEP gradient for breastfeeding, in contrast, provided no evidence of an association with BP and obesity.[137]

5.7.3   Adverse Childhood Experiences

There has been increased interest in how adverse childhood experiences (ACEs), defined as a broad spectrum of traumatic and distressing events that threaten a child's physical, familial, or social safety and security,[138] are related to health outcomes, including to CVD. As ACEs are more likely to be clustered within those from more disadvantaged circumstances, they may also contribute to social inequalities in health.

Findings are, however, somewhat mixed. This may be due, in part, to the variation across studies in the ACEs measured, which can include mistreatment and neglect, exposure to household dysfunction, and physical or sexual abuse, or violence,[139] as well as the approach to modelling. A meta-analysis estimated a doubling of odds of CHD for those with four or more ACEs, but seven of the eight studies were cross-sectional, where ACEs were measured at the same time as assessment of CHD.[140] In contrast in longitudinal studies with ACEs recalled in adulthood and outcomes subsequently determined through electronic health records, there were no associations. In UK Biobank,[141] only specific ACEs—physical, sexual, and emotional abuse, and emotional and physical neglect—were associated with higher risk of CVD and CHD, with associations generally being stronger in women than men. For example, the risk of CHD was 1.48 and 1.20 times higher for women and men, respectively, who experienced physical abuse. This sex difference may be due to women being more susceptible to the deleterious effects of psychosocial stress than men, as ACEs are hypothesised to act through stress-related mechanisms either directly or via poorer psychological health and health related behaviours.

5.8 Later Life

As the proportion of older people in the population rises, understanding CVD into very old age is increasingly important. As described, the incidence of cardiovascular outcomes increases in later life. Women have a higher prevalence of CVD at ages over 80 years and a higher incidence of stroke, while men continue to have a higher incidence of CHD.[142] Ageing is variably associated with cardiovascular risk factors, which have reduced association with outcomes at older ages. For example, BP trends are well characterised through the life course, increasing through to older ages, but there is variability in estimates at ages over 70 years, as shown in Figure 5.2, with declining SBP trends for over a decade prior to death.[143]

Frailty is a state of increased vulnerability to stressors such as infection, which results in accelerated decline.[144] Frailty can be measured objectively by a cumulative deficit count of comorbidities and impairments,[145] or a phenotype approach incorporating exhaustion, slow gait speed, low energy expenditure, unintentional weight loss, and weak grip strength.[146] Prevalent CVD and cardiovascular risk factors are associated with increased risk of frailty, independent of the role of cardiovascular comorbidity within a cumulative deficit model.[147] The Women's Health Initiative Observational Study of 40,657 participants found that CHD and stroke were associated with 47% and 71% increased risk of developing incident frailty, respectively.[148] Cardiovascular risk factors and CVD are also associated with younger onset and accelerated frailty trajectories.[149]

The cardiovascular risk prediction tools are validated at younger ages and pertain to 10-year risk estimation, which is less relevant in older populations. In addition, risk prediction tools are validated in relatively younger cohorts and, therefore, extrapolated risk estimates may be inaccurate. Heart failure and dementia are increasingly common cardiovascular end points in older people, alongside CHD and stroke.

5.9 Conclusions

Although rates have declined, CVD remains an important source of mortality and morbidity, including frailty and increasingly dementia in women as well as men. The standard cardiovascular risk factors are the main causes of disease in women as they are in men. Associations of early growth and nutrition do not appear to exhibit obvious sex differences and underlying mechanisms are still not clearly understood. However, multiple additional exposures from across the life course contribute to risk in women. Among these, adverse pregnancy outcomes demonstrate robust associations, likely indicating underlying susceptibility and may represent an opportunity for early intervention. Understanding the mechanisms underlying the greater social and educational inequalities in CVD in women compared with

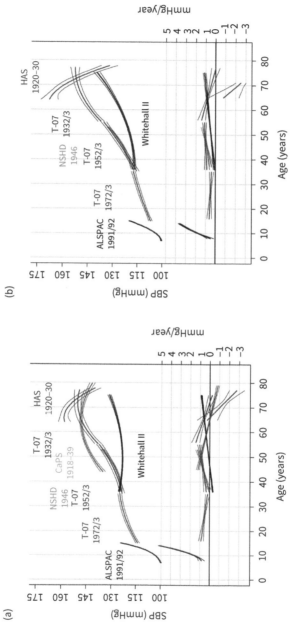

Figure 5.2 Predicted mean systolic blood pressure trajectories in mmHg over the life course.[24] See plate section.

men requires attention, with obesity, blood pressure, smoking behaviours, and potentially response to stress and specific ACEs, as underlying pathways.

Key messages and implications

- Prevention and treatment of classic cardiovascular risk factors across life is key in reducing risk in women, as it is in men, and control of BP may be particularly important.
- Pregnancy may offer an opportunity for early identification of women at risk from subsequent CVD, and the value of subsequent preventive strategies requires consideration.
- Life course socioeconomic and educational inequalities in CVD are wider in women than men, and the underlying pathways likely include inequalities in risk factors across the life course, while a stress pathway is also possible.
- Further research using novel approaches will be needed to elucidate mechanisms relating birthweight and early life body size to CVD in both sexes.

References

1. Roth GA, Mensah GA, Johnson CO, Addolorato G, Ammirati E, Baddour LM, et al. Global burden of cardiovascular diseases and risk factors, 1990–2019: update from the GBD 2019 study. *Journal of the American College of Cardiology*. 2020;76(25):2982–3021.
2. Global Health Data Exchange (GHDx). *2019 global burden of disease results tool*. Seattle: University of Washington; 2022.
3. Timmis A, Townsend N, Gale CP, Torbica A, Lettino M, Petersen SE, et al. European Society of Cardiology: cardiovascular disease statistics 2019. *European Heart Journal*. 2019;41(1):12–85.
4. Mehta LS, Beckie TM, DeVon HA, Grines CL, Krumholz HM, Johnson MN, et al. Acute myocardial infarction in women. *Circulation*. 2016;133(9):916–47.
5. Andersson C, Vasan RS. Epidemiology of cardiovascular disease in young individuals. *Nature Reviews Cardiology*. 2018;15(4):230–40.
6. Bell JA, Santos Ferreira DL, Fraser A, Soares ALG, Howe LD, Lawlor DA, et al. Sex differences in systemic metabolites at four life stages: cohort study with repeated metabolomics. *BMC Medicine*. 2021;19(1):58.
7. Bankhead CR, Lay-Flurrie S, Nicholson BD, Sheppard JP, Gale CP, Liyanage H, et al. Changes in cardiovascular disease monitoring in English primary care during the COVID-19 pandemic: an observational cohort study. *medRxiv*. 2020:2020.12.11.20247742.
8. British Heart Foundation. *Data from: heart and circulatory disease statistics 2022*. British London: Heart Foundation; 2022. [cited 5 July 2022]. Available from: https://www.bhf.org.uk/what-we-do/our-research/heart-statistics/heart-statistics-publications/cardiovascular-disease-statistics-2022.
9. Bartz D, Chitnis T, Kaiser UB, Rich-Edwards JW, Rexrode KM, Pennell PB, et al. Clinical advances in sex- and gender-informed medicine to improve the health of all: a review. *JAMA Internal Medicine*. 2020;180(4):574–83.
10. Benjamin EJ, Muntner P, Alonso A, Bittencourt MS, Callaway CW, Carson AP, et al. Heart disease and stroke statistics 2019 update: a report from the American Heart Association. *Circulation*. 2019;139(10):e56–e528.
11. Virani SS, Alonso A, Benjamin EJ, Bittencourt MS, Callaway CW, Carson AP, et al. Heart disease and stroke statistics 2020 update: a report from the American Heart Association. *Circulation*. 2020;141(9):e139–e596.

12. Seshadri S, Beiser A, Kelly-Hayes M, Kase CS, Au R, Kannel WB, et al. The lifetime risk of stroke. *Stroke*. 2006;37(2):345–50.

13. Bushnell CD, Chaturvedi S, Gage KR, Herson PS, Hurn PD, Jiménez MC, et al. Sex differences in stroke: challenges and opportunities. *Journal of Cerebral Blood Flow & Metabolism*. 2018;38(12):2179–91.

14. Appelros P, Stegmayr B, Terént A. Sex differences in stroke epidemiology. *Stroke*. 2009;40(4):1082–90.

15. Reeves MJ, Bushnell CD, Howard G, Gargano JW, Duncan PW, Lynch G, et al. Sex differences in stroke: epidemiology, clinical presentation, medical care, and outcomes. *Lancet Neurology*. 2008;7(10):915–26.

16. Renoux C, Coulombe J, Li L, Ganesh A, Silver L, Rothwell PM. Confounding by pre-morbid functional status in studies of apparent sex differences in severity and outcome of stroke. *Stroke*. 2017;48(10):2731–8.

17. Reeves MJ, Prager M, Fang J, Stamplecoski M, Kapral MK. Impact of living alone on the care and outcomes of patients with acute stroke. *Stroke*. 2014;45(10):3083–5.

18. Gall SL, Donnan G, Dewey HM, Macdonell R, Sturm J, Gilligan A, et al. Sex differences in presentation, severity, and management of stroke in a population-based study. *Neurology*. 2010;74(12):975–81.

19. Hardy R, Lawlor DA, Kuh D. A life course approach to cardiovascular aging. *Future Cardiology*. 2015;11(1):101–13.

20. Bundy JD, Zhu Z, Ning H, Zhong VW, Paluch AE, Wilkins JT, et al. Estimated impact of achieving optimal cardiovascular health among US Adults on cardiovascular disease events. *Journal of the American Heart Association*. 2021;10(7):e019681.

21. Ference BA, Yoo W, Alesh I, Mahajan N, Mirowska KK, Mewada A, et al. Effect of long-term exposure to lower low-density lipoprotein cholesterol beginning early in life on the risk of coronary heart disease: a Mendelian randomization analysis. *Journal of the American College of Cardiology*. 2012;60(25):2631–9.

22. Stamler J, Wentworth D, Neaton JD. Is relationship between serum cholesterol and risk of premature death from coronary heart disease continuous and graded? Findings in 356,222 primary screenees of the multiple risk factor intervention trial (MRFIT). *JAMA*. 1986;256(20):2823–8.

23. Zhang Y, Vittinghoff E, Pletcher MJ, Allen NB, Zeki Al Hazzouri A, Yaffe K, et al. Associations of blood pressure and cholesterol levels during young adulthood with later cardiovascular events. *Journal of the American College of Cardiology*. 2019;74(3):330–41.

24. Wills AK, Lawlor DA, Matthews FE, Aihie Sayer A, Bakra E, Ben-Shlomo Y, et al. Life course trajectories of systolic blood pressure using longitudinal data from eight UK cohorts. *PLoS Medicine*. 2011;8(6):e1000440.

25. Carvalho JJ, Baruzzi RG, Howard PF, Poulter N, Alpers MP, Franco LJ, et al. Blood pressure in four remote populations in the INTERSALT Study. *Hypertension*. 1989;14(3):238–46.

26. Mills KT, Stefanescu A, He J. The global epidemiology of hypertension. *Nature Reviews Nephrology*. 2020;16(4):223–37.

27. Forouzanfar MH, Alexander L, Anderson HR, Bachman VF, Biryukov S, Brauer M, et al. Global, regional, and national comparative risk assessment of 79 behavioural, environmental and occupational, and metabolic risks or clusters of risks in 188 countries, 1990-2013: a systematic analysis for the Global Burden of Disease Study 2013. *Lancet*. 2015;386(10010):2287–323.

28. Andersson C, Johnson AD, Benjamin EJ, Levy D, Vasan RS. 70-year legacy of the Framingham heart study. *Nature Reviews Cardiology*. 2019;16(11):687–98.

29. Messerli FH, Rimoldi SF, Bangalore S. Changing definition of hypertension in guidelines: how innocent a number game? *European Heart Journal*. 2018;39(24):2241–2.

30. Unger T, Borghi C, Charchar F, Khan NA, Poulter NR, Prabhakaran D, et al. 2020 International Society of Hypertension global hypertension practice guidelines. *Journal of Hypertension*. 2020;38(6). https://www.ahajournals.org/doi/full/10.1161/HYPERTENSIONAHA.120.15026.

31. Mills KT, Bundy JD, Kelly TN, Reed JE, Kearney PM, Reynolds K, et al. Global disparities of hypertension prevalence and control. *Circulation*. 2016;134(6):441–50.

32. Luo D, Cheng Y, Zhang H, Ba M, Chen P, Li H, et al. Association between high blood pressure and long term cardiovascular events in young adults: systematic review and meta-analysis. *BMJ*. 2020;370:m3222.

33. Lewington S, Clasrke R, Qizilbash N, OPeto R, Collins R. Age-specific relevance of usual blood pressure to vascular mortality: a meta-analysis of individual data for one million adults in 61 prospective studies. *Lancet*. 2002;360(9349):1903–13.

34. McCarron P, Smith GD, Okasha M, McEwen J. Blood pressure in young adulthood and mortality from cardiovascular disease. *Lancet*. 2000;355(9213):1430–1.

35. Falkstedt D, Koupil I, Hemmingsson T. Blood pressure in late adolescence and early incidence of coronary heart disease and stroke in the Swedish 1969 conscription cohort. *Journal of Hypertension*. 2008;26(7):1313–20.

36. Gray L, Lee IM, Sesso HD, Batty GD. Blood pressure in early adulthood, hypertension in middle age, and future cardiovascular disease mortality: HAHS (Harvard alumni health study). *Journal of the American College of Cardiology*. 2011;58(23):2396–403.

37. Allen NB, Siddique J, Wilkins JT, Shay C, Lewis CE, Goff DC, et al. Blood pressure trajectories in early adulthood and subclinical atherosclerosis in middle age. *JAMA*. 2014;311(5):490–7.

38. Ghosh AK, Hughes AD, Francis D, Chaturvedi N, Pellerin D, Deanfield J, et al. Midlife blood pressure predicts future diastolic dysfunction independently of blood pressure. *Heart*. 2016;102(17):1380–7.

39. Ghosh AK, Health ObotMRCNSo, Scientific D, Team DC, Hardy RJ, Health ObotMRCNSo, et al. Midlife blood pressure change and left ventricular mass and remodelling in older age in the 1946 British birth cohort study. *European Heart Journal*. 2014;35(46):3287–95.

40. Allen N, Berry JD, Ning H, Horn LV, Dyer A, Lloyd-Jones DM. Impact of blood pressure and blood pressure change during middle age on the remaining lifetime risk for cardiovascular disease. *Circulation*. 2012;125(1):37–44.

41. Ference BA, Julius S, Mahajan N, Levy PD, Williams KA, Flack JM. Clinical effect of naturally random allocation to lower systolic blood pressure beginning before the development of hypertension. *Hypertension*. 2014;63(6):1182–8.

42. Wang H, Li Y, Wang X, Bu J, Yan G, Lou D. Endogenous sex hormone levels and coronary heart disease risk in postmenopausal women: a meta-analysis of prospective studies. *European Journal of Preventive Cardiology*. 2017;24(6):600–11.

43. Mishra SR, Chung H-F, Waller M, Dobson AJ, Greenwood DC, Cade JE, et al. Association between reproductive life span and incident nonfatal cardiovascular disease: a pooled analysis of individual patient data from 12 studies. *JAMA Cardiology*. 2020;5(12):1410–8.

44. Chen X, Liu Y, Sun X, Yin Z, Li H, Liu X, et al. Age at menarche and risk of all-cause and cardiovascular mortality: a systematic review and dose–response meta-analysis. *Menopause*. 2019;26(6):670–6.

45. Magnus MC, Guyatt AL, Lawn RB, Wyss AB, Trajanoska K, Küpers LK, et al. Identifying potential causal effects of age at menarche: a Mendelian randomization phenome-wide association study. *BMC Medicine*. 2020;18(1):71.

46. Au Yeung SL, Jiang C, Cheng KK, Xu L, Zhang W, Lam TH, et al. Age at menarche and cardiovascular risk factors using Mendelian randomization in the Guangzhou Biobank cohort study. *Preventive Medicine*. 2017;101:142–8.

47. Bell JA, Carslake D, Wade KH, Richmond RC, Langdon RJ, Vincent EE, et al. Influence of puberty timing on adiposity and cardiometabolic traits: a Mendelian randomisation study. *PLoS Medicine*. 2018;15(8):e1002641.

48. Zhu D, Chung H-F, Dobson AJ, Pandeya N, Brunner EJ, Kuh D, et al. Type of menopause, age of menopause and variations in the risk of incident cardiovascular disease: pooled analysis of individual data from 10 international studies. *Human Reproduction*. 2020;35(8):1933–43.

49. Sarnowski C, Kavousi M, Isaacs S, Demerath EW, Broer L, Muka T, et al. Genetic variants associated with earlier age at menopause increase the risk of cardiovascular events in women. *Menopause*. 2018;25(4):451–7.

50. Matthews KA, Crawford SL, Chae CU, Everson-Rose SA, Sowers MF, Sternfeld B, et al. Are changes in cardiovascular disease risk factors in midlife women due to chronological aging or to the menopausal transition? *Journal of the American College of Cardiology*. 2009;54(25):2366–73.

51. O'Keeffe LM, Kuh D, Fraser A, Howe LD, Lawlor D, Hardy R. Age at period cessation and trajectories of cardiovascular risk factors across mid and later life. *Heart*. 2020;106(7):499–505.

52. Matthews KA, Gibson CJ, El Khoudary SR, Thurston RC. Changes in cardiovascular risk factors by hysterectomy status with and without oophorectomy: study of women's health across the nation. *Journal of the American College of Cardiology*. 2013;62(3):191–200.

53. Appiah D, Schreiner PJ, Bower JK, Sternfeld B, Lewis CE, Wellons MF. Is surgical menopause associated with future levels of cardiovascular risk factor independent of antecedent levels? The CARDIA study. *American Journal of Epidemiology*. 2015;182(12):991–9.

54. Muka T, Oliver-Williams C, Kunutsor S, Laven JSE, Fauser BCJM, Chowdhury R, et al. Association of age at onset of menopause and time since onset of menopause with cardiovascular outcomes, intermediate vascular traits, and all-cause mortality: a systematic review and meta-analysis. *JAMA Cardiology*. 2016;1(7):767–76.

55. Kok HS, van Asselt KM, van der Schouw YT, van der Tweel I, Peeters PHM, Wilson PWF, et al. Heart disease risk determines menopausal age rather than the reverse. *Journal of the American College of Cardiology*. 2006;47(10):1976–83.

56. Zhu D, Chung H-F, Pandeya N, Dobson AJ, Hardy R, Kuh D, et al. Premenopausal cardiovascular disease and age at natural menopause: a pooled analysis of over 170,000 women. *European Journal of Epidemiology*. 2019;34(3):235–46.

57. Gast G-CM, Pop VJM, Samsioe GN, Grobbee DE, Nilsson PM, Keyzer JJ, et al. Vasomotor menopausal symptoms are associated with increased risk of coronary heart disease. *Menopause*. 2011;18(2):146–51.

58. Thurston RC, Vlachos HEA, Derby CA, Jackson EA, Brooks MM, Matthews KA, et al. Menopausal vasomotor symptoms and risk of incident cardiovascular disease events in SWAN. *Journal of the American Heart Association*. 2021;10(3):e017416.

59. Gast G-CM, Grobbee DE, Pop VJM, Keyzer JJ, Gent CJMW-v, Samsioe GN, et al. Menopausal complaints are associated with cardiovascular risk factors. *Hypertension*. 2008;51(6):1492–8.

60. Zhu D, Chung H-F, Dobson AJ, Pandeya N, Anderson DJ, Kuh D, et al. Vasomotor menopausal symptoms and risk of cardiovascular disease: a pooled analysis of six prospective studies. *American Journal of Obstetrics and Gynecology*. 2020;223(6):898.e1–.e16.

61. Ness RB, Harris T, Cobb J, Flegal KM, Kelsey JL, Balanger A, et al. Number of pregnancies and the subsequent risk of cardiovascular disease. *New England Journal of Medicine*. 1993;328(21):1528–33.

62. Oliver-Williams C, Vladutiu CJ, Loehr LR, Rosamond WD, Stuebe AM. The association between parity and subsequent cardiovascular disease in women: the atherosclerosis risk in communities study. *Journal of Women's Health*. 2019;28(5):721–7.

63. Grinblatt JA. Number of pregnancies and risk of cardiovascular disease. *New England Journal of Medicine*. 1993;329(25):1893–5.

64. Green A, Beral V, Moser K. Mortality in women in relation to their childbearing history. *British Medical Journal*. 1988;297(6645):391–5.

65. Elajami TK, Giuseffi J, Avila MD, Hovnanians N, Mukamal KJ, Parikh N, et al. Parity, coronary heart disease and mortality in the old order Amish. *Atherosclerosis*. 2016;254:14–9.

66. Jacobsen BK, Knutsen SF, Oda K, Fraser GE. Parity and total, ischemic heart disease and stroke mortality: the Adventist health study, 1976–1988. *European Journal of Epidemiology*. 2011;26(9):711–8.

67. Lawlor DA, Emberson JR, Ebrahim S, Whincup PH, Wannamethee SG, Walker M, et al. Is the association between parity and coronary heart disease due to biological effects of pregnancy or adverse lifestyle risk factors associated with child-rearing? *Circulation*. 2003;107(9):1260–4.

68. Hardy R, Lawlor D, Black S, Wadsworth M, Kuh D. Number of children and coronary heart disease risk factors in men and women from a British birth cohort. *BJOG: An International Journal of Obstetrics & Gynaecology*. 2007;114(6):721–30.

69. Kravdal Ø, Tverdal A, Grundy E. The association between parity, CVD mortality and CVD risk factors among Norwegian women and men. *European Journal of Public Health*. 2020;30(6):1133–9.

70. Qureshi AI, Giles WH, Croft JB, Stern BJ. Number of pregnancies and risk for stroke and stroke subtypes. *Archives of Neurology.* 1997;54(2):203–6.

71. Magnus MC, Fraser A, Rich-Edwards JW, Magnus P, Lawlor DA, Håberg SE. Time-to-pregnancy and risk of cardiovascular disease among men and women. *European Journal of Epidemiology.* 2021;36(4):383–91.

72. Bellamy L, Casas J-P, Hingorani AD, Williams DJ. Pre-eclampsia and risk of cardiovascular disease and cancer in later life: systematic review and meta-analysis. *BMJ.* 2007;335(7627):974.

73. Brown MC, Best KE, Pearce MS, Waugh J, Robson SC, Bell R. Cardiovascular disease risk in women with pre-eclampsia: systematic review and meta-analysis. *European Journal of Epidemiology.* 2013;28(1):1–19.

74. Brouwers L, van der Meiden-van Roest A, Savelkoul C, Vogelvang T, Lely A, Franx A, et al. Recurrence of pre-eclampsia and the risk of future hypertension and cardiovascular disease: a systematic review and meta-analysis. *BJOG: An International Journal of Obstetrics & Gynaecology.* 2018;125(13):1642–54.

75. Harskamp RE, Zeeman GG. Preeclampsia: at risk for remote cardiovascular disease. *American Journal of the Medical Sciences.* 2007;334(4):291–5.

76. Catov JM, Wu CS, Olsen J, Sutton-Tyrrell K, Li J, Nohr EA. Early or recurrent preterm birth and maternal cardiovascular disease risk. *Annals of Epidemiology.* 2010;20(8):604–9.

77. Smith GCS, Pell JP, Walsh D. Pregnancy complications and maternal risk of ischaemic heart disease: a retrospective cohort study of 129 290 births. *Lancet.* 2001;357(9273):2002–6.

78. Tanz LJ, Stuart JJ, Williams PL, Rimm EB, Missmer SA, Rexrode KM, et al. Preterm delivery and maternal cardiovascular disease in young and middle-aged adult women. *Circulation.* 2017;135(6):578–89.

79. Davey Smith G, Hyppönen E, Power C, Lawlor DA. Offspring birth weight and parental mortality: prospective observational study and meta-analysis. *American Journal of Epidemiology.* 2007;166(2):160–9.

80. Bellamy L, Casas J-P, Hingorani AD, Williams D. Type 2 diabetes mellitus after gestational diabetes: a systematic review and meta-analysis. *Lancet.* 2009;373(9677):1773–9.

81. Parikh NI, Gonzalez JM, Anderson CAM, Judd SE, Rexrode KM, Hlatky MA, et al. Adverse pregnancy outcomes and cardiovascular disease risk: unique opportunities for cardiovascular disease prevention in women: a scientific statement from the American Heart Association. *Circulation.* 2021;143(18):e902–e916.

82. Okoth K, Chandan JS, Marshall T, Thangaratinam S, Thomas GN, Nirantharakumar K, et al. Association between the reproductive health of young women and cardiovascular disease in later life: umbrella review. *BMJ.* 2020;371:m3502.

83. Xu Z, Li Y, Tang S, Huang X, Chen T. Current use of oral contraceptives and the risk of first-ever ischemic stroke: a meta-analysis of observational studies. *Thrombosis Research.* 2015;136(1):52–60.

84. Xu Z, Yue Y, Bai J, Shen C, Yang J, Huang X, et al. Association between oral contraceptives and risk of hemorrhagic stroke: a meta-analysis of observational studies. *Archives of Gynecology and Obstetrics.* 2018;297(5):1181–91.

85. Glisic M, Shahzad S, Tsoli S, Chadni M, Asllanaj E, Rojas LZ, et al. Association between progestin-only contraceptive use and cardiometabolic outcomes: a systematic review and meta-analysis. *European Journal of Preventive Cardiology.* 2020;25(10):1042–52.

86. Roach RE, Helmerhorst FM, Lijfering WM, Stijnen T, Algra A, Dekkers OM. Combined oral contraceptives: the risk of myocardial infarction and ischemic stroke. *Cochrane Database Systems Reviews.* 2015(8):CD011054.

87. Grady D, Rubin SM, Petitti DB, Fox CS, Black D, Ettinger B, et al. Hormone therapy to prevent disease and prolong life in postmenopausal women. *Annals of Internal Medicine.* 1992;117(12):1016–37.

88. Clarkson TB, Meléndez GC, Appt SE. Timing hypothesis for postmenopausal hormone therapy: its origin, current status, and future. *Menopause.* 2013;20(3):342–53.

89. Nudy M, Chinchilli VM, Foy AJ. A systematic review and meta-regression analysis to examine the 'timing hypothesis' of hormone replacement therapy on mortality, coronary heart disease, and stroke. *International Journal of Cardiology Heart and Vasculature.* 2019;22:123–31.

90. Kim J-E, Chang J-H, Jeong M-J, Choi J, Park J, Baek C, et al. A systematic review and meta-analysis of effects of menopausal hormone therapy on cardiovascular diseases. *Scientific Reports.* 2020;10(1):20631.

91. Backholer K, Peters SAE, Bots SH, Peeters A, Huxley RR, Woodward M. Sex differences in the relationship between socioeconomic status and cardiovascular disease: a systematic review and meta-analysis. *Journal of Epidemiology and Community Health.* 2017;71(6):550–7.

92. Galobardes B, Smith GD, Lynch JW. Systematic review of the influence of childhood socioeconomic circumstances on risk for cardiovascular disease in adulthood. *Annals of Epidemiology.* 2006;16(2):91–104.

93. Hardy R, Kuh D, Langenberg C, Wadsworth MEJ. Birthweight, childhood social class, and change in adult blood pressure in the 1946 British Birth Cohort. *Lancet.* 2003;362(9391):1178–83.

94. Murray ET, Mishra GD, Kuh D, Guralnik J, Black S, Hardy R. Life course models of socioeconomic position and cardiovascular risk factors: 1946 Birth Cohort. *Annals of Epidemiology.* 2011;21(8):589–97.

95. Carter AR, Gill D, Davies NM, Taylor AE, Tillmann T, Vaucher J, et al. Understanding the consequences of education inequality on cardiovascular disease: Mendelian randomisation study. *BMJ.* 2019;365:l1855.

96. Wang Y, Jiao Y, Nie J, O'Neil A, Huang W, Zhang L, et al. Sex differences in the association between marital status and the risk of cardiovascular, cancer, and all-cause mortality: a systematic review and meta-analysis of 7,881,040 individuals. *Global Health Research and Policy.* 2020;5(1):4.

97. Kivimäki M, Kawachi I. Work stress as a risk factor for cardiovascular disease. *Current Cardiology Reports.* 2015;17(9):74.

98. Moorthie S, Babb de Villiers C, Brigden T, Gaynor L, Hall A, Johnson E, et al. *Polygenic scores, risk and cardiovascular disease.* Cambridge: PHG Foundation; 2019.

99. Levy L. Mothers, babies, and disease in later life: By D J P Barker. (Pp 180: £29.95.) London: BMJ Publishing Group, 1994. ISBN 0-7279-0835-9. *Cardiovascular Research.* 1995;29(2):294–5.

100. Wang SF, Shu L, Sheng J, Mu M, Wang S, Tao XY, et al. Birth weight and risk of coronary heart disease in adults: a meta-analysis of prospective cohort studies. *Journal of Developmental Origins of Health and Disease.* 2014;5(6):408–19.

101. Huxley R, Owen CG, Whincup PH, Cook DG, Rich-Edwards J, Smith GD, et al. Is birth weight a risk factor for ischemic heart disease in later life? *American Journal of Clinical Nutrition.* 2007;85(5):1244–50.

102. Mohseni R, Mohammed SH, Safabakhsh M, Mohseni F, Monfared ZS, Seyyedi J, et al. Birth weight and risk of cardiovascular disease incidence in adulthood: a dose-response meta-analysis. *Current Atherosclerosis Reports.* 2020;22(3):12.

103. Fraser A, Lawlor DA. Long-term health outcomes in offspring born to women with diabetes in pregnancy. *Current Diabetes Reports.* 2014;14(5):489.

104. Huxley R, Neil A, Collins R. Unravelling the fetal origins hypothesis: is there really an inverse association between birthweight and subsequent blood pressure? *Lancet.* 2002;360(9334):659–65.

105. Xie YJ, Ho SC, Liu Z-M, Hui SS-C. Birth weight and blood pressure: 'J' shape or linear shape? Findings from a cross-sectional study in Hong Kong Chinese women. *BMJ Open.* 2014;4(9):e005115.

106. Zhang Y, Li H, Liu S-j, Fu G-j, Zhao Y, Xie Y-J, et al. The associations of high birth weight with blood pressure and hypertension in later life: a systematic review and meta-analysis. *Hypertension Research.* 2013;36(8):725–35.

107. Laurén L, Järvelin M-R, Elliott P, Sovio U, Spellman A, McCarthy M, et al. Relationship between birthweight and blood lipid concentrations in later life: evidence from the existing literature. *International Journal of Epidemiology.* 2003;32(5):862–76.

108. Chen L-H, Chen S-S, Liang L, Wang C-L, Fall C, Osmond C, et al. Relationship between birth weight and total cholesterol concentration in adulthood: a meta-analysis. *Journal of the Chinese Medical Association.* 2017;80(1):44–9.

109. Lawlor DA, Owen CG, Davies AA, Whincup PH, Ebrahim S, Cook DG, et al. Sex Differences in the association between birth weight and total cholesterol. A meta-analysis. *Annals of Epidemiology.* 2006;16(1):19–25.

110. Forsén T, Eriksson JG, Tuomilehto J, Osmond C, Barker DJP. Growth in utero and during childhood among women who develop coronary heart disease: longitudinal study. *BMJ*. 1999;319(7222):1403–7.
111. Fall CHD, Vijayakumar M, Barker DJP, Osmond C, Duggleby S. Weight in infancy and prevalence of coronary heart disease in adult life. *BMJ*. 1995;310(6971):17–20.
112. Horikoshi M, Beaumont RN, Day FR, Warrington NM, Kooijman MN, Fernandez-Tajes J, et al. Genome-wide associations for birth weight and correlations with adult disease. *Nature*. 2016;538(7624):248–52.
113. D'Urso S, Wang G, Hwang L-D, Moen G-H, Warrington NM, Evans DM. A cautionary note on using Mendelian randomization to examine the Barker hypothesis and developmental origins of health and disease (DOHaD). *Journal of Developmental Origins of Health and Disease*. 2021;12(5):688–93.
114. Warrington NM, Beaumont RN, Horikoshi M, Day FR, Helgeland Ø, Laurin C, et al. Maternal and fetal genetic effects on birth weight and their relevance to cardio-metabolic risk factors. *Nature Genetics*. 2019;51(5):804–14.
115. Sharp GC, Lawlor DA, Richardson SS. It's the mother! How assumptions about the causal primacy of maternal effects influence research on the developmental origins of health and disease. *Social Science & Medicine*. 2018;213:20–7.
116. van Houten VA, Steegers EA, Witteman JC, Moll HA, Hofman A, Jaddoe VW. Fetal and postnatal growth and blood pressure at the age of 2 years. The generation R study. *Journal of Hypertension*. 2009;27(6):1152–7.
117. Schalekamp-Timmermans S, Cornette J, Hofman A, Helbing WA, Jaddoe VWV, Steegers EAP, et al. In utero origin of sex-related differences in future cardiovascular disease. *Biology of Sex Differences*. 2016;7(1):55.
118. Markopoulou P, Papanikolaou E, Analytis A, Zoumakis E, Siahanidou T. Preterm birth as a risk factor for metabolic syndrome and cardiovascular disease in adult life: a systematic review and meta-analysis. *Journal of Pediatrics*. 2019;210:69–80.e5.
119. Crump C, Sundquist J, Sundquist K. Risk of hypertension into adulthood in persons born prematurely: a national cohort study. *European Heart Journal*. 2019;41(16):1542–50.
120. Cooper R, Atherton K, Power C. Gestational age and risk factors for cardiovascular disease: evidence from the 1958 British Birth Cohort followed to mid-life. *International Journal of Epidemiology*. 2008;38(1):235–44.
121. Parkinson JRC, Hyde MJ, Gale C, Santhakumaran S, Modi N. Preterm birth and the metabolic syndrome in adult life: a systematic review and meta-analysis. *Pediatrics*. 2013;131(4):e1240–e1263.
122. Crump C, Howell EA, Stroustrup A, McLaughlin MA, Sundquist J, Sundquist K. Association of preterm birth with risk of ischemic heart disease in adulthood. *JAMA Pediatrics*. 2019;173(8):736–43.
123. Lewandowski AJ, Augustine D, Lamata P, Davis EF, Lazdam M, Francis J, et al. Preterm heart in adult life. *Circulation*. 2013;127(2):197–206.
124. Paajanen TA, Oksala NKJ, Kuukasjärvi P, Karhunen PJ. Short stature is associated with coronary heart disease: a systematic review of the literature and a meta-analysis. *European Heart Journal*. 2010;31(14):1802–9.
125. Lai FY, Nath M, Hamby SE, Thompson JR, Nelson CP, Samani NJ. Adult height and risk of 50 diseases: a combined epidemiological and genetic analysis. *BMC Medicine*. 2018;16(1):187.
126. Whitley E, Martin RM, Davey Smith G, Holly JMP, Gunnell D. The association of childhood height, leg length and other measures of skeletal growth with adult cardiovascular disease: the Boyd–Orr cohort. *Journal of Epidemiology and Community Health*. 2012;66(1):18–23.
127. Wadsworth M, Hardy R, Paul A, Marshall S, Cole T. Leg and trunk length at 43 years in relation to childhood health, diet and family circumstances; evidence from the 1946 national birth cohort. *International Journal of Epidemiology*. 2002;31(2):383–90.
128. Baker JL, Olsen LW, Sørensen TIA. Childhood body-mass index and the risk of coronary heart disease in adulthood. *New England Journal of Medicine*. 2007;357(23):2329–37.
129. Hardy R, Wadsworth ME, Langenberg C, Kuh D. Birthweight, childhood growth, and blood pressure at 43 years in a British birth cohort. *International Journal of Epidemiology*. 2004;33(1):121–9.

130. Eriksson JG. Early growth and coronary heart disease and type 2 diabetes: findings from the Helsinki Birth Cohort Study (HBCS). *American Journal of Clinical Nutrition*. 2011;94(Suppl 6):1799S–802S.

131. Park MH, Sovio U, Viner RM, Hardy RJ, Kinra S. Overweight in childhood, adolescence and adulthood and cardiovascular risk in later life: pooled analysis of three British birth cohorts. *PLoS ONE*. 2013;8(7):e70684.

132. Norris T, Cole TJ, Bann D, Hamer M, Hardy R, Li L, et al. Duration of obesity exposure between ages 10 and 40 years and its relationship with cardiometabolic disease risk factors: a cohort study. *PLoS Medicine*. 2020;17(12):e1003387.

133. Wills AK, Hardy RJ, Black S, Kuh DJ. Trajectories of overweight and body mass index in adulthood and blood pressure at age 53: the 1946 British Birth Cohort Study. *Journal of Hypertension*. 2010;28(4):679–86.

134. Richardson TG, Sanderson E, Elsworth B, Tilling K, Davey Smith G. Use of genetic variation to separate the effects of early and later life adiposity on disease risk: Mendelian randomisation study. *BMJ*. 2020;369:m1203.

135. Owen CG, Whincup PH, Cook DG. Breast-feeding and cardiovascular risk factors and outcomes in later life: evidence from epidemiological studies. *Proceedings of the Nutrition Society*. 2011;70(4):478–84.

136. Martin RM, Davey Smith G, Mangtani P, Tilling K, Frankel S, Gunnell D. Breastfeeding and cardiovascular mortality: the Boyd Orr cohort and a systematic review with meta-analysis. *European Heart Journal*. 2004;25(9):778–86.

137. Brion M-JA, Lawlor DA, Matijasevich A, Horta B, Anselmi L, Araújo CL, et al. What are the causal effects of breastfeeding on IQ, obesity and blood pressure? Evidence from comparing high-income with middle-income cohorts. *International Journal of Epidemiology*. 2011;40(3):670–80.

138. Suglia SF, Koenen KC, Boynton-Jarrett R, Chan PS, Clark CJ, Danese A, et al. Childhood and adolescent adversity and cardiometabolic outcomes: a scientific statement from the American Heart Association. *Circulation*. 2018;137(5):e15–e28.

139. Godoy LC, Frankfurter C, Cooper M, Lay C, Maunder R, Farkouh ME. Association of adverse childhood experiences with cardiovascular disease later in life: a review. *JAMA Cardiology*. 2021;6(2):228–35.

140. Hughes K, Bellis MA, Hardcastle KA, Sethi D, Butchart A, Mikton C, et al. The effect of multiple adverse childhood experiences on health: a systematic review and meta-analysis. *Lancet Public Health*. 2017;2(8):e356–e366.

141. Soares ALG, Hammerton G, Howe LD, Rich-Edwards J, Halligan S, Fraser A. Sex differences in the association between childhood maltreatment and cardiovascular disease in the UK Biobank. *Heart*. 2020;106(17):1310–6.

142. Yazdanyar A, Newman AB. The burden of cardiovascular disease in the elderly: morbidity, mortality, and costs. *Clinical Geriatric Medicine*. 2009;25(4):563–77, vii.

143. Delgado J, Bowman K, Ble A, Masoli J, Han Y, Henley W, et al. Blood pressure trajectories in the 20 years before death. *JAMA Internal Medicine*. 2018;178(1):93–9.

144. Clegg A, Young J, Iliffe S, Rikkert MO, Rockwood K. Frailty in elderly people. *Lancet*. 2013;381(9868):752–62.

145. Rockwood K, Mitnitski A. Frailty in relation to the accumulation of deficits. *Journals of Gerontology: Series A*. 2007;62(7):722–7.

146. Fried LP, Tangen CM, Walston J, Newman AB, Hirsch C, Gottdiener J, et al. Frailty in older adults: evidence for a phenotype. *The Journals of Gerontology: Series A*. 2001;56(3):M146–M157.

147. Afilalo J. Frailty in patients with cardiovascular disease: why, when, and how to measure. *Current Cardiovascular Risk Reports*. 2011;5(5):467–72.

148. Fugate Woods N, LaCroix AZ, Gray SL, Aragaki A, Cochrane BB, Brunner RL, et al. Frailty: emergence and consequences in women aged 65 and older in the women's health initiative observational study. *Journal of the American Geriatrics Society*. 2005;53(8):1321–30.

149. Raymond E, Reynolds CA, Dahl Aslan AK, Finkel D, Ericsson M, Hägg S, et al. Drivers of frailty from adulthood into old age: results from a 27-year longitudinal population-based study in Sweden. *Journals of Gerontology: Series A*. 2020;75(10):1943–50.

6
A Life Course Approach to Diabetes

Emily Papadimos, Jedidiah Morton, Jessica Harding, and Elizabeth Barr

6.1 Introduction

Type 2 diabetes mellitus (T2DM) has reached epidemic proportions around the world, driven largely by increases in overweight and obesity, sedentary lifestyle, and unhealthy nutrition choices. The global prevalence of diabetes is reported at 10.5%[1] and is projected to rise over the next decade, particularly within regions experiencing economic development, urbanisation, and an ageing population.[2] Global age-standardised data suggest a slightly higher overall prevalence of T2DM among men than women, but this may be region-specific.[3] Sex differences in T2DM rates fluctuate across the lifespan. Females have increased rates of T2DM in youth, whereas males have a higher prevalence of T2DM in midlife.[3] This may be explained by sex differences in insulin regulation, with females demonstrating higher insulin resistance from childhood to midpuberty and males exhibiting greater insulin resistance during late puberty and adulthood.[4]

T2DM is characterised by a dysregulation in glucose and insulin homeostasis, in which insulin resistance contributes to increased hepatic glucose production and reduced glucose uptake in muscle and adipose tissue. Progression to pancreatic beta-cell failure may occur, resulting in relative insulin deficiency. The pathogenesis of T2DM is complex and incorporates genetic, epigenetic, and lifestyle factors which adversely interact with the physical and sociocultural environment.[2]

This chapter focuses on the determinants of T2DM in women and girls across the life course. Although each stage of the life course is considered separately, exposures earlier in life may have upstream consequences that amplify the probability or effects of exposures to increase risks in later life.

6.2 Genetic Determinants of Type 2 Diabetes Risk

While the environment is undoubtedly the primary driver of T2DM risk, it is clear that genetic susceptibility plays a role in the development of T2DM.[5] The relative contribution of genetic compared to environmental factors on the risk of T2DM is, however, difficult to determine because of highly variable estimates of heritability,[5] which itself is dependent on the environment in which it is measured.[6]

The genetic risk for T2DM is made up of many risk loci across the genome, the majority of which are relatively common and have small effect sizes, acting synergistically to predispose

Emily Papadimos, Jedidiah Morton, Jessica Harding, and Elizabeth Barr, *A Life Course Approach to Diabetes* In: *A Life Course Approach to Women's Health*. Second Edition. Edited by: Gita D Mishra, Rebecca Hardy, and Diana Kuh, Oxford University Press.
© Oxford University Press 2023. DOI: 10.1093/oso/9780192864642.003.0006

individuals to the disease.[7,8] Genome-wide association studies (GWAS) have uncovered hundreds of genetic variants that show significant associations with diabetes, obesity, and glucose homeostasis.[7-9] Several of these genetic variants have been functionally characterised and have confirmed and extended our understanding of the pathophysiology of T2DM. For example, one of the first loci associated with T2DM was the *TCF7L2* locus.[10] While much is still unknown about all functions of the transcription factor encoded by *TCF7L2*,[11] one of the major risk alleles at this locus is associated with impaired insulin secretion[12-14]—a pathophysiological pathway through which it and a number of other genetic variants may mediate the risk of T2DM development.[15,16] Further, GWAS have advanced our understanding of genetic influences on peripheral insulin resistance,[9] the phenomenon where peripheral tissues (primarily muscle) become resistant to the actions of insulin in promoting glucose uptake—another central mechanism of T2DM.

Understanding the genetics underpinning susceptibility to T2DM not only is important to characterise the pathophysiology and clinical phenotypes of T2DM but may also inform the development of personalised approaches to early detection and management of T2DM.

6.3 Parent-of-Origin Effects on Offspring Type 2 Diabetes Risk

Parent-of-origin effects are heritable effects that occur when the phenotype of the offspring is dependent on whether transmission of the phenotype originated from the mother or father. In the case of T2DM, it has been shown in many populations that the risk of diabetes in offspring is higher if the mother had diabetes than if the father had diabetes.[17-19]

There has recently been progress in understanding some of the biological mechanisms underpinning this phenomenon. Several mechanisms are likely to contribute, including the intrauterine environment, genomic imprinting, and mitochondrial inheritance. Indeed, several studies[20-22] have shown that the intrauterine environment is strongly associated with offspring risk for T2DM (see Section 6.4.3) but increased maternal transmission of T2DM has also been shown in offspring not exposed to a diabetic intrauterine environment,[23] indicating the contribution of other factors.

Genomic imprinting is an epigenetic phenomenon that causes the expression of genes to bias towards the allele that was inherited from a specific parent. Several genetic variants associated with the risk of T2DM have been shown to have parent-of-origin effects.[24] For example, the maternally expressed genes (i.e. the allele inherited on the maternal chromosome is expressed, while the paternal allele is suppressed) *KLF14* and *KCNQ1* have both been associated with risk for T2DM, but only when carried on the maternal chromosome.[23,25]

Another mechanism that may contribute is matrilineal inheritance of mitochondria. Mitochondria contain their own genome that is inherited from the mother. Mitochondria play an important role in both insulin secretion and insulin sensitivity, and, therefore, it is plausible to hypothesise that mitochondrial inheritance contributes to the excess maternal transmission of T2DM. Indeed, mutations in mitochondrial DNA is the underlying cause of a rare form of monogenic diabetes (maternally inherited diabetes and deafness),[26] and other mutations have been linked to the risk for T2DM.[27-30] Therefore, the matrilineal inheritance of mitochondria may explain some of the excess maternal transmission of T2DM.

6.4 The Effect of the Intrauterine Environment on Offspring Type 2 Diabetes Risk

6.4.1 Developmental Origins of Health and Disease

There is accumulating evidence to support the 'developmental origins of health and disease' hypothesis, the concept that maternal health and intrauterine exposures influence epigenetic and physiological adaptations at critical points of development, creating 'metabolic memory' and predisposing individuals to chronic disease throughout the lifespan.[31] Exposure to maternal hyperglycaemia is considered to alter fetal insulin and glucose metabolism, which may 'program' dysglycaemia later in life.[32,33]

6.4.2 Birth Size

There is evidence that birthweight is associated with the development of diabetes; however, the nature of this association is not clear.[34,35] While low birthweight has been repeatedly associated with risk of diabetes and other metabolic disease in adulthood,[34,36] the effect of macrosomia is less clear and may be mediated by hyperglycaemia in pregnancy and excess maternal weight.[37] Studies have reported either a U- or J-shaped[34] or an inverse linear[36,38,39] association between birthweight and T2DM, and some,[34,40] but not all,[35] studies report a stronger relationship among female offspring.

The association between low birthweight and T2DM in offspring may be a result of fetal maladaptation to prioritise fat stores following a period of adequate nutrition and is hypothesised to cause lifelong dysregulation in glucose and insulin metabolism.[41,42] Accelerated postnatal growth, termed 'catch up growth', is thought to contribute to insulin resistance, thus potentiating adverse metabolic health across the life course.[43] However, healthy nutrition and physical activity modifications in early life may provide an opportunity to prevent the metabolic complications of low birthweight.[44]

6.4.3 Maternal Hyperglycaemia

Diabetes in pregnancy encompasses a spectrum of hyperglycaemia, including preexisting type 1 diabetes mellitus (T1DM) or T2DM, gestational diabetes mellitus (GDM), and overt diabetes first detected in pregnancy.[45] The global prevalence of hyperglycaemia in pregnancy is estimated at 16%, of which 84% is attributed to GDM, 8% to preexisting diabetes, and 8% to overt diabetes first detected in pregnancy.[1]

Animal models demonstrate that exposure to intrauterine hyperglycaemia may have a range of effects,[46] including alterations in hypothalamic neural pathway development and leptin levels (which regulate appetite and energy expenditure),[47] as well as *fetal* islet hyperplasia and hyperinsulinism.[46] These studies showed that while physiological changes were transmitted to the third generation of offspring in female animals, male offspring with impaired glucose tolerance did not appear to transmit these changes to the next generation,[46] suggesting that the effects are specific to maternal hyperglycaemia.

Short-term intrauterine exposure to maternal hyperglycaemia is associated with an increased risk of macrosomia and neonatal adiposity, birth injury including shoulder dystocia, hypoglycaemia, and respiratory distress syndrome, among other complications.[45,48] Maternal diabetes is a key risk factor for macrosomia because of increased placental transfer of glucose and other nutrients from mother to fetus.[49] However, adequate glycaemic management is associated with a reduced rate of severe perinatal outcomes.[48]

Several studies show that maternal hyperglycaemia is associated with an increased risk of obesity during childhood and adolescence.[20,50-56] However, some meta-analyses suggest that this association may not be independent of maternal body mass index (BMI).[20,55-57] Most studies have involved women with GDM rather than women with more severe forms of hyperglycaemia in pregnancy, such as preexisting T1DM or T2DM, which have been demonstrated in some studies to be more strongly associated with offspring obesity.[20,58]

The association between GDM and offspring BMI may not manifest until after 2 years of age,[59-61] although the Hyperglycaemia and Adverse Pregnancy Outcome (HAPO) cohort[27] and another meta-analysis[62] have shown that GDM is associated with an increase in adiposity at earlier ages. The HAPO Study also showed that the association between maternal hyperglycaemia and offspring adiposity appear to continue through to 11 years of age, even after adjusting for maternal BMI.[22] Other studies show that offspring exposed to GDM have a greater likelihood of increased BMI compared to their siblings that experienced a euglycaemic pregnancy, suggesting that intrauterine exposure to diabetes is an important risk factor for increased BMI in childhood, independent of genetic and shared postnatal environmental factors.[47,63] Children exposed to preexisting T2DM are reported to have an even greater risk of developing obesity,[64] T2DM,[65,66] and premature cardiovascular disease[67] compared with children born to mothers with GDM or normoglycaemia. However, the generalisability of these studies may be limited, as most of these studies include First Nations children recruited from US and Canadian populations with high population prevalence of obesity and diabetes.[66,68,69] The excess risk associated with T2DM may be due to dysglycaemia during critical first trimester development and longer exposure to hyperglycaemia for the fetus.[56]

Exposure to maternal hyperglycaemia is associated with development of T2DM in offspring. Youth aged 10–22 years with T2DM were five times more likely to have been exposed to intrauterine GDM than normoglycaemia.[52,70,71] Few studies have examined the long-term risk of glucose intolerance or diabetes in offspring exposed to GDM; although glucose intolerance has been reported to be more than six times higher in offspring aged 20 years and exposed to GDM (versus intrauterine normoglycaemia), the quality of this evidence was impacted by loss to follow-up.[20] Even among mothers with normal glucose tolerance in pregnancy, one standard deviation increase in maternal glucose was associated with higher birthweight and a 1.3-fold greater risk of T2DM.[72] Sibling studies show an almost fourfold increase in diabetes risk and increased likelihood of greater BMI in offspring exposed to intrauterine diabetes compared to siblings born before the mother had developed T2DM.[73] Among First Nations populations in the United States, the prevalence of T2DM was 70% by age 34 years among individuals exposed to intrauterine T2DM, compared to < 15% in children born to euglycaemic mothers.[74]

The extent to which maternal hyperglycaemia is causally linked to the risk of diabetes and obesity in exposed offspring remains unclear,[57] as we are yet to determine the extent to which the effects of intrauterine hyperglycaemia operate, independently of shared genetics, environment, and maternal age. Future studies should account for maternal BMI and the environmental and health behaviours of the mother and child across the life course.

6.4.4 Maternal Adiposity

Even in the absence of GDM, some studies have shown that offspring born to overweight or obese mothers are more likely to have macrosomia[75] and develop metabolic abnormalities later in life.[76] One study showed that prepregnancy obesity was strongly associated with elevated BMI in childhood and that these associations were stronger than those associated with maternal hyperglycaemia or gestational weight gain, though findings may have been limited by a relatively small sample size and few women with GDM.[76] Findings from the SEARCH case-control study showed that maternal diabetes and maternal obesity were independently associated with youth-onset T2DM, and 47% of youth T2DM was estimated to be attributable to both these maternal exposures.[52] Paternal obesity has been associated with offspring T2DM, though the potential biological or social mechanisms and confounding through, for example, the postnatal environment need further exploration.[77] Perinatal weight management may thus be an important modifiable risk factor in the prevention of intergenerational metabolic complications.

6.5 Reproductive Hormones and Type 2 Diabetes Risk

6.5.1 Puberty

Puberty is associated with several significant physiological and metabolic changes. Even among lean healthy children, there is a marked reduction in insulin sensitivity during puberty, leading to increased insulin secretion.[78] Therefore, this dynamic period (similar to pregnancy) may increase the risk of diabetes in susceptible youth with underlying beta-cell dysfunction. In 2009, the prevalence of T2DM among American youth aged 5 to 19 years was 0.24 per 1000.[79] Females had a higher incidence of youth T2DM than males,[79] up to threefold in some populations.[80] The female predominance of youth-onset T2DM[81] has been attributed to increased rates of overweight and obesity in young girls[61] and may reflect the associations between sex steroids and the pathogenesis of youth-onset T2DM.[82] This contrasts with the slight male preponderance seen in adult-onset T2DM.[83]

6.5.2 Timing of Menarche, Menopause, and the Reproductive Period

6.5.2.1 Menarche and Menstrual Cycle
Accumulating data suggest reproductive factors including age at menarche, age of menopause, and menstrual patterns, all related to oestrogen exposure, may influence T2DM risk. Oestrogen may have favourable metabolic effects, including reduced visceral obesity, increased energy expenditure, enhanced insulin secretion and sensitivity, and improved glucose homeostasis.[84] Conversely, oestrogen deficiency adversely affects body fat distribution

and energy expenditure, predisposing an individual to metabolic syndrome and T2DM.[84,85] Interestingly, there appears to be sexually dimorphic associations between testosterone and risk of T2DM; among women, elevated testosterone levels are associated with an increased risk of T2DM, whereas elevated testosterone in men is associated with a lower T2DM risk.[85]

The relationship between age at menarche and risk of T2DM remains unclear, with previous reports suggesting an inverse[86–89] or null association.[90–92] The findings from one meta-analysis showed that early age at menarche was associated with a 22% increased risk of T2DM.[93] Girls with earlier menarche are more likely to be obese;[94] an important driver of adult-related obesity[95] and T2DM risk.[96] Whether elevated prepubertal BMI is a cause or consequence of younger age at menarche is unclear. One study showed that the inverse relationship between age at menarche and adult T2DM was attenuated after adjusting for prepubertal BMI.[87] Another analysis of individual-level pooled data on over 100,000 women showed that adult BMI may be an important effect modifier. Whilst this analysis showed a modest association between earlier age of menarche after adjusting for BMI and other covariates, the association was stronger for women with an adult BMI of ≥25 kg/m^2.[89] Of the Mendelian randomisation studies that aimed to identify causal risk factors for T2DM and cardiometabolic traits; one study reported that age at menarche was inversely associated with T2DM and cardiometabolic disease in adulthood;[97] however, another study reported that an inverse association between age at menarche and T2DM risk was largely attenuated once variants related to either childhood or adult BMI were excluded, indicating that childhood adiposity, rather than pubertal timing itself, may be a stronger risk factor for development of T2DM.[98] Future studies should account for prepubertal BMI[93] and other factors associated with earlier menarche, such as more advantaged socioeconomic position[99,100] and improved nutrition.[99]

In some studies, women who reported irregular or long menstrual cycle length (greater than 40 days) were at increased risk of T2DM compared to women with regular cycles.[91,101–103] These associations were stronger in overweight or obese women,[102] highlighting that weight management may be an important modifiable factor in women with menstrual cycle dysfunction. Clearly, more work is needed to determine the mechanisms by which earlier menarche and atypical menstrual cycle increases the risk of T2DM.

6.5.2.2 Reproductive Duration
One study has shown that in age-adjusted models, women with the shortest (< 30 years) and longest (>45 years) reproductive duration were at greater risk of developing T2DM compared to women with medium-length reproductive durations (36–40 years), with 37% and 23% increased risk, respectively.[103] These associations were partially attenuated when accounting for covariates including baseline BMI, physical activity, and family history of diabetes.[103] However, another study reported no association between reproductive life span and risk of T2DM.[104]

6.5.2.3 Polycystic Ovarian Syndrome
Polycystic ovarian syndrome (PCOS) is characterised by insulin resistance and is associated with reproductive and cardiometabolic disorders, including obesity, central adiposity, and hyperandrogenaemia including elevated free testosterone. A meta-analysis of observational studies showed that women with PCOS have an increased prevalence of impaired glucose tolerance (2.5-times greater) or T2DM (4-times greater) compared to women without PCOS,[105]

but several of the component studies of this meta-analysis were of poorer methodological quality, design, and sample size, and thus there was insufficient evidence to fully examine the role of adiposity in these associations. Mendelian randomisation analysis involving an Asian and European cohort has shown that genetically predicted PCOS was not associated with T2DM, and the authors postulated that the defining attributes of PCOS rather than PCOS per se may play a more important role in the risk of T2DM.[106] Findings from another Mendelian randomisation study support this theory, showing that genetic determinants of higher free testosterone levels were associated with T2DM in women, despite having a protective effect in men.[107] Therefore, while PCOS itself may not directly increase the risk of T2DM, underlying cardiometabolic and reproductive factors, which are often a hallmark of adiposity, may be associated with the development of T2DM in women.[108,109]

6.5.2.4 Menopause

The relationship between menopause and risk of T2DM is somewhat difficult to separate from the effects of ageing alone because women tend to gain weight with age, and the risk for T2DM increases with age.[110] Nevertheless, menopause is associated with changes in body composition (independent of age) including increased visceral fat mass and a reduction in lean body mass,[103,111,112] which are in turn associated with T2DM risk.[113] Women experiencing earlier menopause may be at greater risk of T2DM relative to women experiencing menopause at an older age.[114] However, this association may be at least in part explained by unhealthy lifestyle behaviours, such as smoking and alcohol consumption, which are also associated with an increased likelihood of an earlier onset of menopause.[115,116] Of note, evidence from a meta-analysis of over 100 clinical trials has shown that menopausal hormone therapy, the most common and effective treatment for the symptoms of menopause, is associated with an attenuation of menopausal-related metabolic changes, including a reduction in abdominal fat, HOMA-IR, and a decrease in the risk of T2DM.[117]

Collectively, current evidence suggests that diminishing circulation of reproductive hormones brought about by menopause may be associated with an increased risk for T2DM.[118] Indeed, surgical menopause via a bilateral oophorectomy is associated with adverse effects on glucose and insulin homeostasis,[119] as well as an increased risk of T2DM.[89] However, further studies are required to understand the mechanisms underlying the association between menopause and risk for T2DM, and whether the association between endogenous sex hormones and risk of diabetes operate independently of adiposity.

6.5.3 Hormonal Contraceptive Use and Incidence of T2DM

Worldwide, the use of hormonal contraceptives in women has increased. Hormonal contraceptives are made up of female sex hormones, oestrogen, and progestin (a synthetic form of progesterone), with the most common form being the combined oral contraceptive (COC) pill, though the use of implants and intrauterine devices is increasing.[120] Hormonal contraceptive use has been associated with a two- to sixfold increased risk for venous thrombosis;[121] however, the association with T2DM is less clear.

Observational studies conducted in healthy women have shown that hormonal contraceptives are associated with small changes in carbohydrate metabolism, including decreased glucose tolerance and increased insulin resistance, which are key risk factors for

T2DM.[122,123] The clinical relevance of these findings, however, remains unclear, and most associations have been observed in contraceptives containing oestrogen.[124] Although newer progestins have since been developed, which may have different effects on carbohydrate metabolism, their association with T2DM development is less established. In a 2018 meta-analysis,[125] only 2 of 19 studies reported on progestin-only contraceptive (POC) use and risk of developing T2DM. A case-control study among US Navajo women reported that the odds of T2DM was greater among women who had any history of POC use compared to those who used the COC (3.6 times greater) or no hormonal contraceptive (2.1 times greater), even after adjustment for age and obesity.[126] However, this association was attenuated to the null when further adjustment for GDM history was made.[126] Observational studies of other COCs have similarly shown inconsistent results. For example, a 2020 Finnish study showed that COCs, but not POCs, were significantly associated with T2DM compared to nonhormonal contraceptives,[127] while evidence from the Coronary Artery Risk Development in Young Adults (CARDIA) study found current oral contraceptive pill use was associated with lower mean glucose levels and consequently a lower risk of T2DM.[128] These conflicting results likely arose because of variability in contraceptive type, dose, study populations, and study design, making comparisons difficult. Further, data from observational studies are inherently limited by residual confounding, and thus randomised controlled trials are needed to provide more conclusive evidence of the association between hormonal contraceptive use and T2DM risk.

A 2014 Cochrane review including data from 31 trials reported no major differences in carbohydrate metabolism between different hormonal contraceptives in women without T2DM,[124] though whether this is true in women at high risk for T2DM remains unknown. Further, no trial has compared the hormone contraceptives to a placebo regime—which is not unusual because of ethical concerns—making the task of elucidating true T2DM risk associated with hormonal contraceptive use difficult.

6.6 Gestational Diabetes, Parity, Breastfeeding, and Maternal T2DM Risk

Recent systematic reviews and meta-analyses report that progression to T2DM is almost 10 times higher in women with a history of GDM compared to women who had normoglycaemia during pregnancy,[129] and pooled incidence after GDM is reported to be 26.20 per 1000 person-years.[130] However, both reviews report substantial heterogeneity in postpartum diabetes risk owing to ethnic variation (risk of T2DM being higher in women from non-Europid than Europid populations) and varied uptake of postpartum screening between populations.[129,130]

There is conflicting evidence on the nature of the relationship between parity and maternal T2DM risk. One meta-analysis suggests that a linear dose-response association between increasing parity and higher risk of T2DM.[131] In contrast, another meta-analysis reported a nonlinear dose-response association between increasing parity and risk of T2DM.[132] Several studies have shown that associations between multiparity and risk of diabetes remain, even after adjustment for age, demographics, BMI, lifestyle behaviours and family history of T2DM.[103,133–135] One study showed that mothers with grand multiparity (five or more live births) had a 27% increased risk of developing T2DM compared to mothers having one or two live births.[136] However, a more recent prospective study found that the association between greater parity and risk of T2DM was likely confounded by weight gain,[137] as women who gain excess weight during pregnancy are almost 1.5 times more likely to have diabetes compared to women who gain adequate weight.[138] Interestingly, another study points to the potential confounding factors associated with parenthood rather than female biological mechanisms associated with having children, as this study showed similar associations between number of children and risk of diabetes for men and women.[139] Even in women without diabetes, greater parity has been positively associated with HbA1c levels.[134] Other studies[140] and a large participant-level meta-analysis,[89] however, have shown evidence of a J-shaped association between parity and T2DM risk, with nulliparity and multiparity (≥4 children) being associated with increased diabetes risk, potentially linked to infertility issues, including PCOS, ovulation disorders, and tubal factors.

Physiologic changes that occur during pregnancy may also contribute to the association between parity and T2DM risk. Elevated pregnancy hormones (oestrogen, progesterone, corticosteroids, insulin-like growth factor-1, and human placental lactogen), cytokines, and other mediators[141] can interfere with glucose and insulin metabolism, resulting in peripheral insulin resistance.[104,133] Moreover, in response to progressive insulin resistance and increased insulin secretion during pregnancy, pancreatic beta-cell mass expands to maintain glucose homeostasis, and there are limited studies assessing whether these physiological changes fully reverse following pregnancy.[133]

Growing evidence supports that both breastfeeding[104,142] and increased lifetime breastfeeding duration,[143] including breastfeeding three or more children,[137] is associated with reduced risk of T2DM in the mother, though it is possible that this association is confounded or mediated by weight gain.[144] Increased support for breastfeeding may, therefore, be an important lifestyle factor in addition to maintaining a healthy weight in the prevention of T2DM.

Future studies should include extensive assessment of demographics (including maternal age and socioeconomic status) and physiological and lifestyle changes during pregnancy and the postpartum period to explore which factors mediate the association of parity and development of T2DM.

6.7 Lifestyle Determinants of Type 2 Diabetes

6.7.1 Physical Activity and Sedentary Behaviour

Many studies have investigated the association between physical activity and risk of T2DM, with the large majority of studies reporting an inverse association between the two. However, the amount and type of physical activity needed to reduce the risk of T2DM have been more difficult to ascertain. A 2015 meta-analysis including 81 studies reported that, in general, all subtypes of physical activity appear to be beneficial when comparing high versus low activity, including total physical activity, leisure-time activity, vigorous activity, moderate activity, low-intensity activity, and walking.[145] Further, increasing activity over time, resistance exercise, occupational activity, and cardiorespiratory fitness were also associated with decreased T2DM risk.[145] This meta-analysis also reported that increasing reductions in diabetes risk were observed with up to 5–7 hours of leisure-time, vigorous or low-intensity physical

activity per week, but insufficient evidence was available to determine whether further reductions in T2DM risk could be achieved beyond this range.[145]

A growing body of evidence also points to the effects of sedentary behaviour on T2DM
risk that are independent of physical activity. In a meta-analysis including four studies, a
weak linear association was observed between total sedentary time (in hours) and T2DM risk
after adjustment for physical activity.[146] The association between television viewing time and
T2DM risk appeared to be stronger with a 9% increased risk per hour of viewing time, and
29% of all T2DM incidence cases were estimated to be attributable to television viewing.[146]

6.7.2 Nutrition

In the past few decades, many systematic reviews and meta-analyses have summarised evidence on the associations between dietary behaviours or diet quality indices, food groups,
single foods and beverages, specific macronutrients and micronutrients, and the incidence
of T2DM. To date, strong evidence suggests that higher consumption of whole grains,[147,148]
adherence to a healthy dietary pattern,[147] and exposure to breastfeeding[149] are associated
with a decreased incidence of T2DM. In contrast, a higher intake of red meat,[148] processed
meat,[147,148] and sugar-sweetened beverages[147,148] is associated with an increased incidence
of T2DM.

6.7.3 Smoking and Alcohol

Smoking is an established risk factor for diabetes. Early findings from the Health Professionals
Follow-up Study found that men who smoked 25 or more cigarettes daily were 94% more
likely to develop diabetes compared with nonsmokers.[150] Later studies among women
showed that the strength of the association was slightly lower. In the Nurses' Health Study,
women who smoked 25 or more cigarettes per day were 37% more likely to develop diabetes compared to never smokers.[151] Passive smoke inhalation has also been associated with
a ~30% increased risk for T2DM.[152]

Studies examining the relationship between alcohol consumption and T2DM risk in
women vary widely with some reporting a positive association, a null association, or a U-
shaped or J-shaped relationship.[153] A growing body of evidence suggests that light-to-
moderate alcohol intake may decrease T2DM risk, while high alcohol intake increases T2DM
risk.[153] In the Nurses' Health Study II, those consuming less than 29.9 grams/day of alcohol
(up to almost three cans of beer or three glasses of wine per day) were 20%–58% less likely to
develop diabetes compared to lifelong abstainers, after adjusting for several factors including
dietary intake. However, women consuming 30.0 grams/day or more of liquor (three or more
cans of beer or glasses of wine) showed a 2.5-fold increased risk for developing diabetes
compared to lifelong abstainers.[154] In contrast, the Atherosclerosis Risk in Communities
Study demonstrated no association between alcohol and T2DM risk in middle-aged women
(though high versus low alcohol intake was associated with a 50% increased risk for diabetes in men),[155] and in the National Longitudinal Study of Adolescent Health, frequent alcohol consumption (≥5 drinks, 3–7 days/week) substantially increased T2DM risk by more
than 12 fold in young adults compared to abstainers, though sex-specific results were not

presented.[156] The type of alcohol associated with T2DM risk is not clear, though some evidence suggests that moderate wine consumption, rather than beer and spirits, is associated with T2DM risk reduction;[157,158] however, underlying mechanisms remain unknown.

6.7.4 Stress

The association between stress and T2DM is less clear than other risk factors described in this section owing to the potential bidirectional nature of the relationship, differences in study designs, and forms of ascertainment of stress. To date, most of the work on stress and incident T2DM has concentrated on work-related stress, and the results have been mixed, with the direction of the association dependent on gender, length of follow-up, diabetes ascertainment method, and stress measurement instrument.[159] A meta-analysis of nine studies found no overall association between work-related stress and diabetes,[159] but noted that in the Whitehall II study,[160] women exposed to a combination of job strain and low social support were twice as likely to develop diabetes. Other studies have focused on the relationship between general psychological stress and incident T2DM. A 2016 review included six prospective longitudinal studies (range 10–35 years follow-up) examining the effect between general chronic psychological stress and T2DM risk.[161] Overall, two of six studies found a positive association in women only; three of six in men but not women (one of which was a cohort of only men); and one of six found a positive association in both women and men who had prediabetes.[161] One UK study demonstrated a hazard ratio of 1.33 for incident diabetes after adjustment for age, sex, education, and household income, though this association was attenuated after adjustment for additional confounders.[161] Collectively, these studies support a positive association between chronic psychological stress and incident T2DM, but the link is difficult to assess owing to the aforementioned differences in study design and methods.

6.8 Socioeconomic Position on Type 2 Diabetes Risk

Socioeconomic position is a strong risk factor for T2DM in many countries. In HICs, as well as some LMICs, more disadvantaged socioeconomic position (usually measured by individual or area-level income or educational attainment) is associated with an increased risk of diabetes.[162,163] Further, poorer treatment and outcomes have also been associated with more disadvantaged socioeconomic position among women with diabetes.[164,165]

There are several reasons for the observed associations between socioeconomic position and diabetes risk. Differences in socioeconomic position parallel inequities in the physical environment women are exposed to, as well as working conditions, which in turn impact behavioural and biological outcomes. Accordingly, socioeconomic position and risk for diabetes have been associated with exposure to pollutants and chemicals,[166–170] neighbourhood walkability and green space,[171,172] housing conditions,[173] food access and insecurity,[174–176] and unemployment, insecure work, and shift work.[177–179] Moreover, trials have shown that when aspects of underlying socioeconomic disadvantage (e.g. residing in a neighbourhood with high levels of poverty) are addressed, the risk of T2DM is reduced.[180] Nevertheless, large-scale approaches to tackle diabetes that address underlying socioeconomic inequalities are rarely undertaken, and as income inequality continues to increase in most HICs,[181] these socioeconomic disparities in T2DM risk have increased over time.[182]

Conversely, in many LMICs, diabetes risk is often highest in those with the most advantaged socioeconomic status.[183] In these countries, recent shifts in dietary and physical activity habits towards calorie-dense diets and sedentary lifestyles, initially amongst the most advantaged, are likely important contributing factors to this phenomenon. It might be anticipated that as these countries continue to develop economically, patterns of disease risk will resemble HICs in terms of the socioeconomic gradient for T2DM.[184]

It is worth noting that the effect of socioeconomic status on the risk of disease can often be different for men and women.[185] For example, one study showed that the gradient of risk for the metabolic syndrome by household wealth was steeper in women than men.[186] However, these differences are difficult to generalise, as various countries and regions have distinct social policies and cultural norms that will exacerbate differences between men and women to a greater or lesser degree. Moreover, because traditional gender roles still frequently limit women's access to education and employment, traditional markers of socioeconomic status, such as income and education, may be less appropriate for measuring socioeconomic status in women.

6.9 Conclusion

The burden of diabetes has reached epidemic proportions. There is an excess maternal transmission of diabetes that may be partly attributable to genetic factors, such as mitochondrial inheritance and genomic imprinting, as well as effects from the intrauterine environment. Indeed, the intrauterine environment is an important determinant of adult risk of T2DM, both through fetal undernutrition and intrauterine exposure to maternal diabetes. Additionally, overnutrition, sedentary lifestyles, smoking, alcohol consumption, and increasing rates of diabetes in pregnancy contribute to diabetes risk. Other reproductive factors, such as earlier onset of menarche and menopause, menstrual cycle factors, and GDM may also contribute to risk of T2DM later in life. Therefore, measures to modify lifestyle behaviours, in mothers and children alike, throughout the life course, may be helpful to combat the ongoing rise in T2DM prevalence.

Key messages and implications

- There is increasing evidence to support the intergenerational impact of diabetes during pregnancy on offspring cardiometabolic health and diabetes risk, which may be partly mediated by the intrauterine environment, genomic imprinting, and mitochondrial inheritance.
- There are critical physiological stages in a woman's life that may precipitate, or increase her risk of, diabetes. These stages include during puberty, pregnancy, and menopause, and are crucial time points in which healthy lifestyle behaviours should be encouraged.
- Lifestyle factors that occur across the life course, including reduced physical activity, sedentary behaviour, smoking, alcohol consumption, and stress are also associated with an increased risk of developing diabetes.

> • A woman's risk of diabetes is also influenced by various sociodemographic factors, including the physical environment she is exposed to, her occupation and income, and her food environment.

References

1. International Diabetes Federation. *IDF diabetes atlas, 10th edition.* Brussels: International Diabetes Federation; 2021.
2. Zheng Y, Ley SH, Hu FB. Global aetiology and epidemiology of type 2 diabetes mellitus and its complications. *Nature Reviews Endocrinology.* 2018;14(2):88–98.
3. Huebschmann AG, Huxley RR, Kohrt WM, Zeitler P, Regensteiner JG, Reusch JEB. Sex differences in the burden of type 2 diabetes and cardiovascular risk across the life course. *Diabetologia.* 2019;62(10):1761–72.
4. Sattar N. Gender aspects in type 2 diabetes mellitus and cardiometabolic risk. *Best Practice & Research Clinical Endocrinology & Metabolism.* 2013;27(4):501–7.
5. Willemsen G, Ward KJ, Bell CG, Christensen K, Bowden J, Dalgård C, et al. The concordance and heritability of type 2 diabetes in 34,166 twin pairs from international twin registers: the Discordant Twin (DISCOTWIN) Consortium. *Twin Research and Human Genetics.* 2015;18(6):762–71.
6. Visscher PM, Hill WG, Wray NR. Heritability in the genomics era—concepts and misconceptions. *Nature Reviews Genetics.* 2008;9(4):255–66.
7. Fuchsberger C, Flannick J, Teslovich TM, Mahajan A, Agarwala V, Gaulton KJ, et al. The genetic architecture of type 2 diabetes. *Nature.* 2016;536(7614):41–7.
8. Mahajan A, Taliun D, Thurner M, Robertson NR, Torres JM, Rayner NW, et al. Fine-mapping type 2 diabetes loci to single-variant resolution using high-density imputation and islet-specific epigenome maps. *Nature Genetics.* 2018;50(11):1505–13.
9. Lotta LA, Gulati P, Day FR, Payne F, Ongen H, van de Bunt M, et al. Integrative genomic analysis implicates limited peripheral adipose storage capacity in the pathogenesis of human insulin resistance. *Nature Genetics.* 2017;49(1):17–26.
10. Grant SFA, Thorleifsson G, Reynisdottir I, Benediktsson R, Manolescu A, Sainz J, et al. Variant of transcription factor 7-like 2 (TCF7L2) gene confers risk of type 2 diabetes. *Nature Genetics.* 2006;38(3):320–3.
11. Grant SFA. The *TCF7L2* Locus: a genetic window into the pathogenesis of type 1 and type 2 diabetes. *Diabetes Care.* 2019;42(9):1624.
12. Lyssenko V, Lupi R, Marchetti P, Del Guerra S, Orho-Melander M, Almgren P, et al. Mechanisms by which common variants in the TCF7L2 gene increase risk of type 2 diabetes. *Journal of Clinical Investigation.* 2007;117(8):2155–63.
13. Saxena R, Gianniny L, Burtt NP, Lyssenko V, Giuducci C, Sjögren M, et al. Common single nucleotide polymorphisms in TCF7L2 are reproducibly associated with type 2 diabetes and reduce the insulin response to glucose in nondiabetic individuals. *Diabetes.* 2006;55(10):2890–5.
14. Zhou Y, Park S-Y, Su J, Bailey K, Ottosson-Laakso E, Shcherbina L, et al. TCF7L2 is a master regulator of insulin production and processing. *Human Molecular Genetics.* 2014;23(24):6419–31.
15. Dimas AS, Lagou V, Barker A, Knowles JW, Mägi R, Hivert M-F, et al. Impact of type 2 diabetes susceptibility variants on quantitative glycemic traits reveals mechanistic heterogeneity. *Diabetes.* 2014;63(6):2158.
16. Mahajan A, Wessel J, Willems SM, Zhao W, Robertson NR, Chu AY, et al. Refining the accuracy of validated target identification through coding variant fine-mapping in type 2 diabetes. *Nature Genetics.* 2018;50(4):559–71.
17. Bener A, Yousafzai MT, Al-Hamaq AO, Mohammad A-G, Defronzo RA. Parental transmission of type 2 diabetes mellitus in a highly endogamous population. *World Journal of Diabetes.* 2013;4(2):40–6.

18. Arfa I, Abid A, Malouche D, Ben Alaya N, Azegue TR, Mannai I, et al. Familial aggregation and excess maternal transmission of type 2 diabetes in Tunisia. *Postgraduate Medical Journal.* 2007;83(979):348–51.

19. Alcolado JC, Laji K, Gill-Randall R. Maternal transmission of diabetes. *Diabetic Medicine.* 2002;19(2):89–98.

20. Kawasaki M, Arata N, Miyazaki C, Mori R, Kikuchi T, Ogawa Y, et al. Obesity and abnormal glucose tolerance in offspring of diabetic mothers: a systematic review and meta-analysis. *PLoS ONE.* 2018;13(1):e0190676.

21. The HAPO Study Cooperative Research Group. Hyperglycemia and adverse pregnancy outcome (HAPO) study: associations with neonatal anthropometrics. *Diabetes.* 2009;58(2):453–9.

22. Lowe WL, Jr., Lowe LP, Kuang A, Catalano PM, Nodzenski M, Talbot O, et al. Maternal glucose levels during pregnancy and childhood adiposity in the hyperglycemia and adverse pregnancy outcome follow-up study. *Diabetologia.* 2019;62(4):598–610.

23. Hanson RL, Guo T, Muller YL, Fleming J, Knowler WC, Kobes S, et al. Strong parent-of-origin effects in the association of KCNQ1 variants with type 2 diabetes in American Indians. *Diabetes.* 2013;62(8):2984–91.

24. Lyssenko V, Groop L, Prasad RB. Genetics of type 2 diabetes: it matters from which parent we inherit the risk. *Review of Diabetic Studies.* 2015;12(3-4):233–42.

25. Kong A, Steinthorsdottir V, Masson G, Thorleifsson G, Sulem P, Besenbacher S, et al. Parental origin of sequence variants associated with complex diseases. *Nature.* 2009;462(7275):868–74.

26. Murphy R, Turnbull DM, Walker M, Hattersley AT. Clinical features, diagnosis and management of maternally inherited diabetes and deafness (MIDD) associated with the 3243A>G mitochondrial point mutation. *Diabetic Medicine.* 2008;25(4):383–99.

27. Jiang W, Li R, Zhang Y, Wang P, Wu T, Lin J, et al. Mitochondrial DNA mutations associated with type 2 diabetes mellitus in Chinese Uyghur population. *Scientific Reports.* 2017;7(1):16989.

28. Liou C-W, Chen J-B, Tiao M-M, Weng S-W, Huang T-L, Chuang J-H, et al. Mitochondrial DNA coding and control region variants as genetic risk factors for type 2 diabetes. *Diabetes.* 2012;61(10):2642.

29. Poulton J, Luan JA, Macaulay V, Hennings S, Mitchell J, Wareham NJ. Type 2 diabetes is associated with a common mitochondrial variant: evidence from a population-based case–control study. *Human Molecular Genetics.* 2002;11(13):1581–3.

30. Park KS, Chan JC, Chuang LM, Suzuki S, Araki E, Nanjo K, et al. A mitochondrial DNA variant at position 16189 is associated with type 2 diabetes mellitus in Asians. *Diabetologia.* 2008;51(4):602–8.

31. Fleming TP, Watkins AJ, Velazquez MA, Mathers JC, Prentice AM, Stephenson J, et al. Origins of lifetime health around the time of conception: causes and consequences. *Lancet.* 2018;391(10132):1842–52.

32. McIntyre HD, Catalano P, Zhang C, Desoye G, Mathiesen ER, Damm P. Gestational diabetes mellitus. *Nature Reviews Disease Primers.* 2019;5(1):47.

33. Armengaud JB, Ma RCW, Siddeek B, Visser GHA, Simeoni U. Offspring of mothers with hyperglycaemia in pregnancy: the short term and long-term impact. What is new? *Diabetes Research and Clinical Practice.* 2018;145:155–66.

34. Knop MR, Geng T-T, Gorny AW, Ding R, Li C, Ley SH, et al. Birth weight and risk of type 2 diabetes mellitus, cardiovascular disease, and hypertension in adults: a meta-analysis of 7 646 267 participants from 135 studies. *Journal of the American Heart Association.* 2018;7(23):e008870.

35. Zhao H, Song A, Zhang Y, Zhen Y, Song G, Ma H. The association between birth weight and the risk of type 2 diabetes mellitus: a systematic review and meta-analysis. *Endocrine Journal.* 2018;65(9):923–33.

36. Mi D, Fang H, Zhao Y, Zhong L. Birth weight and type 2 diabetes: a meta-analysis. *Experimental and Therapeutic Medicine.* 2017;14(6):5313–20.

37. Catalano PM. The impact of gestational diabetes and maternal obesity on the mother and her offspring. *Journal of Developmental Origins of Health and Disease.* 2010;1(4):208–15.

38. Birth-Gene Study Working Group. Association of birth weight with type 2 diabetes and glycemic traits: a Mendelian randomization study. *JAMA Network Open.* 2019;2:e1910915.

39. Wang T, Huang T, Li Y, Zheng Y, Manson JE, Hu FB, et al. Low birthweight and risk of type 2 diabetes: a Mendelian randomisation study. *Diabetologia*. 2016;59(9):1920–7.
40. Zimmermann E, Gamborg M, Sørensen TI, Baker JL. Sex differences in the association between birth weight and adult type 2 diabetes. *Diabetes*. 2015;64(12):4220–5.
41. Godfrey KM, Barker DJ. Fetal nutrition and adult disease. *American Journal of Clinical Nutrition*. 2000;71(5 Suppl):1344s–52s.
42. Ross MG, Beall MH. Adult sequelae of intrauterine growth restriction. *Seminars in Perinatology*. 2008;32(3):213–8.
43. Eriksson JG, Forsen T, Tuomilehto J, Osmond C, Barker DJ. Early adiposity rebound in childhood and risk of Type 2 diabetes in adult life. *Diabetologia*. 2003;46(2):190–4.
44. Sauder KA, Bekelman TA, Harrall KK, Glueck DH, Dabelea D. Gestational diabetes exposure and adiposity outcomes in childhood and adolescence: an analysis of effect modification by breastfeeding, diet quality, and physical activity in the EPOCH study. *Pediatric Obesity*. 2019;14(12):e12562.
45. International Association of Diabetes and Pregnancy Study Groups Consensus Panel. International Association of Diabetes and Pregnancy study groups recommendations on the diagnosis and classification of hyperglycemia in pregnancy. *Diabetes Care*. 2010;33(3):676.
46. Fetita L-S, Sobngwi En, Serradas P, Calvo F, Gautier J-FO. Consequences of fetal exposure to maternal diabetes in offspring. *Journal of Clinical Endocrinology & Metabolism*. 2006;91(10):3718–24.
47. Chu AHY, Godfrey KM. Gestational diabetes mellitus and developmental programming. *Annals of Nutrition and Metabolism*. 2020;76(3):4–15.
48. Farahvar S, Walfisch A, Sheiner E. Gestational diabetes risk factors and long-term consequences for both mother and offspring: a literature review. *Expert Review of Endocrinology & Metabolism*. 2019;14(1):63–74.
49. Kamana K, Shakya S, Zhang H. Gestational diabetes mellitus and macrosomia: a literature review. *Annals of Nutrition and Metabolism*. 2015;66(Suppl 2):14–20.
50. Deierlein AL, Siega-Riz AM, Chantala K, Herring AH. The association between maternal glucose concentration and child BMI at age 3 years. *Diabetes Care*. 2011;34(2):480–4.
51. Hillier TA, Pedula KL, Schmidt MM, Mullen JA, Charles MA, Pettitt DJ. Childhood obesity and metabolic imprinting: the ongoing effects of maternal hyperglycemia. *Diabetes Care*. 2007;30(9):2287–92.
52. Dabelea D, Mayer-Davis EJ, Lamichhane AP, D'Agostino RB, Jr., Liese AD, Vehik KS, et al. Association of intrauterine exposure to maternal diabetes and obesity with type 2 diabetes in youth: the SEARCH case-control study. *Diabetes Care*. 2008;31(7):1422–6.
53. Krishnaveni GV, Veena SR, Hill JC, Kehoe S, Karat SC, Fall CHD. Intrauterine exposure to maternal diabetes is associated with higher adiposity and insulin resistance and clustering of cardiovascular risk markers in Indian children. *Diabetes Care*. 2010;33(2):402–4.
54. Silverman BL, Rizzo T, Green OC, Cho NH, Winter RJ, Ogata ES, et al. Long-term prospective evaluation of offspring of diabetic mothers. *Diabetes*. 1991;40(Suppl 2):21–5.
55. Patro Golab B, Santos S, Voerman E, Lawlor DA, Jaddoe VWV, Gaillard R. Influence of maternal obesity on the association between common pregnancy complications and risk of childhood obesity: an individual participant data meta-analysis. *Lancet Child & Adolescent Health*. 2018;2(11):812–21.
56. Kim SY, England JL, Sharma JA, Njoroge T. Gestational diabetes mellitus and risk of childhood overweight and obesity in offspring: a systematic review. *Experimental Diabetes Research*. 2011;2011:541308.
57. Philipps LH, Santhakumaran S, Gale C, Prior E, Logan KM, Hyde MJ, et al. The diabetic pregnancy and offspring BMI in childhood: a systematic review and meta-analysis. *Diabetologia*. 2011;54(8):1957–66.
58. Longmore DK, Barr ELM, Lee IL, Barzi F, Kirkwood M, Whitbread C, et al. Maternal body mass index, excess gestational weight gain, and diabetes are positively associated with neonatal adiposity in the pregnancy and neonatal diabetes outcomes in remote Australia (PANDORA) study. *Pediatric Obesity*. 2019;14(4):e12490.

59. Silverman BL, Rizzo TA, Cho NH, Metzger BE. Long-term effects of the intrauterine environment: the Northwestern University Diabetes in Pregnancy Center. *Diabetes Care.* 1998;21(Suppl 2):B142–B149.

60. Crume TL, Ogden L, Daniels S, Hamman RF, Norris JM, Dabelea D. The impact of in utero exposure to diabetes on childhood body mass index growth trajectories: the EPOCH study. *Journal of Pediatrics.* 2011;158(6):941–6.

61. Zhu Y, Olsen SF, Mendola P, Yeung EH, Vaag A, Bowers K, et al. Growth and obesity through the first 7 y of life in association with levels of maternal glycemia during pregnancy: a prospective cohort study. *American Journal of Clinical Nutrition.* 2016;103(3):794–800.

62. Manerkar K, Harding J, Conlon C, McKinlay C. Maternal gestational diabetes and infant feeding, nutrition and growth: a systematic review and meta-analysis. *British Journal of Nutrition.* 2020;123(11):1201–15.

63. Lawlor DA, Lichtenstein P, Långström N. Association of maternal diabetes mellitus in pregnancy with offspring adiposity into early adulthood: sibling study in a prospective cohort of 280,866 men from 248,293 families. *Circulation.* 2011;123(3):258–65.

64. Hunter WA, Cundy T, Rabone D, Hofman PL, Harris M, Regan F, et al. Insulin sensitivity in the offspring of women with type 1 and type 2 diabetes. *Diabetes Care.* 2004;27(5):1148–52.

65. Meigs JB, Cupples LA, Wilson PW. Parental transmission of type 2 diabetes: the Framingham offspring study. *Diabetes.* 2000;49(12):2201–7.

66. Dabelea D, Knowler WC, Pettitt DJ. Effect of diabetes in pregnancy on offspring: follow-up research in the Pima Indians. *Journal of Maternal-Fetal & Neonatal Medicine.* 2000;9(1):83–8.

67. Yu Y, Arah OA, Liew Z, Cnattingius S, Olsen J, Sorensen HT, et al. Maternal diabetes during pregnancy and early onset of cardiovascular disease in offspring: population based cohort study with 40 years of follow-up. *BMJ (Clinical research ed).* 2019;367:l6398.

68. Bunt JC, Tataranni PA, Salbe AD. Intrauterine exposure to diabetes is a determinant of hemoglobin A(1)c and systolic blood pressure in Pima Indian children. *Journal of Clinical Endocrinology & Metabolism.* 2005;90(6):3225–9.

69. Mendelson M, Cloutier J, Spence L, Sellers E, Taback S, Dean H. Obesity and type 2 diabetes mellitus in a birth cohort of First Nation children born to mothers with pediatric-onset type 2 diabetes. *Pediatr Diabetes.* 2011;12(3 Pt 2):219–28.

70. Holder T, Giannini C, Santoro N, Pierpont B, Shaw M, Duran E, et al. A low disposition index in adolescent offspring of mothers with gestational diabetes: a risk marker for the development of impaired glucose tolerance in youth. *Diabetologia.* 2014;57(11):2413–20.

71. Clausen TD, Mathiesen ER, Hansen T, Pedersen O, Jensen DM, Lauenborg J, et al. High prevalence of type 2 diabetes and pre-diabetes in adult offspring of women with gestational diabetes mellitus or type 1 diabetes: the role of intrauterine hyperglycemia. *Diabetes Care.* 2008;31(2):340–6.

72. Franks PW, Looker HC, Kobes S, Touger L, Tataranni PA, Hanson RL, et al. Gestational glucose tolerance and risk of type 2 diabetes in young Pima Indian offspring. *Diabetes.* 2006;55(2):460–5.

73. Dabelea D, Hanson RL, Lindsay RS, Pettitt DJ, Imperatore G, Gabir MM, et al. Intrauterine exposure to diabetes conveys risks for type 2 diabetes and obesity: a study of discordant sibships. *Diabetes.* 2000;49(12):2208–11.

74. Pettitt DJ, Aleck KA, Baird HR, Carraher MJ, Bennett PH, Knowler WC. Congenital susceptibility to NIDDM. Role of intrauterine environment. *Diabetes.* 1988;37(5):622–8.

75. Catalano PM, Ehrenberg HM. The short- and long-term implications of maternal obesity on the mother and her offspring. *BJOG.* 2006;113(10):1126–33.

76. Catalano PM, Farrell K, Thomas A, Huston-Presley L, Mencin P, de Mouzon SH, et al. Perinatal risk factors for childhood obesity and metabolic dysregulation. *American Journal of Clinical Nutrition.* 2009;90(5):1303–13.

77. Sharp GC, Lawlor DA. Paternal impact on the life course development of obesity and type 2 diabetes in the offspring. *Diabetologia.* 2019;62(10):1802–10.

78. Hannon TS, Janosky J, Arslanian SA. Longitudinal study of physiologic insulin resistance and metabolic changes of puberty. *Pediatric Research.* 2006;60(6):759–63.

79. Pettitt DJ, Talton J, Dabelea D, Divers J, Imperatore G, Lawrence JM, et al. Prevalence of diabetes in U.S. youth in 2009: the SEARCH for diabetes in youth study. *Diabetes Care.* 2014;37(2):402–8.

80. Amed S, Islam N, Sutherland J, Reimer K. Incidence and prevalence trends of youth-onset type 2 diabetes in a cohort of Canadian youth: 2002–2013. *Pediatric Diabetes*. 2018;19(4):630–6.

81. Mayer-Davis EJ, Lawrence JM, Dabelea D, Divers J, Isom S, Dolan L, et al. Incidence trends of type 1 and type 2 diabetes among youths, 2002–2012. *New England Journal of Medicine*. 2017;376(15):1419–29.

82. Copeland KC, Zeitler P, Geffner M, Guandalini C, Higgins J, Hirst K, et al. Characteristics of adolescents and youth with recent-onset type 2 diabetes: the TODAY cohort at baseline. *Journal of Clinical Endocrinology & Metabolism*. 2011;96(1):159–67.

83. Lascar N, Brown J, Pattison H, Barnett AH, Bailey CJ, Bellary S. Type 2 diabetes in adolescents and young adults. *Lancet Diabetes & Endocrinology*. 2018;6(1):69–80.

84. Mauvais-Jarvis F, Clegg DJ, Hevener AL. The role of estrogens in control of energy balance and glucose homeostasis. *Endocrine Reviews*. 2013;34(3):309–38.

85. Ding EL, Song Y, Malik VS, Liu S. Sex differences of endogenous sex hormones and risk of type 2 diabetes: a systematic review and meta-analysis. *JAMA*. 2006;295(11):1288–99.

86. Stöckl D, Döring A, Peters A, Thorand B, Heier M, Huth C, et al. Age at menarche is associated with prediabetes and diabetes in women (aged 32–81 years) from the general population: the KORA F4 study. *Diabetologia*. 2012;55(3):681–8.

87. Pierce MB, Kuh D, Hardy R. The role of BMI across the life course in the relationship between age at menarche and diabetes, in a British birth cohort. *Diabetic Medicine*. 2012;29(5):600–3.

88. He C, Zhang C, Hunter DJ, Hankinson SE, Buck Louis GM, Hediger ML, et al. Age at menarche and risk of type 2 diabetes: results from 2 large prospective cohort studies. *American Journal of Epidemiology*. 2010;171(3):334–44.

89. Pandeya N, Huxley RR, Chung HF, Dobson AJ, Kuh D, Hardy R, et al. Female reproductive history and risk of type 2 diabetes: a prospective analysis of 126,721 women. *Diabetes, Obesity and Metabolism*. 2018;20(9):2103–12.

90. Conway BN, Shu X-O, Zhang X, Xiang Y-B, Cai H, Li H, et al. Age at menarche, the leg length to sitting height ratio, and risk of diabetes in middle-aged and elderly Chinese men and women. *PLoS ONE*. 2012;7(3):e30625.

91. Cooper GS, Ephross SA, Sandler DP. Menstrual patterns and risk of adult-onset diabetes mellitus. *Journal of Clinical Epidemiology*. 2000;53(11):1170–3.

92. Qiu C, Chen H, Wen J, Zhu P, Lin F, Huang B, et al. Associations between age at menarche and menopause with cardiovascular disease, diabetes, and osteoporosis in Chinese Women. *Journal of Clinical Endocrinology & Metabolism*. 2013;98(4):1612–21.

93. Janghorbani M, Mansourian M, Hosseini E. Systematic review and meta-analysis of age at menarche and risk of type 2 diabetes. *Acta Diabetologica*. 2014;51(4):519–28.

94. Bralić I, Tahirović H, Matanić D, Vrdoljak O, Stojanović-Spehar S, Kovačić V, et al. Association of early menarche age and overweight/obesity. *Journal of Pediatric Endocrinology & Metabolism*. 2012;25(1-2):57–62.

95. Simmonds M, Llewellyn A, Owen CG, Woolacott N. Predicting adult obesity from childhood obesity: a systematic review and meta-analysis. *Obesity Reviews*. 2016;17(2):95–107.

96. Eckel RH, Kahn SE, Ferrannini E, Goldfine AB, Nathan DM, Schwartz MW, et al. Obesity and type 2 diabetes: what can be unified and what needs to be individualized? *Journal of Clinical Endocrinology & Metabolism*. 2011;96(6):1654–63.

97. Yuan S, Larsson SC. An atlas on risk factors for type 2 diabetes: a wide-angled Mendelian randomisation study. *Diabetologia*. 2020;63(11):2359–71.

98. Cao M, Cui B. Negative effects of age at menarche on risk of cardiometabolic diseases in adulthood: a Mendelian randomization study. *Journal of Clinical Endocrinology & Metabolism*. 2020;105(2):dgz071.

99. Mishra GD, Cooper R, Tom SE, Kuh D. Early life circumstances and their impact on menarche and menopause. *Women's Health (London)*. 2009;5(2):175–90.

100. Canelón SP, Boland MR. A systematic literature review of factors affecting the timing of menarche: the potential for climate change to impact women's health. *International Journal of Environmental Research and Public Health*. 2020;17(5):1703.

101. Wang Y-X, Shan Z, Arvizu M, Pan A, Manson JE, Missmer SA, et al. Associations of menstrual cycle characteristics across the reproductive life span and lifestyle factors with risk of type 2 diabetes. *JAMA Network Open.* 2020;3(12):e2027928.

102. Solomon CG, Hu FB, Dunaif A, Rich-Edwards J, Willett WC, Hunter DJ, et al. Long or highly irregular menstrual cycles as a marker for risk of type 2 diabetes mellitus. *JAMA.* 2001;286(19):2421–6.

103. LeBlanc ES, Kapphahn K, Hedlin H, Desai M, Parikh NI, Liu S, et al. Reproductive history and risk of type 2 diabetes mellitus in postmenopausal women: findings from the Women's Health Initiative. *Menopause.* 2017;24(1):64–72.

104. Nanri A, Mizoue T, Noda M, Goto A, Sawada N, Tsugane S, et al. Menstrual and reproductive factors and type 2 diabetes risk: the Japan public health center-based prospective study. *Journal of Diabetes Investigation.* 2019;10(1):147–53.

105. Moran LJ, Misso ML, Wild RA, Norman RJ. Impaired glucose tolerance, type 2 diabetes and metabolic syndrome in polycystic ovary syndrome: a systematic review and meta-analysis. *Human Reproduction Update.* 2010;16(4):347–63.

106. Zhu T, Cui J, Goodarzi MO. Polycystic ovary syndrome and risk of type 2 diabetes, coronary heart disease, and stroke. *Diabetes.* 2021;70(2):627–37.

107. Ruth KS, Day FR, Tyrrell J, Thompson DJ, Wood AR, Mahajan A, et al. Using human genetics to understand the disease impacts of testosterone in men and women. *Nature Medicine.* 2020;26(2):252–8.

108. Forslund M, Landin-Wilhelmsen K, Trimpou P, Schmidt J, Brännström M, Dahlgren E. Type 2 diabetes mellitus in women with polycystic ovary syndrome during a 24-year period: importance of obesity and abdominal fat distribution. *Human Reproduction Open.* 2020;2020(1):hoz042.

109. Ding EL, Song Y, Manson JE, Hunter DJ, Lee CC, Rifai N, et al. Sex hormone–binding globulin and risk of type 2 diabetes in women and men. *New England Journal of Medicine.* 2009;361(12):1152–63.

110. Holden SE, Barnett AH, Peters JR, Jenkins-Jones S, Poole CD, Morgan CL, et al. The incidence of type 2 diabetes in the United Kingdom from 1991 to 2010. *Diabetes, Obesity and Metabolism.* 2013;15(9):844–52.

111. Greendale GA, Sternfeld B, Huang M, Han W, Karvonen-Gutierrez C, Ruppert K, et al. Changes in body composition and weight during the menopause transition. *JCI Insight.* 2019;4(5):e124865.

112. Lovejoy JC, Champagne CM, de Jonge L, Xie H, Smith SR. Increased visceral fat and decreased energy expenditure during the menopausal transition. *International Journal of Obesity (London).* 2008;32(6):949–58.

113. Freemantle N, Holmes J, Hockey A, Kumar S. How strong is the association between abdominal obesity and the incidence of type 2 diabetes? *International Journal of Clinical Practice.* 2008;62(9):1391–6.

114. Guo C, Li Q, Tian G, Liu Y, Sun X, Yin Z, et al. Association of age at menopause and type 2 diabetes: a systematic review and dose-response meta-analysis of cohort studies. *Primary Care Diabetes.* 2019;13(4):301–9.

115. Sun L, Tan L, Yang F, Luo Y, Li X, Deng HW, et al. Meta-analysis suggests that smoking is associated with an increased risk of early natural menopause. *Menopause.* 2012;19(2):126–32.

116. Taneri PE, Kiefte-de Jong JC, Bramer WM, Daan NMP, Franco OH, Muka T. Association of alcohol consumption with the onset of natural menopause: a systematic review and meta-analysis. *Human Reproduction Update.* 2016;22(4):516–28.

117. Salpeter SR, Walsh JME, Ormiston TM, Greyber E, Buckley NS, Salpeter EE. Meta-analysis: effect of hormone-replacement therapy on components of the metabolic syndrome in postmenopausal women. *Diabetes, Obesity and Metabolism.* 2006;8(5):538–54.

118. Mauvais-Jarvis F, Manson JE, Stevenson JC, Fonseca VA. Menopausal hormone therapy and type 2 diabetes prevention: evidence, mechanisms, and clinical implications. *Endocrine Reviews.* 2017;38(3):173–88.

119. Pirimoglu ZM, Arslan C, Buyukbayrak EE, Kars B, Karsidag YK, Unal O, et al. Glucose tolerance of premenopausal women after menopause due to surgical removal of ovaries. *Climacteric.* 2011;14(4):453–7.

120. Howard B, Grubb E, Lage MJ, Tang B. Trends in use of and complications from intrauterine contraceptive devices and tubal ligation or occlusion. *Reprod Health*. 2017;14(1):70.

121. van Hylckama Vlieg A, Helmerhorst FM, Vandenbroucke JP, Doggen CJ, Rosendaal FR. The venous thrombotic risk of oral contraceptives, effects of oestrogen dose and progestogen type: results of the MEGA case-control study. *BMJ (Clinical Research Ed)*. 2009;339:b2921.

122. Dorflinger LJ. Metabolic effects of implantable steroid contraceptives for women. *Contraception*. 2002;65(1):47–62.

123. Kahn HS, Curtis KM, Marchbanks PA. Effects of injectable or implantable progestin-only contraceptives on insulin-glucose metabolism and diabetes risk. *Diabetes Care*. 2003;26(1):216–25.

124. Lopez LM, Grimes DA, Schulz KF. Steroidal contraceptives: effect on carbohydrate metabolism in women without diabetes mellitus. *Cochrane Database of Systematic Reviews*. 2014(4):CD006133.

125. Glisic M, Shahzad S, Tsoli S, Chadni M, Asllanaj E, Rojas LZ, et al. Association between progestin-only contraceptive use and cardiometabolic outcomes: a systematic review and meta-analysis. *European Journal of Preventive Cardiology*. 2018;25(10):1042–52.

126. Kim C, Seidel KW, Begier EA, Kwok YS. Diabetes and depot medroxyprogesterone contraception in Navajo women. *Archives of Internal Medicine*. 2001;161(14):1766–71.

127. Mosorin ME, Haverinen A, Ollila MM, Nordstrom T, Jokelainen J, Keinanen-Kiukaanniemi S, et al. Current use of combined hormonal contraception is associated with glucose metabolism disorders in perimenopausal women. *European Journal of Endocrinology*. 2020;183(6):619–26.

128. Kim C, Siscovick DS, Sidney S, Lewis CE, Kiefe CI, Koepsell TD, et al. Oral contraceptive use and association with glucose, insulin, and diabetes in young adult women: the CARDIA study. Coronary artery risk development in young adults. *Diabetes Care*. 2002;25(6):1027–32.

129. Vounzoulaki E, Khunti K, Abner SC, Tan BK, Davies MJ, Gillies CL. Progression to type 2 diabetes in women with a known history of gestational diabetes: systematic review and meta-analysis. *BMJ (Clinical Research Ed)*. 2020;369:m1361.

130. Li Z, Cheng Y, Wang D, Chen H, Chen H, Ming WK, et al. Incidence rate of type 2 diabetes mellitus after gestational diabetes mellitus: A systematic review and meta-analysis of 170,139 women. *Journal of Diabetes Research*. 2020;2020:3076463.

131. Guo P, Zhou Q, Ren L, Chen Y, Hui Y. Higher parity is associated with increased risk of type 2 diabetes mellitus in women: a linear dose-response meta-analysis of cohort studies. *Journal of Diabetes and Its Complications*. 2017;31(1):58–66.

132. Li P, Shan Z, Zhou L, Xie M, Bao W, Zhang Y, et al. Mechanisms in endocrinology: parity and risk of type 2 diabetes: a systematic review and dose-response meta-analysis. *European Journal of Endocrinology*. 2016;175(5):R231–R245.

133. Tian Y, Shen L, Wu J, Chen W, Yuan J, Yang H, et al. Parity and the risk of diabetes mellitus among Chinese women: a cross-sectional evidence from the Tongji-Dongfeng cohort study. *PLoS ONE*. 2014;9(8):e104810.

134. Mueller NT, Mueller NJ, Odegaard AO, Gross MD, Koh WP, Yuan JM, et al. Higher parity is associated with an increased risk of type-II diabetes in Chinese women: the Singapore Chinese health study. *BJOG*. 2013;120(12):1483–9.

135. Kritz-Silverstein D, Barrett-Connor E, Wingard DL. The effect of parity on the later development of non-insulin-dependent diabetes mellitus or impaired glucose tolerance. *New England Journal of Medicine*. 1989;321(18):1214–19.

136. Nicholson WK, Asao K, Brancati F, Coresh J, Pankow JS, Powe NR. Parity and risk of type 2 diabetes: the atherosclerosis risk in communities study. *Diabetes Care*. 2006;29(11):2349–54.

137. Luo J, Hendryx M, LeBlanc ES, Shadyab AH, Qi L, Sealy-Jefferson S, et al. Associations between parity, breastfeeding, and risk of maternal type 2 diabetes among postmenopausal women. *Obstetrics and Gynecology*. 2019;134(3):591–9.

138. Al Mamun A, Mannan M, O'Callaghan MJ, Williams GM, Najman JM, Callaway LK. Association between gestational weight gain and postpartum diabetes: evidence from a community based large cohort study. *PLoS ONE*. 2013;8(12):e75679.

139. Peters SA, Yang L, Guo Y, Chen Y, Bian Z, Millwood IY, et al. Parenthood and the risk of diabetes in men and women: a 7 year prospective study of 0.5 million individuals. *Diabetologia*. 2016;59(8):1675–82.

140. Hanley AJ, McKeown-Eyssen G, Harris SB, Hegele RA, Wolever TM, Kwan J, et al. Association of parity with risk of type 2 diabetes and related metabolic disorders. *Diabetes Care*. 2002;25(4):690–5.

141. Cruz NG, Sousa LP, Sousa MO, Pietrani NT, Fernandes AP, Gomes KB. The linkage between inflammation and type 2 diabetes mellitus. *Diabetes Research and Clinical Practice*. 2013;99(2):85–92.

142. Horta BL, de Lima NP. Breastfeeding and type 2 diabetes: systematic review and meta-analysis. *Current Diabetes Reports*. 2019;19(1):1.

143. Aune D, Norat T, Romundstad P, Vatten LJ. Breastfeeding and the maternal risk of type 2 diabetes: a systematic review and dose-response meta-analysis of cohort studies. *Nutrition, Metabolism and Cardiovascular Diseases*. 2014;24(2):107–15.

144. Jäger S, Jacobs S, Kröger J, Fritsche A, Schienkiewitz A, Rubin D, et al. Breast-feeding and maternal risk of type 2 diabetes: a prospective study and meta-analysis. *Diabetologia*. 2014;57(7):1355–65.

145. Aune D, Norat T, Leitzmann M, Tonstad S, Vatten LJ. Physical activity and the risk of type 2 diabetes: a systematic review and dose-response meta-analysis. *European Journal of Epidemiology*. 2015;30(7):529–42.

146. Patterson R, McNamara E, Tainio M, de Sa TH, Smith AD, Sharp SJ, et al. Sedentary behaviour and risk of all-cause, cardiovascular and cancer mortality, and incident type 2 diabetes: a systematic review and dose response meta-analysis. *European Journal of Epidemiology*. 2018;33(9):811–29.

147. Bellou V, Belbasis L, Tzoulaki I, Evangelou E. Risk factors for type 2 diabetes mellitus: an exposure-wide umbrella review of meta-analyses. *PLoS ONE*. 2018;13(3):e0194127.

148. Schwingshackl L, Hoffmann G, Lampousi AM, Knuppel S, Iqbal K, Schwedhelm C, et al. Food groups and risk of type 2 diabetes mellitus: a systematic review and meta-analysis of prospective studies. *European Journal of Epidemiology*. 2017;32(5):363–75.

149. Horta BL, de Lima NP. Breastfeeding and type 2 diabetes: systematic review and meta-analysis. *Current Diabetes Reports*. 2019;19(1):1.

150. Rimm EB, Chan J, Stampfer MJ, Colditz GA, Willett WC. Prospective study of cigarette smoking, alcohol use, and the risk of diabetes in men. *BMJ (Clinical Research Ed)*. 1995;310(6979):555–9.

151. Rimm EB, Manson JE, Stampfer MJ, Colditz GA, Willett WC, Rosner B, et al. Cigarette smoking and the risk of diabetes in women. *American Journal of Public Health*. 1993;83(2):211–14.

152. Wang Y, Ji J, Liu YJ, Deng X, He QQ. Passive smoking and risk of type 2 diabetes: a meta-analysis of prospective cohort studies. *PLoS ONE*. 2013;8(7):e69915.

153. Polsky S, Akturk HK. Alcohol consumption, diabetes risk, and cardiovascular disease within diabetes. *Current Diabetes Reports*. 2017;17(12):136.

154. Wannamethee SG, Camargo CA, Jr., Manson JE, Willett WC, Rimm EB. Alcohol drinking patterns and risk of type 2 diabetes mellitus among younger women. *Archives of Internal Medicine*. 2003;163(11):1329–36.

155. Kao WH, Puddey IB, Boland LL, Watson RL, Brancati FL. Alcohol consumption and the risk of type 2 diabetes mellitus: atherosclerosis risk in communities study. *American Journal of Epidemiology*. 2001;154(8):748–57.

156. Liang W, Chikritzhs T. Alcohol consumption during adolescence and risk of diabetes in young adulthood. *BioMed Research International*. 2014;2014:795741.

157. Hodge AM, English DR, O'Dea K, Giles GG. Alcohol intake, consumption pattern and beverage type, and the risk of type 2 diabetes. *Diabetic Medicine*. 2006;23(6):690–7.

158. Rasouli B, Ahlbom A, Andersson T, Grill V, Midthjell K, Olsson L, et al. Alcohol consumption is associated with reduced risk of type 2 diabetes and autoimmune diabetes in adults: results from the Nord-Trondelag health study. *Diabetic Medicine*. 2013;30(1):56–64.

159. Cosgrove MP, Sargeant LA, Caleyachetty R, Griffin SJ. Work-related stress and type 2 diabetes: systematic review and meta-analysis. *Occupational Medicine (London)*. 2012;62(3):167–73.

160. Heraclides A, Chandola T, Witte DR, Brunner EJ. Psychosocial stress at work doubles the risk of type 2 diabetes in middle-aged women: evidence from the Whitehall II study. *Diabetes Care*. 2009;32(12):2230–5.

161. Joseph JJ, Golden SH. Cortisol dysregulation: the bidirectional link between stress, depression, and type 2 diabetes mellitus. *Annals of the New York Academy of Sciences*. 2017;1391(1):20–34.

162. Agardh E, Allebeck P, Hallqvist J, Moradi T, Sidorchuk A. Type 2 diabetes incidence and socio-economic position: a systematic review and meta-analysis. *International Journal of Epidemiology*. 2011;40(3):804–18.

163. Anjana RM, Deepa M, Pradeepa R, Mahanta J, Narain K, Das HK, et al. Prevalence of diabetes and prediabetes in 15 states of India: results from the ICMR-INDIAB population-based cross-sectional study. *Lancet Diabetes & Endocrinology*. 2017;5(8):585–96.

164. Bijlsma-Rutte A, Rutters F, Elders PJM, Bot SDM, Nijpels G. Socio-economic status and HbA(1c) in type 2 diabetes: a systematic review and meta-analysis. *Diabetes/Metabolism Research and Reviews*. 2018;34(6):e3008.

165. Rawshani A, Svensson A-M, Zethelius B, Eliasson B, Rosengren A, Gudbjörnsdottir S. Association between socioeconomic status and mortality, cardiovascular disease, and cancer in patients with type 2 diabetes. *JAMA Internal Medicine*. 2016;176(8):1146–54.

166. Hajat A, Hsia C, O'Neill MS. Socioeconomic disparities and air pollution exposure: a global review. *Current Environmental Health Reports*. 2015;2(4):440–50.

167. Tessum CW, Apte JS, Goodkind AL, Muller NZ, Mullins KA, Paolella DA, et al. Inequity in consumption of goods and services adds to racial–ethnic disparities in air pollution exposure. *Proceedings of the National Academy of Sciences*. 2019;116(13):6001.

168. Thayer KA, Heindel JJ, Bucher JR, Gallo MA. Role of environmental chemicals in diabetes and obesity: a National Toxicology Program workshop review. *Environmental Health Perspectives*. 2012;120(6):779–89.

169. Evangelou E, Ntritsos G, Chondrogiorgi M, Kavvoura FK, Hernández AF, Ntzani EE, et al. Exposure to pesticides and diabetes: a systematic review and meta-analysis. *Environment International*. 2016;91:60–8.

170. Jaacks LM, Staimez LR. Association of persistent organic pollutants and non-persistent pesticides with diabetes and diabetes-related health outcomes in Asia: a systematic review. *Environment International*. 2015;76:57–70.

171. Chandrabose M, Rachele JN, Gunn L, Kavanagh A, Owen N, Turrell G, et al. Built environment and cardio-metabolic health: systematic review and meta-analysis of longitudinal studies. *Obesity Reviews*. 2019;20(1):41–54.

172. Twohig-Bennett C, Jones A. The health benefits of the great outdoors: a systematic review and meta-analysis of greenspace exposure and health outcomes. *Environmental Research*. 2018;166:628–37.

173. Schootman M, Andresen EM, Wolinsky FD, Malmstrom TK, Miller JP, Yan Y, et al. The effect of adverse housing and neighborhood conditions on the development of diabetes mellitus among middle aged African Americans. *American Journal of Epidemiology*. 2007;166(4):379–87.

174. Ahern M, Brown C, Dukas S. A national study of the association between food environments and county-level health outcomes. *Journal of Rural Health*. 2011;27(4):367–79.

175. Auchincloss AH, Diez Roux AV, Mujahid MS, Shen M, Bertoni AG, Carnethon MR. Neighborhood resources for physical activity and healthy foods and incidence of type 2 diabetes mellitus: the multi-ethnic study of atherosclerosis. *Archives of Internal Medicine*. 2009;169(18):1698–704.

176. Seligman HK, Bindman AB, Vittinghoff E, Kanaya AM, Kushel MB. Food insecurity is associated with diabetes mellitus: results from the National Health Examination and Nutrition Examination Survey (NHANES) 1999–2002. *Journal of General Internal Medicine*. 2007;22(7):1018–23.

177. Varanka-Ruuska T, Rautio N, Lehtiniemi H, Miettunen J, Keinänen-Kiukaanniemi S, Sebert S, et al. The association of unemployment with glucose metabolism: a systematic review and meta-analysis. *International Journal of Public Health*. 2018;63(4):435–46.

178. Gan Y, Yang C, Tong X, Sun H, Cong Y, Yin X, et al. Shift work and diabetes mellitus: a meta-analysis of observational studies. *Occupational & Environmental Medicine*. 2015;72(1):72–8.

179. Ferrie JE, Virtanen M, Jokela M, Madsen IEH, Heikkilä K, Alfredsson L, et al. Job insecurity and risk of diabetes: a meta-analysis of individual participant data. *CMAJ*. 2016;188(17–18):E447–E55.

180. Ludwig J, Sanbonmatsu L, Gennetian L, Adam E, Duncan GJ, Katz LF, et al. Neighborhoods, obesity, and diabetes—a randomized social experiment. *New England Journal of Medicine*. 2011;365(16):1509–19.

181. Cingano F. *Trends in income inequality and its impact on economic growth, OECD social, employment and migration Working Papers No. 163.* Paris: OECD Publishing; 2014.

182. Beckles GL, Chou CF. Disparities in the prevalence of diagnosed diabetes—United States, 1999–2002 and 2011–2014. *Morbidity and Mortality Weekly Report.* 2016;65(45):1265–9.

183. Seiglie JA, Marcus M-E, Ebert C, Prodromidis N, Geldsetzer P, Theilmann M, et al. Diabetes prevalence and its relationship with education, wealth, and BMI in 29 low- and middle-income countries. *Diabetes Care.* 2020;43(4):767.

184. Jones-Smith JC, Gordon-Larsen P, Siddiqi A, Popkin BM. Is the burden of overweight shifting to the poor across the globe? Time trends among women in 39 low- and middle-income countries (1991–2008). *International Journal of Obesity (2005).* 2012;36(8):1114–20.

185. O'Neil A, Russell JD, Thompson K, Martinson ML, Peters SAE. The impact of socioeconomic position (SEP) on women's health over the lifetime. *Maturitas.* 2020;140:1–7.

186. Perel P, Langenberg C, Ferrie J, Moser K, Brunner E, Marmot M. Household wealth and the metabolic syndrome in the Whitehall II study. *Diabetes Care.* 2006;29(12):2694.

7

A Life Course Approach to Musculoskeletal Ageing

Rachel Cooper, Kate A. Ward, and Avan Aihie Sayer

7.1 Introduction

Impairments to musculoskeletal health and function are a key threat to healthy ageing.[1] Adverse age-related changes in musculoskeletal structure and function that generally occur from midlife onwards, including declines in bone strength, loss of muscle mass and function, and degeneration of cartilage, can ultimately lead to clinical diagnoses of osteoporosis, sarcopenia, and osteoarthritis, respectively.[2–4] These three age-related clinical conditions are leading contributors to the burden of disease and disability in all world regions;[5,6] evidence suggests that their burden has been increasing in recent decades[6,7] for a number of reasons including global population ageing.

Alongside their impacts on individuals and their families, osteoporosis, sarcopenia, and osteoarthritis also have major societal implications. These are related to the high costs of care associated with the treatment and management of the conditions and also the myriad of other outcomes, including mobility disability, falls, and fragility fractures, that they precipitate.[8–13]

Unfortunately, a considerable gap between the scale of the burden of age-related musculoskeletal conditions and the allocation of research funding for the study of these conditions has been reported.[14] This likely reflects the fact that the importance of musculoskeletal health and function for overall health and disease has arguably been underappreciated for many years.[15] However, this is changing as musculoskeletal health across life is shown to be important for a number of contemporaneous policy and research priorities on population health. The first example of this is multimorbidity, currently a strategic priority for global health research.[16] Characterising meaningful clusters of different health conditions is an important preliminary aim of multimorbidity research. Although this work is still in its relative infancy, it has already been shown that musculoskeletal conditions are frequently found in multimorbidity[17] and are an important component of some of the most commonly identified clusters.[16,18] A second example is research highlighting the importance of musculoskeletal health and function for surgical outcomes. There is compelling evidence that people with poorer musculoskeletal function presurgery, experience less favourable postsurgical outcomes.[19] This has prompted considerable interest in the concept of prehabilitation[20,21] with intervention studies now underway to assess the impact of a range of presurgical interventions to improve musculoskeletal function on surgical outcomes in different patient groups including people requiring cancer treatment. Prompted by the COVID-19 pandemic,

Rachel Cooper, Kate A. Ward, and Avan Aihie Sayer, *A Life Course Approach to Musculoskeletal Ageing* In: *A Life Course Approach to Women's Health*. Second Edition. Edited by: Gita D Mishra, Rebecca Hardy, and Diana Kuh, Oxford University Press.
© Oxford University Press 2023. DOI: 10.1093/oso/9780192864642.003.0007

in 2020, it was also proposed that this concept could be extended to consider the role that improving the population's fitness, including their musculoskeletal health and function, may be able to play in mitigating the effects of future infectious disease epidemics.[22]

Taken together, evidence of the many direct and indirect impacts of age-related musculoskeletal conditions provides a compelling case for needing to understand their aetiology and identify preventive and treatment strategies across life. To do this, it is first important to understand the basic descriptive epidemiology of these conditions and, in the context of this book, to consider differences between women and men. As osteoporosis, sarcopenia, and osteoarthritis are all conditions typically resulting from age-related changes in musculoskeletal structure and function, it is unsurprising that prevalence of all three conditions generally increases with age. These increases are seen in both women and men. However, at any one particular age, women have higher prevalence of osteoporosis and osteoarthritis (at two of the three most common sites, the knee and hand, but not the hip) than men.[23,24] On average, women have weaker muscle strength and lower muscle mass than men at all life stages,[25] but as these differences have usually been taken into account when establishing sex-specific cut-points to identify sarcopenia, gender differences in the prevalence of sarcopenia are often not observed or reported.[3,26]

Since the term *life course epidemiology* was coined in 1997, there has been a steady increase in the number of studies using a life course approach to investigate musculoskeletal conditions (see Figure 7.1). There have been a number of excellent summaries and reviews

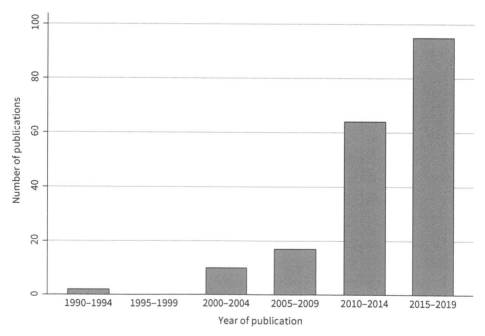

Figure 7.1 Number of publications identified in a Medline search of papers (published 1990–2019) that include the term *life course* in their title or abstract plus at least one of the following terms in any field: *musculoskeletal, sarcopenia, osteoporosis, osteoarthritis, muscle, bone, joints, cartilage,* and *fracture*. Note: This is an update of a search originally conducted in 2015.[38] Of 6311 papers indexed in Medline between 1990 and February 2021 that used the term *life course* in their title or abstract, 200 included a listed musculoskeletal term.

of evidence on life course epidemiological approaches to musculoskeletal ageing,[27-32] not least the chapter and accompanying commentary in the previous edition of this book[33,34] and relevant chapters in other books in the life course approach to health series.[35-37] In this chapter, we aim to provide an update on recent developments in this continually evolving field of study. In addition, we aim to assess the extent to which empirical evidence generated by taking a life course approach to the study of musculoskeletal ageing is being translated into policy and practice.

7.2 Definitions

Inconsistencies in evidence can arise because of variations in definitions, diagnostic criteria, and the methods of ascertainment of outcomes employed in different studies. It is, therefore, important to briefly summarise recent developments on definitions. Perhaps most noteworthy are the major advances that have been made with regards to sarcopenia. In 2016, sarcopenia was assigned an ICD-10 code (M62.84),[39] giving it similar clinical status to osteoporosis and osteoarthritis. This reflects major efforts since the early 2000s to highlight the clinical importance of age-related changes in muscle and work towards agreement on diagnostic criteria for sarcopenia.

There are challenges associated with achieving consensus on diagnostic criteria for all three musculoskeletal conditions. In the case of osteoporosis, the key challenge is that bone strength cannot be directly measured in vivo, and while there are a range of surrogate measures of bone strength, many of these have limitations.[36] Despite this, in 1994 the World Health Organization (WHO) were able to agree on an operational definition of osteoporosis which has been widely applied ever since.[40] However, it is important to acknowledge that as this definition is based on data for white postmenopausal women, its application in other populations may not be optimal.[41]

Parallels have been drawn between the work and debates currently ongoing to establish universal agreement on an operational definition of sarcopenia with those that led up to the agreement of the WHO's operational definition of osteoporosis.[41] Like the WHO diagnostic criteria for osteoporosis—bone mineral density (BMD) -2.5 standard deviations or more below the mean for a young adult—it has been proposed that sarcopenia should be diagnosed when muscle mass and/or strength fall below cut-points established using normative data for healthy young adults.[3,42] While debate continues on the specific muscle parameters to be used, the recommended methods of measuring these parameters, and the cut-points to be applied when defining sarcopenia,[43] progress in the last decade has been promising.

With work continuing towards universal agreement on an operational definition of sarcopenia, the hope is to remove barriers to further progress in research and clinical practice. Such barriers have been documented in the study of osteoarthritis. Perhaps reflecting its complex pathology and heterogeneous symptomatology, different clinical organisations promote different definitions of osteoarthritis and recommend different diagnostic criteria leading to calls for greater standardisation and uniformity.[4,44] Further complicating the study of osteoarthritis and adding to these calls for standardisation is evidence of a high degree of discordance between reports of joint pain (a key symptom used for diagnosis) and pathological indicators of osteoarthritis detected by radiography. For example, in a review on knee osteoarthritis, the majority of studies included in a data synthesis reported that the proportion of people with knee pain who were found to have radiographic osteoarthritis was < 50%, and, likewise, the proportion of people with radiographic osteoarthritis who reported knee pain was as low as 15% in one study and < 50% in many studies.[45]

7.3 Changes in Relevant Phenotypes Across Life

Osteoporosis, sarcopenia, and osteoarthritis typically do not become clinically manifest until later in life. As for many other age-related conditions, their study from a life course perspective is thus aided by the identification of phenotypes that capture meaningful inter- and intraindividual variability predictive of future clinical risk at different life stages. By understanding the changes in these phenotypes across life, identifying when clinically significant changes are most likely to occur and the key drivers of these changes, the aim is to identify when and how to intervene across life to maximise opportunities to prevent the onset of age-related musculoskeletal conditions, and the many adverse outcomes they precipitate.

As cases of osteoporosis and sarcopenia are identified by applying cut-points to continuous measures of BMD, muscle mass, and strength, respectively, and meaningful variation in these measures can be captured at different life stages, these two age-related musculoskeletal outcomes lend themselves to study from a life course perspective. Over the last 20 years, more studies in a wider range of settings have been able to take advantage of advances in musculoskeletal imaging[36] and functional testing to capture data on many relevant bone and muscle parameters at different life stages. As a result of these methodological advances and major collaborative initiatives to harmonise and pool data from different studies, our ability to model and understand life course trajectories of bone and muscle has improved greatly. So, while there are still no studies capturing relevant musculoskeletal measures in the same individuals across all life stages, there are now: i) a number of population-based studies spanning wide age-ranges,[46–51] and ii) sufficient studies with comparable bone and/or muscle measures, many with repeat data, covering different life stages that can be concatenated.[25,52]

These have provided empirical evidence that bone and muscle parameters of relevance to osteoporosis and sarcopenia, respectively, follow a 'typical' life course trajectory—a developmental phase from infancy through to early adulthood when peak levels are reached, a phase in early to midadulthood during which peak is maintained, followed by a degenerative phase from midlife into old age (see Figure 7.2).[25,49] While mean levels at any one particular life stage have been shown to vary by sex, ethnicity, and country,[48,53,54] the general shape of observed mean trajectories is remarkably consistent.

Much research on osteoporosis and sarcopenia justifiably focuses on age-related declines from midlife.[55,56] However, empirical life course data clearly demonstrate that whether or not an older individual falls below established cut-points is a function not only of the timing of onset and rate of decline they have experienced since midlife but also their pattern of development in early life and the peak level they attained in early adulthood. This point is emphasised in a theoretical analysis that aimed to estimate the relative contributions of peak BMD, menopause, and rate of BMD loss to women's osteoporosis risk, peak BMD was found to be the most important contributor.[57] Factors shown to influence bone and muscle during any phase of life are, therefore, expected to impact future risk of osteoporosis and sarcopenia.

As an increasing number of studies collect repeat measures of bone and muscle phenotypes within the same individuals over multiple life stages, there will be more opportunities

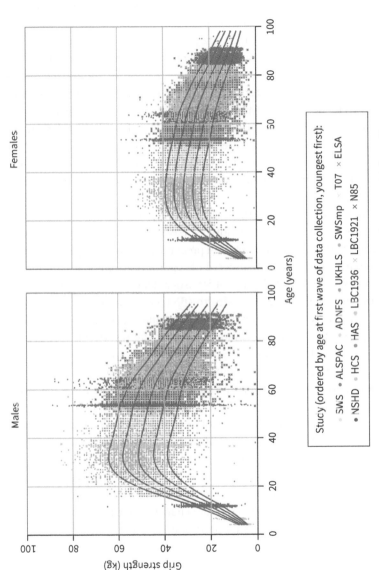

Figure 7.2 Cross-cohort centile curves for grip strength using data from 12 British studies.

Centiles shown 10th, 25th, 50th, 75th, and 90th percentiles are shown. The studies include ADNFS Allied Dunbar National Fitness Survey, ALSPAC Avon Longitudinal Study of Parents and Children, ELSA English Longitudinal Study of Ageing, HAS Hertfordshire Ageing Study, HCS Hertfordshire Cohort Study, LBC1921 and LBC1936 Lothian Birth Cohorts of 1921 and 1936, N85 Newcastle 85+ Study, NSHD Medical Research Council National Survey of Health and Development, SWS Southampton Women's Survey, SWSmp Mothers and Their Partners From the SWS, T-07 West of Scotland Twenty-07 Study, UKHLS Understanding Society: the UK Household Panel Study. See plate section.

Source: Richard M Dodds, et al. 2014. Grip Strength across the life course: normative data from twelve British studies. *PLoS ONE*, 9(12):e113637.

to try and distinguish age from cohort and period effects, which is often not possible using data from existing studies. It will also become possible to undertake further detailed investigations of intraindividual changes and the heterogeneity between individuals in patterns of age-related change.[58] In addition, as measures of bone and muscle are integrated into more life course studies that also capture data on the structure and function of other body systems, it will be possible to do further work to elucidate how age-related changes in bones, muscles, and joints relate to age-related changes in measures such as cognition, mental health, and neurological, cardio-metabolic, and respiratory function. As the number of studies with data that can be used to chart these changes from earlier life grows, it is hoped that we will be able to establish the extent to which changes in one body system precede, interact, and may even precipitate changes in other body systems. This information will improve our understanding of the acquisition sequence of different long-term conditions (i.e. the life course development of multimorbidity) and aid identification of the most suitable targets for preventive intervention. For example, could there be novel opportunities to reduce the risk of sarcopenia by targeting people who have recently been diagnosed with type 2 diabetes or vice versa? Or could there even be opportunities to intervene earlier, when adverse changes in glycosylated haemoglobin or muscle function are first detected, that prevent development of both diabetes and sarcopenia?

As diagnosis of osteoarthritis is not straightforward and debate continues about the main mechanisms underlying its development,[59] phenotypes have not yet been identified that would allow us to chart and better understand relevant preclinical changes across life prior to the manifestation of osteoarthritis. This has hampered life course research on osteoarthritis. However, research has shown the potential value of Statistical Shape Modelling of joints,[60] and a Foundation for the National Institutes of Health (FNIH) Osteoarthritis Biomarkers Consortium has recently reported on a number of imaging and biochemical biomarkers related to cartilage morphometry, collagen degradation, and bone resorption that predict osteoarthritis progression.[61] While the main purpose of the FNIH work has been to aid treatment development,[62] it is possible that these biomarkers could also be used to chart important changes occurring across life even before the onset of symptoms or clinical diagnosis of osteoarthritis. Work to identify biomarkers is not restricted to the study of osteoarthritis. Recognising that imaging and functional testing cannot be conducted in all environments, as they often involve the use of expensive equipment that is not portable, and these techniques may not capture all clinically relevant changes in bone and muscle, work is also ongoing to identify biomarkers of osteoporosis and sarcopenia.[63,64] As such work progresses and these measures are adopted in more studies, we would expect to see even greater opportunity to gain an improved understanding of the clinically relevant changes occurring across life prior to the manifestation of age-related musculoskeletal conditions.

7.4 Factors Across Life Associated with Musculoskeletal Ageing

7.4.1 Genetic Factors

Findings from heritability studies indicate that a proportion of the observed variation in risk of developing osteoporosis, sarcopenia, and osteoarthritis is inherited. Estimates of heritability range from 50% to 85% for BMD,[2] 30% to 85% for muscle strength, 45% to 90% for muscle mass,[65] and 40% to 80% for osteoarthritis.[4] Each year, as large genome-wide association studies identify additional loci, further progress is made towards better understanding the contributions of specific genetic variants to all three age-related musculoskeletal conditions[65–69] and to their shared genetic aetiology.[70,71]

For the last decade, there has been growing interest in epigenetics and the potential for work in this area to provide important novel insights on the mechanisms underlying development of many age-related conditions.[67,68,72] However, the full potential of this research is still to be realised for musculoskeletal conditions. There are likely to be many interesting developments in this area in the coming decade as new technologies are advanced, methods standardised, and it becomes easier to measure DNA methylation, histone deacetylation, and microRNAs in relevant tissue samples (i.e. bone, muscle, and cartilage).[67,73]

7.4.2 Oestrogen Exposure

One lifetime exposure that clearly distinguishes women from men is oestrogen, and so, oestrogen exposure is often proposed as an explanation for gender differences in many health outcomes. This includes osteoporosis, sarcopenia, and osteoarthritis because: i) the timing of onset or acceleration of age-related declines in musculoskeletal structure and function coincide with the timing of menopause; ii) there are plausible mechanisms by which the changes in endogenous hormone levels women experience during menopause could detrimentally impact on bone, muscle, and joints; and iii) menopausal hormone therapy has been shown to be an effective prophylactic and therapeutic treatment for osteoporosis in peri- and postmenopausal women and was widely prescribed for this reason until its adverse effects on cardiovascular disease and some cancers were identified (see Chapter 4, Section 4.5.2).[2]

Menopause is just one of a number of factors that contributes to a woman's lifetime exposure to oestrogen. Associations between the factors contributing to oestrogen exposure from adolescence onwards, including timing of menarche, childbearing, exogenous hormone use (oral contraceptives and hormone replacement therapy), and type and timing of menopause have been most comprehensively studied in relation to osteoporosis risk. Studies have consistently shown that later age at menarche and earlier age at menopause, both of which contribute to reduced lifetime exposure to oestrogen, are associated with lower BMD and increased risk of osteoporosis.[74,75] Mendelian randomization (MR) studies have also recently provided evidence to suggest that the age at menarche-BMD association may be causal.[76] However, whether there are associations between other reproductive characteristics, such as parity and breastfeeding, and osteoporosis is less clear perhaps because these characteristics not only contribute to lifetime oestrogen exposure but also indicate other social and biological factors.

Recent reviews of the associations between indicators of lifetime oestrogen exposure and osteoarthritis suggest that there is some evidence of links with menarche, parity, menopause, and exogenous hormone use.[77,78] However, the findings are not conclusive, and authors of these published reviews[77,78] highlighted a number of methodological limitations that need to be addressed in future studies. These limitations include important differences in outcome definition (as discussed in Section 7.2), and when studying menopause, a reliance on cross-sectional studies comparing pre-, peri-, and postmenopausal women, which do not allow effects of menopause to be distinguished from the effects of age. Similar limitations are found in the handful of studies that have investigated associations between indicators of lifetime oestrogen exposure and sarcopenia or muscle mass and strength.[79-81] This highlights the need for more high-quality life course research to elucidate the potential role of lifetime oestrogen exposure in explaining gender differences in osteoarthritis and key characteristics of muscle used to define sarcopenia.

7.4.3   Growth

In the first edition of this book, relationships of growth, during earlier phases of life (from intrauterine and early postnatal periods through to peak height attainment in late adolescence), with osteoporosis and muscle mass and strength were described.[33] Based on findings from seminal life course studies, many UK based, that had data on size at birth and/or repeat measures of body size across infancy, childhood, and adolescence, and musculoskeletal outcomes in adulthood, it was concluded that poor growth in utero and during childhood was associated with increased risk of osteoporosis and sarcopenia in later life. There are a number of plausible mechanisms relating to the acquisition of peak bone and muscle strength that could explain these associations.[33,35,36] Since the publication of the first edition of this book, other chapters in the life course series[35,36] have described the accumulation of further evidence from studies in different world regions. Taken together, this body of evidence demonstrates the importance of promoting healthy growth in utero and early life to ensure the attainment of maximal peak bone and muscle strength and prevent osteoporosis and sarcopenia in later life.[82-87] These life course findings have informed the development of a number of interventions to improve maternal nutritional status, especially in countries where there are concerns about the nutritional status of women of reproductive age.[88-90] However, which nutritional interventions are most effective, and whether these translate into long-term benefits for the growth and musculoskeletal health of offspring is still to be established.[91,92]

7.4.4   Obesity

Over the last 20 years, the prevalence of obesity has continued to increase in most world regions,[93] and earlier onset of overweight and obesity has been documented in more recently born cohorts (as described in more detail in Chapter 16).[94] Understanding the associations of overweight and obesity across life with osteoporosis, sarcopenia, and osteoarthritis, and the implications of this for future generations of older adults, has thus become increasingly urgent.

Evidence of an important role for obesity in the development of age-related musculoskeletal conditions is most compelling for osteoarthritis. Studies have consistently shown that obesity is strongly associated with increased risk of knee osteoarthritis,[95] and there is also moderate evidence of associations between obesity and hip and hand osteoarthritis.[96,97] A number of potential explanations for these associations have been proposed including altered mechanical loading of the joints and chronic inflammation.

Using measures of body mass index (BMI) prospectively ascertained between ages 2 and 53 years in the MRC National Survey of Health and Development (NSHD), a life course perspective to the study of this association was added. In the NSHD, the effects of overweight and obesity on risk of knee osteoarthritis were found to accumulate from adolescence in women and from early adulthood in men, possibly reflecting earlier onset of fat mass accrual in women than men.[98] This complements findings from a large case-control study—Genetics of Osteoarthritis and Lifestyle (GOAL)—which examined associations between retrospective estimates of lifetime weight, assessed using body shape diagrams, and osteoarthritis.[99] Results from this study suggested that the earlier the onset of overweight in adulthood, the greater the odds of both knee and hip osteoarthritis, with some evidence of stronger associations in women than men for knee osteoarthritis. Utilising MR with UK Biobank data, evidence that associations between BMI and both knee and hip osteoarthritis are causal has recently been presented.[100] This adds further support to calls already being made by organisations, including Public Health England and Versus Arthritis, for obesity prevention strategies to be implemented across life to reduce risk of osteoarthritis.[101]

The role of lifetime obesity in the development of osteoporosis is less clear. For many years, it was widely believed that obesity was protective against osteoporosis, in part, because of beneficial effects of increased loading on bone, and because, in postmenopausal women, adipose tissue is a key source of endogenous oestrogen. This is supported by consistent evidence of associations between higher BMI and greater BMD at different ages across life in many different settings.[86,102] While MR analyses provide evidence to suggest that positive associations between BMI, fat mass, and BMD are causal,[76] findings of increased risk of fracture in women who are morbidly obese[103] have highlighted that extreme obesity may also have adverse effects on bone microarchitecture that require further investigation.[104,105]

The association between obesity and sarcopenia is complex—there are plausible reasons to expect changes with age in the scale and direction of associations between obesity and muscle mass and strength that may vary by sex.[106] Existing evidence, predominantly based on smaller, cross-sectional physiological studies, suggests that adiposity has both anabolic and catabolic effects on muscle—in earlier adulthood, increased loading associated with a higher BMI may promote muscle growth and function, especially among men, but by later adulthood, these compensatory mechanisms become less effective, and the catabolic effects of chronic low-grade inflammation and fat infiltration of muscle manifest. This, along with the limitations of using BMI to assess adiposity when it also captures muscle mass, likely explains inconsistencies in current life course findings.[107,108] To be able to clearly establish the implications of the increasing prevalence of obesity and earlier onset of obesity in younger generations on future sarcopenia risk, further research with more rigorous assessment of body composition is required. Ideally, we need to better characterise the associations between adiposity and muscle size, function, and quality at different life stages and formally assess whether associations vary by age and sex. This research would benefit from studies that have measured body fat percentage and fat mass and have ascertained a range of different parameters of muscle, including indicators of muscle quality such as fat infiltration.

7.4.5 Behavioural Risk Factors

There is a growing body of evidence demonstrating the potentially important role of behavioural risk factors across life, including physical activity, smoking, alcohol consumption, and dietary intake, in the development of osteoporosis, sarcopenia, and osteoarthritis. For brevity, we focus on the two that are arguably most important: diet quality and physical activity.

Optimising diet quality and nutrient intake across life is considered to be a key component of many disease prevention strategies, including those targeting age-related musculoskeletal conditions.[101] This is based on observational and experimental evidence reporting on associations between certain dietary patterns and intake of specific food groups, nutrients, and vitamins, and musculoskeletal outcomes.[109-112] Added to which are the important roles of maternal diet in promoting optimal growth of offspring and of a healthy, balanced diet in preventing obesity. However, as highlighted in reviews of the evidence on nutrition across life and osteoporosis, sarcopenia, and osteoarthritis,[109-111] while available studies do demonstrate some relevant associations at different life stages, there are still few studies with longitudinal dietary data that allow for a detailed examination of these associations from a life course perspective.[112-114] Taken together with recent findings from MR analyses of limited evidence of causal associations between vitamin D, milk intake, serum calcium, and BMD,[76] this suggests the need for more life course studies with longitudinal data on dietary patterns and nutritional status, and further causal inference work to interrogate associations found. Owing in part to the acknowledged methodological challenges of studying nutrition in observational studies, this ideally would be complemented by intervention studies to improve dietary intake, quality, and nutritional status with longer term follow-up. Most existing intervention studies have relatively short follow-up periods, and even where benefits are observed on musculoskeletal phenotypes, it is not usually clear whether these translate into reduced risk of osteoporosis, sarcopenia, and osteoarthritis in the longer term.

Many national and international physical activity guidelines now specifically recommend that people of all ages engage in muscle and bone strengthening activities.[115-118] This reflects: (i) growing recognition among policymakers that improving and maintaining musculoskeletal health across life is important, and (ii) the fact that intervention studies have consistently demonstrated that specific exercise regimes, namely those that incorporate weight-bearing activity and resistance training, are most effective at promoting or minimising loss of bone and muscle strength, respectively. As these benefits are observed in intervention studies of children and adults across the full age range, cumulative benefits of engaging in these types of activity would be expected. Although cumulative associations between self-reported leisure time physical activity across adulthood and bone and muscle outcomes have been investigated in some studies, these have not assessed specific types of activity.[119-122] As cumulative associations of leisure time physical activity across adulthood with bone health and grip strength were not observed among women in some of these analyses,[120,122] this suggests that even active women may not be engaging in sufficient levels of the right types of physical activity as part of their usual routines to maximise benefits for their musculoskeletal health. This was confirmed in a study using accelerometers to capture potentially osteogenic vertical impacts that found that many older people, especially women, were experiencing very limited high impact, weight-bearing physical activity as part of their daily lives.[123] This highlights the clear value of making specific recommendations on bone and muscle strengthening activities in physical activity guidelines. While this has been achieved in the latest guidelines, the challenge now is to ensure that these are as widely communicated as other recommendations.[124] As the benefits of muscle and bone strengthening activities at different ages were highlighted in public health documents produced in 2020 to support people's health and well-being during national lockdowns, this suggests progress on this is being made.[125]

Additional insights on physical activity in relation to musculoskeletal health have been gained in recent years with the advent of affordable research-grade wearable accelerometers. While much of this research thus far is cross-sectional, studies relating accelerometry data to musculoskeletal health have been conducted on participants at different life stages. In addition, studies are beginning to emerge examining longitudinal profiles of physical activity derived from repeat accelerometry data in relation to bone that highlight important variations in patterns of activity over time that are differentially associated with outcomes.[126]

Perhaps more important than the insights gained from accelerometers on physical activity are the advances in our understanding of the importance of sedentary behaviour, which had been difficult to characterise reliably using self-report data. Although it has been argued that further evidence is required before specific recommendations on sedentary behaviour can be made[127] using accelerometry data, associations of increased sedentary time with poorer musculoskeletal health independent of time spent active are being reported,[119,128] and general advice on reducing sedentary time, specifically sitting, is now being included in physical activity guidelines.[115] With concerns about the widespread impacts of the strategies taken to suppress the community transmission of COVID-19, including national lockdowns and 'stay at home' orders, on sedentariness and the long-term implications of the resultant deconditioning,[129,130] promoting reductions in sedentary time and participation in specific types of activity beneficial for musculoskeletal health among all age groups has recently become increasingly urgent.

7.4.6 Sociodemographic Factors

Although there is insufficient space to provide a detailed overview of life course research on socioeconomic position, ethnicity, and other sociodemographic factors, it is essential to acknowledge the importance of these influences. This is not least because many of the other factors discussed in this chapter are socioeconomically patterned and vary by ethnicity.

Over the course of 2020, the global COVID-19 pandemic provided a powerful reminder, should one have been needed, of the important implications of inequalities in health driven by socioeconomic disadvantage, ethnicity, age, and gender. As the full scale and reach of the impact of the COVID-19 pandemic is realised, it is going to be important to identify strategies to reduce the stark inequalities in health across life that have been exacerbated in many countries over the last 2 years.[131,132]

Reducing inequalities in age-related musculoskeletal conditions is likely to require action at every life stage. This is especially as there is evidence among women that there are cumulative associations between socioeconomic adversity across life and lower muscle mass in early old age,[133] and that socioeconomic position in earlier life may be associated with age-related declines in grip strength.[134] However, as most research on socioeconomic inequalities in age-related musculoskeletal conditions to date has focused on older adults who have been assessed on only one or a limited number of occasions, further work in studies covering different life stages and with repeat outcome measures is ideally required to elucidate how socioeconomic position relates to different musculoskeletal phenotypes at different life stages and their changes with age. This additional information would aid identification of the timing and design of the most effective strategies for reducing lifetime socioeconomic inequalities in age-related musculoskeletal conditions in current and future generations of older adults. Alongside which is the call for more quantitative research on inequalities that acknowledges its complexity and takes an intersectional approach.[135,136] This would involve taking account of different drivers of inequality including ethnicity, age, and gender, as well as lifetime socioeconomic position within the same models in recognition of the fact that there may be important interactions between these different drivers of inequality and, their impacts are unlikely to be simply additive. So far, life course studies of inequalities in health outcomes including age-related musculoskeletal conditions have tended to focus on single drivers of inequality despite the complementary insights and valuable information to guide strategies on reducing inequalities likely to be provided by an intersectional approach.

7.5 Conclusions

Many national and international organisations are now using a life course framework to develop their strategies on the prevention of age-related musculoskeletal conditions and the promotion of healthy ageing.[101,137] This is testament to the research using a life course approach conducted over the last few decades demonstrating that opportunities may exist at each and every life stage to prevent the onset of age-related musculoskeletal conditions, and the many other adverse outcomes they precipitate. In this chapter, we have summarised recent key findings on genetics, oestrogen, growth, obesity, diet, physical activity, and sociodemographic factors. However, there is still much to elucidate in relation to these life course risk factors and others that existing and new studies will be well positioned to address in the coming years as they embrace further technological and methodological advancements.

Key messages and implications

- Osteoporosis, sarcopenia, and osteoarthritis pose major threats to healthy ageing and are leading contributors to the burden of disease and disability in all world regions especially among women.
- A life course approach has provided new insights on the epidemiology of osteoporosis, sarcopenia, and osteoarthritis.
- Opportunities may exist at each and every life stage to prevent the onset of age-related musculoskeletal conditions and the many adverse outcomes they precipitate.
- Life course findings on growth, obesity, nutrition, physical activity, and sedentariness are informing policy and practice.
- Using a life course framework will be essential to reduce inequalities in age-related musculoskeletal conditions in current and future generations of older adults.

References

1. Briggs AM, Cross MJ, Hoy DG, Sanchez-Riera L, Blyth FM, Woolf AD, et al. Musculoskeletal health conditions represent a global threat to healthy aging: a report for the 2015 World Health Organization World Report on Ageing and Health. *Gerontologist*. 2016;56(Suppl 2):S243–S255.

2. Compston JE, McClung MR, Leslie WD. Osteoporosis. *Lancet*. 2019;393(10169):364–76.

3. Cruz-Jentoft AJ, Sayer AA. Sarcopenia. *Lancet*. 2019;393(10191):2636–46.

4. Hunter DJ, Bierma-Zeinstra S. Osteoarthritis. *Lancet*. 2019;393(10182):1745–59.

5. GBD 2019 Diseases and Injuries Collaborators. Global burden of 369 diseases and injuries in 204 countries and territories, 1990–2019: a systematic analysis for the Global Burden of Disease Study 2019. *Lancet*. 2020;396:1204–22.

6. Sebbag E, Felten R, Sagez F, Sibilia J, Devilliers H, Arnaud L. The world-wide burden of musculoskeletal diseases: a systematic analysis of the World Health Organization Burden of Diseases database. *Annals of the Rheumatic Diseases*. 2019;78(6):844–8.

7. Safiri S, Kolahi AA, Smith E, Hill C, Bettampadi D, Mansournia MA, et al. Global, regional and national burden of osteoarthritis 1990-2017: a systematic analysis of the Global Burden of Disease Study 2017. *Annals of the Rheumatic Diseases*. 2020;79(6):819–28.

8. Borgstrom F, Karlsson L, Ortsater G, Norton N, Halbout P, Cooper C, et al. Fragility fractures in Europe: burden, management and opportunities. *Archives of Osteoporosis*. 2020;15(1):59.

9. Mohd-Tahir NA, Li SC. Economic burden of osteoporosis-related hip fracture in Asia: a systematic review. *Osteoporos International*. 2017;28(7):2035–44.

10. Aziziyeh R, Amin M, Habib M, Garcia Perlaza J, Szafranski K, McTavish RK, et al. The burden of osteoporosis in four Latin American countries: Brazil, Mexico, Colombia, and Argentina. *Journal of Medical Economics*. 2019;22(7):638–44.

11. Norman K, Otten L. Financial impact of sarcopenia or low muscle mass—a short review. *Clinical Nutrition*. 2019;38(4):1489–95.

12. Puig-Junoy J, Ruiz Zamora A. Socio-economic costs of osteoarthritis: a systematic review of cost-of-illness studies. *Seminars in Arthritis and Rheumatism*. 2015;44(5):531–41.

13. Xie F, Kovic B, Jin X, He X, Wang M, Silvestre C. Economic and humanistic burden of osteoarthritis: a systematic review of large sample studies. *Pharmacoeconomics*. 2016;34(11):1087–100.

14. Lewis R, Gomez Alvarez CB, Rayman M, Lanham-New S, Woolf A, Mobasheri A. Strategies for optimising musculoskeletal health in the 21(st) century. *BMC Musculoskeletal Disorders*. 2019;20(1):164.

15. Wolfe RR. The underappreciated role of muscle in health and disease. *American Journal of Clinical Nutrition*. 2006;84(3):475–82.

16. Academy of Medical Sciences. *Multimorbidity: a priority for global health research*. London: Academy of Medical Sciences; 2018.

17. Duffield SJ, Ellis BM, Goodson N, Walker-Bone K, Conaghan PG, Margham T, et al. The contribution of musculoskeletal disorders in multimorbidity: implications for practice and policy. *Best Practice & Research Clinical Rheumatology*. 2017;31(2):129–44.

18. Whitty CJ. Harveian Oration 2017: triumphs and challenges in a world shaped by medicine. *Clinical Medicine (London)*. 2017;17(6):537–44.

19. Jones K, Gordon-Weeks A, Coleman C, Silva M. Radiologically determined sarcopenia predicts morbidity and mortality following abdominal surgery: a systematic review and meta-analysis. *World Journal of Surgery*. 2017;41(9):2266–79.

20. West MA, Wischmeyer PE, Grocott MPW. Prehabilitation and nutritional support to improve perioperative outcomes. *Current Anesthesiology Reports*. 2017;7(4):340–9.

21. Durrand J, Singh SJ, Danjoux G. Prehabilitation. *Clinical Medicine (London)*. 2019;19(6):458–64.

22. Silver JK. Prehabilitation could save lives in a pandemic. *BMJ*. 2020;369:m1386.

23. Cawthon PM. Gender differences in osteoporosis and fractures. *Clinical Orthopaedics and Related Research*. 2011;469(7):1900–5.

24. Srikanth VK, Fryer JL, Zhai G, Winzenberg TM, Hosmer D, Jones G. A meta-analysis of sex differences prevalence, incidence and severity of osteoarthritis. *Osteoarthritis and Cartilage*. 2005;13(9):769–81.

25. Dodds RM, Syddall HE, Cooper R, Benzeval M, Deary IJ, Dennison EM, et al. Grip strength across the life course: normative data from twelve British studies. *PLoS ONE*. 2014;9(12):e113637.

26. Mayhew AJ, Amog K, Phillips S, Parise G, McNicholas PD, de Souza RJ, et al. The prevalence of sarcopenia in community-dwelling older adults, an exploration of differences between studies and within definitions: a systematic review and meta-analyses. *Age and Ageing*. 2019;48(1):48–56.

27. Harvey N, Dennison E, Cooper C. Osteoporosis: a lifecourse approach. *Journal of Bone and Mineral Research*. 2014;29(9):1917–25.
28. Kuh D, Karunananthan S, Bergman H, Cooper R. A life-course approach to healthy ageing: maintaining physical capability. *Proceedings of the Nutrition Society*. 2014:73(2):237–48.
29. Dodds RM, Roberts HC, Cooper C, Sayer AA. The epidemiology of sarcopenia. *Journal of Clinical Densitometry*. 2015;18(4):461–6.
30. Curtis E, Litwic A, Cooper C, Dennison E. Determinants of muscle and bone aging. *Journal of Cellular Physiology*. 2015;230(11):2618–25.
31. Ferrucci L, Cooper R, Shardell M, Simonsick EM, Schrack JA, Kuh D. Age-related change in mobility: perspectives from life course epidemiology and geroscience. *Journal of Gerontology Medical Sciences*. 2016;71:1184–94.
32. Shaw SC, Dennison EM, Cooper C. Epidemiology of sarcopenia: determinants throughout the lifecourse. *Calcified Tissue International*. 2017;101(3):229–47.
33. Bassey J, Sayer AA, Cooper C. A life course approach to musculoskeletal ageing: muscle strength, osteoporosis, and osteoarthritis. In: Kuh D, Hardy R, eds. *A life course approach to women's health*. 1st edition. Oxford: Oxford University Press; 2002. pp. 141–54.
34. Cauley J. Commentary on 'A life course approach to musculoskeletal ageing: muscle strength, osteoporosis, and osteoarthritis'. In: Kuh D, Hardy R, eds. *A life course approach to women's health*. Oxford: Oxford University Press; 2002. pp. 154–60.
35. Sayer AA, Cooper C. A life course approach to biological ageing. In: Kuh D, Ben-Shlomo Y, eds. *A life course approach to chronic disease epidemiology*. 2nd edition. Oxford: Oxford University Press; 2004. pp. 306–23.
36. Ward KA, Adams JE, Prentice A, Sayer AA, Cooper C. A life course approach to healthy musculoskeletal ageing. In: Kuh D, Cooper R, Hardy R, Richards M, Ben-Shlomo Y, eds. *A life course approach to healthy ageing*. Oxford: Oxford University Press; 2014. pp. 162–76.
37. Cooper R, Hardy R, Sayer AA, Kuh D. A life course approach to physical capability. In: Kuh D, Cooper R, Hardy R, Richards M, Ben-Shlomo Y, eds. *A life course approach to healthy ageing*. Oxford: Oxford University Press; 2014. pp. 16–31.
38. Ben-Shlomo Y, Cooper R, Kuh D. The last two decades of life course epidemiology, and its relevance for research on ageing. *International Journal of Epidemiology*. 2016;45(4):973–88.
39. Anker SD, Morley JE, von Haehling S. Welcome to the ICD-10 code for sarcopenia. *Journal of Cachexia, Sarcopenia and Muscle*. 2016;7(5):512–4.
40. World Health Organization. *Assessment of fracture risk and its application to screening for postmenopausal osteoporosis. Report of a WHO study group*. Geneva: World Health Organization; 1994. WHO Technical Report Series 843.
41. Bijlsma AY, Meskers CG, Westendorp RG, Maier AB. Chronology of age-related disease definitions: osteoporosis and sarcopenia. *Ageing Research Reviews*. 2012;11(2):320–4.
42. Cruz-Jentoft AJ, Bahat G, Bauer J, Boirie Y, Bruyere O, Cederholm T, et al. Sarcopenia: revised European consensus on definition and diagnosis. *Age and Ageing*. 2019;48(1):16–31.
43. Cawthon PM. Recent progress in sarcopenia research: a focus on operationalizing a definition of sarcopenia. *Current Osteoporosis Reports*. 2018;16(6):730–7.
44. Kraus VB, Blanco FJ, Englund M, Karsdal MA, Lohmander LS. Call for standardized definitions of osteoarthritis and risk stratification for clinical trials and clinical use. *Osteoarthritis and Cartilage*. 2015;23(8):1233–41.
45. Bedson J, Croft PR. The discordance between clinical and radiographic knee osteoarthritis: a systematic search and summary of the literature. *BMC Musculoskeletal Disorders*. 2008;9:116.
46. Spruit MA, Sillen MJ, Groenen MT, Wouters EF, Franssen FM. New normative values for handgrip strength: results from the UK Biobank. *Journal of the American Medical Directors Association*. 2013;14(10):775e5–e11.
47. Peterson MD, Krishnan C. Growth charts for muscular strength capacity with quantile regression. *American Journal of Preventive Medicine*. 2015;49(6):935–8.
48. Leong DP, Teo KK, Rangarajan S, Kutty VR, Lanas F, Hui C, et al. Reference ranges of handgrip strength from 125,462 healthy adults in 21 countries: a prospective urban rural epidemiologic (PURE) study. *Journal of Cachexia, Sarcopenia and Muscle*. 2016;7(5):535–46.

49. Metter EJ, Conwit R, Tobin J, Fozard JL. Age-associated loss of power and strength in the upper extremities in women and men. *Journals of Gerontology Series A-Biological Sciences and Medical Sciences.* 1997;52(5):B267–B76.

50. Vianna LC, Oliveira RB, Araujo CG. Age-related decline in handgrip strength differs according to gender. *Journal of Strength and Conditioning Research.* 2007;21(4):1310–14.

51. Lauretani F, Bandinelli S, Griswold ME, Maggio M, Semba R, Guralnik JM, et al. Longitudinal changes in BMD and bone geometry in a population-based study. *Journal of Bone and Mineral Research.* 2008;23(3):400–8.

52. Cooper R, Hardy R, Sayer AA, Ben-Shlomo Y, Birnie K, Cooper C, et al. Age and gender differences in physical capability levels from mid-life onwards: the harmonisation and meta-analysis of data from eight UK cohort studies. *PLoS ONE.* 2011;6(11):e27899.

53. Dodds RM, Syddall HE, Cooper R, Kuh D, Cooper C, Sayer AA. Global variation in grip strength: a systematic review and meta-analysis of normative data. *Age and Ageing.* 2016;45(2):209–16.

54. Silva AM, Shen W, Heo M, Gallagher D, Wang Z, Sardinha LB, et al. Ethnicity-related skeletal muscle differences across the lifespan. *American Journal of Human Biology.* 2010;22(1):76–82.

55. Frederiksen H, Hjelmborg J, Mortensen J, Mcgue M, Vaupel JW, Christensen K. Age trajectories of grip strength: cross-sectional and longitudinal data among 8,342 Danes aged 46 to 102. *Annals of Epidemiology.* 2006;16(7):554–62.

56. Mitchell WK, Williams J, Atherton P, Larvin M, Lund J, Narici M. Sarcopenia, dynapenia, and the impact of advancing age on human skeletal muscle size and strength; a quantitative review. *Frontiers in Physiology.* 2012;3:260.

57. Hernandez CJ, Beaupre GS, Carter DR. A theoretical analysis of the relative influences of peak BMD, age-related bone loss and menopause on the development of osteoporosis. *Osteoporosis International.* 2003;14(10):843–7.

58. Hoekstra T, Rojer AGM, van Schoor NM, Maier AB, Pijnappels M. Distinct trajectories of individual physical performance measures across 9 years in 60- to 70-year-old adults. *Journal of Gerontology Medical Sciences.* 2020;75(10):1951–9.

59. Aspden RM, Saunders FR. Osteoarthritis as an organ disease: from the cradle to the grave. *European Cells and Materials.* 2019;37:74–87.

60. Gregory JS, Waarsing JH, Day J, Pols HA, Reijman M, Weinans H, et al. Early identification of radiographic osteoarthritis of the hip using an active shape model to quantify changes in bone morphometric features: can hip shape tell us anything about the progression of osteoarthritis? *Arthritis & Rheumatology.* 2007;56(11):3634–43.

61. Hunter DJ, Deveza LA, Collins JE, Losina E, Nevitt MC, Roemer FW, et al. Multivariable modeling of biomarker data from the phase 1 Foundation for the NIH Osteoarthritis Biomarkers Consortium. *Arthritis Care & Research (Hoboken).* 2022;74(7):1142–53.

62. Kraus VB, Karsdal MA. Osteoarthritis: current molecular biomarkers and the way forward. *Calcified Tissue International.* 2021;109(3):329–38.

63. Parveen B, Parveen A, Vohora D. Biomarkers of osteoporosis: an update. *Endocrine, Metabolic & Immune Disorders - Drug Targets.* 2019;19(7):895–912.

64. Cawthon PM, Blackwell T, Cummings SR, Orwoll ES, Duchowny KA, Kado DM, et al. Muscle mass assessed by the D3-creatine dilution method and incident self-reported disability and mortality in a prospective observational study of community-dwelling older men. *Journal of Gerontology Medical Sciences.* 2021;76(1):123–30.

65. Tan LJ, Liu SL, Lei SF, Papasian CJ, Deng HW. Molecular genetic studies of gene identification for sarcopenia. *Human Genetics.* 2012;131(1):1–31.

66. Jones G, Trajanoska K, Santanasto AJ, Stringa N, Kuo CL, Atkins JL, et al. Genome-wide meta-analysis of muscle weakness identifies 15 susceptibility loci in older men and women. *Nature Communications.* 2021;12(1):654.

67. Reynard LN, Barter MJ. Osteoarthritis year in review 2019: genetics, genomics and epigenetics. *Osteoarthritis and Cartilage.* 2020;28(3):275–84.

68. Yang TL, Shen H, Liu A, Dong SS, Zhang L, Deng FY, et al. A road map for understanding molecular and genetic determinants of osteoporosis. *Nature Reviews Endocrinology.* 2020;16(2):91–103.

69. Pilling LC, Joehanes R, Kacprowski T, Peters M, Jansen R, Karasik D, et al. Gene transcripts associated with muscle strength: a CHARGE meta-analysis of 7,781 persons. *Physiological Genomics*. 2016;48(1):1–11.

70. Karasik D, Cohen-Zinder M. The genetic pleiotropy of musculoskeletal aging. *Frontiers in Physiology*. 2012;3:303.

71. Hackinger S, Trajanoska K, Styrkarsdottir U, Zengini E, Steinberg J, Ritchie GRS, et al. Evaluation of shared genetic aetiology between osteoarthritis and bone mineral density identifies SMAD3 as a novel osteoarthritis risk locus. *Human Molecular Genetics*. 2017;26(19):3850–8.

72. Saul D, Kosinsky RL. Epigenetics of aging and aging-associated diseases. *International Journal of Molecular Sciences*. 2021;22(1):401.

73. Voisin S, Harvey NR, Haupt LM, Griffiths LR, Ashton KJ, Coffey VG, et al. An epigenetic clock for human skeletal muscle. *Journal of Cachexia, Sarcopenia and Muscle*. 2020;11(4):887–98.

74. Kuh D, Muthuri S, Cooper R, Moore A, Mackinnon K, Cooper C, et al. Menopause, reproductive life, hormone replacement therapy, and bone phenotype at age 60–64 years: a British birth cohort. *Journal of Clinical Endocrinology and Metabolism*. 2016;101(10):3827–37.

75. Kuh D, Muthuri SG, Moore A, Cole TJ, Adams JE, Cooper C, et al. Pubertal timing and bone phenotype in early old age: findings from a British birth cohort study. *International Journal of Epidemiology*. 2016;45(4):1113–24.

76. Zheng J, Frysz M, Kemp JP, Evans DM, Davey Smith G, Tobias JH. Use of Mendelian randomization to examine causal inference in osteoporosis. *Frontiers in Endocrinology (Lausanne)*. 2019;10:807.

77. Hussain SM, Cicuttini FM, Alyousef B, Wang Y. Female hormonal factors and osteoarthritis of the knee, hip and hand: a narrative review. *Climacteric*. 2018;21(2):132–9.

78. Nguyen UDT, Saunders FR, Martin KR. Sex difference in OA: is estrogen to be blamed? *European Journal of Rheumatology*. 2021;[in press 26 April 2021].

79. Cooper R, Mishra G, Clennell S, Guralnik J, Kuh D. Menopausal status and physical performance in midlife: findings from a British birth cohort study. *Menopause*. 2008;15(6):1079–85.

80. da Camara SM, Zunzunegui MV, Pirkle C, Moreira MA, Maciel AC. Menopausal status and physical performance in middle aged women: a cross-sectional community-based study in Northeast Brazil. *PLoS ONE*. 2015;10(3):e0119480.

81. Sipila S, Tormakangas T, Sillanpaa E, Aukee P, Kujala UM, Kovanen V, et al. Muscle and bone mass in middle-aged women: role of menopausal status and physical activity. *Journal of Cachexia, Sarcopenia and Muscle*. 2020;11(3):698–709.

82. Dodds R, Denison HJ, Ntani G, Cooper R, Cooper C, Sayer AA, et al. Birth weight and muscle strength: a systematic review and meta-analysis. *Journal of Nutrition, Health & Aging*. 2012;16(7):609–15.

83. Schlussel MM, Vaz JS, Kac G. Birth weight and adult bone mass: a systematic literature review. *Osteoporosis International*. 2010;21(12):1981–91.

84. Baird J, Kurshid MA, Kim M, Harvey N, Dennison E, Cooper C. Does birthweight predict bone mass in adulthood? A systematic review and meta-analysis. *Osteoporosis International*. 2011;22(5):1323–34.

85. Martinez-Mesa J, Restrepo-Mendez MC, Gonzalez DA, Wehrmeister FC, Horta BL, Domingues MR, et al. Life-course evidence of birth weight effects on bone mass: systematic review and meta-analysis. *Osteoporosis International*. 2013;24(1):7–18.

86. Tandon N, Fall CH, Osmond C, Sachdev HP, Prabhakaran D, Ramakrishnan L, et al. Growth from birth to adulthood and peak bone mass and density data from the New Delhi birth cohort. *Osteoporosis International*. 2012;23(10):2447–59.

87. Bann D, Wills A, Cooper R, Hardy R, Aihie SA, Adams J, et al. Birth weight and growth from infancy to late adolescence in relation to fat and lean mass in early old age: findings from the MRC National Survey of Health and Development. *International Journal of Obesity (London)*. 2014;38(1):69–75.

88. World Health Organization. *Essential nutrition actions: improving maternal, newborn, infant and young child health and nutrition*. Geneva: World Health Organization; 2013.

89. Scientific Advisory Committee on Nutrition. *The influence of maternal, fetal and child nutrition on the development of chronic disease in later life*. London: The Stationery Office; 2011.

90. Ward KA, Jarjou L, Prentice A. Long-term effects of maternal calcium supplementation on childhood growth differ between males and females in a population accustomed to a low calcium intake. *Bone*. 2017;103:31–8.

91. Ramakrishnan U, Imhoff-Kunsch B, Martorell R. Maternal nutrition interventions to improve maternal, newborn, and child health outcomes. *Nestle Nutrition Institute Workshop Series*. 2014;78:71–80.

92. Bhutta ZA, Das JK, Rizvi A, Gaffey MF, Walker N, Horton S, et al. Evidence-based interventions for improvement of maternal and child nutrition: what can be done and at what cost? *Lancet*. 2013;382(9890):452–77.

93. NCD Risk Factor Collaboration. Trends in adult body-mass index in 200 countries from 1975 to 2014: a pooled analysis of 1698 population-based measurement studies with 19.2 million participants. *Lancet*. 2016;387:1377–96.

94. Johnson W, Li L, Kuh D, Hardy R. How has the age-related process of overweight or obesity development changed over time? Co-ordinated analyses of individual participant data from five United Kingdom birth cohorts. *PLoS Medicine*. 2015;12(5):e1001828.

95. Zheng H, Chen C. Body mass index and risk of knee osteoarthritis: systematic review and meta-analysis of prospective studies. *BMJ Open*. 2015;5(12):e007568.

96. Lievense AM, Bierma-Zeinstra SM, Verhagen AP, van Baar ME, Verhaar JA, Koes BW. Influence of obesity on the development of osteoarthritis of the hip: a systematic review. *Rheumatology (Oxford)*. 2002;41(10):1155–62.

97. Jiang L, Xie X, Wang Y, Wang Y, Lu Y, Tian T, et al. Body mass index and hand osteoarthritis susceptibility: an updated meta-analysis. *International Journal of Rheumatic Diseases*. 2016;19(12):1244–54.

98. Wills AK, Black S, Cooper R, Coppack RJ, Hardy R, Martin KR, et al. Life course body mass index and risk of knee osteoarthritis at the age of 53 years: evidence from the 1946 British birth cohort study. *Annals of Rheumatic Diseases*. 2012;71(5):655–60.

99. Holliday KL, McWilliams DF, Maciewicz RA, Muir KR, Zhang W, Doherty M. Lifetime body mass index, other anthropometric measures of obesity and risk of knee or hip osteoarthritis in the GOAL case-control study. *Osteoarthritis & Cartilage*. 2011;19(1):37–43.

100. Funck-Brentano T, Nethander M, Moverare-Skrtic S, Richette P, Ohlsson C. Causal factors for knee, hip, and hand osteoarthritis: a Mendelian randomization study in the UK Biobank. *Arthritis & Rheumatology*. 2019;71(10):1634–41.

101. Department of Health and Social Care, Public Health England, and Versus Arthritis. *Musculoskeletal health: a 5 year strategic framework for prevention across the lifecourse*. London: Department of Health and Social Care, Public Health England, and Versus Arthritis; 2019. PHE publications gateway number: GW-477.

102. Felson DT, Zhang Y, Hannan MT, Anderson JJ. Effects of weight and body mass index on bone mineral density in men and women: the Framingham study. *Journal of Bone and Mineral Research*. 1993;8(5):567–73.

103. Cawsey S, Padwal R, Sharma AM, Wang X, Li S, Siminoski K. Women with severe obesity and relatively low bone mineral density have increased fracture risk. *Osteoporosis International*. 2015;26(1):103–11.

104. Gkastaris K, Goulis DG, Potoupnis M, Anastasilakis AD, Kapetanos G. Obesity, osteoporosis and bone metabolism. *Journal of Musculoskeletal and Neuronal Interactions*. 2020;20(3):372–81.

105. Oliveira MC, Vullings J, van de Loo FAJ. Osteoporosis and osteoarthritis are two sides of the same coin paid for obesity. *Nutrition*. 2020;70:110486.

106. Tomlinson DJ, Erskine RM, Morse CI, Winwood K, Onambele-Pearson G. The impact of obesity on skeletal muscle strength and structure through adolescence to old age. *Biogerontology*. 2016;17(3):467–83.

107. Stenholm S, Sallinen J, Koster A, Rantanen T, Sainio P, Heliovaara M, et al. Association between obesity history and hand grip strength in older adults-exploring the roles of inflammation and insulin resistance as mediating factors. *Journal of Gerontology Medical Sciences*. 2011;66(3):341–8.

108. Cooper R, Hardy R, Bann D, Aihie SA, Ward KA, Adams JE, et al. Body mass index from age 15 years onwards and muscle mass, strength, and quality in early old age: findings from the

MRC National Survey of Health and Development. *Journal of Gerontology Medical Sciences*. 2014;69:1253–9.

109. Ward K. Symposium 2: vitamins in muscular and skeletal function musculoskeletal phenotype through the life course: the role of nutrition. *Proceedings of the Nutrition Society*. 2012;71(1):27–37.

110. Robinson S, Cooper C, Aihie SA. Nutrition and sarcopenia: a review of the evidence and implications for preventive strategies. *Journal of Aging Research*. 2012;2012:510801.

111. Thomas S, Browne H, Mobasheri A, Rayman MP. What is the evidence for a role for diet and nutrition in osteoarthritis? *Rheumatology (Oxford)*. 2018;57(Suppl 4):iv61–iv74.

112. Ward KA, Prentice A, Kuh DL, Adams JE, Ambrosini GL. Life course dietary patterns and bone health in later life in a British birth cohort study. *Journal of Bone and Mineral Research*. 2016;31(6):1167–76.

113. Mulla UZ, Cooper R, Mishra GD, Kuh D, Stephen AM. Adult macronutrient intake and physical capability in the MRC National Survey of Health and Development. *Age and Ageing*. 2013;42(1):81–7.

114. Robinson SM, Westbury LD, Cooper R, Kuh D, Ward K, Syddall HE, et al. Adult lifetime diet quality and physical performance in older age: findings from a British birth cohort. *Journal of Gerontology Medical Sciences*. 2018;73(11):1532–7.

115. UK Government Department of Health & Social Care. *UK Chief Medical Officers' physical activity guidelines*. London: UK Government Department of Health & Social Care; 2019.

116. US Department of Health and Human Services. *Physical activity guidelines for Americans, 2nd edition*. Washington, DC: US Department of Health and Human Services; 2018.

117. World Health Organisation. *Global recommendations on physical activity for health*. Geneva: World Health Organisation; 2010.

118. Beck BR, Daly RM, Singh MA, Taaffe DR. Exercise and Sports Science Australia (ESSA) position statement on exercise prescription for the prevention and management of osteoporosis. *Journal of Science and Medicine in Sport*. 2017;20(5):438–45.

119. Bann D, Kuh D, Wills AK, Adams J, Brage S, Cooper R. Physical activity across adulthood in relation to fat and lean body mass in early old age: findings from the Medical Research Council National Survey of Health and Development, 1946–2010. *American Journal of Epidemiology*. 2014;179(10):1197–207.

120. Cooper R, Mishra GD, Kuh D. Physical activity across adulthood and physical performance in midlife: findings from a British birth cohort. *American Journal of Preventive Medicine*. 2011;41(4):376–84.

121. Dodds R, Kuh D, Aihie SA, Cooper R. Physical activity levels across adult life and grip strength in early old age: updating findings from a British birth cohort. *Age and Ageing*. 2013;42(6):794–8.

122. Muthuri SG, Ward KA, Kuh D, Elhakeem A, Adams JE, Cooper R. Physical activity across adulthood and bone health in later life: the 1946 British birth cohort. *Journal of Bone and Mineral Research*. 2019;34(2):252–61.

123. Hannam K, Deere KC, Hartley A, Clark EM, Coulson J, Ireland A, et al. A novel accelerometer-based method to describe day-to-day exposure to potentially osteogenic vertical impacts in older adults: findings from a multi-cohort study. *Osteoporosis International*. 2017;28(3):1001–11.

124. Strain T, Fitzsimons C, Kelly P, Mutrie N. The forgotten guidelines: cross-sectional analysis of participation in muscle strengthening and balance & co-ordination activities by adults and older adults in Scotland. *BMC Public Health*. 2016;16(1):1108.

125. Public Health England. *Health and wellbeing at home—advice and resources for everyone spending more time indoors. [Internet]*. London: Housing Learning and Improvement Network; 2020 [updated 15 June 2020; cited 27 March 2021]. Available from: https://publichealthengland.exposure.co/health-and-wellbeing-at-home.

126. Elhakeem A, Heron J, Tobias JH, Lawlor DA. Physical activity throughout adolescence and peak hip strength in young adults. *JAMA Network Open*. 2020;3(8):e2013463.

127. Stamatakis E, Ekelund U, Ding D, Hamer M, Bauman AE, Lee IM. Is the time right for quantitative public health guidelines on sitting? A narrative review of sedentary behaviour research paradigms and findings. *British Journal of Sports Medicine*. 2019;53(6):377–82.

128. Cooper R, Stamatakis E, Hamer M. Associations of sitting and physical activity with grip strength and balance in mid-life: 1970 British cohort study. *Scandinavian Journal of Medicine & Science in Sports.* 2020;30(12):2371–81.
129. Narici M, De Vito G, Franchi M, Paoli A, Moro T, Marcolin G, et al. Impact of sedentarism due to the COVID-19 home confinement on neuromuscular, cardiovascular and metabolic health: physiological and pathophysiological implications and recommendations for physical and nutritional countermeasures. *European Journal of Sport Science.* 2021;21(4);614–35.
130. Kirwan R, McCullough D, Butler T, Perez de Heredia F, Davies IG, Stewart C. Sarcopenia during COVID-19 lockdown restrictions: long-term health effects of short-term muscle loss. *Geroscience.* 2020;42(6):1547–78.
131. Bambra C, Riordan R, Ford J, Matthews F. The COVID-19 pandemic and health inequalities. *Journal of Epidemiology and Community Health.* 2020;74(11):964–8.
132. Perry BL, Aronson B, Pescosolido BA. Pandemic precarity: COVID-19 is exposing and exacerbating inequalities in the American heartland. *Proceedings of the National Academy of Sciences of the United States of America.* 2021;118(8):e2020685118.
133. Bann D, Cooper R, Wills AK, Adams J, Kuh D. Socioeconomic position across life and body composition in early old age: findings from a British birth cohort study. *Journal of Epidemiology and Community Health.* 2014;68(6):516–23.
134. Kuh D, Hardy R, Blodgett JM, Cooper R. Developmental factors associated with decline in grip strength from midlife to old age: a British birth cohort study. *BMJ Open.* 2019;9(5):e025755.
135. Bauer GR. Incorporating intersectionality theory into population health research methodology: challenges and the potential to advance health equity. *Social Science & Medicine.* 2014;110:10–7.
136. Agenor M. Future directions for incorporating intersectionality into quantitative population health research. *American Journal of Public Health.* 2020;110(6):803–6.
137. Beard J, Officer A, Cassels A. *World report on ageing and health.* Geneva: World Health Organization; 2015.

8

A Life Course Approach to Lung Function Impairment and COPD

Dinh S. Bui and Shyamali C. Dharmage

8.1 Introduction to the Lungs and COPD

The main function of the lungs is to exchange gas to meet the metabolic demands of the body. Through the gas exchange process, oxygen is absorbed into the bloodstream while carbon dioxide is excreted from the bloodstream. Breathing and gas exchange ensure the sufficient supply of oxygen to every tissue and cell in the body. Good lung function is essential for good general health and longevity.

The lungs are primarily constructed by airways and parenchymal lung tissues.[1] Large airways are divided into small airways, which end up with the alveoli. While airways are primarily responsible for the ventilation of the air during breathing, alveoli are functional units for gas exchange. Alveoli are 'air sacs' in which gases exchange through the alveola-capillary membrane. The breathing process is supported by a continuous layer of epithelial cells that line the airways, together with other components of the proximal and distal airway tract, including endothelial and mesenchymal cells, as well as the structural components of the airway walls made up of airway smooth muscle cells and other proteins (e.g. collagens, elastins). As foreign particles and environmental pathogens are inhaled during the process of respiration, airway fluid and components of the airway tract act not only as a physical and mechanical barrier to potential trauma and damage but also as a functional immunological interface, playing a specialised and active role in immunity and host defence.

Airways and alveoli can be influenced at multiple windows by different risk factors throughout the life course, causing lung impairments and chronic lung disease. Accumulating evidence suggests that sex impacts the incidence, susceptibility, and severity of several lung diseases. This is not surprising given sex influences both lung development and physiology (see Section 8.2.3). Impaired lung function imposes a significant health burden. Lung function deficits at any period throughout the life course including impaired lung function in childhood,[2] reduced lung function growth, lower lung function levels in early adulthood,[3,4] and accelerated lung function decline in adulthood[5,6] are associated with all-cause mortality.[5-9] Moreover, impaired lung function is associated with subsequent chronic lung diseases and cardiovascular disorders in late adulthood, which creates further health burdens.[3,10]

One common form of lung function impairment is chronic obstructive deficits that subsequently lead to chronic obstructive pulmonary disease (COPD), the focus of this chapter.

Dinh S. Bui and Shyamali C. Dharmage, *A Life Course Approach to Lung Function Impairment and COPD* In: *A Life Course Approach to Women's Health*. Second Edition. Edited by: Gita D Mishra, Rebecca Hardy, and Diana Kuh, Oxford University Press.
© Oxford University Press 2023. DOI: 10.1093/oso/9780192864642.003.0008

Obstruction of the airways is typically caused by airway inflammation, thickness and remodelling, excessive mucus production, and alveoli destruction. Obstruction of the airways can affect ventilation and, ultimately, lung function capacity. Airway obstruction can be fully or partly reversible or irreversible with the administration of a bronchodilator, a type of medication that relaxes the muscles surrounding the airways. Nonreversible airway obstruction, measured using spirometry (a common breathing test that assesses how well the lungs work), is a criterion for COPD diagnosis.

COPD is now a significant public health problem worldwide. An estimated 392 million people are currently affected by COPD globally,[11] and the prevalence of COPD is predicted to increase in the coming decades because of ageing of the world's population and continued exposure to risk factors.[12] COPD is currently the third leading cause of death, contributing to over three million deaths annually worldwide.[13,14]

There are clear differences between the sexes when it comes to lungs and lung function impairment. Males and females have different lung anatomy (i.e. structure; e.g. difference in diameter of airways) and physiology (i.e. functioning; e.g. difference in lung volume), and aetiology of chronic lung diseases, particularly COPD. Specifically, COPD risk factor exposures, susceptibility to insults, and severity/prognosis of COPD are highly sex specific. The substantial influence of reproductive factors and events through the lifespan on lung health in females is another distinction. Details of such sex differences are discussed in Sections 8.2.3 and 8.3.2.

8.2 The Changes in Lung Function Across the Life Course and COPD

An overview of lung function across the life course and COPD are presented in Sections 8.1 and 8.2. Sex differences are then discussed in Section 8.3.

8.2.1 Life Course of Lung Function

Lung function can be assessed with several tests, of which spirometry is the most common. Spirometry measures dynamic lung volumes and ventilatory capacity of the lungs and assesses how effectively and quickly the lungs can be filled or emptied. Parameters from a spirometry test include forced expiratory volume in the first second (FEV_1), forced vital capacity (FVC), FEV_1/FVC ratio, forced expiratory flow over the middle half of the FVC ($FEF_{25\%-75\%}$), and peak expiratory flow rate (PEF) (see Table 8.1 for definitions).

As spirometry parameters are dependent on sex, age, height, and ethnicity, they are often standardised to the healthy population using reference equations (e.g. GLI reference equations[15]), giving predicted values, percent of predicted values, and z-scores for spirometry parameters (see Table 8.1 for definitions).

Across the life course, there are distinct physiological phases of lung function changes. Lung development takes place from the early weeks of gestation and spans to the early postnatal years.[16] The lungs then expand through childhood to adolescence and early adulthood and ends with peak lung function attained around 20–25 years of age. During early to midadulthood, there is a plateau phase when lung function is relatively stable. The plateau

Table 8.1 Parameters of a spirometry test for lung function and statistical terminology

Spirometry Parameter	Measurement
Forced expiratory volume in the first second (FEV$_1$)	The volume of air expired in the first second with maximal expiration (a forced manoeuvre) after a full inspiration and a physiological measure of elastic recoil and patent airways
Forced vital capacity (FVC)	The maximal volume of air expired during a forced manoeuvre and a physiological measure of reduced lung volume, gas trapping, or poor test effort
FEV$_1$/FVC ratio	The magnitude of airflow obstruction
Forced expiratory flow over the middle half of the FVC (FEF$_{25\%-75\%}$)	The average flow of air expired during the middle half of a forced manoeuvre
Peak expiratory flow rate (PEF)	The maximal flow of air during a forced manoeuvre
Statistical terminology	**Definition**
Predicted value	The mean value of the population of the same age, sex, height, and ethnicity
Percent of predicted value	The percentage of the observed value out of its predicted value
Z-score	The number of standard deviations one observed value deviates from the population mean or its predicted value (i.e. z-score has a mean of 0; 68% of the population falls in one standard deviation or z-score between -1 and 1; 95% within approximately two standard deviations or z-score between −1.96 and 1.96)

phase is followed by a decline phase from mid to late adulthood, in which lung function declines gradually with ageing. The combination of these phases, so-called lifetime lung function patterns or trajectories, determine lung function outcomes in older age.

Exposure to risk factors may result in lung impairment at different physiological phases throughout the life course. These include impaired lung development, reduced lung growth, suboptimal peak lung function, early decline, and accelerated decline. Individuals may have their own profile of exposures across the life course and thus have their own distinct lifetime lung function trajectory.

There has been significant research interest in lifetime lung function trajectories. Impaired lung function at one or more life stages is associated with subsequent chronic lung diseases, particularly COPD.[10,17,18] These diseases are commonly only diagnosed in older age when lung function impairment has already reached a critical threshold. Lifetime lung function trajectories can provide valuable information on the pathogenesis of the disease. Although information on the lifetime lung function trajectory can guide optimal treatment and management of chronic lung diseases, particularly COPD, it has been difficult to research because of a lack of studies with longitudinal lung function data throughout life. Recently, the Tasmanian Longitudinal Health Study was the first to provide unique information on population lung function trajectories from the first to the sixth decade of life.[19] This study reported six distinct lung function trajectories (see Figure 8.1) and provided insights into lung function trajectories leading to COPD.[19]

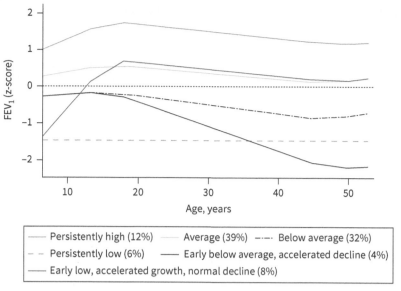

Figure 8.1 Lung function trajectories leading to COPD (reproduced from Bui et al., 2018,[19] with permission). FEV_1 was presented in z-scores (standardised for age, height, and sex), with a z-score of zero representing the population average. Individuals in the 'average' trajectory had lung function levels around the population average (z-score around 0) at any time. Individuals in the 'persistently low' trajectory had low childhood lung function, which then grew and declined at the population average rate. Individuals in the 'persistently high' trajectory had high childhood lung function, which then grew and declined at the population average rate. Individuals in the 'early low, accelerated growth, normal decline' trajectory had low childhood lung function, which then grew at a greater rate than the population average rate, but declined at the population average rate. Individuals in the 'early below average, accelerated decline' trajectory had childhood lung function below the population average and lung function declined at a greater rate than the population average rate. Individuals in the 'below average' trajectory had childhood lung function below the population average, which then grew and declined at the population average rate. Three trajectories, namely 'persistently low', 'early below average, accelerated decline', and 'below average', had increased risk of developing COPD by age 53 years. See plate section.

8.2.2 Life Course Perspective of Chronic Obstructive Pulmonary Disease

COPD is defined as 'a common, preventable and treatable disease that is characterised by persistent respiratory symptoms and airflow limitation that is due to airway and/or alveolar abnormalities usually caused by significant exposure to noxious particles or gases'.[12] As the hallmark of COPD, airflow limitation (fixed airflow obstruction) is defined as the ratio of postbronchodilator force expiratory volume in the first second to forced vital capacity (FEV_1/ FVC) below a certain cut-off (e.g. 0.7 or lower limit of normal derived from reference equations). COPD is often diagnosed in patients aged in their sixties when their lung function impairment reaches these conventional thresholds.

The traditional view is that COPD is a disease of adult male smokers with accelerated lung function decline as the hallmark.[20] However, these dogmas of COPD have since been overturned. Smoking is no longer the only risk factor for COPD, and many other risk factors are now known to contribute.[21] Moreover, it is now recognised that COPD can develop from both an accelerated lung function decline in adulthood and/or a reduced lung function level before early adult life.[17,19]

COPD is now increasingly viewed from a life course point of view. Although COPD often manifests and is diagnosed in older age, it is only the end product of lung function impairments throughout life. Landmark studies on lung function trajectories have provided novel evidence to support the role of lifetime lung function impairments in COPD.[17,19] For example, three different lung function trajectories have been found to be associated with COPD with two of them having lower lung function from childhood (see Figure 8.1).[19] Moreover, there is recent interest in 'early COPD', which is now a new field of research. *Early COPD* refers to the point when lung function impairment that leads to later life COPD first commences. It has also been shown that a number of risk factors operating throughout life can increase the risk of COPD development (see Section 8.3.1).

8.2.3 Lungs and COPD: Sex Differences

There are major differences in lung anatomy and physiology and natural history of lung function between the sexes. Females have smaller lungs and airways than males, and for any given age and height, lung function levels are lower in females than males.[22] Moreover, lung function reaches the maximally attained level, and the plateau phase earlier in females (around 20 years) than in males (around 25 years). These biological discrepancies may partly contribute to increased susceptibility and have implications for the pathology and progression of chronic lung diseases and lung deficits in females.[23]

The pathogenesis and prognosis of COPD in females differ from those in males. Females are more likely to develop COPD at a younger age[23] and females also appear to have more severe COPD, increased reactivity and narrowing of the airways, more shortness of breath, and lower self-reported health status and quality of life compared to males with COPD.[24–26] COPD appears to have sex-specific phenotypes, with small airways disease being more common in female COPD, and emphysema being more common in male COPD.[25] Moreover, females with severe COPD are more likely to have a poorer prognosis with greater risk of hospitalisation and death from respiratory failure and comorbidities compared to males with severe COPD.[27]

COPD in females has become an emerging public health issue. Until recently, COPD was considered a disease of males, and COPD in females was neglected for decades. However, it is now evident that COPD in females is also highly prevalent and has substantial burden. A recent large systematic review and meta-analysis on sex-specific COPD included 156 population-based studies and reported a global COPD prevalence of 6.16% in females compared to 9.23% in males.[28] Although the global prevalence of COPD is still lower in females than in males, this difference is no longer significant in many developed countries.[28,29] Notably, there is some evidence for a more rapid increase in the prevalence and mortality of COPD in females than in males in recent decades.[30,31] It is believed that the increase in morbidity and mortality from COPD in females drove the overall increase seen in the population as a whole over the past decades.[32]

Despite the increasing prevalence and burden of COPD in females, COPD in females is still undertreated. This is partly because COPD is more commonly underdiagnosed in females than in males.[33,34] Spirometry tests, which are needed for COPD diagnosis, and referrals to pulmonologists are less commonly ordered for females than males at clinics[23] and the long-lasting perception of COPD as a male disease among healthcare workers may contribute to this underdiagnosis.[23]

In summary, COPD is now recognised to be sex specific. COPD in females is characterised by its own pattern of risk factors, disease pathogenesis, presentation, and prognosis as well as by disparity in diagnosis and treatment (see Figure 8.2).[35]

8.3 Life Course Risk Factors for Lung Function Impairment and COPD

8.3.1 Risk factors for Lung Function Deficits and COPD Throughout the Life Course

It is believed that genetic and environmental factors and their interactions all contribute to lung function deficits and COPD (see Figure 8.3). Individuals may be exposed to environmental risk factors at any life stage, which can cause not only acute but also long-term lung impairment.

During adulthood, exposures can cause accelerated lung function decline and subsequent COPD. While smoking is an established risk factor for lung function decline and COPD,[36] the contribution of other adult exposures and clinical conditions including occupational exposures,[37] air pollution,[38,39] asthma,[36,40] and obesity[39] is now evident. Moreover, adult risk factors also interact in a multiplicative manner, augmenting the adverse effect of each other. An example is the interaction between adult smoking and asthma on COPD.[41] Notably, genetic factors and early life exposures may increase the susceptibility to the impact of adult exposures on lung function decline and COPD.[39] Besides an accelerated rate of lung function decline, it is proposed that adult exposures may be associated with a shortened plateau phase and earlier commencement of the decline phase. Although there are suggestions of such associations for smoking and asthma,[42] factors influencing the plateau phase are still poorly understood.

Exposures during childhood and adolescence influence lung function growth leading to suboptimal peak lung function in early adulthood. Childhood asthma, particularly persistent asthma, is a major factor associated with reduced lung function growth.[43] Respiratory infections are another risk factor for reduced lung function growth.[44] There is also strong evidence from longitudinal studies for the association between indoor and/or ambient air pollution exposure and reduced lung function growth.[45,46] Similarly, exposure to environmental tobacco smoke and active smoking during adolescence adversely affect lung function growth.[47,48]

A number of factors in utero can affect lung development. Parental smoking, particularly maternal smoking during gestation, is a well-established risk factor for impaired lung function in infancy and childhood.[49] Maternal diet and nutrition also play an important role, with a high-fat maternal diet associated with impaired lung development.[50] Similarly, air pollution exposure during gestation has been found to adversely affect lung development.[51,52]

TOBACCO USE

Prevalence:
- Varies by location
- Equal to men in some countries
- Increasing in many developing countries

In women with COPD there is evidence of:
- Greater harm vs men for same level of tobacco smoke exposure
- Greater benefits of smoking cessation
- More difficulty with smoking cessation vs men

OCCUPATIONAL EXPOSURES

Women now work more frequently in traditionally male occupations

In some locations, women are more likely than men to be exposed to risks from unregulated 'cottage' industries, such as fish smoking and textile working

NON-OCCUPATIONAL EXPOSURES

Biomass fuel exposure greater as a result of more domestic responsibilities

UNDER-DIAGNOSIS AND SUBOPTIMAL TREATMENT

Women with COPD are more likely to be misdiagnosed, potentially leading to suboptimal treatment

COPD DISEASE PRESENTATION

Women are generally younger, smoke less and have lower BMI than men
Evidence of more dyspnea

SOCIOECONOMIC STATUS

Women with COPD are likely to be of lower socioeconomic status than men

COPD DISEASE PRESENTATION

Differential burden of comobidities in women vs men
More asthma, osteoporosis and depression vs men
Evidence of greater psychological impairment in women vs men

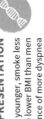

Figure 8.2 Distinct characteristics of COPD in females (reproduced from Jenkin et al.,[35] with permission).

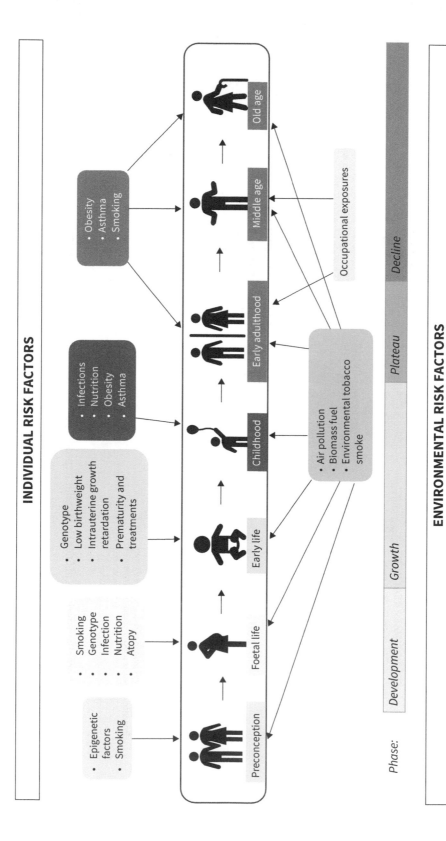

INDIVIDUAL RISK FACTORS

- Epigenetic factors
- Smoking

- Smoking
- Genotype
- Infection
- Nutrition
- Atopy

- Genotype
- Low birthweight
- Intrauterine growth retardation
- Prematurity and treatments

- Infections
- Nutrition
- Obesity
- Asthma

- Obesity
- Asthma
- Smoking

Preconception | Foetal life | Early life | Childhood | Early adulthood | Middle age | Old age

ENVIRONMENTAL RISK FACTORS

- Air pollution
- Biomass fuel
- Environmental tobacco smoke

Occupational exposures

Phase: Development | Growth | Plateau | Decline

Figure 8.3 Life course risk factors for lung function deficits and COPD (Courtesy of Dr Raisa Cassim, the University of Melbourne). See plate section.

There is emerging evidence for the adverse effect of preconception exposures on respiratory health in offspring. Maternal occupational exposure to indoor cleaning and paternal exposure to welding before conception have been found to be associated with an increased risk of childhood asthma in offspring.[53,54] Similarly, an association between exposure to air pollution before age 18 years in mothers and childhood asthma in their offspring was reported.[55,56] Fathers smoking during their own adolescence and mothers' exposure to tobacco smoke during their own gestation are associated with asthma in offspring.[54] Epigenetic changes in relation to preconception exposures are proposed as a mechanism for these associations. However, more research is needed to establish robust evidence.

8.3.2 Specific Risk and Increased Susceptibility in Females

8.3.2.1 Different Contribution of Major Exposures in Females

The contribution of major risk factors for lung function deficits and COPD in females is different from that in males (Figure 8.3). Females are more commonly exposed to some risk factors but less commonly exposed to other factors. Clear differences are seen between the sexes for major risk factors including smoking, occupational exposure, and indoor air pollution.

Smoking has been a long-established risk factor for lung function impairment and COPD, but its role among genders is changing. Smoking has been constantly highly prevalent in males and, as such, has been the major risk factor for male COPD. In fact, COPD has been long considered as a disease of adult male smokers.[20] In contrast, the role of smoking in female COPD was previously relatively minimal as smoking prevalence was much lower in females than in males. However, the number of ever smoking females has increased in recent decades in many countries.[57] This age-period-cohort effect increase has contributed to a sharp rise in total COPD prevalence and made smoking a major risk factor for female COPD.

Indoor air pollution exposure, particularly from biomass burning, is a major risk factor for lung function deficits and COPD in females. A meta-analysis revealed that females exposed to biomass smoke had a 2.65-fold increase in COPD risk.[58] Approximately three billion people still rely on biomass as an energy source globally; however, females are much more commonly exposed and affected than males.[59] This is particularly an issue in LMICs where biomass is widely used for cooking and heating, and women are responsible for cooking and spend more time indoors.[59] In these countries, biomass smoke exposure is a main contributing factor of female COPD.[21] Promisingly, trials in LMICs have provided evidence that improved cooking fuels and kitchen ventilation reduced the rate of lung function decline and incidence of COPD in females.[58,60–62]

High-risk occupational exposure is another major contributing factor to poor lung health and COPD in females. Females are vulnerable as they are the main labour force in some of the high-risk industries in many countries. For example, three quarters of the global garment workforce are female.[63] In Australia, 86% of the hairdressing workforce and 93% of hair and beauty salon assistants are female.[64] Females are also more likely to be exposed from occupational and domestic cleaning.[65] Studies have shown that workers in the garment industry, particularly in LMICs, are exposed to high levels of dusts and have an increased risk of accelerated lung function decline and COPD.[66] Workers in the hair and beauty industry are highly exposed to dusts, fumes, and solvents, and such exposures are associated with higher risk of impaired lung function and COPD.[67,68] Similarly, exposure to chemicals from occupational and domestic cleaning is associated with accelerated rate of lung function decline and COPD in females.[69] In addition to the high-risk traditionally female industries, females now work more frequently in traditionally male occupations (e.g. construction, mining, and transportation), leading to higher COPD burden.

8.3.2.2 Increased Susceptibility for Risk Factors in Females

It is suggested that females may be more susceptible to the impact of some risk factors compared to males, which highlights the importance of understanding female-specific risk factors for COPD. There is evidence from a systematic review that female smokers had a more rapid rate of lung function decline than male smokers even though they smoked less.[70] The loss of lung function per pack-year of smoking was found to be greater in females than males.[27] Similarly, in individuals with COPD who had a low level of smoking exposure, female gender was associated with worse lung function and more severe disease.[30] Similar to cigarette smoke, it is postulated that females are also more susceptible to the adverse impacts of other environmental exposures such as biomass smoke and occupational exposures. Such heightened susceptibility in females may be explained by different mechanisms. Biologically, the difference in cigarette metabolism between the sexes may contribute to an increased female susceptibility.[71] Moreover, females have anatomically smaller lungs and airways, which leads to a greater exposure per unit area for a given amount of cigarette smoke, thus leading to more deleterious effects.[72] More recently, it has been hypothesised that sex hormones play an important role in the heightened susceptibility to lung function impairment and COPD in females.[22,73] This hypothesis is biologically plausible given the substantial changes in sex hormones during the life course in females and that these are putative mediators of respiratory health, and regulate bronchodilation, cell proliferation, and inflammation.

8.4 The Role of Reproductive Exposures in Lung Function Impairment and COPD in Females

The sex hormone hypothesis has been investigated using observational markers of endogenous and exogenous hormonal exposures, such as age at menarche, age at menopause, the use of exogenous hormones (e.g. hormonal contraceptives and menopausal hormone therapy (MHT)), menstrual irregularity, pregnancy, and polycystic ovary syndrome. While some associations have been recorded, the exact mechanisms underpinning the associations between reproductive exposures and respiratory outcomes in women remains unclear. Overall, it has been hypothesised that these associations stem from a combination of intrinsic or genetic differences, response to environmental stimuli, and, perhaps most importantly, sex hormone signalling effects.[24,74] To this point, there is further biological evidence to suggest that the actions of sex hormones and other reproductive factors, including corresponding receptors and coregulators, can have widespread effects on a range of cellular pathways and functions throughout the body.[24,75-77]

Until recently, the link between related reproductive exposures and respiratory health has been mainly investigated using observational designs. There has been recent interest to apply Mendelian randomization (MR) study design to explore these associations. These MR studies have supported, as well as contradicted, some observational findings. Overall, we know little about these reproductive event indicators in relation to lung function deficits and

COPD risk. The existing knowledge on the associations between reproductive events related to major hormonal changes and lung function and COPD are described Sections 8.4.1–8.4.3.

8.4.1 Menarche

Adolescence is an important period that is accompanied by significant sex-dependent changes (e.g. puberty and rapid growth), and it is also a critical period for the maturation of lung function (see Section 8.2.1). Two key epidemiological studies, the European Community Respiratory Health Survey and Tasmanian Longitudinal Health Study,[78,79] have suggested that women reporting early menarche are at a higher risk of impaired adult lung function patterns that are related to both obstructive and restrictive lung disease. On the other hand, the Tasmanian Longitudinal Health Study also found that those who reach menarche early have had better lung function in childhood. Confirming these observational findings, a MR study showed that genetic proxies for early age at menarche are associated with improved adolescent lung function but impaired adult lung function.[80] However, it is not known whether those with early menarche are able to reach the optimal peak lung function and whether they reach the peak earlier than those with normal menarche, which warrants further investigation. Studies investigating age at menarche in relation to COPD are particularly scarce. The UK Biobank study indicated that late menarche, categorised as over 15 years of age, but not early menarche (age < 12 years), was associated with higher risk of COPD-related hospitalisation or death.[81]

8.4.2 Menopause

Studies have suggested that the menopausal transition (e.g. menopausal status, age at menopause) is associated with changes in respiratory health outcomes. The majority of studies investigating the relationship between menopausal status and objective lung function outcomes have documented postmenopausal status to be associated with reduced non-obstructive, but not obstructive, lung function deficits.[82–87] Contrary to observational findings, a MR study found genetic proxies for early menopause (before the age of 45 years) was associated with a reduced risk of obstructive lung function deficits, compared to normal menopause (45–55 years).[88] Further studies are warranted to better understand the inconsistency between the two types of studies and to investigate the underlying mechanisms and role of female sex hormones. There is only limited research into the direct link between menopause and COPD. The UK Biobank study reported an association between early menopause (age < 47) and increased risk of COPD-related hospitalisation or death.[81]

8.4.3 Exogenous Hormones: Hormonal Contraceptives and Menopausal Hormone Therapy

Few observational or intervention studies have investigated the associations between hormonal contraceptives and MHT and respiratory health outcomes, including lung function parameters. In this limited literature, the study methods and quality, collection of exposure data (e.g. duration of use, age at use), and parameters used to assess lung function outcomes are highly inconsistent. A recent systematic review deemed the experimental studies on MHT to be heterogenous, of low quality, and of bias.[89]

Although only a few studies have been conducted, most—including small experimental studies—have found evidence of a slight beneficial effect of hormonal contraceptive use and MHT on various lung function measures.[90–96] In observational studies, these associations were independent of potential confounders that are associated with both the use of hormones and lung function.[97] It has been proposed that the type of MHT preparation (e.g. oestrogen-progesterone or oestrogen-only) may influence the extent to which it may impact lung function parameters. Given the limited collection of literature, further work is needed to truly begin to understand the relationship between exogenous hormonal use and lung function parameters.

8.5 Life Course Approach for Lung Health

Lung function in older age is the end product of lung function throughout the life course. The lungs pass through different physiological phases of development and decline, and impairment can be acquired at one or more phases, creating distinct longitudinal trajectories. When studying COPD, it is important to take a life course approach. In other words, in addition to COPD diagnosis at a time in older age, it is of importance to examine the lifetime lung function trajectories that lead to COPD. This knowledge would help identify COPD phenotypes, optimise diagnosis and management, and inform drug development.

Exposures to risk factors can happen at different stages throughout the life course, and their impact on lifetime lung function is complex. In fact, the combination of timing, type, duration, and severity of exposures determine the adverse impact of risk factors.[98] Some early life exposures have long-term impacts on later life, even without ongoing exposures.[99] Moreover, early life exposures can interact with adulthood exposures.[39] This creates a complex web of exposures throughout the life course. For example, many reproductive health events, such as menarche, menopause, and hormonal use, all affect lung function and COPD. Thus, a life course approach that comprehensively considers the profile of lifetime exposures or 'exposome' is needed for risk prediction and COPD phenotyping.

8.6 Conclusions

COPD, an adverse outcome of lung function impairment, is a prevalent and burdensome public health problem. A more rapid increase in the prevalence and mortality of COPD in females has been observed in recent decades, and it is now believed that the increase in female COPD morbidity and mortality actually drove the overall increase seen in the population as a whole over the past decades. These sex-specific observations may be related to both the increasing exposure to harmful factors and the high susceptibility to these risk factors in females, which has led to hypotheses that sex hormones interact with environmental exposures and influence respiratory health. Biological knowledge of the reproductive system components, including their hormonal elements, clearly support the potential for sex hormones to modulate physiological and immunological functions of the respiratory system. Given the complexity of lifetime lung function trajectories, the natural history of COPD, and profiles of lifetime adverse exposures, it is necessary to adopt a life course approach to combat the increasing global burden of COPD. In the context of promoting women's health, the potential causal factors of heightened susceptibility in females should be further investigated to help develop female-specific COPD interventions.

Key messages and implications

- There are distinct developmental and physiological phases of lung function throughout the life course, and exposure to risk factors in one or more phases may result in lung impairment and subsequent lung diseases, particularly COPD.
- Accumulating evidence shows that females have more exposure to some major risk factors for COPD and increased susceptibility to others; however, as it is still viewed as a disease for males, COPD remains underdiagnosed and undertreated in females.
- A limited number of studies have shown that early menarche and early menopause are associated with altered lung function; however, the impact of female reproductive events on lung function trajectories across the life course requires further investigation.

References

1. Cotes JE, Chinn DJ, Miller MR. *Lung function: physiology, measurement and application in medicine*. Oxford: Blackwell Publishing; 2006.
2. Meszaros D, Dharmage SC, Matheson MC, Venn A, Wharton CL, Johns DP, et al. Poor lung function and tonsillectomy in childhood are associated with mortality from age 18 to 44. *Respiratory Medicine*. 2010;104(6):808–15.
3. Agusti A, Noell G, Brugada J, Faner R. Lung function in early adulthood and health in later life: a transgenerational cohort analysis. *Lancet Respiratory Medicine*. 2017;5(12):935–45.
4. Vasquez MM, Zhou M, Hu C, Martinez FD, Guerra S. Low lung function in young adult life is associated with early mortality. *American Journal of Respiratory and Critical Care Medicine*. 2017;195(10):1399–401.
5. Mannino DM, Reichert MM, Davis KJ. Lung function decline and outcomes in an adult population. *American Journal of Respiratory and Critical Care Medicine*. 2006;173(9):985–90.
6. Mannino DM, Davis KJ. Lung function decline and outcomes in an elderly population. *Thorax*. 2006;61(6):472–7.
7. Ryan G, Knuiman MW, Divitini ML, James A, Musk AW, Bartholomew HC. Decline in lung function and mortality: the Busselton Health Study. *Journal of Epidemiology and Community Health*. 1999;53(4):230–4.
8. Baughman P, Marott JL, Lange P, Martin CJ, Shankar A, Petsonk EL, et al. Combined effect of lung function level and decline increases morbidity and mortality risks. *European Journal of Epidemiology*. 2012;27(12):933–43.
9. Schunemann HJ, Dorn J, Grant BJ, Winkelstein WJ, Trevisan M. Pulmonary function is a long-term predictor of mortality in the general population: 29-year follow-up of the Buffalo Health Study. *Chest*. 2000;118(3):656–64.
10. Agarwal SK, Heiss G, Barr RG, Chang PP, Loehr LR, Chambless LE, et al. Airflow obstruction, lung function, and risk of incident heart failure: the Atherosclerosis Risk in Communities (ARIC) Study. *European Journal of Heart Failure*. 2012;14(4):414–22.

11. Adeloye D, Song P, Zhu Y, Campbell H, Sheikh A, Rudan I; NIHR RESPIRE Global Respiratory Health Unit. Global, regional, and national prevalence of, and risk factors for, chronic obstructive pulmonary disease (COPD) in 2019: a systematic review and modelling analysis. *The Lancet Respiratory Medicine.* 2022;10(5):447–58.

12. Global Initiative for Chronic Obstructive Lung Disease (GOLD). *Global strategy for the diagnosis, management, and prevention of chronic obstructive pulmonary disease.* Global Initiative for Chronic Obstructive Lung Disease.

13. Global Burden of Disease 2016 Causes of Death Collaborators. Global, regional, and national age-sex specific mortality for 264 causes of death, 1980–2016: a systematic analysis for the Global Burden of Disease Study 2016. *Lancet.* 2017;390(10100):1151–210.

14. World Health Organization. *The top 10 causes of death.* [Internet]. World Health Organization; 2020 [Cited 01 March 2023]. Available from: https://www.who.int/news-room/fact-sheets/detail/the-top-10-causes-of-death

15. Quanjer PH, Stanojevic S, Cole TJ, Baur X, Hall GL, Culver BH, et al. Multi-ethnic reference values for spirometry for the 3–95 year age range: the global lung function 2012 equations: report of the Global Lung Function Initiative (GLI), ERS Task Force to establish improved lung function reference values. *European Respiratory Journal.* 2012;40(6):1324–43.

16. Merkus PJ, ten Have-Opbroek AA, Quanjer PH. Human lung growth: a review. *Pediatric Pulmonology.* 1996;21(6):383–97.

17. Lange P, Celli B, Agustí A, Boje Jensen G, Divo M, Faner R, et al. Lung-function trajectories leading to chronic obstructive pulmonary disease. *New England Journal of Medicine.* 2015;373(2):111–22.

18. Engstrom G, Melander O, Hedblad B. Population-based study of lung function and incidence of heart failure hospitalisations. *Thorax.* 2010;65(7):633–8.

19. Bui DS, Lodge CJ, Burgess JA, Lowe AJ, Perret J, Bui MQ, et al. Childhood predictors of lung function trajectories and future COPD risk: a prospective cohort study from the first to the sixth decade of life. *Lancet Respiratory medicine.* 2018;6(7):535–44.

20. Fletcher C, Peto R. The natural history of chronic airflow obstruction. *British Medical Journal.* 1977;1(6077):1645–8.

21. Salvi SS, Barnes PJ. Chronic obstructive pulmonary disease in non-smokers. *Lancet.* 2009;374(9691):733–43.

22. LoMauro A, Aliverti A. Sex differences in respiratory function. *Breathe (Sheffield, England).* 2018;14(2):131–40.

23. Gut-Gobert C, Cavaillès A, Dixmier A, Guillot S, Jouneau S, Leroyer C, et al. Women and COPD: do we need more evidence? *European Respiratory Review: An Official Journal of the European Respiratory Society.* 2019;28(151):180055.

24. Townsend EA, Miller VM, Prakash YS. Sex differences and sex steroids in lung health and disease. *Endocrine Reviews.* 2012;33(1):1–47.

25. Martinez FJ, Curtis JL, Sciurba F, Mumford J, Giardino ND, Weinmann G, et al. Sex differences in severe pulmonary emphysema. *American Journal of Respiratory and Critical Care Medicine.* 2007;176(3):243–52.

26. Camp PG, Coxson HO, Levy RD, Pillai SG, Anderson W, Vestbo J, et al. Sex differences in emphysema and airway disease in smokers. *Chest.* 2009;136(6):1480–8.

27. Prescott E, Bjerg AM, Andersen PK, Lange P, Vestbo J. Gender difference in smoking effects on lung function and risk of hospitalization for COPD: results from a Danish longitudinal population study. *European Respiratory Journal.* 1997;10(4):822–7.

28. Ntritsos G, Franek J, Belbasis L, Christou MA, Markozannes G, Altman P, et al. Gender-specific estimates of COPD prevalence: a systematic review and meta-analysis. *International Journal of Chronic Obstructive Pulmonary Disease.* 2018;13:1507–14.

29. Mannino DM, Buist AS. Global burden of COPD: risk factors, prevalence, and future trends. *Lancet.* 2007;370(9589):765–73.

30. Sørheim IC, Johannessen A, Gulsvik A, Bakke PS, Silverman EK, DeMeo DL. Gender differences in COPD: are women more susceptible to smoking effects than men? *Thorax.* 2010;65(6):480–5.

31. Aryal S, Diaz-Guzman E, Mannino DM. Influence of sex on chronic obstructive pulmonary disease risk and treatment outcomes. *International Journal of Chronic Obstructive Pulmonary Disease*. 2014;9:1145–54.

32. Barnes PJ. Sex differences in chronic obstructive pulmonary disease mechanisms. *American Journal of Respiratory and Critical Care Medicine*. 2016;193(8):813–4.

33. Ancochea J, Miravitlles M, García-Río F, Muñoz L, Sánchez G, Sobradillo V, et al. Underdiagnosis of chronic obstructive pulmonary disease in women: quantification of the problem, determinants and proposed actions. *Archivos de bronconeumologia*. 2013;49(6):223–9.

34. Chapman KR, Tashkin DP, Pye DJ. Gender bias in the diagnosis of COPD. *Chest*. 2001;119(6):1691–5.

35. Jenkins CR, Chapman KR, Donohue JF, Roche N, Tsiligianni I, Han MK. Improving the management of COPD in women. *Chest*. 2017;151(3):686–96.

36. James AL, Palmer LJ, Kicic E, Maxwell PS, Lagan SE, Ryan GF, et al. Decline in lung function in the Busselton Health Study: the effects of asthma and cigarette smoking. *American Journal of Respiratory and Critical Care Medicine*. 2005;171(2):109–14.

37. Liao S-Y, Lin X, Christiani DC. Occupational exposures and longitudinal lung function decline. *American Journal of Industrial Medicine*. 2015;58(1):14–20.

38. Rice MB, Ljungman PL, Wilker EH, Dorans KS, Gold DR, Schwartz J, et al. Long-term exposure to traffic emissions and fine particulate matter and lung function decline in the Framingham heart study. *American Journal of Respiratory and Critical Care Medicine*. 2015;191(6):656–64.

39. Bui DS, Perret JL, Walters EH, Abramson MJ, Burgess JA, Bui MQ, et al. Lifetime risk factors for pre- and post-bronchodilator lung function decline. A population-based study. *Annals of the American Thoracic Society*. 2020;17(3):302–12.

40. Lange P, Parner J, Vestbo J, Schnohr P, Jensen G. A 15-year follow-up study of ventilatory function in adults with asthma. *New England Journal of Medicine*. 1998;339(17):1194–200.

41. Perret JL, Dharmage SC, Matheson MC, Johns DP, Gurrin LC, Burgess JA, et al. The interplay between the effects of lifetime asthma, smoking, and atopy on fixed airflow obstruction in middle age. *American Journal of Respiratory and Critical Care Medicine*. 2013;187(1):42–8.

42. McGeachie MJ, Yates KP, Zhou X, Guo F, Sternberg AL, Van Natta ML, et al. Patterns of growth and decline in lung function in persistent childhood asthma. *New England Journal of Medicine*. 2016;374(19):1842–52.

43. Lodge CJ, Lowe AJ, Allen KJ, Zaloumis S, Gurrin LC, Matheson MC, et al. Childhood wheeze phenotypes show less than expected growth in FEV1 across adolescence. *American Journal of Respiratory and Critical Care Medicine*. 2014;189(11):1351–8.

44. Bakke PS. Factors affecting growth of FEV1. *Monaldi Arch Chest Dis*. 2003;59(2):103–7.

45. Gauderman WJ, Avol E, Gilliland F, Vora H, Thomas D, Berhane K, et al. The effect of air pollution on lung development from 10 to 18 years of age. *New England Journal of Medicine*. 2004;351(11):1057–67.

46. Rojas-Martinez R, Perez-Padilla R, Olaiz-Fernandez G, Mendoza-Alvarado L, Moreno-Macias H, Fortoul T, et al. Lung function growth in children with long-term exposure to air pollutants in Mexico City. *American Journal of Respiratory and Critical Care Medicine*. 2007;176(4):377–84.

47. Schultz ES, Hallberg J, Andersson N, Thacher JD, Pershagen G, Bellander T, et al. Early life determinants of lung function change from childhood to adolescence. *Respiratory Medicine*. 2018;139:48–54.

48. Allinson JP, Hardy R, Donaldson GC, Shaheen SO, Kuh D, Wedzicha JA. Combined impact of smoking and early-life exposures on adult lung function trajectories. *American Journal of Respiratory and Critical Care Medicine*. 2017;196(8):1021–30.

49. Stocks J, Dezateux C. The effect of parental smoking on lung function and development during infancy. *Respirology*. 2003;8(3):266–85.

50. Heyob KM, Mieth S, Sugar SS, Graf AE, Lallier SW, Britt RD, Jr., et al. Maternal high-fat diet alters lung development and function in the offspring. *American Journal of Physiology Lung Cellular and Molecular Physiology*. 2019;317(2):L167–L174.

51. Jedrychowski WA, Perera FP, Maugeri U, Mroz E, Klimaszewska-Rembiasz M, Flak E, et al. Effect of prenatal exposure to fine particulate matter on ventilatory lung function of preschool children of non-smoking mothers. *Paediatric and Perinatal Epidemiology.* 2010;24(5):492–501.

52. Morales E, Garcia-Esteban R, de la Cruz OA, Basterrechea M, Lertxundi A, de Dicastillo MD, et al. Intrauterine and early postnatal exposure to outdoor air pollution and lung function at preschool age. *Thorax.* 2015;70(1):64–73.

53. Tjalvin G, Igland J, Benediktsdóttir B, Dharmage S, Forsberg B, Holm M, et al. Maternal preconception exposure to cleaning agents and disinfectants and offspring asthma. *European Respiratory Journal.* 2020;56(Suppl 64):3142.

54. Svanes C, Koplin J, Skulstad SM, Johannessen A, Bertelsen RJ, Benediktsdottir B, et al. Father's environment before conception and asthma risk in his children: a multi-generation analysis of the Respiratory Health in Northern Europe Study. *International Journal of Epidemiology.* 2017;46(1):235–45.

55. Kuiper IN, Markevych I, Accordini S, Bertelsen RJ, Bråbäck L, Christensen JH, et al. Associations of preconception exposure to air pollution and greenness with offspring asthma and hay fever. *International Journal of Environmental Research and Public Health.* 2020;17(16):5828.

56. Kuiper IN, Svanes C, Markevych I, Heinrich J, Halvorsen T, Bertelsen RJ, et al. Preconception air pollution exposure and early onset asthma and hay fever in the offspring. *European Respiratory Journal.* 2019;54(Suppl 63):PA4453.

57. Jafari A, Rajabi A, Gholian-Aval M, Peyman N, Mahdizadeh M, Tehrani H. National, regional, and global prevalence of cigarette smoking among women/females in the general population: a systematic review and meta-analysis. *Environmental Health and Preventive Medicine.* 2021;26(1):5.

58. Pathak U, Gupta NC, Suri JC. Risk of COPD due to indoor air pollution from biomass cooking fuel: a systematic review and meta-analysis. *International Journal of Environmental Health Research.* 2020;30(1):75–88.

59. Rehfuess E, Mehta S, Prüss-Ustün A. Assessing household solid fuel use: multiple implications for the Millennium Development Goals. *Environ Health Perspect.* 2006;114(3):373–8.

60. Smith-Sivertsen T, Díaz E, Pope D, Lie RT, Díaz A, McCracken J, et al. Effect of reducing indoor air pollution on women's respiratory symptoms and lung function: the RESPIRE Randomized Trial, Guatemala. *American Journal of Epidemiology.* 2009;170(2):211–20.

61. Romieu I, Riojas-Rodríguez H, Marrón-Mares AT, Schilmann A, Perez-Padilla R, Masera O. Improved biomass stove intervention in rural Mexico: impact on the respiratory health of women. *American Journal of Respiratory and Critical Care Medicine.* 2009;180(7):649–56.

62. Zhou Y, Zou Y, Li X, Chen S, Zhao Z, He F, et al. Lung function and incidence of chronic obstructive pulmonary disease after improved cooking fuels and kitchen ventilation: a 9-year prospective cohort study. *PLoS Medicine.* 2014;11(3):e1001621.

63. Clean Cloths Campaign. *Made by women: gender, the global garment industry and the movement for women workers' rights.* Available from: https://ecommons.cornell.edu/handle/1813/99675.

64. *Hair and beauty salon assistants* [Internet]. [Accessed 1 June 2021] [updated cited Available from: https://joboutlook.gov.au/occupations/hair-and-beauty-salon-assistants?occupationCode= 451812.

65. Archangelidi O, Sathiyajit S, Consonni D, Jarvis D, De Matteis S. Cleaning products and respiratory health outcomes in occupational cleaners: a systematic review and meta-analysis. *Occupational and Environmental Medicine.* 2020;Online ahead of print.

66. Lai PS, Christiani DC. Long-term respiratory health effects in textile workers. *Current Opinion in Pulmonary Medicine.* 2013;19(2):152–7.

67. Nemer M, Kristensen P, Nijem K, Bjertness E, Skare Ø, Skogstad M. Lung function and respiratory symptoms among female hairdressers in Palestine: a 5-year prospective study. *BMJ Open.* 2015;5(10):e007857.

68. Quiros-Alcala L, Pollack AZ, Tchangalova N, DeSantiago M, Kavi LKA. Occupational exposures among hair and nail salon workers: a scoping review. *Current Environmental Health Reports.* 2019;6(4):269–85.

69. Svanes Ø, Bertelsen RJ, Lygre SHL, Carsin AE, Antó JM, Forsberg B, et al. Cleaning at home and at work in relation to lung function decline and airway obstruction. *American Journal of Respiratory and Critical Care Medicine*. 2018;197(9):1157–63.

70. Gan WQ, Man SF, Postma DS, Camp P, Sin DD. Female smokers beyond the perimenopausal period are at increased risk of chronic obstructive pulmonary disease: a systematic review and meta-analysis. *Respiratory Research*. 2006;7(1):52.

71. Ben-Zaken Cohen S, Paré PD, Man SF, Sin DD. The growing burden of chronic obstructive pulmonary disease and lung cancer in women: examining sex differences in cigarette smoke metabolism. *American Journal of Respiratory and Critical Care Medicine*. 2007;176(2):113–20.

72. Han MK, Postma D, Mannino DM, Giardino ND, Buist S, Curtis JL, et al. Gender and chronic obstructive pulmonary disease: why it matters. *American Journal of Respiratory and Critical Care Medicine*. 2007;176(12):1179–84.

73. Buist AS, McBurnie MA, Vollmer WM, Gillespie S, Burney P, Mannino DM, et al. International variation in the prevalence of COPD (the BOLD Study): a population-based prevalence study. *Lancet*. 2007;370(9589):741–50.

74. Postma DS. Gender differences in asthma development and progression. *Gender Medicine*. 2007;4(Suppl B):S133–S146.

75. Cunningham M, Gilkeson G. Estrogen receptors in immunity and autoimmunity. *Clinical Reviews in Allergy & Immunology*. 2011;40(1):66–73.

76. Zhang P, Zein J. Novel insights on sex-related differences in asthma. *Current Allergy and Asthma Reports*. 2019;19(10):44.

77. Ticconi C, Pietropolli A, Piccione E. Estrogen replacement therapy and asthma. *Pulmonary Pharmacology & Therapeutics*. 2013;26(6):617–23.

78. Campbell B, Simpson JA, Bui DS, Lodge CJ, Lowe AJ, Matheson MC, et al. Early menarche is associated with lower adult lung function: a longitudinal cohort study from the first to sixth decade of life. *Respirology*. 2020;25(3):289–97.

79. Macsali F, Real FG, Plana E, Sunyer J, Anto J, Dratva J, et al. Early age at menarche, lung function, and adult asthma. *American Journal of Respiratory and Critical Care Medicine*. 2011;183(1):8–14.

80. Gill D, Sheehan NA, Wielscher M, Shrine N, Amaral AFS, Thompson JR, et al. Age at menarche and lung function: a Mendelian randomization study. *European Journal of Epidemiology*. 2017;32(8):701–10.

81. Tang R, Fraser A, Magnus MC. Female reproductive history in relation to chronic obstructive pulmonary disease and lung function in UK biobank: a prospective population-based cohort study. *BMJ Open*. 2019;9(10):e030318.

82. Real FG, Svanes C, Omenaas ER, Antò JM, Plana E, Jarvis D, et al. Lung function, respiratory symptoms, and the menopausal transition. *Journal of Allergy and Clinical Immunology*. 2008;121(1):72–80.e3.

83. Campbell B, Davis SR, Abramson MJ, Mishra G, Handelsman DJ, Perret JL, et al. Menopause, lung function and obstructive lung disease outcomes: a systematic review. *Climacteric: The Journal of the International Menopause Society*. 2018;21(1):3–12.

84. Hayatbakhsh MR, Najman JM, O'Callaghan MJ, Williams GM, Paydar A, Clavarino A. Association between smoking and respiratory function before and after menopause. *Lung*. 2011;189(1):65–71.

85. Amaral AF, Strachan DP, Gómez Real F, Burney PG, Jarvis DL. Lower lung function associates with cessation of menstruation: UK Biobank data. *European Respiratory Journal*. 2016;48(5):1288–97.

86. Songür N, Aydin ZD, Oztürk O, Sahin U, Khayri U, Bircan A, et al. Respiratory symptoms, pulmonary function, and reproductive history: Isparta Menopause and Health Study. *Journal of Women's Health (2002)*. 2010;19(6):1145–54.

87. Triebner K, Matulonga B, Johannessen A, Suske S, Benediktsdóttir B, Demoly P, et al. Menopause is associated with accelerated lung function decline. *American Journal of Respiratory and Critical Care Medicine*. 2017;195(8):1058–65.

88. van der Plaat DA, Pereira M, Pesce G, Potts JF, Amaral AFS, Dharmage SC, et al. Age at menopause and lung function: a Mendelian randomisation study. *European Respiratory Journal*. 2019;54(4):1802421.

89. McCleary N, Nwaru BI, Nurmatov UB, Critchley H, Sheikh A. Endogenous and exogenous sex steroid hormones in asthma and allergy in females: a systematic review and meta-analysis. *Journal of Allergy and Clinical Immunology.* 2018;141(4):1510–13.e8.

90. Resmi SS, Samuel E, Kesavachandran C, Shashidhar S. Effect of oral contraceptives on respiratory function. *Indian Journal of Physiology and Pharmacology.* 2002;46(3):361–6.

91. Strinić T, Eterović D. Oral contraceptives improve lung mechanics. *Fertility and Sterility.* 2003;79(5):1070–3.

92. Kumar P, Singh S, Singh U, Verma P. Oral contraceptive pills decrease pulmonary airway resistance in healthy north Indian women. *Indian Journal of Medical Sciences.* 2011;65(2):64–8.

93. Triebner K, Accordini S, Calciano L, Johannessen A, Benediktsdóttir B, Bifulco E, et al. Exogenous female sex steroids may reduce lung ageing after menopause: a 20-year follow-up study of a general population sample (ECRHS). *Maturitas.* 2019;120:29–34.

94. Pata O, Atiş S, Utku Oz A, Yazici G, Tok E, Pata C, et al. The effects of hormone replacement therapy type on pulmonary functions in postmenopausal women. *Maturitas.* 2003;46(3):213–8.

95. Stipic I, Polasek O, Vulic M, Punda H, Grandic L, Strinic T. Estrogen replacement therapy improves pulmonary function in postmenopausal women with genital prolapse. *Rejuvenation Research.* 2012;15(6):596–600.

96. Cevrioglu AS, Fidan F, Unlu M, Yilmazer M, Orman A, Fenkci IV, et al. The effects of hormone therapy on pulmonary function tests in postmenopausal women. *Maturitas.* 2004;49(3):221–7.

97. Carlson CL, Cushman M, Enright PL, Cauley JA, Newman AB. Hormone replacement therapy is associated with higher FEV1 in elderly women. *American Journal of Respiratory and Critical Care Medicine.* 2001;163(2):423–8.

98. Kallapur SG, Ikegami M. Physiological consequences of intrauterine insults. *Paediatric Respiratory Reviews.* 2006;7(2):110–6.

99. Dratva J, Zemp E, Dharmage SC, Accordini S, Burdet L, Gislason T, et al. Early life origins of lung ageing: early life exposures and lung function decline in adulthood in two European cohorts aged 28–73 years. *PloS One.* 2016;11(1):e0145127.

9

Depression and Psychological Distress

Barbara Maughan

9.1 Introduction

Depression is a common mental health disorder, estimated to affect more than 300 million people globally.[1] It is characterised by feelings of sadness, guilt and low self-worth, a loss of enjoyment, disturbed sleep and appetite, fatigue and poor concentration, and hopelessness about the future.[1,2] Depressive phenomena can be viewed as indicators of categorically defined disorders or dimensional markers of an underlying continuum of distress.[2] Depression is often recurrent, causes distress, reduces quality of life, and impairs functioning; in the latest World Health Organization Global Burden of Disease study, it ranked as the largest contributor to disease-related disability worldwide. For women, these findings are especially salient because, from early adolescence onwards, women are roughly twice as likely as men to experience depression.[3]

A complex array of factors—biological, psychological, and social—are now known to contribute to vulnerability to depressive disorders. Some arise very early in the life course, some cumulate across development, and yet others occur much more proximally to the onset of a specific depressive episode. This chapter provides a brief account of recent evidence on these varying patterns of risk, and on current thinking on how they may combine. Given women's increased vulnerability to depression, it also examines how far women and men vary in their exposure or susceptibility to these well-established risks, and whether any female-specific risks have been identified. To set the scene, it begins by sketching in epidemiological findings on the developmental 'profile' of depressive disorders across age, along with other key features of the epidemiological picture.

9.2 Depression Across the Life Course

Many mental health problems are now known to onset early in the life course, and depression is no exception. Clinically significant depression is rare in childhood but shows a sharp rise in incidence early in the teens. Figure 9.1 illustrates these trends with data from the Dunedin Multidisciplinary Study of Health and Development, a longitudinal birth cohort study that has tracked the 1-year prevalence of depression in the same representative age-cohort of young people from age 9 years into adulthood.[4,5] Rates of depression are low in prepubertal children, and in line with other studies that estimate prevalence at approximately 1% of preschoolers and school-aged children,[6] with little evidence of gender differences. Two

Barbara Maughan, *Depression and Psychological Distress* In: *A Life Course Approach to Women's Health*. Second Edition.
Edited by: Gita D Mishra, Rebecca Hardy, and Diana Kuh, Oxford University Press. © Oxford University Press 2023.
DOI: 10.1093/oso/9780192864642.003.0009

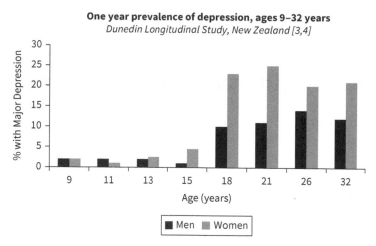

Figure 9.1 One-year prevalence of depression in males and females aged 9–32 years in the Dunedin Multidisciplinary Study of Health and Development (data presented with permission from Professor Terrie Moffitt[4,5]). See plate section.

key changes then take place in the early teens. First, levels of depression begin to rise in both sexes, and second, that rise is stronger in girls than in boys, so that by late adolescence, the female preponderance typical of the adult years is already clearly established. Similar findings have now been reported in many other community samples[7] and in large-scale register-based studies of young people seeking treatment for depression.[8]

Following this adolescent rise, new onsets of depression continue across the adult years and into older age. Retrospective reports place median ages at onset in the mid-20s.[9] The point prevalence of depressive episodes rises steadily across the adult years, peaking in the early 60s in women, before declining in older age.[1] Although depression is primarily an episodic disorder, it also often recurs and for some individuals, it can become chronic; estimates of lifetime prevalence vary, but generally lie between 10% and 20%.[9] By no means do all individuals with clinically significant depression seek or receive treatment. Treatments for mild depression often centre on psychological therapies; pharmacotherapy (often in combination with psychological treatments) can be effective in more severe cases, though there are marked individual differences in response.

The gender gap in rates of depression that emerges in early adolescence persists across the life course. Adult women are consistently about twice as likely as men to report unipolar depression,[10] though the gap may narrow in older age.[11] A variety of checks suggest that these gender differences are unlikely to be artefactual.[3] Some particular forms of depression-related illnesses (premenstrual dysphoric disorder, postpartum depression, and postmenopausal depression and anxiety) are specific to women, but they only account for a small proportion of the gender disparity. Longitudinal studies find few gender differences in rates of recurrence, remission, or chronicity, suggesting that the female excess may largely reflect higher rates of new onsets.[12-14] Adult women are also at increased risk of dysthymia (a less severe but more chronic lowering of mood), though not of bipolar disorders (less common conditions involving both manic and depressive episodes). Although women are more likely than men to attempt suicide, the risk of completed suicide is much higher in men.[15] Historical trends in depression have been difficult to establish, because both diagnostic criteria and assessment methods have changed over time. A recent meta-analysis of studies using comparable assessment methods has, however, pointed to an increasing trend in levels of both major depressive episodes and mean depression symptom levels;[16] some studies suggest that these rising trends are most marked among late-adolescent and young adult women. These groups also seem to have been especially susceptible to the psychological sequelae of the COVID-19 pandemic.[17]

Two other features of the epidemiological picture are important by way of background. First, Major Depressive disorder (MDD) is phenotypically heterogeneous, and investigators are examining a range of different approaches to subtyping.[2] At the same time, depression shows high levels of both concurrent and longitudinal comorbidity with other psychiatric disorders, in particular anxiety.[2] As a result, although the risk pathways discussed below have been examined in relation to (variously defined) depression and depressive episodes, many may in practice be much less specific.

9.3 Vulnerability and Risk for Depression in Adolescence and Adult Life

Depression has been described a 'prototypical' multifactorial disorder,[18] with replicated evidence of associations with genetic, neural, psychological, cognitive, and social and environmental risks.[2] Many theoretical models postulate accumulations of risk factors across the life course, beginning very early in development.[19] Methodologically, such long-term processes are inevitably difficult to track—a task made more challenging by the fact that any specific early influence might plausibly be carried forward via a variety of biological, psychological, and social pathways. In addition, much early evidence on the role of adverse exposures in childhood relied on retrospective reports, potentially subject to problems of recall and bias. As prospective cohorts have matured, empirical tests have increasingly been possible using these more robust designs; wherever possible, prospective evidence of this kind is highlighted in the sections that follow.

9.3.1 Genetic Influences

Depression is a familial disorder, with part of that familiality reflecting heritable risks. Adult twin studies estimate the heritability of MDD at 30%–40%,[20] with the great majority of the remaining variance attributable to individual-specific environmental risks. Twin studies in adolescence paint a similar picture, but depression in prepubertal children seems less heritable and more strongly associated with psychosocial adversity.[21] In older age, although evidence from genetically sensitive designs is limited, a family history of depression may be less strongly predictive than in younger age groups, and a past history of depression may also decline in predictive power with age.[11]

Genome-wide association studies have confirmed that depression is highly polygenic,[20] and identified links with genes involved in neuronal growth, synaptic function, and inflammation. Genetic risks for depression overlap with genetic liability to a number of other psychiatric disorders, and to personality characteristics such as neuroticism. Recent findings[22] suggest that polygenic risk scores (PRS) for depression, anxiety, and neuroticism are associated with both the severity and the rate of change in depression symptoms across adolescence and begin to be clearly associated with higher symptom scores between the ages of 12 and 14 years. If replicated, these findings suggest that genetic liability may contribute to the adolescent rise in depression, whether through effects on biological and hormonal pathways impacting adolescent brain development or an increase in gene-environment correlations with environmental stressors in the early teens.

Two aspects of gene-environment interplay have attracted particular attention: first, that genetic risks affect variations in *sensitivity* to environmental stressors (gene-environment interaction), and second, that heritable factors affect *exposure* to adverse environments (gene-environment correlation), influencing the extent to which individuals 'select' themselves into environments with increased levels of risk.[23] Both are important from a life course perspective. Early gene-environment interaction studies produced somewhat inconsistent findings, but recent PRS studies suggest that genetic factors may be associated with variations in vulnerability to both childhood adversity and adult social disadvantage and may also interact with potential 'protective' factors, including social support and physical exercise.[20]

9.3.2 Prenatal and Early Life Exposures

Stress exposure plays a central role in many aetiological models for depression, and recent years have seen an explosion of interest in the part that very early adverse exposures—in utero and in the immediately postnatal period—may play in risk for later mental health. The fetal period is one of rapid neurobiological development, and early brain development appears highly susceptible to prenatal stressors which, in combination with genetic liabilities and later postnatal exposures, may increase vulnerability to depression.[19] There is now robust meta-analytic evidence for associations between a range of pre- and early postnatal exposures and subsequent depression risk, spanning indicators such as maternal age, maternal smoking in pregnancy, prenatal maternal stress, and both pre- and postnatal maternal depression.[24] Some studies point to links between low birthweight, as a marker of uterine development, and depression, though the evidence in this area is more mixed.[25]

Although many of the mechanisms involved here remain to be clarified, it seems likely that pathways via impacts on hypothalamic-pituitary-adrenal (HPA) axis functioning, brain development, and DNA methylation will prove important.[19] The HPA axis is the body's primary stress response system (see Chapter 14). When the maternal HPA axis is activated, it produces hormones like cortisol. When these hormones cross the placenta in high concentrations, it can disrupt the fetus's developing brain and HPA axis. It can also result in epigenetic changes, such as to DNA methylation.[26] These structural and functional changes can persist into adulthood and increase susceptibility to mental health problems across the life course.[27]

In addition, there are pointers to sex differences in these early processes. This may be partly related to differences in the way male and female placentae respond to stress.[28] Female placentae and fetuses are more responsive, which reduces their early mortality but increases their later risk of affective disorders.[29] For example, girls but not boys exposed to elevated maternal cortisol during pregnancy were more likely to have a fearful temperament in infancy and anxiety in preadolescence.[30] Sex differences have also been found in the brain development of children exposed to maternal stress during pregnancy,[29] such as increased amygdala volume in girls compared to boys.[30] There is evidence that female fetuses may be more vulnerable to the long-term effects of exposure to prenatal depression, whereas maternal postnatal depression is more strongly associated with risk for late-adolescent depression in males.[31]

9.3.3 Childhood Adversities

Beyond these very early exposures, an extensive body of evidence has documented links between adverse childhood experiences (ACEs) and vulnerability to physical and mental health problems, including depression, later in life. A recent umbrella review estimated that exposure to ACEs is associated with a doubling of the risk for common mental disorders and suicide.[32] Physical, sexual, and emotional abuse and neglect are among the most widely studied ACEs, but other family-related stressors have also been implicated, along with chronic exposure to poverty in childhood and factors outside the family such as bullying, victimisation, and depriving institutional care. Early evidence based on retrospective reports is increasingly being confirmed in prospective studies. Using data from the 1958 British birth cohort, for example, investigators have recently documented associations between childhood adversities (assessed between ages 7 and 16 years) and an increased risk for low mood that persisted across the adult years and was still evident at midlife.[33] Retrospective data suggest that childhood adversities continue to be associated with new onsets of depression even in older age.[34]

Exposure to early adversity is common: almost a fifth of participants in the 1958 British birth cohort study were exposed to one childhood adversity, and 7% to two or more. By no means all individuals exposed to such stressors will, of course, develop depression, and a variety of factors—including the type, severity, and timing of early exposures—appear to affect the likelihood of long-term effects.[35] Childhood adversities often overlap, meaning that additive or interactive effects may also be implicated, and there are clearly individual differences in susceptibility to such early risks, reflecting a range of individual characteristics, impacts of prior exposures, and heritable influences.[35]

How might early experience affect vulnerability to later psychiatric disturbance? Studies of the short-term impact of abuse in childhood point to effects on multiple developmental systems including emotion regulation, attachment security, quality of peer relationships, and the development of the self-system.[35] Each of these might plausibly contribute to risk for depression and low mood. Documented neurobiological effects include dysregulation of HPA axis functioning, dysfunctions in autoimmune processes, structural and functional brain changes, and epigenetic effects including altered DNA methylation.[36–38] In addition, for girls in particular, a number of early adversities predict earlier pubertal maturation, providing a further pathway for the carry-forward of effects of early adversity specific to girls.[39]

A variety of mechanisms have been proposed as contributing to longer-term impacts, including continuities in 'external' environmental adversity and stress generation, along with effects on 'internal' psychological and neurobiological pathways.[2] Current findings point to a complex interweaving of effects across the life course, implicating many domains of risk.[2] While much progress has been made in elucidating these pathways, key questions remain. Does early adversity convey a general susceptibility to psychological distress, or a more latent vulnerability only activated in the face of later stressors? How specific are the effects involved, both in terms of developmental pathways and psychopathological outcomes? How do genetic vulnerabilities play into these pathways? And, especially pertinent from the perspective of women's health, are childhood adversities more strongly predisposing factors for depression in women than in men? To date, there is little evidence for marked gender differences in associations between early adversity and later mental health,[32] and there are few gender differences in exposure to most types of early risk. In one case, however—sexual abuse—exposure is clearly more common among girls,[40] suggesting that early abusive experiences may play a significant role in contributing to women's increased vulnerability to depression.

9.3.4 Life Stage Influences

9.3.4.1 Adolescence

The sharp rise in depression in teens suggests that adolescence may be a further key developmental 'window' for evolving risk. The early adolescent years are marked by changes in young people's social roles, in relationships with parents and peers, and in patterns of self and social cognitions, as well as by the major biological changes of puberty and continuing maturation of the developing brain.

The pubertal transition involves an extended period of neuroendocrine changes associated with changes in neural, cognitive, emotional, social, and sexual development. Individuals vary in both the timing and the tempo of these changes, and risk for adolescent depression shows links with pubertal development independent of chronological age.[41] Both more advanced pubertal development and pubertal timing seem important here, with early developmental timing relative to peers especially salient for girls.[12,42,43] In one study, for example, girls in the earliest quintile of pubertal timing were up to six times more likely to be depressed than later developers in early to midadolescence.[44] Although puberty is a biological process, the effects of early pubertal timing may be socially and psychologically mediated, whether via the disparity between early maturers' physical development and their cognitive and social skills, or the effects of body objectification.[39,45]

Increases in sex steroids have been linked to organisational effects on brain structure and function in adolescence, but teasing out specific effects of hormonal influences on risk for psychopathology has proved challenging. There are pointers that rising oestrogen levels are associated with rises in negative affect in the early teens, and one recent study found that testosterone showed independent links with depression in girls across the 9–16-year age range, perhaps consistent with reports of sex-differentiated impacts of testosterone on brain regions often implicated in emotional and cognitive processing of experience.[44]

Adolescent changes in the 'social brain' may also be implicated.[46] Social cognitions, including self-perceptions and mentalising capacities, change across the adolescent years, with factors such as self-esteem—well-established as both a predictor and an outcome of depression—showing specific declines in girls.[47] Relations with peers and romantic partners also take on increasing importance in the teens. Peer rejection and bullying victimisation are strong predictors of emotional difficulties in adolescence, with effects that may persist to adult life.[48,49] Close, supportive friendships are typically protective against threats to well-being, but there is also evidence that co-rumination—intensive dyadic discussion of problems with one close friend—is more common among girls than boys, and can be associated with an increase in internalising symptoms.[50] There are widespread concerns that social media may be accentuating a range of these risks, though current evidence is inconclusive.[51]

9.3.4.2 Pregnancy and Menopause

Possible impacts of hormonal influences have also been examined at later stages in the life course. Premenstrual dysphoric disorder has been linked with heightened sensitivity to fluctuating concentrations of reproductive hormones,[52] and a hormone-sensitive subtype of postpartum depression has also been proposed.[53] The rise in oestrogen levels in pregnancy is not, however, accompanied by any marked decrease in depression, and falling oestrogen levels at the menopause do not appear to be associated with any increase in depression. Indeed, although the menopause was long assumed to carry increased risk for low mood,[54] both the broader epidemiological literature and studies specific to the menopausal years have now shown that this view may be misplaced. In the 1946 British birth cohort, for example, repeated assessments between ages 47 and 52 years showed no association between menopausal status and levels of psychological symptoms for the majority of women, though some subgroups did show increases at the start of the menopause,[55] and hormone therapy users also had higher levels of symptomatology.[56]

9.3.4.3 Older Age

Additional, age-related influences are implicated in risk for depression later in the life course. Epidemiological data suggest that half or more of late-life depressions represent first onsets after age 60,[11] and that older age is a consistent risk factor for poorer depression course.[57] Broad categories of risk for late-life depression include stressors that occur more frequently in older age, such as bereavement and caregiving, along with declines in social engagement and meaningful activities, and losses in social support.[11,57] In addition, age-related biological risks seem especially salient. Late-life depression commonly occurs in the context of medical and neurological illness, with elevated rates of depression reported in patients with cardiovascular disease and diabetes, and in neurological conditions including Parkinson's disease and stroke.[11] A variety of aetiological pathways—including the possibility of shared genetic and other risks, as well as reactions to illness—has been proposed in each case.[11] Late-life depression also shows strong overlaps with dementia, with proposals that the two disorders may reflect a common cause, and that depression may constitute a prodromal stage in some individuals.[58] And although the pathophysiology of late-life depression remains poorly understood, investigators have proposed that microvascular dysfunction may constitute one key mechanism,[59] that may help account for observed overlaps with apathy, cognitive dysfunction, dementia, and stroke.

9.3.4.4 Life Events and Difficulties

Acute stressful life events and longer-term difficulties play a key role in the immediate precipitation of many first episodes of depression.[60] Experiences involving loss, humiliation, or 'entrapment'—breakdowns in relationships, for example, or being caught in a poor job or an unhappy marriage—seem central to these effects. Exposure to stressful events markedly increases the risk of a depressive episode in the immediately succeeding weeks or months, and for individuals who are depressed, experiencing stressors is associated with a longer duration of illness and a higher likelihood of relapse. Acute events—especially those centring on relationship difficulties and personal disappointments—are also important risk factors for depression in adolescence; girls appear to experience more interpersonal stressors than boys in the teens, and may also be more susceptible to them.[3] As noted above, the nature of life stressors changes in older age, with health-related disability and loss of close social contacts among the most common precursors of first onsets of depression, although ongoing difficulties account for most episodes.[34]

Do men and women differ in exposure or response to life stressors? Findings on exposure vary, but there are pointers that women and girls may experience higher levels of both acute stressors and longer-term adverse conditions than males.[3] Sexual abuse, interpersonal violence, and sexual victimisation are all more common among women than men, and women may face low status, disadvantaged life circumstances, and stresses associated with caring roles more frequently than their male counterparts.[2] Losses or interpersonal problems involving close loved ones seem equally likely to provoke depression in both sexes.[61] Where differences have been noted, however, is in relation to 'network' events involving a broader circle of kin and friends.[62–64] These do seem more salient for women, perhaps reflecting biologically and culturally influenced tendencies to involvement in affiliative, nurturing roles.

9.3.4.5 Individual Vulnerability Factors: Personality, Cognitive Styles, and Prior Disorder

A variety of personality characteristics, cognitive styles, and coping strategies also show strong links with depression. Among personality features, neuroticism shows the most consistent links and shares genetic variance with depression.[65] Personality characteristics might affect risk for depression in a variety of ways: adult studies have shown, for example, that neuroticism is associated with differential risk of exposure to life events, with variations in perceptions of the severity of events, and with variations in vulnerability to event-related psychological distress.[65]

Cognitive theories of depression highlight the negative attributional styles and cognitive biases seen in many depressed individuals, whereby the self, the future, and the world are viewed in negative, dysfunctional ways.[60] Depressed people often see themselves as unworthy and undesirable, expect failure and rejection, and interpret their experiences as confirming those expectations. These cognitive schemas are argued to be acquired from early experience, and to be activated by exposure to experiences of rejection or deprivation later in life.[66] There is little clear evidence of gender differences in attributional styles, but coping styles—the ways in which individuals respond to an initial lowering of mood—do appear to differ. Here, evidence suggests that men tend to use more active coping strategies, distracting themselves through involvement in activities, while women have a more ruminative style, more likely to prolong depressed mood.[67,68] Neurocognitive studies suggest that variations of this kind may have implications for differential activation of brain regions associated with depression.[69]

One further set of individually based precursors lies in the realm of early onset psychiatric disorders. As noted earlier, depression is frequently comorbid with anxiety, and there has been considerable interest in the developmental patterning of these disorders earlier in development. Although diagnoses of depression are rare before puberty, prepubertal anxiety is more common, and shows a clear female excess.[3] First onset of anxiety disorders typically occurs in childhood and early adolescence—well before the main rise in rates of depression—and prospective studies have confirmed that preexisting anxiety disorders function as strong risks for the onset of depression in adolescence and early adulthood.[12,70,71] How far these associations reflect shared risk factors or other aetiological mechanisms remains to be clarified. In addition, girls with conduct problems and other 'externalising' difficulties may also be at increased risk of depression, whether because they often follow stress-prone life pathways, or as a result of prior comorbidity with depression or other vulnerability factors.[72]

9.3.5 Social and Cultural Influences

In addition to these individually based influences, epidemiological findings suggest that broader social factors are also implicated in risk for depression. Disadvantaged socioeconomic position is associated with a higher prevalence of affective disorders, and though part of this association may reflect selection effects, some causal influences also seem likely to be involved.[73] In addition, the degree of structural gender equality (measured by factors such as political participation, economic autonomy, and reproductive rights) is associated with variations in the degree of gender differences in depression.[3]

Rates of depression also vary by marital and partnership status. In general, marriage shows 'protective' effects against low mood, while higher rates of distress are found among the separated, widowed, and divorced.[74] Importantly, these marital status effects also vary by gender: the excess of depression in women is most marked among the married, less notable among the widowed and divorced, and least evident among adults who remain single.[75] Young married women looking after small children seem especially at risk, as do single mothers. This suggests that aspects of social roles may contribute to risk for depression, whether through role overload or underload,[3] through overinvestment in a limited number of roles, or through the value (or lack of it) that individuals attach to the social categories they occupy. This last possibility is underscored by findings that gender differences are much less marked in cultural groups where a high value is typically placed on caring and homemaker roles. Women frequently combine childcare with work outside the home. In general, employment has been found to be beneficial for psychological health, providing interest, fulfilment, and social contacts as well as access to financial rewards. Not unexpectedly, however, these benefits vary between men and women, and among women in different social circumstances: the advantages of work are less marked for married than for single women, weaker if they have children, and weakest of all for those with children of preschool age.[3] Once again, role strain and role overload have been argued to be key contributors to these effects.

9.4 Integrating the Evidence

As this brief overview suggests, a complex array of factors, reflecting distinct risk domains and arising at different developmental periods, has been implicated in risk for depression. Linking these diverse elements into more integrated, comprehensive life course models of risk is challenging. Much research continues to focus on individual risk domains, and few individual studies have the capacity to test associations among more than a subset of the elements potentially involved. We conclude by outlining illustrative findings from some studies that have begun to move in this direction.

Given the importance of the early adolescent years for first onsets of depression, investigators are examining multidomain risk models in adolescent samples with the aim of informing preventive interventions. One recent study, tracking a community sample of girls across the early to midteens, identified depressive symptoms, rumination, parental mood disorder, and parental criticism as independent predictors of first onset of depression.[76] Depressive symptoms, low extraversion, poor peer relationships, and a blunted neural response to rewards predicted depressive disorders that, even at this early stage in development, showed a chronic or recurrent course.

Later in the life course, path modelling of data from an adult twin sample[20] and the 1946 British birth cohort[77] have taken a more explicitly developmental approach to examining risks for adult depressive episodes. Both converged in finding recent stressors the most powerful individual predictors, along with prior depressive episodes, whether in adulthood or in the teens. The twin study identified potentially wide-ranging impacts of genetic influences, with high genetic risk for depression being correlated with other childhood risks (disturbed family environment, childhood sexual abuse, and parental loss), and predicting to both neuroticism and adult exposure to traumatic events. A subsequent study of opposite-sex twin pairs[64] found that neuroticism and indicators of the quality and continuity of interpersonal relationships (parental warmth, divorce, social support, and marital satisfaction) were more important predictors of depression in women than in men. The birth cohort study identified two separate pathways of influence from childhood risks, one running via early deprivation and parental divorce to low social position in adult life, the second from low birthweight through early neurodevelopment to adolescent emotional problems, and thence to an adult episode. Both studies point to the possibility of multiple risk pathways to the same final outcome and paint a picture of the accumulation of risk factors across the life course in the manner of developmental cascades.

9.5 Conclusions

Depression places a heavy burden on individuals, families, and the wider society. As we have seen, that burden has been increasing in recent decades and falls disproportionately on women. Vulnerability to depressive disorders reflects a complex range of influences, acting and interacting throughout the life course; women's increased vulnerability may reflect contributions from many differing risk domains. Developmentally oriented research has been important in highlighting the role of very early risks and identifying adverse early exposures that can inform prevention efforts in pregnancy and childhood and school-based programmes in the teens. Building and testing comprehensive life course models of risk for depression is challenging, and a range of different developmental pathways may be involved. As prospective cohorts mature, the base for elaborating such models is increasing. The availability of DNA samples, polygenic risk indicators, and epigenetic data within such cohorts holds the promise that genetic factors—likely implicated in risk throughout the life course—can be incorporated into life course models more fully and flexibly than in the past. And as psychiatry sets out on the path of developing prediction models for clinical practice, insights from life course research will form one key element in efforts to reduce the heavy burdens of depression.

Key messages and implications

- Depression is a common, often recurrent disorder associated with wide-ranging impairments in functioning.
- From early adolescence onwards, women are roughly twice as likely as men to experience depression.
- Depression is a multifactorial disorder, with influences from genetic, biological, psychological, and social risks across development.
- Women's increased vulnerability is likely to reflect contributions from a range of differing influences.
- Life course models may need to incorporate a number of different developmental pathways.

References

1. World Health Organization. *Depression and other common mental disorders: global health estimates*. Geneva: World Health Organization; 2017. WHO/MSD/MER/2017.2.
2. Herrman H, Patel V, Kieling C, Berk M, Buchweitz C, Cuijpers P, et al. Time for united action on depression: a Lancet–World Psychiatric Association Commission. *Lancet*. 2022;399(10328):957–1022.
3. Kuehner C. Why is depression more common among women than among men? *Lancet Psychiatry*. 2017;4(2):146–58.
4. Moffitt TE. *Personal communication*. 2001.
5. Hankin BL, Abramson LY, Moffitt TE, Silva PA, McGee R, Angell KE. Development of depression from preadolescence to young adulthood: emerging gender differences in a 10-year longitudinal study. *Journal of Abnormal Psychology (1965)*. 1998;107(1):128–40.
6. Vasileva M, Graf RK, Reinelt T, Petermann U, Petermann F. Research review: a meta-analysis of the international prevalence and comorbidity of mental disorders in children between 1 and 7 years. *Journal of Child Psychology and Psychiatry*. 2021;62(4):372–81.
7. Avenevoli SP, Swendsen JP, He J-PMS, Burstein MP, Merikangas KRP. Major Depression in the National Comorbidity Survey–Adolescent Supplement: Prevalence, Correlates, and Treatment. *Journal of the American Academy of Child and Adolescent Psychiatry*. 2015;54(1):37–44.e2.
8. Dalsgaard S, Thorsteinsson E, Trabjerg BB, Schullehner J, Plana-Ripoll O, Brikell I, et al. Incidence rates and cumulative incidences of the full spectrum of diagnosed mental disorders in childhood and adolescence. *Journal of the American Academy of Child and Adolescent Psychiatry*. 2019;77(2):155–64.
9. Kessler RC, Bromet EJ. The epidemiology of depression across cultures. *Annual Review of Public Health*. 2013;34(1):119–38.
10. Salk RH, Hyde JS, Abramson LY. Gender differences in depression in representative national samples: meta-analyses of diagnoses and symptoms. *Psychological Bulletin*. 2017;143(8):783–822.
11. Fiske A, Wetherell JL, Gatz M. Depression in older adults. *Annual Review of Clinical Psychology*. 2009;5(1):363–89.
12. Kuehner C. Gender differences in unipolar depression: an update of epidemiological findings and possible explanations. *Acta Psychiatrica Scandinavica*. 2003;108(3):163–74.
13. Hardeveld F, Spijker J, De Graaf R, Nolen WA, Beekman ATF. Prevalence and predictors of recurrence of major depressive disorder in the adult population. *Acta Psychiatrica Scandinavica*. 2010;122(3):184–91.

14. Mackenzie CSPD, El-Gabalawy RMA, Chou K-LPD, Sareen JMD. Prevalence and predictors of persistent versus remitting mood, anxiety, and substance disorders in a national sample of older adults. *American Journal of Geriatric Psychiatry*. 2014;22(9):854–65.

15. World Health Organization. *Preventing suicide: a global imperative*. Geneva: World Health Organization; 17 August 2014.

16. Moreno-Agostino D, Wu Y-T, Daskalopoulou C, Hasan MT, Huisman M, Prina M. Global trends in the prevalence and incidence of depression: a systematic review and meta-analysis. *Journal of Affective Disorders*. 2021;281:235–43.

17. Pierce M, McManus S, Hope H, Hotopf M, Ford T, Hatch SL, et al. Mental health responses to the COVID-19 pandemic: a latent class trajectory analysis using longitudinal UK data. *Lancet Psychiatry*. 2021;8(7):610–9.

18. Kendler KS, Gardner CO, Prescott CA. Toward a comprehensive developmental model for major depression in women. *American Journal of Psychiatry*. 2002;159(7):1133–45.

19. Van den Bergh BRH, van den Heuvel MI, Lahti M, Braeken M, de Rooij SR, Entringer S, et al. Prenatal developmental origins of behavior and mental health: the influence of maternal stress in pregnancy. *Neuroscience and Biobehavioral Reviews*. 2020;117:26–64.

20. Kendall KM, Van Assche E, Andlauer TFM, Choi KW, Luykx JJ, Schulte EC, et al. The genetic basis of major depression. *Psychological Medicine*. 2021;51(13):2217–30.

21. Rice F. Genetics of childhood and adolescent depression: Insights into etiological heterogeneity and challenges for future genomic research. *Genome Medicine*. 2010;2(9):68.

22. Kwong ASF, Morris TT, Pearson RM, Timpson NJ, Rice F, Stergiakouli E, et al. Polygenic risk for depression, anxiety and neuroticism are associated with the severity and rate of change in depressive symptoms across adolescence. *Journal of Child Psychology and Psychiatry*. 2021;62(12):1462–74.

23. Rutter M, Silberg J. Gene-environment interplay in relation to emotional and behavioral disturbance. *Annual Review of Psychology*. 2002;53(1):463–90.

24. Su Y, D'Arcy C, Meng X. Research review: developmental origins of depression—a systematic review and meta-analysis. *Journal of Child Psychology and Psychiatry*. 2021;62(9):1050–66.

25. Orri M, Pingault J-B, Turecki G, Nuyt A-M, Tremblay RE, Côté SM, et al. Contribution of birth weight to mental health, cognitive and socioeconomic outcomes: two-sample Mendelian randomisation. *British Journal of Psychiatry*. 2021;219(3):507–14.

26. Beijers R, Buitelaar JK, Weerth Cd. Mechanisms underlying the effects of prenatal psychosocial stress on child outcomes: beyond the HPA axis. *European Child and Adolescent Psychiatry*. 2014;23(10):943–56.

27. Van den Bergh BRH, Dahnke R, Mennes M. Prenatal stress and the developing brain: risks for neurodevelopmental disorders. *Developmental Psychopathology*. 2018;30(3):743–62.

28. Glover V, Hill J. Sex differences in the programming effects of prenatal stress on psychopathology and stress responses: an evolutionary perspective. *Physiology and Behavior*. 2012;106(5):736–40.

29. Sandman CA, Glynn LM, Davis EP. *Fetal development*. Cham: Springer International Publishing; 2016. pp. 229–65.

30. Sandman CA, Glynn LM, Davis EP. Is there a viability–vulnerability tradeoff? Sex differences in fetal programming. *Journal of Psychosomatic Research*. 2013;75(4):327–35.

31. Quarini C, Pearson RM, Stein A, Ramchandani PG, Lewis G, Evans J. Are female children more vulnerable to the long-term effects of maternal depression during pregnancy? *Journal of Affective Disorders*. 2015;189:329–35.

32. Sahle BW, Reavley NJ, Li W, Morgan AJ, Yap MBH, Reupert A, et al. The association between adverse childhood experiences and common mental disorders and suicidality: an umbrella review of systematic reviews and meta-analyses. *European Child and Adolescent Psychiatry*. 2021:31, 1489-1499

33. Selous C, Kelly-Irving M, Maughan B, Eyre O, Rice F, Collishaw S. Adverse childhood experiences and adult mood problems: evidence from a five-decade prospective birth cohort. *Psychological Medicine*. 2020;50(14):2444–51.

34. Falkingham J, Evandrou M, Qin M, Vlachantoni A. Accumulated lifecourse adversities and depressive symptoms in later life among older men and women in England: a longitudinal study. *Ageing and Society*. 2020;40(10):2079–105.
35. Nelson CA, Bhutta ZA, Burke Harris N, Danese A, Samara M. Adversity in childhood is linked to mental and physical health throughout life. *British Medical Journal*. 2020;371:m3048.
36. Jawahar MC, Murgatroyd C, Harrison EL, Baune BT. Epigenetic alterations following early postnatal stress: A review on novel aetiological mechanisms of common psychiatric disorders. *Clinical Epigenetics*. 2015;7(1):122
37. Nemeroff CB. Paradise lost: the neurobiological and clinical consequences of child abuse and neglect. *Neuron*. 2016;89(5):892–909.
38. Teicher MH, Samson JA. Annual research review: enduring neurobiological effects of childhood abuse and neglect. *Journal of Child Psychology and Psychiatry*. 2016;57(3):241–66.
39. Graber JA. Pubertal timing and the development of psychopathology in adolescence and beyond. *Hormones and Behavior*. 2013;64(2):262–9.
40. Stoltenborgh M, Bakermans-Kranenburg MJ, Alink LRA, van Ijzendoorn MH. The prevalence of child maltreatment across the globe: review of a series of meta-analyses. *Child Abuse Review*. 2015;24(1):37–50.
41. Lewis G, Ioannidis K, van Harmelen AL, Neufeld S, Stochl J, Lewis G, et al. The association between pubertal status and depressive symptoms and diagnoses in adolescent females: a population-based cohort study. *PLoS ONE*. 2018;13(6):e0198804.
42. Hankin BL, Young JF, Abela JRZ, Smolen A, Jenness JL, Gulley LD, et al. Depression from childhood into late adolescence: influence of gender, development, genetic susceptibility, and peer stress. *Journal of Abnormal Psychology*. 2015;124(4):803–16.
43. Patton GCMD, Olsson CPD, Bond LPD, Toumbourou JWP, Carlin JBP, Hemphill SAP, et al. Predicting female depression across puberty: a two-nation longitudinal study. *Journal of the American Academy of Child and Adolescent Psychiatry*. 2008;47(12):1424–32.
44. Copeland WE, Worthman C, Shanahan L, Costello EJ, Angold A. Early pubertal timing and testosterone associated with higher levels of adolescent depression in girls. *Journal of the American Academy of Child and Adolescent Psychiatry*. 2019;58(12):1197–206.
45. Hyde JS, Mezulis AH, Abramson LY. The ABCs of depression: integrating affective, biological, and cognitive models to explain the emergence of the gender difference in depression. *Psychological Review*. 2008;115(2):291–313.
46. Pfeifer JH, Allen NB. Puberty initiates cascading relationships between neurodevelopmental, social, and internalizing processes across adolescence. *Biological Psychiatry*. 2021;89(2):99–108.
47. Baldwin SA, Hoffmann JP. The dynamics of self-esteem: a growth-curve analysis. *Journal of Youth and Adolescence*. 2002;31(2):101–13.
48. Copeland WE, Wolke D, Angold A, Costello EJ. Adult psychiatric outcomes of bullying and being bullied by peers in childhood and adolescence. *Journal of the American Academy of Child and Adolescent Psychiatry*. 2013;70(4):419–26.
49. Platt B, Cohen Kadosh K, Lau JY. The role of peer rejection in adolescent depression. *Depression Anxiety*. 2013;30(9):809–21.
50. Rose AJ, Rudolph KD. A review of sex differences in peer relationship processes: potential trade-offs for the emotional and behavioral development of girls and boys. *Psychological Bulletin*. 2006;132(1):98–131.
51. Valkenburg PM, Meier A, Beyens I. Social media use and its impact on adolescent mental health: an umbrella review of the evidence. *Current Opinion in Psychology*. 2022;44:58–68.
52. Hantsoo L, Epperson CN. Premenstrual dysphoric disorder: epidemiology and treatment. *Current Psychiatry Reports*. 2015;17(11):87.
53. Schiller CE, Meltzer-Brody S, Rubinow DR. The role of reproductive hormones in postpartum depression. *CNS Spectrums*. 2015;20(1):48–59.
54. Freeman EW. Associations of depression with the transition to menopause. *Menopause*. 2010;17(4):823–7.

55. Mishra GD, Kuh D. Health symptoms during midlife in relation to menopausal transition: British prospective cohort study. *British Medical Journal*. 2012;344(7846):16.
56. Kuh D, Hardy R, Rodgers B, Wadsworth MEJ. Lifetime risk factors for women's psychological distress in midlife. *Social Science and Medicine*. 2002;55(11):1957–73.
57. Schaakxs R, Comijs HC, Lamers F, Kok RM, Beekman ATF, Penninx BWJH. Associations between age and the course of major depressive disorder: a 2-year longitudinal cohort study. *Lancet Psychiatry*. 2018;5(7):581–90.
58. Mirza SSMD, Wolters FJMD, Swanson SAS, Koudstaal PJP, Hofman AP, Tiemeier HP, et al. 10-year trajectories of depressive symptoms and risk of dementia: a population-based study. *Lancet Psychiatry*. 2016;3(7):628–35.
59. Empana J-P, Boutouyrie P, Lemogne C, Jouven X, van Sloten TT. Microvascular contribution to late-onset depression: mechanisms, current evidence, association with other brain diseases, and therapeutic perspectives. *Biological Psychiatry (1969)*. 2021;90(4):214–25.
60. Hammen C. Risk factors for depression: an autobiographical review. *Annual Review of Clinical Psychology*. 2018;14(1):1–28.
61. Maciejewski PK, Prigerson HG, Mazure CM. Sex differences in event-related risk for major depression. *Psychological Medicine*. 2001;31(4):593–604.
62. Hakulinen C, Elovainio M, Pulkki-Råback L, Virtanen M, Kivimäki M, Jokela M. Personality and depressive symptoms: individual participant meta-analysis of 10 cohort studies. *Depression and Anxiety*. 2015;32(7):461–70.
63. Leach LS, Christensen H, Mackinnon AJ, Windsor TD, Butterworth P. Gender differences in depression and anxiety across the adult lifespan: the role of psychosocial mediators. *Social Psychiatry and Psychiatric Epidemiology*. 2008;43(12):983–98.
64. Kendler KS, Gardner CO. Sex differences in the pathways to major depression: a study of opposite-sex twin pairs. *American Journal of Psychiatry*. 2014;171(4):426–35.
65. Ormel J, Jeronimus BF, Kotov R, Riese H, Bos EH, Hankin B, et al. Neuroticism and common mental disorders: meaning and utility of a complex relationship. *Clinical Psychology Review*. 2013;33(5):686–97.
66. Hammen C. Risk factors for depression: an autobiographical review. *Annual Review of Clinical Psychology*. 2018;14:1–28.
67. Rood L, Roelofs J, Bögels SM, Nolen-Hoeksema S, Schouten E. The influence of emotion-focused rumination and distraction on depressive symptoms in non-clinical youth: a meta-analytic review. *Clinical Psychology Review*. 2009;29(7):607–16.
68. Johnson DP, Whisman MA. Gender differences in rumination: a meta-analysis. *Personality and Individual Differences*. 2013;55(4):367–74.
69. Heller W. Gender differences in depression: perspectives from neuropsychology. *Journal of Affective Disorders*. 1993;29(2–3):129–43.
70. Davies SJC, Pearson RM, Stapinski L, Bould H, Christmas DM, Button KS, et al. Symptoms of generalized anxiety disorder but not panic disorder at age 15 years increase the risk of depression at 18 years in the Avon Longitudinal Study of Parents and Children (ALSPAC) Cohort Study. *Psychological Medicine*. 2016;46(1):73–85.
71. Asselmann E, Wittchen H-U, Lieb R, Höfler M, Beesdo-Baum K. Associations of fearful spells and panic attacks with incident anxiety, depressive, and substance use disorders: a 10-year prospective-longitudinal community study of adolescents and young adults. *Journal of Psychiatric Research*. 2014;55(1):8–14.
72. Konrad K, Kohls G, Baumann S, Bernhard A, Martinelli A, Ackermann K, et al. Sex differences in psychiatric comorbidity and clinical presentation in youths with conduct disorder. *Journal of Child Psychlogy and Psychiatry*. 2021;63(2):218–28.
73. Colman I, Ataullahjan A. Life course perspectives on the epidemiology of depression. *Canadian Journal of Psychiatry*. 2010;55(10):622–32.
74. Grundström J, Konttinen H, Berg N, Kiviruusu O. Associations between relationship status and mental well-being in different life phases from young to middle adulthood. *SSM Population Health*. 2021;14:100774.

75. Bulloch AGM, Williams JVA, Lavorato DH, Patten SB. The depression and marital status relationship is modified by both age and gender. *Journal of Affective Disorders*. 2017;223:65–8.

76. Michelini G, Perlman G, Tian Y, Mackin DM, Nelson BD, Klein DN, et al. Multiple domains of risk factors for first onset of depression in adolescent girls. *Journal of Affective Disorders*. 2021;283:20–9.

77. Colman I, Jones PB, Kuh D, Weeks M, Naicker K, Richards M, et al. Early development, stress and depression across the life course: pathways to depression in a national British birth cohort. *Psychological Medicine*. 2014;44(13):2845–54.

10
Cognition Function and Dementia
A Life Course Perspective

Erin E. Sundermann, Sarah J. Banks, and Carlos Araujo Menendez

10.1 Introduction

Dementia is a collective term for neurodegenerative diseases characterised by impairment of
at least two brain functions (e.g. memory loss and judgement) that is severe enough to interfere with daily function. Although rates of dementia are rising due to the ageing of the population, the age-specific incidence of dementia is decreasing in many countries likely because
of improvements in health care and lifestyle factors such as education and diet.[1] This trend
supports the role of modifiable risk factors across the lifespan in the risk of dementia. Based
on the evidence thus far, the 2020 Lancet Commission on dementia prevention identified
12 potentially modifiable risk factors that account for about 40% of global dementia cases,
including less education, hypertension, hearing impairment, smoking, obesity, depression,
physical inactivity, diabetes, low social contact, excessive alcohol consumption, traumatic
brain injury, and air pollution.[2] Notably, these factors represent risks across the life course
suggesting that public policy, health care programs, and individually tailored interventions
are all important in reducing dementia risk, particularly in LMICs where changes to the environment and health care will reap the most benefit.[2]

There are multiple types of dementia including AD, vascular, frontotemporal, dementia
with Lewy Bodies, and Parkinson's disease type. AD is the most common type contributing
to 60%–70% of dementia cases.[3] More than 6 million Americans are currently living with
AD dementia in the United States, and these rates are expected to increase with the ageing of
the baby boomers to 13 million in 2050.[4] Of these cases, two thirds are women,[4] signalling a
critical sex difference in AD. AD is a progressive neurodegenerative disease that leads to loss
of daily function because of memory loss, thinking and reasoning deficits, and behavioural
changes. The precursor stage to dementia is termed mild cognitive impairment (MCI), in
which cognitive impairment is observed on clinical tests; however, this impairment is not severe enough to impact daily functioning. Similar to dementia, there are multiple subtypes of
MCI with the amnestic MCI (aMCI) subtype characterised by episodic memory impairment
and most likely to lead to AD dementia specifically.

The hallmark brain changes in AD include the deposition of extracellular senile plaques
composed of amyloid-b (Aβ) protein, intracellular neurofibrillary tangles composed of ab-
normally phosphorylated tau protein, and neurodegeneration.[5] However, there is substantial heterogeneity in AD pathology, with most cases having some degree of mixed pathology
from different dementia types. These pathological brain changes are known to occur up to a

Erin E. Sundermann, Sarah J. Banks, and Carlos Araujo Menendez, *Cognition Function and Dementia* In: *A Life Course Approach to
Women's Health*. Second Edition. Edited by: Gita D Mishra, Rebecca Hardy, and Diana Kuh, Oxford University Press.
© Oxford University Press 2023. DOI: 10.1093/oso/9780192864642.003.0010

decade before the emergence of cognitive deficits, and this lag period is likely mediated by differences in brain resiliency or cognitive reserve.[6] Although pathological brain changes in AD have been well defined, the cause of the disease and effective treatment remains elusive.

10.2 Sex Differences in AD Rates

It is well known that women bear the greatest burden of AD, and this chapter will examine this sex disparity through a lifespan lens that will consider the contributions of life-long sex differences in brain structure and function and reproductive ageing and gender-related socio-cultural factors. In discussing sex/gender, it is important to note that *sex* refers to biological differences between males and females that primarily result from gonadal hormones and sex chromosome (XX versus XY) differences. *Gender* is a social construct referring to how one identifies themselves that can be influenced by environmental, social, and cultural factors. A limitation of this classification is its often-binary nature in research fails to capture the fluidity and diversity that can occur for both sex and gender within and among individuals.

The higher frequency of AD in women is well-established; however, whether women are at higher risk for AD after adjusting for their longer lifespan remains controversial. Studies account for this sex difference in longevity by measuring the incidence of AD or the proportion of individuals who develop AD at a given age. Multiple large-scale epidemiological studies have found a higher age-specific incidence rate of AD in women versus men,[7-10] suggesting that the higher prevalence of AD in women goes beyond their longevity. Some robust evidence for a significantly higher incident rate in women versus men is from the EURODEM study: a large-pooled analysis of four European, population-based studies of individuals aged 65 years and older. With over 28,000 person-years of follow-up and 528 incident dementia cases, the EURODEM study reported that cumulative risk of AD was about two times higher in women versus men at age 85 years, and this difference increased as age increased.[8] However, multiple studies in the United States and globally have reported no sex difference[11-13] or even the reverse sex difference (higher AD risk in men versus women) in the UK-based Cognitive Function and Ageing Study,[14] making this view controversial and perhaps dependent on the age distribution of the sample and the geographic region of the study. Regardless of whether women are truly at higher risk for AD, this chapter describes evidence for sex/gender differences in multiple aspects of AD, including risk factors, diagnostic accuracy, clinical trajectory, and pathological burden, and understanding these differences can provide mechanistic clues into disease aetiology and provide insights into risk reduction and intervention strategies that are optimal for each sex.

10.3 Sex Differences in Cognitive Function Throughout the Lifespan

There are well-established sex differences in cognitive abilities across the lifespan. Women tend to excel at tasks involving verbal and fine motor skills and processing speed.[15-20] In terms of verbal skills, the female advantage in verbal memory (memory for verbally presented material, e.g. stories, word lists) has been reliably demonstrated across the adult lifespan,[21] as well as in children.[22,23] Conversely, there is a male advantage in visuospatial abilities and this advantage is seen across the lifespan including among children.[23,24] Because these sex differences are often observed across the lifespan, most take a behavioural endocrinological approach to these differences and believe that they primarily reflect organisational effects of sex hormones or the permanent effects of sex steroid hormones on brain structure and function in utero.

In addition to the organisational effects of sex hormones, there are activational effects describing the immediate effects of sex hormones on the body that vary based on the current levels of circulating hormones. The activational effects of sex hormones on brain function are believed to be superimposed on the organisational effects. This notion stems from studies demonstrating changes in cognitive function congruent with changes in sex hormone levels. In a randomised clinical trial of hormone therapy (oestrogen alone or oestrogen-androgen combination) for women who underwent surgical menopause because of benign disease (e.g. ovarian cysts), decreases in verbal memory performance were reported postsurgery in women receiving placebo treatment, whereas women who received hormone therapy maintained verbal memory performance.[25] Changes in cognitive function have also been observed across the menstrual cycle in women, whereby cognitive performance during the high-oestrogen phase of the menstrual cycle improved on cognitive abilities favouring females (i.e. fine motor coordination and processing speed) and declined on cognitive abilities favouring males (i.e. visuospatial ability) as compared to the low-oestrogen phase.[26] A formative study of transsexuals found that testosterone treatment in female-to-male transsexuals enhanced performance on male-favouring tasks (i.e. visuospatial function). In contrast, antiandrogen treatment in combination with oestrogen therapy did not influence performance on either male- or female-favouring tasks in male-to-female transsexuals.[27]

In older age, some degree of cognitive decline is consistently observed in both sexes and across cognitive domains; however, sex differences have been observed in the rate of cognitive decline. A study of cognitively normal older adults (mean age of 64 to 70 years) from the Baltimore Study of Longitudinal Aging examined trajectories of various cognitive measures across a mean follow-up period of 5 to 9 years (N = 1065 to 2127).[28] It found a more accelerated decline for men on measures of global mental status, perceptuomotor speed and integration, and visuospatial ability, but there were no cognitive tasks in which women showed a more accelerated decline. These findings suggest that women may be more resilient to age-related cognitive decline than men.[28]

10.4 Female Verbal Memory Advantage: Implications for AD Trajectory and Diagnosis

Although the female advantage in verbal memory is functionally beneficial, it may have disadvantages in terms of early detection of AD. This is because clinical tests of verbal memory are a key component of aMCI and AD diagnostic criteria, and the normative data for these tests typically account for differences in verbal memory performance by age and/or education, but not sex, which could have clinical implications for the clinical detection of aMCI and AD. It is possible that the female advantage in verbal memory may enhance women's ability to compensate for advancing disease burden and maintain what is considered 'normal' memory performance on clinical testing. In support of this theory, studies found that the female advantage in verbal memory is sustained even in samples of men and women with evidence of moderate AD pathology (hippocampal atrophy, brain glucose hypometabolism, and Aβ plaque burden).[29-31] Moreover, women demonstrate a greater burden of pathological tau—the AD pathology most closely tethered to clinical symptoms[32,33]—than men early in the AD trajectory.[34-39] The female verbal memory advantage appears to persist even through this elevated pathological burden.[40,41] Critically, the female advantage might mask underlying brain pathology particularly in earlier disease stages, which has implications for early detection and intervention. A delayed onset of clinically evident verbal memory impairment would limit the opportunity for early diagnosis and intervention when our currently available interventions are most likely to be effective and life planning is better implemented.

The impressive resilience shown by women during the earlier phases of the AD continuum cannot persist as the disease spreads. In fact, after MCI diagnosis, women demonstrate a decline in cognition which is two times faster than men.[42] It has been hypothesised that the cognitive trajectory of AD in women resembles a waterfall effect, whereby women are better able to sustain normal cognitive function than men in prodromal AD stages, but as AD pathology becomes more advanced, women are no longer able to compensate and accelerated cognitive decline begins. In keeping with a more aggressive clinical trajectory in later stages of the AD trajectory, a study of 141 autopsy cases with antemortem cognitive data found that AD pathology is more likely to be clinically expressed as dementia in women than in men.[43] The shifting profile of sex differences in AD trajectory suggests a sex-specific balance of brain-related resilience and risk factors that change over the course of AD and stresses the importance of considering disease stage when investigating sex differences.

10.5 Sex Differences in Pathophysiological Brain Changes in AD

10.5.1 Sex Differences in Tau Burden

It is well-evidenced that pathological tau levels, the principal component of the AD-related neurofibrillary tangles, are elevated in women versus men in AD.[34-39] However, why this is the case is largely unknown. Spread of tau is thought to occur via a prion-like mechanism involving transfer of abnormal tau seeds from a 'donor cell' to a 'recipient cell'.[44] Because of this propagation pattern, interconnected brain regions with high levels of synaptic connectivity appear to pave a path for the spread of tau.[45] Shokouhi and colleagues[46] examined whether the network connectivity patterns of regional tau deposition among brain regions differ by sex. They found that higher network density and number of direct regional connections in women versus men may favour accelerated brain-wide tau spread and, in turn, greater tau burden.[46]

There may be other biological differences for why women show more tau. While we do not know why pathological tau accumulates exactly, the potential involvement of inflammation, vascular dysfunction, hormones, or changes in the blood-brain barrier could all contribute. An important link has been demonstrated between testosterone and tau, such that low testosterone predicts higher tau levels, regardless of sex, but particularly in those at higher genetic risk for AD through the apolipoprotein-ε e4 allele.[39] These findings suggest that women may be predisposed to tau by way of lower testosterone levels, particularly among those at higher genetic risk for AD.

10.5.2 Sex Differences in Brain Function

One biological sex difference that may be relevant to AD is in brain metabolism. Glucose is the primary fuel source for the brain, and we can use PET imaging to measure the amount of glucose metabolism in the brain as a proxy for brain energy utilisation. Thus, low glucose metabolism reflects low brain efficiency and dysfunction. There is evidence of higher levels of brain glucose metabolism in women versus men among healthy adults and in the early stages of AD.[31,47–51] Among 1259 (44% women) cognitively normal, aMCI and AD dementia participants, Sundermann et al. examined whether this female metabolic advantage was sustained in AD and whether it represents a brain resilience mechanism that enables women to sustain their memory function despite AD brain changes.[52] As expected, they found that brain metabolism was significantly higher in women versus men with the exception of those without advanced AD pathology burden. Concurrent with higher brain metabolism, these women also showed a cognitive advantage over men that extended past verbal memory to more global cognition; however, this female cognitive advantage was eliminated when accounting for the higher brain metabolism in these women.[52] These findings suggest that the higher brain metabolic function in women helps to explain the female cognitive advantage in earlier AD stages possibly by conferring cognitive resilience against early AD pathology.[52]

10.6 AD Risk Factors in Women

AD risk factors occur across the lifespan. This section highlights some risk factors that occur both in early and mid to late life. Many of these risk factors show sex/gender disparities in different ways: i) risk factors that are equally common in women and men but have a stronger effect in one sex/gender group, ii) risk factors that have a similar effect in women and men but are more common in one sex/gender, and iii) risk factors restricted to one sex (e.g. pregnancy, menopause).

10.6.1 Early Life Risk Factors

Early life risk factors include low education and other socioeconomic and environmental factors such as poverty, barriers to health care, and air pollution that are particularly prevalent in LMICs. Early life risk factors can also include biological factors such as birthweight and whether or not one was breastfed. While birthweight and being breastfed are each associated with academic achievement, cognitive function, and intellectual performance in childhood, even with adjustment for parental socioeconomic position (SEP),[53–56] it is unclear if these effects remain in old age. To the best of our knowledge, only three studies have examined the association between breastfeeding and cognitive ability in old age with two of those studies among men only.[57–59] The only study thus far that included women in their sample of adults at least 70 years old reported that being breastfed in infancy is associated with higher IQ in older age, which is thought to confer cognitive reserve in the face of dementia-related pathology. However, this association was accounted for once adjusting for SEP in childhood,[58] and sex differences in the association were not examined. Regarding the association between birthweight and cognition, the largest study on the topic was done in the Swedish Twin

Registry (N = 35,191) by Mosing et al.[60] They found that low birthweight was a risk factor for late-life cognitive dysfunction and dementia, even after adjusting for gestational age, prenatal covariates (e.g. parity of mother, age of mother at birth), SES at birth, and education level.[60]

10.6.2 Cardiovascular Risk Factors

Our brains are massively vascularised organs and the role of vascular disease either as a central mechanism of AD or a promoting factor is widely acknowledged.[61,62] The delicate myriad of small vessels in the brain tend to deteriorate with ageing, but this is hastened by risk factors such as obesity,[63] lack of physical activity,[64] hypercholesterolemia, hypertension, and diabetes.[65] These vascular risk factors do not impact men and women equally. Large epidemiological studies point to a critical period in the fourth and fifth decade of life, when hypertension appears to pose a higher risk for late-onset dementia in women than men.[66,67] Sedentary behaviour has been associated with greater pathological tau[68-79] and worse cognitive function;[80-85] however, several studies, including meta-analyses,[86,87] report that the association with worse cognitive function is either stronger in women[86-89] or female- specific.[90-92] Obesity is another vascular risk factor for dementia, especially midlife obesity,[93] while later-life obesity has a less clear relationship with dementia, possibly because of the potential for reverse causation whereby the weight loss that occurs in the preclinical phase makes higher BMI appear protective.[94] Sex differences have been detected with obesity, seeming to be a stronger risk factor for AD in women[95] potentially as a function of inflammation.[96]

10.6.3 Depression

Depression represents another highly prevalent and often underdiagnosed or undertreated risk factor for AD.[97] Depression is twice as common in women than men[98] (see Chapter 9 for further details). Despite this, the Baltimore Longitudinal Study of Aging showed that midlife symptoms of depression were more of a risk factor for Alzheimer's in men compared with women.[99] Another study found similar levels of risk for men and women with midlife depression for later onset of all-cause dementia.[100] There is evidence to suggest that depression could be part of a behavioural prodrome for AD, and this seems to be especially the case in women who develop depressive symptoms in late life.[101] Thus, the data are mixed and depending on timing, midlife versus late life, of symptoms, there may be a differential effect of sex.

10.6.4 APOE4

A genetic isoform (ε4 allele) of the apolipoprotein E gene (APOE) is an example of a risk factor that is equally prevalent in men and women, but evidence suggests a more adverse effect of the genetic variant in women. APOE-ε4 is the most common genetic risk factor for late-onset AD.[102,103] The gene codes for a plasma protein involved in lipoprotein synthesis and cholesterol transport. The human APOE gene exists as three polymorphic alleles, ε2, ε3, and ε4, with frequencies in the global population of 8.4%, 77.9%, and 13.7%, respectively.[104] While the infrequent ε2 allele has a protective effect against AD, the ε4 allele increases risk and the ε3 allele is risk neutral. The presence of one allele (APOE4 heterozygotes) increases the risk of AD approximately threefold, while presence of two alleles (APOE4 homozygotes) increases risk approximately ninefold.[105] Cross-sectional, longitudinal. and meta-analytic studies indicate that APOE4 confers a greater risk for AD in women than in men[36,104,106–111] even when adjusting for longevity.[110] The more deleterious effect of APOE4 in women versus men has been shown to be driven more so by ε3/ε4 heterozygotes than ε4/ε4 homozygotes.[107,108] Specifically, a meta-analysis by Farrer et al.[104] showed that, compared to the ε3/ε3 genotype, the ε3/ε4 genotype was associated with a 4-fold increased risk of AD in women and a 1.5-fold increased risk in men. As with most sex differences in AD, the underlying mechanism of the stronger APOE4 effect in women remains unclear. Sex hormones likely contribute given that oestrogen plays a critical role in the regulation of APOE expression in the brain.[112]

10.7 Female-Specific AD Risk and Protective Factors

Given that reproductive hormones are a central determinant of sex differences in brain structure and function,[113,114] it is important to consider factors that influence lifetime exposure to these hormones when understanding sex differences in AD. At the cellular level, oestrogen facilitates synaptogenesis,[115] long-term potentiation in the hippocampus,[116] and survival of new neurons,[117] while reducing the formation of β-amyloid.[118,119] An important consideration for brain and cognitive ageing is how long and to what degree was the brain exposed to the neuroprotective effects of oestradiol throughout a women's lifetime. While both sexes experience reproductive ageing, this process is more complex in women with a constellation of hormone-altering events including menopause, pregnancy, breastfeeding, and the use of oral contraceptives (OC) and hormone therapies (HT). As these factors contribute to the lifetime degree of oestrogen exposure and help determine the hormonal milieu of the brain, growing evidence indicates that they may be female-specific risk and protective factors that influence the pathological processes that lead to AD.[120] More recently, studies have attempted to mathematically combine reproductive history factors into an index of cumulative oestrogen exposure and, so far, this index has shown inverse relationships with AD risk[121] but not consistently.[122]

10.7.1 Menopause

Multiple studies have shown associations between early menopause due to either natural causes or medical intervention and poorer cognitive function in later life and/or increased risk of AD.[123–127] Other studies reported an association of longer reproductive span (time span from menarche to menopause) with lower risk of AD or all-cause dementia.[121,127,128] In the largest study to date to examine female reproductive factors in relation to dementia risk, Yoo et al. used the Korean National Health Insurance System database to identify 4,696,633 postmenopausal women without dementia at baseline and with data on reproductive factors from a self-administered questionnaire.[127] They found a 21% reduction in risk of dementia for women with a menopausal age ≥55 years compared to women with a menopausal age < 40 years. Similarly, they found a 19% reduction in risk of dementia for women with a reproductive span of ≥40 years compared those with a reproductive span < 30 years. However, findings have been inconsistent, with another study reporting an association of longer reproductive span with higher dementia risk[129] and others reporting no association.[122,130] These inconsistencies in the literature may be partly explained by the fact that the reproductive span is complicated by a number of factors that can alter the degree of oestrogen exposure influencing lifetime endocrine exposure, including exogenous hormone use and reproductive history (e.g. OC, hormone therapy, and pregnancy). Thus, it is challenging to determine whether there is a causal effect between reproductive span and AD risk. A Mendelian randomization study attempted to address the causality question using publicly available summary statistics based on individuals of European ancestry from the MRC Integrative Epidemiology Unit genome-wide association studies database.[131] They found no significant causal relationship between the genetically determined age at menarche or age at menopause and AD risk; however, higher age at menarche was significantly associated with lower BMI, suggesting that reproductive span proxies may influence AD risk indirectly through other health factors.[131]

Studies have also examined menopause in relation to neuroimaging biomarkers of AD. In a study of cognitively normal participants aged approximately 52 years including 99 women and 29 men, Schelbaum et al. found that postmenopausal women showed lower grey matter volume in AD-sensitive brain regions compared to men, and peri- and postmenopausal women showed lower grey matter volume in the temporal cortex compared to premenopausal women.[132] Among postmenopausal women, longer reproductive span was associated with higher grey matter volume in temporal and frontal cortices and precuneus.[132] In a MRI and PET study of 121 (70% women) cognitively normal midlife-to-older participants aged 40–65 years, postmenopausal status was a strong predictor, second to female sex, of higher Aβ deposition, lower brain glucose metabolism, and lower grey and white matter volumes.[133]

10.7.2 Hormone Therapy

Despite well-established findings of the neuroprotective effects of endogenous oestrogen, the effect of HT is complicated and controversial. In the 1990s, a series of observational studies showed a protective effect of HT on AD risk in menopausal women. This evidence was promising and led to the first randomised clinical trial of the effects of HT on dementia risk in older (aged ≥65 years) postmenopausal women, conducted by The Women's Health Initiative Memory Study (WHIMS). Specifically, WHIMS investigated the impact of conjugated equine oestrogen (CEE) in women with prior hysterectomy over age 65 and the impact of CEE combined with progesterone therapy (medroxyprogesterone acetate [MPA]) in naturally postmenopausal women over age 65.[134,135] The trials were surprisingly stopped prematurely because of a lack of evidence that CEE lowered the risk of all-cause dementia in postmenopausal women with prior hysterectomy[134] and combination CEE/MPA actually doubled the risk for all-cause dementia among naturally postmenopausal women.[135] This finding came as a shock to many researchers since none of the prior observational studies reported an increased risk in dementia with HT and impelled a push to identify what was different about this clinical trial compared to the observational studies. Since the WHIMS trial was limited to women age 65 and older, whereas most of the earlier observational studies were in women who were closer to the menopause transition, the possibility of a critical window of time for the beneficial effects of HT on the brain was raised with that critical period being during the menopause transition or soon after.[136-139] The critical window hypothesis is supported by rodent models that find improved performance on a spatial memory task when HT use is initiated immediately after ovariectomy in female rats but not when initiation was delayed 10 months.[140] However, findings from more two randomised controlled trials in recently postmenopausal women were not supportive of the critical window hypothesis. The Kronos Early Estrogen Prevention Study (KEEPS) (N = 727) and The Early vs Late Intervention Trial with Estradiol (ELITE) (N = 567) found that HT use did not benefit cognition in recently postmenopausal women.[141,142] Importantly, these studies also did not find a negative effect of HT use on cognition. More follow-up data will need to be collected in these cohorts in order to adequately assess HT in relation to dementia risk.

10.7.3 Pregnancy

Pregnancy is a significant event in women's reproductive history that leads to large fluctuations in sex hormone levels as well as changes to immunological factors.[143,144] While oestrogen levels elevate during pregnancy, the more long-lasting effect of pregnancy is a decrease in lifetime oestrogen levels of about ~22% postpregnancy.[145] Large epidemiological studies have found that multiparity, or multiple pregnancies that reach viable gestational age, is associated with an increased risk of all-cause dementia and AD,[122,146-148] as well as cognitive decline[147,149,150] and earlier age of onset of sporadic AD,[151] suggesting that these hormonal changes may have long-lasting impacts on brain health and risk of neurodegenerative diseases. In particular, grand multiparity (>5 pregnancies) increased dementia risk by 30% compared to women with less than four pregnancies.[147,149] However, results are highly inconsistent with another group reporting a beneficial effect of pregnancy on AD risk.[152] The authors proposed that the reduction in AD risk may be due to an improvement in immunoregulation caused by T-regulatory cells that dramatically rise during the first trimester and continue to gradually increase for at least a year postpartum.[153-155] Parity has also shown a relationship to AD neuropathology. Schelbaum et al. found that number of children and pregnancies were positively associated with grey matter volume predominantly in temporal and frontal cortices and precuneus, and these associations were independent of age, APOE4 status, and midlife health factors.[132] Beeri et al. found that greater number of children was associated with increased neuropathologic lesions of AD and neuritic plaques in female postmortem cases.[156] Jung et al. found that grand multiparity was associated with reduced overall brain and hippocampal volume, but not with Aβ pathology or white matter hyperintensities.[157] The inconsistent findings may be attributed to studies not accounting for age at first pregnancy and breastfeeding history and/or examining gravity (total number of pregnancies regardless of length) versus parity. Future studies should account for factors that may confound the relationship between pregnancy and AD, such as age at first pregnancy, history of breastfeeding, and incomplete pregnancies.

10.7.4 Oral Contraceptives

While the cognitive effects of menopausal HT have been studied extensively, few investigations have examined how altering natural ovarian hormone production in premenopausal women through hormone-based treatments impacts brain health. Considering that over 100 million women use worldwide use OC,[158] this question has weighty public health significance. The minimal evidence so far has suggested both acute and long-term effects of OC use on cognitive and brain function. In terms of acute effects, Mordecai et al.[159] found that OC users showed enhanced verbal memory during the active versus inactive pill phase. In terms of long-term effects, large community-based studies have found lower risk of dementia[127] or better cognitive function[160,161] in previous OC users versus never users. Neuroimaging studies have also found links between OCs and brain structure/function outcomes. In the Schelbaum et al. study, past OC use was associated with higher grey matter volume mostly in the temporal and frontal cortices and precuneus, independent of age and APOE4 status and midlife health factors.[132] In another structural and functional MRI study, OC users demonstrated larger grey matter volume in certain brain regions compared to nonusers,[162,163] as well as stronger activation in the right-hemispheric task-specific areas during a word generation task.[164] Findings thus far hint at a beneficial effect of OC use on the brain; however, these studies are merely scratching the surface of the potential consequences of ovarian hormone suppression on the brain, which are likely influenced by a myriad of factors including OC formulation, age at initiation, and length of use.

10.8 Gender and Sociocultural Risk Factors for AD

Thus far, we have mostly discussed sex-related biological factors that likely contribute to AD risk; however, gender-related factors are likely to play a role as well. For example, low education is an example of an AD risk factor that has a similar harmful effect in men and women but is historically more common in women, given fewer opportunities for higher education in women versus men in older generations. However, this trend has actually reversed in younger generations with more women in graduate-level programs than men in the United States.[165] Low physical activity, particularly during midlife, is another risk factor for AD that tends to be more common in women versus men. Although time spent in exercise does not differ by gender, women are less likely to engage in rigorous exercise than men, and this is thought to be due, in part, to the different work, family and parenting roles typically occupied by men and women.[166] Nonmarried status, either because one never married or is widowed, is one of the few, if not only, risk factors for AD that appears to have a more adverse effect in men compared to women.[9,167,168] One contributing factor to this disparity may be the societal and cultural demands on women to adopt the role of a family caregiver (e.g. scheduling doctor's appointments, providing a nutritious diet)[169] and sometimes at the expense of their own health. Additionally, single women are more likely than single men to have regular visits with healthcare providers.[170]

10.9 Conclusions

In addition to AD rates, critical sex differences have been reported in disease risk factors, diagnosis, clinical trajectory, and pathology burden. The reasons for these sex differences remain elusive but are likely multifactorial and include a combination of differences related to gender (e.g. education) and biological sex. The findings described in this chapter illustrate the importance of having a life course perspective when considering risk of AD in women versus men. For example, the life-long female advantage in verbal memory can have critical implications for the presentation and diagnosis of AD considering that clinical tests of verbal memory are a key component of MCI and AD diagnosis and the norms for these tests typically do not adjust for this sex difference. Research into the harmful consequences of non-sex-adjusted norms has begun to motivate change in normative data development. For example, the Mayo's Older Americans Normative Studies recently revised their norms for the commonly used Rey Auditory Verbal Learning Test by including a sex adjustment.

Given well-documented effects of sex hormones on the brain, there is a critical need for research to consider the influence that female reproductive history has on the ageing brain. Although often overlooked by dementia research that is focused on late-life brain health, we argue that factors related to female reproductive history are an important consideration for brain ageing as they alter the length of time and the degree to which the brain is exposed to the neuroprotective effects of sex hormones throughout the lifetime. An emerging appreciation for the influence of sex on health processes and outcomes and an awareness of over-reliance on male animals and cells in biomedical research led to policy implementation by the National Institute of Health (NIH). Since 2016, the NIH requires the consideration of sex as a biological variable in NIH-funded research. Policies such as this can only improve the value of biomedical science in that discovery of sex differences in disease outcomes can advance the development of risk assessments and therapeutic strategies that are optimal for each sex and serve as a window into causal pathways of disease.

Key messages and implications

- Women have an advantage in verbal memory over men; however, this may mask early clinical detection of amnestic MCI and AD dementia.
- The principal component of the AD-related neurofibrillary tangles, tau, is more elevated in women than in men.
- More research is needed to establish the relationship between reproductive factors (e.g. age at menopause, hormone therapy, and pregnancy characteristics) and risk of AD.

References

1. Wu Y-T, Beiser AS, Breteler MMB, Fratiglioni L, Helmer C, Hendrie HC, et al. The changing prevalence and incidence of dementia over time—current evidence. *Nature Reviews Neurology*. 2017;13(6):327–39.

2. Livingston G, Huntley J, Sommerlad A, Ames D, Ballard C, Banerjee S, et al. Dementia prevention, intervention, and care: 2020 report of the Lancet Commission. *Lancet.* 2020;396(10248):413–46.

3. World Health Organization. *World Health Organization—dementia key facts* [Internet]. Geneva: World Health Organization; 2021 [updated 2 September 2021; cited 26 May 2022]. Available from: https://www.who.int/news-room/fact-sheets/detail/dementia.

4. Alzheimer's Association. 2020 Alzheimer's disease facts and figures. *Alzheimer's & Dementia.* 2020;16(3):391–460.

5. Jack CR, Knopman DS, Jagust WJ, Petersen RC, Weiner MW, Aisen PS, et al. Tracking pathophysiological processes in Alzheimer's disease: an updated hypothetical model of dynamic biomarkers. *Lancet Neurology.* 2013;12(2):207–16.

6. Stern Y. Cognitive Reserve and Alzheimer Disease. *Alzheimer Disease & Associated Disorders.* 2006;20(2):112–17.

7. Gao S, Hendrie HC, Hall KS, Hui S. The relationships between age, sex, and the incidence of dementia and Alzheimer disease: a meta-analysis. *Archives of General Psychiatry.* 1998;55(9):809–15.

8. Andersen K, Launer LJ, Dewey ME, Letenneur L, Ott A, Copeland JRM, et al. Gender differences in the incidence of AD and vascular dementia. *EURODEM Studies.* 1999;53(9):1992.

9. Miech RA, Breitner JCS, Zandi PP, Khachaturian AS, Anthony JC, Mayer L. Incidence of AD may decline in the early 90s for men, later for women. *Cache County Study.* 2002;58(2):209–18.

10. Ott A, Breteler MMB, Harskamp FV, Stijnen T, Hofman A. Incidence and risk of dementia: the Rotterdam Study. *American Journal of Epidemiology.* 1998;147(6):574–80.

11. Katz MJ, Lipton RB, Hall CB, Zimmerman ME, Sanders AE, Verghese J, et al. Age-specific and sex-specific prevalence and incidence of mild cognitive impairment, dementia, and Alzheimer dementia in blacks and whites: a report from the Einstein Aging Study. *Alzheimer Disease & Associated Disorders.* 2012;26(4):335–43.

12. Fiest KM, Jetté N, Roberts JI, Maxwell CJ, Smith EE, Black SE, et al. The prevalence and incidence of dementia: a systematic review and meta-analysis. *Canadian Journal of Neurological Sciences/ Journal Canadien des Sciences Neurologiques.* 2016;43(S1):S3–S50.

13. Mielke M, Vemuri P, Rocca W. Clinical epidemiology of Alzheimer's disease: assessing sex and gender differences. *Clinical Epidemiology.* 2013;6:37–48.

14. Matthews FE, Arthur A, Barnes LE, Bond J, Jagger C, Robinson L, et al. A two-decade comparison of prevalence of dementia in individuals aged 65 years and older from three geographical areas of England: results of the Cognitive Function and Ageing Study I and II. *Lancet.* 2013;382(9902):1405–12.

15. Halari R, Hines M, Kumari V, Mehrotra R, Wheeler M, Ng V, et al. Sex differences and individual differences in cognitive performance and their relationship to endogenous gonadal hormones and gonadotropins. *Behavioral Neuroscience.* 2005;119:104–17.

16. Mann VA, Sasanuma S, Sakuma N, Masaki S. Sex differences in cognitive abilities: a cross-cultural perspective. *Neuropsychologia.* 1990;28(10):1063–77.

17. Schmidt SL, Oliveira RM, Rocha FOR, Abreu-Villaca Y. Influences of handedness and gender on the grooved pegboard test. *Brain and Cognition.* 2000;44(3):445–54.

18. Kramer JH, Delis DC, Daniel M. Sex differences in verbal learning. *Journal of Clinical Psychology.* 1988;44(6):907–15.

19. Snow WG, Weinstock J. Sex differences among non-brain-damaged adults on the Wechsler adult intelligence scales: a review of the literature. *Journal of Clinical and Experimental Neuropsychology.* 1990;12(6):873–86.

20. Weiss EM, Ragland JD, Brensinger CM, Bilker WB, Deisenhammer EA, Delazer M. Sex differences in clustering and switching in verbal fluency tasks. *Journal of the International Neuropsychological Society.* 2006;12(4):502–9.

21. Van Der Elst WIM, Van Boxtel MPJ, Van Breukelen GJP, Jolles J. Rey's verbal learning test: normative data for 1855 healthy participants aged 24–81 years and the influence of age, sex, education, and mode of presentation. *Journal of the International Neuropsychological Society.* 2005;11(3):290–302.

22. Kramer JH, Delis DC, Kaplan E, O'Donnell L, Prifitera A. Developmental sex differences in verbal learning. *Neuropsychology.* 1997;11:577–84.

23. Mous SE, Schoemaker NK, Blanken LME, Thijssen S, van der Ende J, Polderman TJC, et al. The association of gender, age, and intelligence with neuropsychological functioning in young typically developing children: the Generation R Study. *Applied Neuropsychology: Child*. 2017;6(1):22–40.

24. Kimura D, Hampson E. Neural and hormonal mechanisms mediating sex differences in cognition. In: Vernon PA, ed. *Biological approaches to the study of human intelligence*. Norwood, NJ: Ablex Publishing; 1993. pp. 375–97.

25. Sherwin BB. Estrogen and/or androgen replacement therapy and cognitive functioning in surgically menopausal women. *Psychoneuroendocrinology*. 1988;13(4):345–57.

26. Hampson E. Variations in sex-related cognitive abilities across the menstrual cycle. *Brain and Cognition*. 1990;14(1):26–43.

27. Slabbekoorn D, van Goozen SHM, Megens J, Gooren LJG, Cohen-Kettenis PT. Activating effects of cross-sex hormones on cognitive functioning: a study of short-term and long-term hormone effects in transsexuals. *Psychoneuroendocrinology*. 1999;24(4):423–47.

28. McCarrey AC, An Y, Kitner-Triolo MH, Ferrucci L, Resnick SM. Sex differences in cognitive trajectories in clinically normal older adults. *Psychology and Aging*. 2016;31(2):166–75.

29. Sundermann EE, Biegon A, Rubin LH, Lipton RB, Mowrey W, Landau S, et al. Better verbal memory in women than men in MCI despite similar levels of hippocampal atrophy. *Neurology*. 2016;86(15):1368–76.

30. Sundermann EE, Biegon A, Rubin LH, Lipton RB, Landau S, Maki PM, et al. Does the female advantage in verbal memory contribute to underestimating Alzheimer's disease pathology in women versus men? *Journal of Alzheimer's Disease*. 2017;56:947–57.

31. Sundermann EE, Maki PM, Rubin LH, Lipton RB, Landau S, Biegon A. Female advantage in verbal memory. *Evidence of Sex-Specific Cognitive Reserve*. 2016;87(18):1916–24.

32. Ossenkoppele R, Schonhaut DR, Schöll M, Lockhart SN, Ayakta N, Baker SL, et al. Tau PET patterns mirror clinical and neuroanatomical variability in Alzheimer's disease. *Brain*. 2016;139(5):1551–67.

33. Lowe VJ, Wiste HJ, Senjem ML, Weigand SD, Therneau TM, Boeve BF, et al. Widespread brain tau and its association with ageing, Braak stage and Alzheimer's dementia. *Brain*. 2017;141(1):271–87.

34. Buckley RF, Mormino EC, Rabin JS, Hohman TJ, Landau S, Hanseeuw BJ, et al. Sex differences in the association of global amyloid and regional tau deposition measured by positron emission tomography in clinically normal older adults. *JAMA Neurology*. 2019;76(5):542–51.

35. Hohman TJ, Dumitrescu L, Barnes LL, Thambisetty M, Beecham G, Kunkle B, et al. Sex-specific association of apolipoprotein e with cerebrospinal fluid levels of Tau. *JAMA Neurology*. 2018;75(8):989–98.

36. Altmann A, Tian L, Henderson VW, Greicius MD, Investigators AsDNI. Sex modifies the APOE-related risk of developing Alzheimer disease. *Annals of Neurology*. 2014;75(4):563–73.

37. Oveisgharan S, Arvanitakis Z, Yu L, Farfel J, Schneider JA, Bennett DA. Sex differences in Alzheimer's disease and common neuropathologies of aging. *Acta Neuropathologica*. 2018;136(6):887–900.

38. Buckley RF, Scott MR, Jacobs HIL, Schultz AP, Properzi MJ, Amariglio RE, et al. Sex mediates relationships between regional tau pathology and cognitive decline. *Annals of Neurology*. 2020;88(5):921–32.

39. Sundermann EE, Panizzon MS, Chen X, Andrews M, Galasko D, Banks SJ, et al. Sex differences in Alzheimer's-related tau biomarkers and a mediating effect of testosterone. *Biology of Sex Differences*. 2020;11(1):33.

40. Caldwell JZK, Cummings JL, Banks SJ, Palmqvist S, Hansson O. Cognitively normal women with Alzheimer's disease proteinopathy show relative preservation of memory but not of hippocampal volume. *Alzheimer's Research & Therapy*. 2019;11(1):109.

41. Digma LA, Madsen JR, Rissman RA, Jacobs DM, Brewer JB, Banks SJ, et al. Women can bear a bigger burden: ante- and post-mortem evidence for reserve in the face of tau. *Brain Communications*. 2020;2(1).

42. Lin KA, Choudhury KR, Rathakrishnan BG, Marks DM, Petrella JR, Doraiswamy PM, et al. Marked gender differences in progression of mild cognitive impairment over 8 years. *Alzheimer's & Dementia: Translational Research & Clinical Interventions*. 2015;1(2):103–10.

43. Barnes LL, Wilson RS, Bienias JL, Schneider JA, Evans DA, Bennett DA. Sex differences in the clinical manifestations of Alzheimer disease pathology. *Archives of General Psychiatry*. 2005;62(6):685–91.

44. Ayers JI, Giasson BI, Borchelt DR. Prion-like spreading in tauopathies. *Biological Psychiatry*. 2018;83(4):337–46.

45. Ahmed Z, Cooper J, Murray TK, Garn K, McNaughton E, Clarke H, et al. A novel in vivo model of tau propagation with rapid and progressive neurofibrillary tangle pathology: the pattern of spread is determined by connectivity, not proximity. *Acta Neuropathologica*. 2014;127(5):667–83.

46. Shokouhi S, Taylor WD, Albert K, Kang H, Newhouse PA, Initiative TAsDN. In vivo network models identify sex differences in the spread of tau pathology across the brain. *Alzheimer's & Dementia: Diagnosis, Assessment & Disease Monitoring*. 2020;12(1):e12016.

47. Andreason PJ, Zametkin AJ, Guo AC, Baldwin P, Cohen RM. Gender-related differences in regional cerebral glucose metabolism in normal volunteers. *Psychiatry Research*. 1994;51(2):175–83.

48. Hu Y, Xu Q, Li K, Zhu H, Qi R, Zhang Z, et al. Gender differences of brain glucose metabolic networks revealed by FDG-PET: evidence from a large cohort of 400 young adults. *PLoS ONE*. 2013;8(12):e83821.

49. Perneczky R, Drzezga A, Diehl-Schmid J, Li Y, Kurz A. Gender differences in brain reserve. *Journal of Neurology*. 2007;254(10):1395.

50. Braque Caballero MÁ, Brendel M, Delker A, Ren J, Rominger A, Bartenstein P, et al. Mapping 3-year changes in gray matter and metabolism in Aβ-positive nondemented subjects. *Neurobiology of Aging*. 2015;36(11):2913–24.

51. Goyal MS, Blazey TM, Su Y, Couture LE, Durbin TJ, Bateman RJ, et al. Persistent metabolic youth in the aging female brain. *Proceedings of the National Academy of Sciences*. 2019;116(8):3251–5.

52. Sundermann EE, Maki PM, Reddy S, Bondi MW, Biegon A, Initiative ftAsDN. Women's higher brain metabolic rate compensates for early Alzheimer's pathology. *Alzheimer's & Dementia: Diagnosis, Assessment & Disease Monitoring*. 2020;12(1):e12121.

53. Horta BL, Loret de Mola C, Victora CG. Breastfeeding and intelligence: a systematic review and meta-analysis. *Acta Paediatrica*. 2015;104(S467):14–9.

54. Heinonen K, Räikkönen K, Pesonen A-K, Kajantie E, Andersson S, Eriksson JG, et al. Prenatal and postnatal growth and cognitive abilities at 56 months of age: a longitudinal study of infants born at term. *Pediatrics*. 2008;121(5):e1325–e1333.

55. Veena SR, Krishnaveni GV, Wills AK, Kurpad AV, Muthayya S, Hill JC, et al. Association of birthweight and head circumference at birth to cognitive performance in 9- to 10-year-old children in South India: prospective birth cohort study. *Pediatric Research*. 2010;67(4):424–9.

56. Kramer MS, Aboud F, Mironova E, Vanilovich I, Platt RW, Matush L, et al. Breastfeeding and child cognitive development: new evidence from a large randomized trial. *Archives of General Psychiatry*. 2008;65(5):578–84.

57. Rantalainen V, Lahti J, Henriksson M, Kajantie E, Mikkonen M, Eriksson JG, et al. Association between breastfeeding and better preserved cognitive ability in an elderly cohort of Finnish men. *Psychological Medicine*. 2018;48(6):939–51.

58. Gale CR, Martyn CN. Breastfeeding, dummy use, and adult intelligence. *Lancet*. 1996;347(9008):1072–5.

59. Elwood PC, Pickering J, Gallacher JEJ, Hughes J, Davies D. Long term effect of breast feeding: cognitive function in the Caerphilly cohort. *Journal of Epidemiology and Community Health*. 2005;59(2):130–3.

60. Mosing MA, Lundholm C, Cnattingius S, Gatz M, Pedersen NL. Associations between birth characteristics and age-related cognitive impairment and dementia: a registry-based cohort study. *PLoS Medicine*. 2018;15(7):e1002609.

61. Sweeney MD, Montagne A, Sagare AP, Nation DA, Schneider LS, Chui HC, et al. Vascular dysfunction—the disregarded partner of Alzheimer's disease. *Alzheimer's & Dementia*. 2019;15(1):158–67.

62. Luchsinger JA, Mayeux R. Cardiovascular risk factors and Alzheimer's disease. *Current Atherosclerosis Reports*. 2004;6(4):261–6.

63. Jagust W, Harvey D, Mungas D, Haan M. Central obesity and the aging brain. *Archives of Neurology*. 2005;62(10):1545–8.

64. Rabin JS, Klein H, Kirn DR, Schultz AP, Yang H-S, Hampton O, et al. Associations of physical activity and β-amyloid with longitudinal cognition and neurodegeneration in clinically normal older adults. *JAMA Neurology.* 2019;76(10):1203–10.

65. Sims-Robinson C, Kim B, Rosko A, Feldman EL. How does diabetes accelerate Alzheimer disease pathology? *Nature Reviews Neurology.* 2010;6(10):551–9.

66. Debette S, Seshadri S, Beiser A, Au R, Himali JJ, Palumbo C, et al. Midlife vascular risk factor exposure accelerates structural brain aging and cognitive decline. *Neurology.* 2011;77(5):461–8.

67. Mayeda ER, Glymour MM, Quesenberry CP, Whitmer RA. Inequalities in dementia incidence between six racial and ethnic groups over 14 years. *Alzheimer's & Dementia.* 2016;12(3):216–24.

68. Wang C, Holtzman DM. Bidirectional relationship between sleep and Alzheimer's disease: role of amyloid, tau, and other factors. *Neuropsychopharmacology.* 2020;45(1):104–20.

69. Wu H, Dunnett S, Ho Y-S, Chang RC-C. The role of sleep deprivation and circadian rhythm disruption as risk factors of Alzheimer's disease. *Frontiers in Neuroendocrinology.* 2019;54:100764.

70. Tapia-Rojas C, Aranguiz F, Varela-Nallar L, Inestrosa NC. Voluntary running attenuates memory loss, decreases neuropathological changes and induces neurogenesis in a mouse model of Alzheimer's disease. *Brain Pathology.* 2016;26(1):62–74.

71. Brown BM, Rainey-Smith SR, Dore V, Peiffer JJ, Burnham SC, Laws SM, et al. Self-reported physical activity is associated with tau burden measured by positron emission tomography. *Journal of Alzheimer's Disease.* 2018;63:1299–305.

72. Ning S, Jorfi M. Beyond the sleep-amyloid interactions in Alzheimer's disease pathogenesis. *Journal of Neurophysiology.* 2019;122(1):1–4.

73. Leem Y-H, Lee Y-I, Son H-J, Lee S-H. Chronic exercise ameliorates the neuroinflammation in mice carrying NSE/htau23. *Biochemical and Biophysical Research Communications.* 2011;406(3):359–65.

74. Brown BM, Peiffer J, Rainey-Smith SR. Exploring the relationship between physical activity, beta-amyloid and tau: a narrative review. *Ageing Research Reviews.* 2019;50:9–18.

75. Law LL, Rol RN, Schultz SA, Dougherty RJ, Edwards DF, Koscik RL, et al. Moderate intensity physical activity associates with CSF biomarkers in a cohort at risk for Alzheimer's disease. *Alzheimer's & Dementia: Diagnosis, Assessment & Disease Monitoring.* 2018;10(1):188–95.

76. Laws SM, Gaskin S, Woodfield A, Srikanth V, Bruce D, Fraser PE, et al. Insulin resistance is associated with reductions in specific cognitive domains and increases in CSF tau in cognitively normal adults. *Scientific Reports.* 2017;7(1):9766.

77. Starks EJ, Patrick O'Grady J, Hoscheidt SM, Racine AM, Carlsson CM, Zetterberg H, et al. Insulin resistance is associated with higher cerebrospinal fluid tau levels in asymptomatic APOE ε4 carriers. *Journal of Alzheimer's Disease.* 2015;46:525–33.

78. Bubu OM, Pirraglia E, Andrade AG, Sharma RA, Gimenez-Badia S, Umasabor-Bubu OQ, et al. Obstructive sleep apnea and longitudinal Alzheimer's disease biomarker changes. *Sleep.* 2019;42(6):zsz048.

79. Winer JR, Mander BA, Helfrich RF, Maass A, Harrison TM, Baker SL, et al. Sleep as a potential biomarker of tau and β-amyloid burden in the human brain. *Journal of Neuroscience.* 2019;39(32):6315–24.

80. Sofi F, Valecchi D, Bacci D, Abbate R, Gensini GF, Casini A, et al. Physical activity and risk of cognitive decline: a meta-analysis of prospective studies. *Journal of Internal Medicine.* 2011;269(1):107–17.

81. Karssemeijer EGA, Aaronson JA, Bossers WJ, Smits T, Olde Rikkert MGM, Kessels RPC. Positive effects of combined cognitive and physical exercise training on cognitive function in older adults with mild cognitive impairment or dementia: a meta-analysis. *Ageing Research Reviews.* 2017;40:75–83.

82. Northey JM, Cherbuin N, Pumpa KL, Smee DJ, Rattray B. Exercise interventions for cognitive function in adults older than 50: a systematic review with meta-analysis. *British Journal of Sports Medicine.* 2018;52(3):154–60.

83. Rosenberg A, Ngandu T, Rusanen M, Antikainen R, Bäckman L, Havulinna S, et al. Multidomain lifestyle intervention benefits a large elderly population at risk for cognitive decline and dementia regardless of baseline characteristics: the FINGER trial. *Alzheimer's & Dementia.* 2018;14(3):263–70.

84. Kivipelto M, Solomon A, Ahtiluoto S, Ngandu T, Lehtisalo J, Antikainen R, et al. The Finnish Geriatric Intervention Study to Prevent Cognitive Impairment and Disability (FINGER): study design and progress. *Alzheimer's & Dementia*. 2013;9(6):657–65.
85. Eikelenboom P, van Exel E, Hoozemans JJM, Veerhuis R, Rozemuller AJM, van Gool WA. Neuroinflammation—an early event in both the history and pathogenesis of Alzheimer's disease. *Neurodegenerative Diseases*. 2010;7(1-3):38–41.
86. Colcombe S, Kramer AF. Fitness effects on the cognitive function of older adults: a meta-analytic study. *Psychological Science*. 2003;14(2):125–30.
87. Barha CK, Davis JC, Falck RS, Nagamatsu LS, Liu-Ambrose T. Sex differences in exercise efficacy to improve cognition: a systematic review and meta-analysis of randomized controlled trials in older humans. *Frontiers in Neuroendocrinology*. 2017;46:71–85.
88. Laurin D, Verreault R, Lindsay J, MacPherson K, Rockwood K. Physical activity and risk of cognitive impairment and dementia in elderly persons. *Archives of Neurology*. 2001;58(3):498–504.
89. Dufouil C, Seshadri S, Chêne G. Cardiovascular risk profile in women and dementia. *Journal of Alzheimer's Disease*. 2014;42:S353–S363.
90. Ho SC, Woo J, Sham A, Chan SG, Yu AL. A 3-year follow-up study of social, lifestyle and health predictors of cognitive impairment in a Chinese older cohort. *International Journal of Epidemiology*. 2001;30(6):1389–96.
91. Barha CK, Hsiung G-YR, Best JR, Davis JC, Eng JJ, Jacova C, et al. Sex difference in aerobic exercise efficacy to improve cognition in older adults with vascular cognitive impairment: secondary analysis of a randomized controlled trial. *Journal of Alzheimer's Disease*. 2017;60:1397–410.
92. Barha CK, Best JR, Rosano C, Yaffe K, Catov JM, Liu-Ambrose T, et al. Sex-specific relationship between long-term maintenance of physical activity and cognition in the Health ABC Study: potential role of hippocampal and dorsolateral prefrontal cortex volume. *Journals of Gerontology: Series A*. 2019;75(4):764–70.
93. Whitmer RA, Gunderson EP, Barrett-Connor E, Quesenberry CP, Yaffe K. Obesity in middle age and future risk of dementia: a 27 year longitudinal population based study. *BMJ*. 2005;330(7504):1360.
94. Barrett-Connor E, Edelstein SL, Corey-Bloom J, Wiederholt WC. Weight loss precedes dementia in community-dwelling older adults. *Journal of the American Geriatrics Society*. 1996;44(10):1147–52.
95. Hayden KM, Zandi PP, Lyketsos CG, Khachaturian AS, Bastian LA, Charoonruk G, et al. Vascular risk factors for incident Alzheimer disease and vascular dementia: the Cache County Study. *Alzheimer Disease & Associated Disorders*. 2006;20(2):93–100.
96. Moser VA, Pike CJ. Obesity and sex interact in the regulation of Alzheimer's disease. *Neuroscience & Biobehavioral Reviews*. 2016;67:102–18.
97. Green RC, Cupples LA, Kurz A, Auerbach S, Go R, Sadovnick D, et al. Depression as a risk factor for Alzheimer disease: the MIRAGE Study. *Archives of Neurology*. 2003;60(5):753–9.
98. Angst J, Merikangas K. The depressive spectrum: diagnostic classification and course. *Journal of Affective Disorders*. 1997;45(1):31–40.
99. Dal Forno G, Palermo MT, Donohue JE, Karagiozis H, Zonderman AB, Kawas CH. Depressive symptoms, sex, and risk for Alzheimer's disease. *Annals of Neurology*. 2005;57(3):381–7.
100. Saczynski JS, Beiser A, Seshadri S, Auerbach S, Wolf PA, Au R. Depressive symptoms and risk of dementia. *Framingham Heart Study*. 2010;75(1):35–41.
101. Kim D, Wang R, Kiss A, Bronskill SE, Lanctot KL, Herrmann N, et al. Depression and increased risk of Alzheimer's dementia: longitudinal analyses of modifiable risk and sex-related factors. *American Journal of Geriatric Psychiatry*. 2021;29(9):917–26.
102. Corder EH, Ghebremedhin E, Taylor MG, Thal DR, Ohm TG, H. B. The biphasic relationship between regional brain senile plaque and neurofibrillary tangle distributions: modification by age, sex, and APOE polymorphism. *Annals of the New York Academy of Sciences*. 2004;1019:24–8.
103. Saunders AM, Strittmatter WJ, Schmechel D, St. George-Hyslop PH, Pericak-Vance MA, Joo SH, et al. Association of apolipoprotein E allele ε4 with late-onset familial and sporadic Alzheimer's disease. *Neurology*. 1993;43(8):1467.

104. Farrer LA, Cupples LA, Haines JL, Hyman B, Kukull WA, Mayeux R, et al. Effects of age, sex, and ethnicity on the association between apolipoprotein E genotype and Alzheimer disease: a meta-analysis. *JAMA*. 1997;278:1349–56.

105. Kuusisto J, Koivisto K, Kervinen K, Mykkanen L, Helkala E-L, Vanhanen M, et al. Association of apolipoprotein E phenotypes with late onset Alzheimer's disease: population based study. *BMJ*. 1994;309(6955):636–8.

106. Bretsky PM, Buckwalter JG, Seeman TE, Miller CA, Poirier J, Schellenberg GD, et al. Evidence for an interaction between apolipoprotein E genotype, gender, and Alzheimer disease. *Alzheimer Disease & Associated Disorders*. 1999;13(4):216–21.

107. Payami H, Montee KR, Kaye JA, Bird TD, Yu C-E, Wijsman EM, et al. Alzheimer's disease, apolipoprotein E4, and gender. *JAMA*. 1994;271(17):1316–17.

108. Poirier J, Bertrand P, Poirier J, Kogan S, Gauthier S, Poirier J, et al. Apolipoprotein E polymorphism and Alzheimer's disease. *Lancet*. 1993;342(8873):697–9.

109. Breitner JCS, Wyse BW, Anthony JC, Welsh-Bohmer KA, Steffens DC, Norton MC, et al. APOE-ε4 count predicts age when prevalence of AD increases, then declines. *Cache County Study*. 1999;53(2):321.

110. Payami H, Zareparsi S, Montee KR, Sexton GJ, Kaye JA, Bird TD, et al. Gender difference in apolipoprotein E-associated risk for familial Alzheimer disease: a possible clue to the higher incidence of Alzheimer disease in women. *American Journal of Human Genetics*. 1996;58(4):803–11.

111. Neu SC, Pa J, Kukull W, Beekly D, Kuzma A, Gangadharan P, et al. Apolipoprotein E genotype and sex risk factors for Alzheimer disease: a meta-analysis. *JAMA Neurology*. 2017;74(10):1178–89.

112. Struble RG, Rosario ER, Kircher ML, Ludwig SM, McAdamis PJ, Watabe K, et al. Regionally specific modulation of brain apolipoprotein E in the mouse during the estrous cycle and by exogenous 17β estradiol. *Experimental Neurology*. 2003;183(2):638–44.

113. Vadakkadath Meethal S, Atwood CS. Alzheimer's disease: the impact of age-related changes in reproductive hormones. *Cellular and Molecular Life Sciences CMLS*. 2005;62(3):257–70.

114. Marrocco J, McEwen BS. Sex in the brain: hormones and sex differences. *Dialogues in Clinical Neuroscience*. 2016;18(4):373–83.

115. Woolley CS, McEwen BS. Roles of estradiol and progesterone in regulation of hippocampal dendritic spine density during the estrous cycle in the rat. *Journal of Comparative Neurology*. 1993;336(2):293–306.

116. Foy MR, Henderson VW, Berger TW, Thompson RF. Estrogen and neural plasticity. *Current Directions in Psychological Science*. 2000;9(5):148–52.

117. Tanapat P, Hastings NB, Reeves AJ, Gould E. Estrogen stimulates a transient increase in the number of new neurons in the dentate gyrus of the adult female rat. *Journal of Neuroscience*. 1999;19(14):5792–801.

118. Goodman Y, Bruce AJ, Cheng B, Mattson MP. Estrogens attenuate and corticosterone exacerbates excitotoxicity, oxidative injury, and amyloid β-peptide toxicity in hippocampal neurons. *Journal of Neurochemistry*. 1996;66(5):1836–44.

119. Petanceska SS, Nagy V, Frail D, Gandy S. Ovariectomy and 17β-estradiol modulate the levels of Alzheimer's amyloid β peptides in brain. *Neurology*. 2000;54(12):2212–17.

120. Peterson A, Tom SE. A lifecourse perspective on female sex-specific risk factors for later life cognition. *Current Neurology and Neuroscience Reports*. 2021;21(9):46.

121. Fox M, Berzuini C, Knapp LA. Cumulative estrogen exposure, number of menstrual cycles, and Alzheimer's risk in a cohort of British women. *Psychoneuroendocrinology*. 2013;38(12):2973–82.

122. Prince MJ, Acosta D, Guerra M, Huang Y, Jimenez-Velazquez IZ, Llibre Rodriguez JJ, et al. Reproductive period, endogenous estrogen exposure and dementia incidence among women in Latin America and China: a 10/66 population-based cohort study. *PLoS ONE*. 2018;13(2):e0192889.

123. Kuh D, Cooper R, Moore A, Richards M, Hardy R. Age at menopause and lifetime cognition: Findings from a British Birth Cohort Study. *Neurology*. 2018;90(19):e1673–e1681.

124. Georgakis MK, Beskou-Kontou T, Theodoridis I, Skalkidou A, Petridou ET. Surgical menopause in association with cognitive function and risk of dementia: a systematic review and meta-analysis. *Psychoneuroendocrinology*. 2019;106:9–19.

125. Ryan J, Scali J, Carrière I, Amieva H, Rouaud O, Berr C, et al. Impact of a premature menopause on cognitive function in later life. *BJOG*. 2014;121(13):1729–39.

126. Rocca WA, Grossardt BR, Shuster LT. Oophorectomy, estrogen, and dementia: a 2014 update. *Molecular and Cellular Endocrinology*. 2014;389(1):7–12.

127. Yoo JE, Shin DW, Han K, Kim D, Won H-S, Lee J, et al. Female reproductive factors and the risk of dementia: a nationwide cohort study. *European Journal of Neurology*. 2020;27(8):1448–58.

128. Gilsanz P, Lee C, Corrada MM, Kawas CH, Quesenberry CP, Whitmer RA. Reproductive period and risk of dementia in a diverse cohort of health care members. *Neurology*. 2019;92(17):e2005–e2014.

129. Geerlings MI, Ruitenberg A, Witteman JCM, van Swieten JC, Hofman A, van Duijn CM, et al. Reproductive period and risk of dementia in postmenopausal women. *JAMA*. 2001;285(11):1475–81.

130. Paganini-Hill A, Corrada MM, Kawas CH. Prior endogenous and exogenous estrogen and incident dementia in the 10th decade of life: the 90+ Study. *Climacteric*. 2020;23(3):311–15.

131. Li M, Lin J, Liang S, Chen Z, Bai Y, Long X, et al. The role of age at menarche and age at menopause in Alzheimer's disease: evidence from a bidirectional mendelian randomization study. *Aging*. 2021;13(15):19722–49.

132. Schelbaum E, Loughlin L, Jett S, Zhang C, Jang G, Malviya N, et al. Association of reproductive history with brain MRI biomarkers of dementia risk in midlife. *Neurology*. 2021;97(23):e2328–e2339.

133. Rahman A, Schelbaum E, Hoffman K, Diaz I, Hristov H, Andrews R, et al. Sex-driven modifiers of Alzheimer risk: A Multimodality Brain Imaging Study. *Neurology*. 2020;95(2):e166–e178.

134. Shumaker SA, Legault C, Kuller L, Rapp SR, Thal L, Lane DS, et al. Conjugated equine estrogens and incidence of probable dementia and mild cognitive impairment in postmenopausal women: the Women's Health Initiative Memory Study. *JAMA*. 2004;291(24):2947–58.

135. Shumaker SA, Legault C, Rapp SR, Thal L, Wallace RB, Ockene JK, et al. Estrogen plus progestin and the incidence of dementia and mild cognitive impairment in postmenopausal women: the Women's Health Initiative Memory Study—a randomized controlled trial. *JAMA*. 2003;289(20):2651–62.

136. Henderson VW. Estrogen-containing hormone therapy and Alzheimer's disease risk: understanding discrepant inferences from observational and experimental research. *Neuroscience*. 2006;138(3):1031–9.

137. Maki PM. Hormone therapy and cognitive function: is there a critical period for benefit? *Neuroscience*. 2006;138(3):1027–30.

138. Resnick SM, Henderson VW. Hormone therapy and risk of Alzheimer disease: a critical time. *JAMA*. 2002;288(17):2170–2.

139. Sano M, Bell K, Jacobs D. Cognitive effects of estrogens in women with cardiac disease: what we do not know. *American Journal of Medicine*. 2002;113(7):612–13.

140. Gibbs RB. Long-term treatment with estrogen and progesterone enhances acquisition of a spatial memory task by ovariectomized aged rats. *Neurobiology of Aging*. 2000;21(1):107–16.

141. Henderson VW, St. John JA, Hodis HN, McCleary CA, Stanczyk FZ, Shoupe D, et al. Cognitive effects of estradiol after menopause: A Randomized Trial of the Timing Hypothesis. *Neurology*. 2016;87(7):699–708.

142. Gleason CE, Dowling NM, Wharton W, Manson JE, Miller VM, Atwood CS, et al. Effects of hormone therapy on cognition and mood in recently postmenopausal women: findings from the randomized, controlled KEEPS–Cognitive and Affective Study. *PLoS Medicine*. 2015;12(6):e1001833.

143. Dashe JS, Bloom SL, Spong CY, Hoffman BL. *Williams obstetrics*. New York: McGraw Hill Professional; 2018.

144. Mor G, Aldo P, Alvero AB. The unique immunological and microbial aspects of pregnancy. *Nature Reviews Immunology*. 2017;17(8):469–82.

145. Bernstein L, Pike MC, Ross RK, Judd HL, Brown JB, Henderson BE. Estrogen and sex hormone-binding globulin levels in nulliparous and parous women. *Journal of the National Cancer Institute*. 1985;74(4):741–5.

146. Bae JB, Lipnicki DM, Han JW, Sachdev PS, Kim TH, Kwak KP, et al. Parity and the risk of incident dementia: a COSMIC study. *Epidemiology and Psychiatric Sciences*. 2020;29:e176.

147. Jang H, Bae JB, Dardiotis E, Scarmeas N, Sachdev PS, Lipnicki DM, et al. Differential effects of completed and incomplete pregnancies on the risk of Alzheimer disease. *Neurology*. 2018;91(7):e643–e651.

148. Ptok U, Barkow K, Heun R. Fertility and number of children in patients with Alzheimer's disease. *Archives of Women's Mental Health*. 2002;5(2):83–6.

149. Li F-D, He F, Chen T-R, Xiao Y-Y, Lin S-T, Shen W, et al. Reproductive history and risk of cognitive impairment in elderly women: A cross-sectional study in Eastern China. *Journal of Alzheimer's Disease*. 2016;49:139–47.

150. McLay RN, Pauline M, Maki PM, Lyketsos CG. Nulliparity and late menopause are associated with decreased cognitive decline. *Journal of Neuropsychiatry and Clinical Neurosciences*. 2003;15(2):161–7.

151. Sobow T, Kloszewska IK. Modulation of age at onset in late-onset sporadic Alzheimer's disease by estrogen-related factors: the age of menopause and number of pregnancies. *German Journal of Psychiatry*. 2003;6.

152. Fox M, Berzuini C, Knapp LA, Glynn LM. Women's pregnancy life history and Alzheimer's risk: can immunoregulation explain the link? *American Journal of Alzheimer's Disease & Other Dementias*. 2018;33(8):516–26.

153. Heikkinen J, Möttönen M, Alanen A, Lassila O. Phenotypic characterization of regulatory T cells in the human decidua. *Clinical & Experimental Immunology*. 2004;136(2):373–8.

154. Lima J, Martins C, Nunes G, Sousa M-J, Branco JC, Borrego L-M. Regulatory T cells show dynamic behavior during late pregnancy, delivery, and the postpartum period. *Reproductive Sciences*. 2017;24(7):1025–32.

155. Somerset DA, Zheng Y, Kilby MD, Sansom DM, Drayson MT. Normal human pregnancy is associated with an elevation in the immune suppressive CD25+ CD4+ regulatory T-cell subset. *Immunology*. 2004;112(1):38–43.

156. Beeri MS, Rapp M, Schmeidler J, Reichenberg A, Purohit DP, Perl DP, et al. Number of children is associated with neuropathology of Alzheimer's disease in women. *Neurobiology of Aging*. 2009;30(8):1184–91.

157. Jung JH, Lee GW, Lee JH, Byun MS, Yi D, Jeon SY, et al. Multiparity, brain atrophy, and cognitive decline. *Frontiers in Aging Neuroscience*. 2020;12:159.

158. Rivera R, Yacobson I, Grimes D. The mechanism of action of hormonal contraceptives and intrauterine contraceptive devices. *American Journal of Obstetrics and Gynecology*. 1999;181(5):1263–9.

159. Mordecai KL, Rubin LH, Maki PM. Effects of menstrual cycle phase and oral contraceptive use on verbal memory. *Hormones and Behavior*. 2008;54(2):286–93.

160. Song X, Wu J, Zhou Y, Feng L, Yuan J-M, Pan A, et al. Reproductive and hormonal factors and risk of cognitive impairment among Singapore Chinese women. *American Journal of Obstetrics and Gynecology*. 2020;223(3):410.e1–.e23.

161. Egan KR, Gleason CE. Longer duration of hormonal contraceptive use predicts better cognitive outcomes later in life. *Journal of Women's Health*. 2012;21(12):1259–66.

162. Pletzer B, Kronbichler M, Aichhorn M, Bergmann J, Ladurner G, Kerschbaum HH. Menstrual cycle and hormonal contraceptive use modulate human brain structure. *Brain Research*. 2010;1348:55–62.

163. De Bondt T, Jacquemyn Y, Van Hecke W, Sijbers J, Sunaert S, Parizel PM. Regional gray matter volume differences and sex-hormone correlations as a function of menstrual cycle phase and hormonal contraceptives use. *Brain Research*. 2013;1530:22–31.

164. Rumberg B, Baars A, Fiebach J, Ladd ME, Forsting M, Senf W, et al. Cycle and gender-specific cerebral activation during a verb generation task using fMRI: comparison of women in different cycle phases, under oral contraception, and men. *Neuroscience Research*. 2010;66(4):366–71.

165. Ryan CL, Siebens J. *Educational attainment in the United States: 2009. Current population reports*. Washington, DC: United States Census Bureau; 1 February 2012. pp. 20–566.

166. Nomaguchi KM, Bianchi SM. Exercise time: gender differences in the effects of marriage, parenthood, and employment. *Journal of Marriage and Family*. 2004;66(2):413–30.

167. Pankratz VS, Roberts RO, Mielke MM, Knopman DS, Jack CR, Geda YE, et al. Predicting the risk of mild cognitive impairment in the Mayo Clinic Study of Aging. *Neurology*. 2015;84(14):1433–42.

168. van Gelder BM, Tijhuis M, Kalmijn S, Giampaoli S, Nissinen A, Kromhout D. Marital status and living situation during a 5-year period are associated with a subsequent 10-year cognitive decline in older men: the FINE study. *Journals of Gerontology: Series B*. 2006;61(4):P213–P219.

169. National Alliance for Caregiving. *Caregiving in the U.S. 2009*. Washington, DC: AARP Research; December 2009.

170. Mielke MM. Sex and gender differences in Alzheimer's disease dementia. *Psychiatr Times*. 2018;35(11):14–17.

11
The Life Course Epidemiology of Breast Cancer

Lauren C. Houghton, Nancy Potischman, and Rebecca Troisi

11.1 Introduction

Tumours develop in stages, with considerable variation in growth velocity before clinical detection. Multiple exposures over an individual's lifetime are likely to be important in tumour initiation and progression, but only since the early 1990s has research focused on those measured during periods other than adulthood. For a few decades, interest has expanded to factors that may act in utero or very early in life. Linking risk factors that operate at different developmental periods may advance our understanding of the origins of breast cancer and its development.

Life course epidemiology, however, is profoundly challenging. Ideally, large cohorts of people with serial data could be leveraged to assess factors across life stages. Existing cohorts generally begin observation in adulthood when cancer rates start to rise. Cohorts that capture exposures in earlier time periods require many years of follow-up to accrue sufficient numbers of cases to study. Record linkage studies, largely from the Scandinavian countries, have successfully used data from health and other registers to obtain exposure information over meaningful time frames. These large population-based datasets also address the relative rarity of cancer compared with other chronic diseases. Cancer is generally less amenable than other chronic diseases to the use of intermediate outcomes, for example, hypertension for cardiovascular disease or haemoglobin A1C for diabetes, which occur earlier and are more prevalent or can be measured on all participants. The lack of intermediate markers for breast cancer also has limited the usefulness of younger cohorts, although greater mammographic density and high-risk parenchymal patterns of breast tissue have been used,[1] and studies are investigating the utility of other biomarkers such as nipple aspirate fluid.[2]

Despite these obstacles, evidence now suggests that early life exposures could be as important in the aetiology of breast cancer as those acting in adult life. We will briefly review the established adult risk factors for breast cancer, followed by a more in-depth assessment of the evidence for factors occurring in increasingly earlier life stages, from the woman's own pregnancy characteristics, to adolescence, childhood, infancy, and her own experience while in utero. Some factors naturally span life stages (e.g. diet and nutrition and height and weight). Finally, we will consider the aetiology of breast cancer in a life course framework in which

Lauren C. Houghton, Nancy Potischman, and Rebecca Troisi, *The Life Course Epidemiology of Breast Cancer* In: *A Life Course Approach to Women's Health*. Second Edition. Edited by: Gita D Mishra, Rebecca Hardy, and Diana Kuh, Oxford University Press.
© Oxford University Press 2023. DOI: 10.1093/oso/9780192864642.003.0011

risk factors occurring at each life stage are linked to investigate possible pathways from early life events to adulthood and subsequent occurrence of breast cancer.

11.2 Adult Risk Factors

Increasing age is the strongest influence on breast cancer risk. Family history of breast cancer in a first-degree relative accounts for < 10% of all breast cancers,[3] while migrant studies demonstrate that the vast amount of breast cancer incidence is explained by the environment (i.e. nongenetic factors).[4] Much of the population attributable risk percent for breast cancer is explained by reproductive factors, including early onset of menarche, late age at first birth, nulliparity, low parity, and late age at menopause.[5] For example, lactation for long durations may reduce risk,[6–9] while oestrogen and progestogen-containing contraceptives[10] and menopausal therapies[11] are associated with an elevated risk. Demographic and lifestyle factors associated with an elevated breast cancer risk include having never been married,[12] higher socioeconomic position,[13] adult weight gain,[14] inactivity or low physical activity,[14] alcohol consumption,[15] and smoking.[16] As summarised by the International Agency for Research on Cancer (IARC),[17] there is some evidence in humans for environmental contaminants, including dieldrin, digoxin, and ethylene oxide, and for night shift work, though associations may be stronger for exposures occurring during periods of breast development.[18-20] We cover pregnancy factors (see Section 11.3) that have been less studied in relation to the mother's breast cancer risk, and then in the subsequent section (see Section 11.4), we review factors progressively earlier in life, starting with adolescence and working back to a woman's own in utero environment.

11.3 The Woman's Pregnancy

Greater parity protects against the mother's breast cancer risk, but the effect depends on age at pregnancy and tumour subtype.[21] Pregnancy increases risk, mainly of oestrogen receptor (ER) negative tumours, for several years following delivery, while if the pregnancy occurs at a young age, long-term risk of ER-positive tumours is reduced.[22] To provide benefit, the pregnancy must be full-term, as miscarriages do not provide equivalent protection;[23] it is unclear if gestational length of a pregnancy resulting in a live birth is associated with risk.[24] A positive history of preeclampsia has been linked to an approximate 20% reduction in maternal breast cancer risk;[25] hypertension diagnosed before pregnancy and gestational hypertension also show some protection.[26] One study demonstrated a marked reduction with elevated mean arterial pressure (MAP)[27] and systolic blood pressure increases from mid-to-late pregnancy below the diagnostic criterion for hypertension (i.e. in normotensive pregnancies).[28] Characteristics of the placenta, including weight,[29] diameter, and maternal floor infarctions,[30] may also be involved with maternal breast cancer risk. Other complications have been studied less because of methodological issues or infrequency of occurrence.[30] Diethylstilbestrol (DES), a synthetic oestrogen that was administered during pregnancy, has been associated with a small increase in risk of breast cancer in the mother.[31]

11.4 Adolescence and Early Life

11.4.1 Adolescence

The association with ionising and gamma radiation provides evidence of a critical window of susceptibility for breast cancer development. Epidemiological data are consistent with a linear relationship in which the excess risk of breast cancer is proportional to radiation dose, but the greatest effects are observed in women under the age of 20 years, whereas in women over 50 years, there is no association.[32]

Data suggest that several other breast cancer risk factors may operate during adolescence, including body size and diet.[33–35] Greater adolescent body weight, likely a proxy for a variety of nutritional, physical activity, and endocrine variables, appears protective for premenopausal[36] and postmenopausal breast cancer[37–39] and greater height is positively associated with risk.[40] Adolescent body size depends on growth during earlier time periods and can be highly correlated with adult body size (see Section 11.6 for a more detailed discussion).

11.4.1.1 Adolescent and Childhood Nutrition and Diet
Results of the few breast cancer studies that have assessed adolescent diet retrospectively from adults have been generally weak and inconsistent.[41–43] Adolescent consumption of fat[31,34] and red meat[44] has been positively associated with premenopausal breast cancer risk, while high intakes of fruit,[45] and fruit and vegetables appear protective.[42,46] In contrast, greater childhood consumption of dairy was not related to increased breast cancer risk,[45] although there was a suggestion of differences in associations by hormone receptor status of the tumour; this requires further evaluation.

11.4.1.2 Adolescent Physical Activity
High levels of physical activity during ages 5–19 years were associated with reduced breast cancer risk in The Sister Study, with more pronounced reductions for ER-positive tumours, especially for activity at earlier ages (5–12 years).[47] In the Nurses' Health Study, physical activity between ages 14 and 22 years appeared to be modestly protective for premenopausal breast cancer, with adjustment for adult physical activity, and slightly stronger for ER-negative tumours and in younger premenopausal women; there was no association with postmenopausal breast cancer.[48] In the Breast Cancer Family Registry,[37] adolescent physical activity was not associated with risk, whereas, being physically active as an adult was consistently associated with lower breast cancer risk, regardless of the degree of inactivity or activity in adolescence. For those who were inactive as adults, there was no association between being active (versus inactive) in adolescence with breast cancer risk.[49] Thus, currently the evidence for a protective effect on breast cancer is more consistent for adult activity than for activity earlier in life.

11.4.2 Puberty

Puberty is not one event but rather a series of physical changes—menarche (first menstrual period), thelarche (onset of breast development), pubarche (onset of pubic hair development), and adrenarche (full maturation of the adrenal gland);[50] these changes are also discussed in Chapter 2. These pubertal events may have independent associations with breast cancer or the relation between them, known as tempo, may also be implicated in risk.

11.4.2.1 Menarche
Earlier age at menarche is one of the most established pubertal risk factors for breast cancer.[51-54] There is a lower limit to how early menarche can occur, and in the United States and other HICs, the population average age at menarche, which formerly decreased over time, seems to have stabilised since the 1960s to age 12 years.[55] However, the onset of puberty, namely breast development, continues to decline.

11.4.2.2 Thelarche
Many breast cancer studies have established that early age at menarche is associated with increased risk, but it is more likely that thelarche (i.e. breast development) begins the pubertal window of breast tissue susceptibility.[56] Thelarche, typically the first sign of puberty, occurs 2–4 years before menarche. Earlier versus later recalled age at thelarche has been associated with a 20% increased risk of breast cancer (the same magnitude of association as earlier versus later menarche), independent of the effect of menarche.[57]

11.4.2.3 Tempo
Assessing both age and tempo of pubertal development prospectively in longitudinal studies is preferable because misclassification in recalled pubertal timing may attenuate the association with breast cancer risk. Using longitudinal assessment of thelarche and menarche in children and following participants into their mid-twenties, the Dietary Intervention Study in Children follow-up study demonstrated that a longer pubertal tempo (i.e. greater number of months between thelarche and menarche) was associated with increased breast density,[58] a marker for increased breast cancer risk. In addition, longer pubertal tempo has been positively associated with breast cancer risk, independent of either age at thelarche or menarche.[57] The elongation and branching of ductal structures in the breast, which increase rates of proliferating cells, mostly occurs during this time. Longer pubertal tempo may allow a wider window of susceptibility as vulnerable breast tissue is exposed to carcinogenic stimuli.

11.4.3 Prenatal and Infant

A woman's own birth weight has been positively associated with breast cancer risk and is only modestly attenuated by other maternal or pregnancy factors, including maternal age, birth order[59] and daughter's adult breast cancer risk factors,[60] or not at all.[61-66] New methods for analysing these data suggest that genetically-predicted birth weight is not positively associated with increased breast cancer risk, but leaves open the question as to whether the higher birth weight and increased breast cancer risk observed in observational studies are due to increases in birth weight from nongenetic factors, such as maternal hormones and nutrition.[67]

Overall, breast cancer risk appears to be increased in twins, but whether the risk is higher in dizygotic compared with monozygotic twins and singletons is unclear.[68] Modestly increased risks have been observed for daughters born to older mothers in some studies[69] and with increasing paternal age.[70] A positive effect of maternal age on daughter's risk does not appear to be modified by birth order,[71] and studies that have investigated birth order as a main effect have shown no relation with breast cancer risk.[69]

Daughter's risk related to her having been breastfed was evaluated in early studies of breast cancer in which investigators hypothesised that a viral agent could be transmitted through breast milk. These studies[72–74] found little association between having been breastfed with risk, however, and do not support the viral hypothesis. Nor did a large case-control study,[75] showing that risk was not elevated in breastfed daughters whose mother later developed breast cancer. In subsequent studies included in a meta-analysis, having been breastfed was not associated with overall breast cancer risk, although there was a reduced risk of premenopausal breast cancer in women who had been breastfed.[66] One of the drawbacks of assessing breastfeeding in high-income populations is the limited variability in the prevalence and duration of breastfeeding.

Most studies have shown no consistent association for the daughters between gestational age at birth and risk of breast cancer.[60,65] Results are also inconsistent for placental weight, gestational age or prematurity, and exposure to the mother's pregnancy hypertension or preeclampsia.[76]

Daughters exposed to DES in utero have a slightly elevated risk of premenopausal, but generally not postmenopausal, breast cancer.[77] In a study linking birth and cancer registry records in Sweden,[78] an increased risk was noted for infants who experienced jaundice. Several studies have assessed whether season of birth affects breast cancer risk in daughters with some showing an increase in risk resulting from births occurring at certain times of the year; however, the effect is small and inconsistent.[79–81] Studies provide little evidence that maternal smoking during pregnancy[82–85] or exposure to passive smoking[82] affects daughter's risk of breast cancer.

11.5 Life Course Methods

The preceding sections suggest that the aetiology of breast cancer likely includes effects that act at, and accumulate through, several stages of life. Ideally, statistical modelling should consider and incorporate this timing to describe complicated causal relationships and interactions between factors. However, most studies of early life risk factors, like those of adult risk factors, have used traditional methods to estimate effects on breast cancer risk, when possible, adjusting for established adult risk factors. For a full understanding of the aetiology of breast cancer, a life course perspective—and not just the collection of life course data—is necessary. Studies should be focused on identifying 'pathways of disease'[86] and establishing how prenatal and early life risk factors interact with those operating in adulthood. An example of linking risk factors across time for premenopausal breast cancer is demonstrated in Figure 11.1. For instance, is the increased breast cancer risk associated with early age at menarche owing to a longer period of breast exposure to endogenous oestrogens, because menarche is a marker of permanent structural changes to the breast that occur with exposures during breast development, or because of correlations with prepubertal growth rates? If the latter, to what extent are the effects of rapid prenatal and postnatal growth modified by changes in body size in adult life? The analysis of body size across the life course is an excellent example of how such methods can be applied to identify appropriate timing for intervention.

Chain of Risk Model of Body Size and Breast Cancer Risk

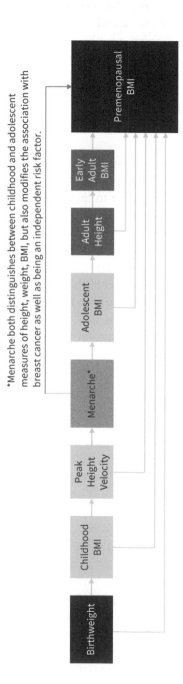

*Menarche both distinguishes between childhood and adolescent measures of height, weight, BMI, but also modifies the association with breast cancer as well as being an independent risk factor.

■ Variables measured in studies of both childhood and adulthood growth and breast cancer
■ Growth measured only in childhood and/or adolescence
■ Growth measured only in adulthood

Figure 11.1 Chain of risk model of body size over the life course and premenopausal breast cancer risk. See plate section.

11.6 Weight, BMI, and Height Across the Life Course

A recent pooled analysis of 20 prospective studies demonstrated positive linear associations between adult height and premenopausal and postmenopausal breast cancer risk,[87] while adult BMI at cohort baseline (age range 18–93 years) was strongly inversely associated with premenopausal risk, and strongly positively and nonlinearly associated with postmenopausal risk. The height and BMI findings were adjusted for established risk factors and mainly observed for receptor-positive tumours.

In the pooled analysis, early adult BMI (at 18–20 years) showed inverse linear associations for premenopausal and postmenopausal breast cancer risk with stronger associations for receptor-negative tumours.[87] Weight gain from early (18–20 years) to later adulthood was associated with increased risk of postmenopausal breast cancer, stronger for receptor-positive tumours, and among women who were leaner in early adulthood.[87] Women who were heavier in early adulthood generally had reduced premenopausal risk, independent of later weight gain. Weight loss over this period has been associated with reduced risk.[35]

There is evidence from the Copenhagen School Health Record Registry that childhood BMI at age 14 years is inversely associated with breast cancer risk, predominantly premenopausal cancer;[37] an inverse association also was suggested for BMI at ages 7 and 13, with mainly postmenopausal cancer.[88] Compared with children with an average increase in BMI between ages 7 and 13, those who had a greater than average increase had a lower breast cancer risk (predominantly premenopausal).[37]

While the above studies focus on body size in either adulthood or childhood, a life course approach to the association between body size and breast cancer risk would ideally have prospective measures across the life course. A recent study in the Women's Health Initiative used recalled self-report of birth weight and weights at ages 18, 35, and 50 years, and measures of height and weight at baseline to conclude that the association between low birth weight (< 6 lbs) and decreased breast cancer risk was mediated by adult height (44%) and weight (21%).[89] Another study, that does have prospectively measured childhood growth at multiple ages, found that height velocity at age 4–7 years and age 11–15 years and body mass index velocity at age 2–4 years increased risk, particularly in women with early menarche (age < 12.5 years).[90] Clearly, these associations are complex and additional studies that measure childhood, adolescent, and adult height and weight are needed to determine how much growth in height and weight mediates the association between birth weight and risk.

The positive association between adult height and breast cancer risk is consistent with the hypothesis that factors that promote growth in childhood are positively associated with breast cancer risk. The results of studies that benefited from detailed information on growth patterns suggest that high growth velocity further supports an association between a relatively early growth spurt and greater breast cancer risk compared with reaching maximal height at a later point during adolescent development.[91]

De Stavola and colleagues[92] showed that high birth weight was related to breast cancer risk, but only for girls with high growth velocity in childhood, as indicated by greater height measured at age 7 years. Another study, however, found no interaction between birth weight and body mass index at ages 7 to 15 with risk of breast cancer.[62] These studies, using longitudinal information from birth throughout childhood and adolescence, present useful models for evaluations of the interactions among early risk factors and for potential evaluations among risk factors identified throughout the life course.

Height, like puberty, can be broken into component parts, leg length and sitting height, the former having been considered a marker of nutrition. In adult women, leg length does not seem to be more strongly associated with breast cancer among postmenopausal women than sitting height.[93] Leg length measured in childhood was positively associated with mortality from breast cancer in the Boyd Orr prospective study but was statistically significant only for women whose leg length was measured in the prepubertal period, that is, before age 8 years.[94]

11.7 Life Course Models: Chain Reaction, Accumulation, Critical Window

Several theories have sought to provide a framework for how exposures and biological mechanisms during life interact to subsequently result in breast cancer.[95] Breast tumours could culminate from a chain of biologically linked events (i.e. the 'chains of risk model'), or from cumulative effects of one factor or a set of independent risk factors (i.e. the 'accumulation model'). Windows of susceptibility also may be critical. For example, the Pike model predicts that the breast will be most susceptible to carcinogens at early ages.[96] Increased breast cancer risk associated with exposure to ionising radiation before menarche but not later in life is in support of this.[97] The period between puberty and first birth may set the stage for later disease.[98]

The original hypothesis put forth by Trichopoulos (1990)[99] stated that a high endogenous oestrogen environment underlies an elevated risk of breast cancer, and recent studies suggest that androgens,[100] insulin, and insulin-like growth factors may also be important.[101–103] During puberty, there is a substantial increase in circulating steroid hormone concentrations and the timing of puberty represents the first dose of oestrogen in the accumulative oestrogen hypothesis for breast cancer. However, puberty is driven by underlying hormonal changes, including androgens, as well as oestrogens, and is not one event, but rather a series of physiological changes. It is also when the breast undergoes rapid development and may have heightened vulnerability to carcinogenic effects.[56] Rather than framing puberty as merely the beginning of oestrogenic exposure, puberty can be considered as a window of susceptibility or a critical exposure period. The next major event in breast development is pregnancy, with the possibility of irreversible changes to breast structure and to circulating hormone concentrations after the first pregnancy.[104] Epigenetic changes in utero, in puberty, or during pregnancy could also result in a change in later endogenous risk factors, like circulating hormones. In any case, the seeds of cancer are likely already planted at this point, and adult exposures such as increasing weight and subsequently higher steroid hormone concentrations, merely drive tumour progression. The last major breast event is menopause when the breast involutes and appears to become less susceptible to carcinogenic insult. Clemmensen's hook highlights that breast cancer incidence rates do not rise exponentially with advancing age: the increase in rates, while still substantial, begins to slow before age 50 years, coinciding with menopause.[105]

11.8 Conclusion

The numerous early life and adult risk factors that are associated with breast cancer demonstrate the utility of taking a life course perspective to understanding its aetiology. Yet because of the lack of longitudinal data on sufficient numbers of women that span all the periods that we touched upon in this chapter, the field is still in its infancy when it comes to methodology. Pathway analyses,[88] such as those we illustrated using the example of height and weight in Figure 11.1, are still rare in comparison to the majority of studies that examine independent risk factors during isolated periods of the life course. Applying the evolving theories and methods of life course epidemiology to Scandinavian data resources may be fruitful in identifying the interaction of risk factors across the life course. Pooled analyses may provide large enough numbers of cases to investigate specific hypothesised pathways and distinguish causal pathways and accumulation of risk factors from critical period effects. Many aspects of this research can be conducted by examining the influence of early life events on other risk factors or intermediary events without the need for long-term longitudinal data. Further, with the advancements in molecular characterisation of breast cancer tumours, we need more studies that compare the life course epidemiology of the different breast cancer subtypes (oestrogen receptor–positive (ER+), progesterone receptor-positive (PR+), epidermal growth factor receptor 2–positive (HER2+), or triple-negative cancers (ER-/PR-/HER2-). For example, after menarche, the type of associations of reproductive factors with triple-negative breast cancers diverges from oestrogen-driven cancers. Also, more studies with racial and ethnically diverse populations are needed in that the distribution of risk factors and breast cancer subtypes may differ to those in the white populations in HICs that have been predominantly studied to date.

Considerable work has been accomplished in the last few decades to characterise risk factors occurring many years before breast cancer occurs. The next steps will involve continuing to study the underlying biology of how these factors work together to affect breast cancer development years later.

Key messages and implications

- Breast cancer development is likely the culmination of multiple exposures across an individual's lifetime, beginning from the prenatal period with some factors, such as body size and nutrition, and spanning different developmental periods.
- Adolescence is a critical time for breast cancer exposures as timing of pubertal events can affect breast tissue development, increasing its vulnerability to later life tumour formation.
- Whilst research has significantly advanced our understanding of breast cancer risk factors and aetiology, more complex analyses are required to determine how timing of developmental events and growth velocity contribute to tumour formation and breast cancer subtypes.

References

1. Gastounioti A, Conant EF, Kontos D. Beyond breast density: a review on the advancing role of parenchymal texture analysis in breast cancer risk assessment. *Breast Cancer Research*. 2016;18(1):91.

2. Jiwa N, Gandhewar R, Chauhan H, Ashrafian H, Kumar S, Wright C, et al. Diagnostic accuracy of nipple aspirate fluid cytology in asymptomatic patients: a meta-analysis and systematic review of the literature. *Annals of Surgical Oncology*. 2021;28(7):3751–60.

3. Hemminki K, Granström C, Czene K. Attributable risks for familial breast cancer by proband status and morphology: a nationwide epidemiologic study from Sweden. *International Journal of Cancer*. 2002;100(2):214–9.

4. Hoover RN. That recognised risk factors can explain past and present international differences in breast cancer incidence: misconceptions 5. *British Journal of Cancer*. 2012;107(3):408–10.

5. Tamimi RM, Spiegelman D, Smith-Warner SA, Wang M, Pazaris M, Willett WC, et al. Population attributable risk of modifiable and nonmodifiable breast cancer risk factors in postmenopausal breast cancer. *American Journal of Epidemiology*. 2016;184(12):884–93.

6. Ambrosone CB, Higgins MJ. Relationships between breast feeding and breast cancer subtypes: lessons learned from studies in humans and in mice. *Cancer Research*. 2020;80(22):4871–7.

7. Collaborative Group on Hormonal Factors in Breast Cancer. Breast cancer and breastfeeding: collaborative reanalysis of individual data from 47 epidemiological studies in 30 countries, including 50302 women with breast cancer and 96973 women without the disease. *Lancet*. 2002;360:187–95.

8. Cabrera L, Trapero I. Evaluation of the effectiveness of breastfeeding as a factor in the prevention of breast cancer. *Endocrine, Metabolic & Immune Disorders—Drug Targets*. 2022;22(1):15–25.

9. Migliavacca Zucchetti B, Peccatori FA, Codacci-Pisanelli G. Pregnancy and lactation: risk or protective factors for breast cancer? In: Alipour S, Omranipour R, eds. *Diseases of the breast during pregnancy and lactation* . Cham: Springer International Publishing; 2020. pp. 195–7.

10. Mørch LS, Skovlund CW, Hannaford PC, Iversen L, Fielding S, Lidegaard Ø. Contemporary hormonal contraception and the risk of breast cancer. *New England Journal of Medicine*. 2017;377(23):2228–39.

11. Collaborative Group on Hormonal Factors in Breast Cancer. Type and timing of menopausal hormone therapy and breast cancer risk: individual participant meta-analysis of the worldwide epidemiological evidence. *Lancet*. 2019;394:1159–68.

12. Li M, Han M, Chen Z, Tang Y, Ma J, Zhang Z, et al. Does marital status correlate with the female breast cancer risk? A systematic review and meta-analysis of observational studies. *PLoS ONE*. 2020;15(3):e0229899.

13. Klassen AC, Smith KC. The enduring and evolving relationship between social class and breast cancer burden: a review of the literature. *Cancer Epidemiology*. 2011;35(3):217–34.

14. Chan DSM, Abar L, Cariolou M, Nanu N, Greenwood DC, Bandera EV, et al. World Cancer Research Fund International: Continuous Update Project—systematic literature review and meta-analysis of observational cohort studies on physical activity, sedentary behavior, adiposity, and weight change and breast cancer risk. *Cancer Causes & Control*. 2019;30(11):1183–200.

15. Liu Y, Nguyen N, Colditz GA. Links between alcohol consumption and breast cancer: a look at the evidence. *Women's Health*. 2015;11(1):65–77.

16. Macacu A, Autier P, Boniol M, Boyle P. Active and passive smoking and risk of breast cancer: a meta-analysis. *Breast Cancer Research and Treatment*. 2015;154(2):213–24.

17. International Agency for Research on Cancer. *List of classifications by cancer sites with sufficient or limited evidence in humans, IARC monographs volumes 1–132*. Geneva: World Health Organization; 2022.

18. Gehlert S and Clanton M on behalf of the Shift Work Breast Cancer Strategic Advisory Group. Shift work and breast cancer. *International Journal of Environmental Research and Public Health*. 2020;17:9544.

19. Rodgers KM, Udesky JO, Rudel RA, Brody JG. Environmental chemicals and breast cancer: an updated review of epidemiological literature informed by biological mechanisms. *Environmental Research*. 2018;160:152–82.

20. Terry MB, Michels KB, Brody JG, Byrne C, Chen S, Jerry DJ, et al. Environmental exposures during windows of susceptibility for breast cancer: a framework for prevention research. *Breast Cancer Research*. 2019;21(1):96.

21. Nichols HB, Schoemaker MJ, Cai J, Xu J, Wright LB, Brook MN, et al. Breast cancer risk after recent childbirth. *Annals of Internal Medicine*. 2019;170(1):22–30.

22. Behrens I, Basit S, Jensen A, Lykke JA, Nielsen LP, Wohlfahrt J, et al. Hypertensive disorders of pregnancy and subsequent risk of solid cancer—a nationwide cohort study. *International Journal of Cancer*. 2016;139(1):58–64.

23. National Cancer Institute. *Summary report: Early Reproductive Events and Breast Cancer Workshop* [Internet]. Maryland: National Cancer Institute; 2010 [updated 12 January 2010; cited 18 May 2021]. Available from: https://www.cancer.gov/types/breast/abortion-miscarriage-risk#summary-report.

24. Albrektsen G, Heuch I, Hansen S, Kvåle G. Breast cancer risk by age at birth, time since birth and time intervals between births: exploring interaction effects. *British Journal of Cancer*. 2005;92(1):167–75.

25. Nechuta S, Paneth N, Velie EM. Pregnancy characteristics and maternal breast cancer risk: a review of the epidemiologic literature. *Cancer Causes & Control*. 2010;21(7):967–89.

26. Troisi R, Gulbech Ording A, Grotmol T, Glimelius I, Engeland A, Gissler M, et al. Pregnancy complications and subsequent breast cancer risk in the mother: a Nordic population-based case–control study. *International Journal of Cancer*. 2018;143(8):1904–13.

27. Richardson BE, Peck JD, Wormuth JK. Mean arterial pressure, pregnancy-induced hypertension, and preeclampsia: evaluation as independent risk factors and as surrogates for high maternal serum α-fetoprotein in estimating breast cancer risk. *Cancer Epidemiology, Biomarkers & Prevention*. 2000;9(12):1349–55.

28. Cohn BA, Cirillo PM, Christianson RE, van den Berg BJ, Siiteri PK. Placental characteristics and reduced risk of maternal breast cancer. *Journal of the National Cancer Institute*. 2001;93(15):1133–40.

29. Cnattingius S, Torrång A, Ekbom A, Granath F, Petersson G, Lambe M. Pregnancy characteristics and maternal risk of breast cancer. *JAMA*. 2005;294(19):2474–80.

30. Tsilidis KK, Kasimis JC, Lopez DS, Ntzani EE, Ioannidis JPA. Type 2 diabetes and cancer: umbrella review of meta-analyses of observational studies. *BMJ*. 2015;350:g7607.

31. Titus-Ernstoff L, Hatch EE, Hoover RN, Palmer J, Greenberg ER, Ricker W, et al. Long-term cancer risk in women given diethylstilbestrol (DES) during pregnancy. *British Journal of Cancer*. 2001;84(1):126–33.

32. Ronckers CM, Erdmann CA, Land CE. Radiation and breast cancer: a review of current evidence. *Breast Cancer Research*. 2004;7(1):21.

33. Brinton LA, Devesa SA. Etiology and pathogenesis of breast cancer. Epidemiologic factors. In: Harris J, Morrow M, Lippman M, Hellman S, eds. *Diseases of the breast*. Philadelphia: Lippincott-Raven; 1996. pp. 159–8.

34. Linos E, Willett WC, Cho E, Frazier L. Adolescent diet in relation to breast cancer risk among premenopausal women. *Cancer Epidemiology, Biomarkers & Prevention*. 2010;19(3):689–96.

35. Willett WC. Diet and breast cancer. *Journal of Internal Medicine*. 2001;249(5):395–411.

36. Furer A, Afek A, Sommer A, Keinan-Boker L, Derazne E, Levi Z, et al. Adolescent obesity and midlife cancer risk: a population-based cohort study of 2.3 million adolescents in Israel. *Lancet Diabetes & Endocrinology*. 2020;8(3):216–25.

37. Ahlgren M, Melbye M, Wohlfahrt J, Sørensen TIA. Growth patterns and the risk of breast cancer in women. *New England Journal of Medicine*. 2004;351(16):1619–26.

38. Fortner RT, Katzke V, Kühn T, Kaaks R. Obesity and breast cancer. In: Pischon T, Nimptsch K, eds. *Obesity and cancer*. Cham: Springer International Publishing; 2016. pp. 43–65.

39. Rosner B, Eliassen AH, Toriola AT, Chen WY, Hankinson SE, Willett WC, et al. Weight and weight changes in early adulthood and later breast cancer risk. *International Journal of Cancer*. 2017;140(9):2003–14.

40. Zhang B, Shu X-O, Delahanty RJ, Zeng C, Michailidou K, Bolla MK, et al. Height and breast cancer risk: evidence from prospective studies and Mendelian randomization. *Journal of the National Cancer Institute*. 2015;107(11).

41. Hislop TG, Coldman AJ, Elwood JM, Brauer G, Kan L. Childhood and recent eating patterns and risk of breast cancer. *Cancer Detection and Prevention*. 1986;9(1–2):47–58.

42. Potischman N, Swanson CA, Hoover RN, Brinton LA, Weiss HA, Coates RJ, et al. Diet during adolescence and risk of breast cancer among young women. *Journal of the National Cancer Institute*. 1998;90(3):226–33.

43. Pryor M, Slattery ML, Robison LM, Egger M. Adolescent diet and breast cancer in Utah. *Cancer Research*. 1989;49(8):2161–7.

44. Linos E, Willett WC, Cho E, Colditz G, Frazier LA. Red meat consumption during adolescence among premenopausal women and risk of breast cancer. *Cancer Epidemiology, Biomarkers & Prevention*. 2008;17(8):2146–51.

45. Farvid MS, Eliassen AH, Cho E, Chen WY, Willett WC. Dairy consumption in adolescence and early adulthood and risk of breast cancer. *Cancer Epidemiology, Biomarkers & Prevention*. 2018;27(5):575–84.

46. Romieu, II, Amadou A, Chajes V. The role of diet, physical activity, body fatness, and breastfeeding in breast cancer in young women: epidemiological evidence. *Rev Invest Clin*. 2017;69(4):193–203.

47. Niehoff NM, White AJ, Sandler DP. Childhood and teenage physical activity and breast cancer risk. *Breast Cancer Research and Treatment*. 2017;164(3):697–705.

48. Boeke CE, Eliassen AH, Oh H, Spiegelman D, Willett WC, Tamimi RM. Adolescent physical activity in relation to breast cancer risk. *Breast Cancer Research and Treatment*. 2014;145(3):715–24.

49. Kehm RD, Genkinger JM, MacInnis RJ, John EM, Phillips K-A, Dite GS, et al. Recreational physical activity is associated with reduced breast cancer risk in adult women at high risk for breast cancer: a cohort study of women selected for familial and genetic risk. *Cancer Research*. 2020;80(1):116–25.

50. Houghton LC, Cooper GD, Bentley GR, Booth M, Chowdhury OA, Troisi R, et al. A migrant study of pubertal timing and tempo in British-Bangladeshi girls at varying risk for breast cancer. *Breast Cancer Research*. 2014;16(6):469.

51. Anderson KN, Schwab RB, Martinez ME. Reproductive risk factors and breast cancer subtypes: a review of the literature. *Breast Cancer Research and Treatment*. 2014;144(1):1–10.

52. Barnard ME, Boeke CE, Tamimi RM. Established breast cancer risk factors and risk of intrinsic tumor subtypes. *Biochimica et Biophysica Acta (BBA)—Reviews on Cancer*. 2015;1856(1):73–85.

53. Fuhrman BJ, Moore SC, Byrne C, Makhoul I, Kitahara CM, Berrington de González A, et al. Association of the age at menarche with site-specific cancer risks in pooled data from nine cohorts. *Cancer Research*. 2021;81(8):2246–55.

54. Yang XR, Sherman ME, Rimm DL, Lissowska J, Brinton LA, Peplonska B, et al. Differences in risk factors for breast cancer molecular subtypes in a population-based study. *Cancer Epidemiology, Biomarkers & Prevention*. 2007;16(3):439–43.

55. Lee Y, Styne D. Influences on the onset and tempo of puberty in human beings and implications for adolescent psychological development. *Hormones and Behavior*. 2013;64(2):250–61.

56. Fenton SE. Endocrine-disrupting compounds and mammary gland development: early exposure and later life consequences. *Endocrinology*. 2006;147(6):s18–s24.

57. Bodicoat DH, Schoemaker MJ, Jones ME, McFadden E, Griffin J, Ashworth A, et al. Timing of pubertal stages and breast cancer risk: the Breakthrough Generations Study. *Breast Cancer Research*. 2014;16(1):R18.

58. Houghton LC, Jung S, Troisi R, LeBlanc ES, Snetselaar LG, Hylton NM, et al. Pubertal timing and breast density in young women: a prospective cohort study. *Breast Cancer Research*. 2019;21(1):122.

59. Silva IDS, Stavola BD, McCormack V, Collaborative Group on Pre-Natal Risk, Factors Subsequent Risk of Breast, Cancer. Birth size and breast cancer risk: re-analysis of individual participant data from 32 studies. *PLOS Medicine*. 2008;5:e193.

60. Sanderson M, Daling JR, Doody DR, Malone KE. Perinatal factors and mortality from breast cancer. *Cancer Epidemiology, Biomarkers & Prevention*. 2006;15(10):1984–7.

61. Andersson SW, Bengtsson C, Hallberg L, Lapidus L, Niklasson A, Wallgren A, et al. Cancer risk in Swedish women: the relation to size at birth. *British Journal of Cancer*. 2001;84(9):1193–8.

62. Hilakivi-Clarke L, Forsén T, Eriksson JG, Luoto R, Tuomilehto J, Osmond C, et al. Tallness and overweight during childhood have opposing effects on breast cancer risk. *British Journal of Cancer*. 2001;85(11):1680–4.

63. Innes K, Byers T, Schymura M. Birth characteristics and subsequent risk for breast cancer in very young women. *American Journal of Epidemiology*. 2000;152(12):1121–8.

64. Michels KB, Trichopoulos D, Robins JM, Rosner BA, Manson JE, Hunter DJ, et al. Birthweight as a risk factor for breast cancer. *Lancet*. 1996;348(9041):1542–6.

65. Sanderson M, Williams MA, White E, Daling JR, Holt VL, Malone KE, et al. Validity and reliability of subject and mother reporting of perinatal factors. *American Journal of Epidemiology*. 1998;147(2):136–40.

66. Vatten LJ, Mæhle BO, Lund Nilsen TI, Tretli S, Hsieh Cc, Trichopoulos D, et al. Birth weight as a predictor of breast cancer: a case-control study in Norway. *British Journal of Cancer*. 2002;86(1):89–91.

67. Kar SP, Andrulis IL, Brenner H, Burgess S, Chang-Claude J, Considine D, et al. The association between weight at birth and breast cancer risk revisited using Mendelian randomisation. *European Journal of Epidemiology*. 2019;34(6):591–600.

68. Troisi R, Potischman N, Hoover RN. Exploring the underlying hormonal mechanisms of prenatal risk factors for breast cancer: a review and commentary. *Cancer Epidemiology, Biomarkers & Prevention*. 2007;16(9):1700–12.

69. Park SK, Kang D, McGlynn KA, Garcia-Closas M, Kim Y, Yoo KY, et al. Intrauterine environments and breast cancer risk: meta-analysis and systematic review. *Breast Cancer Research*. 2008;10(1):R8.

70. Hemminki K, Kyyronen P. Parental age and risk of sporadic and familial cancer in offspring: implications for germ cell mutagenesis. *Epidemiology*. 1999;10(6):747–51.

71. Rothman KJ, MacMahon B, Lin TM, Lowe CR, Mirra AP, Ravnihar B, et al. Maternal age and birth rank of women with breast cancer. *Journal of the National Cancer Institute*. 1980;65(4):719–22.

72. Bucalossi P, Veronesi U. Some observations on cancer of the breast in mothers and daughters. *British Journal of Cancer*. 1957;11(3):337–47.

73. Henderson BE, Powell D, Rosario I, Keys C, Hanisch R, Young M, et al. An epidemiologic study of breast cancer. *Journal of the National Cancer Institute*. 1974;53(3):609–14.

74. Tokuhata GK. Morbidity and mortality among offspring of breast cancer mothers. *American Journal of Epidemiology*. 1969;89(2):139–53.

75. Titus-Ernstoff L, Egan KM, Newcomb PA, Baron JA, Stampfer M, Greenberg ER, et al. Exposure to breast milk in infancy and adult breast cancer risk. *Journal of the National Cancer Institute*. 1998;90(12):921–4.

76. Troisi R, Bjørge T, Gissler M, Grotmol T, Kitahara CM, Myrtveit Sæther SM, et al. The role of pregnancy, perinatal factors and hormones in maternal cancer risk: a review of the evidence. *Journal of Internal Medicine*. 2018;283(5):430–45.

77. Palmer JR, Hatch EE, Rosenberg CL, Hartge P, Kaufman RH, Titus-Ernstoff L, et al. Risk of breast cancer in women exposed to diethylstilbestrol in utero: preliminary results (United States). *Cancer Causes & Control*. 2002;13(8):753–8.

78. Ekbom A, Adami H-O, Hsieh C-C, Lipworth L, Trichopoulos D. Intrauterine environment and breast cancer risk in women: a population-based study. *Journal of the National Cancer Institute*. 1997;89(1):71–6.

79. Kristoffersen S, Hartveit F. Is a woman's date of birth related to her risk of developing breast cancer? *Oncology Reports*. 2000;7(2):245–52.

80. Severson RK, Davis S. Breast cancer incidence and month of birth: evidence against an etiologic association. *European Journal of Cancer and Clinical Oncology*. 1987;23(7):1067–70.

81. Yuen J, Ekbom A, Trichopoulos D, Hsieh CC, Adami HO. Season of birth and breast cancer risk in Sweden. *British Journal of Cancer*. 1994;70(3):564–8.

82. Sanderson M, Williams MA, Daling JR, Holt VL, Malone KE, Self SG, et al. Maternal factors and breast cancer risk among young women. *Paediatric and Perinatal Epidemiology*. 1998;12(4):397–407.

83. Sanderson M, Williams MA, Malone KE, Stanford JL, Emanuel I, White E, et al. Perinatal factors and risk of breast cancer. *Epidemiology*. 1996;7(1):34–7.

84. Sandler DP, Everson RB, Wilcox AJ, Browder JP. Cancer risk in adulthood from early life exposure to parents' smoking. *American Journal of Public Health*. 1985;75(5):487–92.

85. Weiss HA, Potischman NA, Brinton LA, Brogan D, Coates RJ, Gammon MD, et al. Prenatal and perinatal risk factors for breast cancer in young women. *Epidemiology*. 1997;8(2):181–7.

86. Mishra GD, Cooper R, Kuh D. A life course approach to reproductive health: theory and methods. *Maturitas*. 2010;65(2):92–7.

87. van den Brandt PA, Ziegler RG, Wang M, Hou T, Li R, Adami H-O, et al. Body size and weight change over adulthood and risk of breast cancer by menopausal and hormone receptor status: a pooled analysis of 20 prospective cohort studies. *European Journal of Epidemiology*. 2021;36(1):37–55.

88. Andersen ZJ, Baker JL, Bihrmann K, Vejborg I, Sørensen TIA, Lynge E. Birth weight, childhood body mass index, and height in relation to mammographic density and breast cancer: a register-based cohort study. *Breast Cancer Research*. 2014;16(1):R4.

89. Luo J, Chen X, Manson JE, Shadyab AH, Wactawski-Wende J, Vitolins M, et al. Birth weight, weight over the adult life course and risk of breast cancer. *International Journal of Cancer*. 2020;147(1):65–75.

90. De Stavola BL, dos Santos Silva I, McCormack V, Hardy RJ, Kuh DJ, Wadsworth MEJ. Childhood Growth and Breast Cancer. *American Journal of Epidemiology*. 2004;159(7):671–82.

91. Li CI, Malone KE, White E, Daling JR. Age when maximum height is reached as a risk factor for breast cancer among young U.S. women. *Epidemiology*. 1997;8(5):559–65.

92. Stavola BLD, Hardy R, Kuh D, Silva IDS, Wadsworth M, Swerdlow AJ. Birthweight, childhood growth and risk of breast cancer in a British cohort. *British Journal of Cancer*. 2000;83(7):964–8.

93. Mellemkjær L, Christensen J, Frederiksen K, Baker JL, Olsen A, Sørensen TIA, et al. Leg length, sitting height and postmenopausal breast cancer risk. *British Journal of Cancer*. 2012;107(1):165–8.

94. Gunnell DJ, Davey Smith G, Frankel S, Nonchiral K, Braddon FE, Pemberton J, et al. Childhood leg length and adult mortality: follow up of the Carnegie (Boyd Orr) Survey of Diet and Health in Pre-War Britain. *Journal of Epidemiology and Community Health*. 1998;52(3):142–52.

95. Hardy R, Potischman P, Kuh D. Life course approach to research in women's health. 2013. In: *Women and health, 2nd edition*. [Internet]. Amsterdam: Elsevier.

96. Pike MC, Karlo MD, Henderson BE, Casagrande JT, Hoel DG. 'Hormonal' risk factors, 'breast tissue age' and the age-incidence of breast cancer. *Nature*. 1983;303(5920):767–70.

97. Tokunaga M, Land CE, Yamamoto T, Asano M, Tokuoka S, Ezaki H, et al. Incidence of female breast cancer among atomic bomb survivors, Hiroshima and Nagasaki, 1950–1980. *Radiation Research*. 1987;112(2):243–72.

98. Colditz GA, Frazier AL. Models of breast cancer show that risk is set by events of early life: prevention efforts must shift focus. *Cancer Epidemiology, Biomarkers & Prevention*. 1995;4(5):567–71.

99. Trichopoulos D. Hypothesis: does breast cancer originate in utero? *Lancet*. 1990;335(8695):939–40.

100. Liao DJ, Dickson RB. Roles of androgens in the development, growth, and carcinogenesis of the mammary gland. *Journal of Steroid Biochemistry and Molecular Biology*. 2002;80(2):175–89.

101. Bohlke K, Cramer DW, Trichopoulos D, Mantzoros CS. Insulin-like growth factor-I in relation to premenopausal ductal carcinoma in situ of the breast. *Epidemiology*. 1998;9(5):570–3.

102. Bruning PF, Bonfrèr JMG, van Noord PAH, Hart AAM, de Jong-Bakker M, Nooijen WJ. Insulin resistance and breast-cancer risk. *International Journal of Cancer*. 1992;52(4):511–6.

103. Hankinson SE, Willett WC, Colditz GA, Hunter DJ, Michaud DS, Deroo B, et al. Circulating concentrations of insulin-like growth factor I and risk of breast cancer. *Lancet*. 1998;351(9113):1393–6.

104. Sivaraman L, Medina D. Hormone-induced protection against breast cancer. *Journal of Mammary Gland Biology and Neoplasia*. 2002;7(1):77–92.

105. Clemmesen J. Carcinoma of the breast; results from statistical research. *British Journal of Radiology*. 1948;21(252):583–90.

12
Gynaecological Cancers

A Life Course Perspective

Susan J. Jordan and Penelope M. Webb

12.1 Introduction

Gynaecological cancer includes all cancers arising in the female reproductive tract from the vulva to the ovary. The most common are those of the endometrium (lining) of the uterus, the ovary (mainly epithelial cancers), and the cervix, although the relative frequency varies geographically. In countries with a very high Human Development Index (a summary measure of life expectancy, education, and income indicators developed by the United Nations Development Programme), uterine cancer is the most common (age-standardised incidence rate (ASR_{world}) 15.9 per 100,000), and cervical cancer is less common (ASR_{world} 9.1/100,000), but this is reversed in countries with a low Human Development Index (ASR_{world} 2.9 and 27.2, respectively).[1] Ovarian cancer is slightly more common in high-income than in low-income countries (ASR_{world} 8.3 versus 5.1/100,000).[1] The differences likely reflect socioeconomically driven variation in nongenetic risk factor prevalence and access to cervical cancer screening. In the following sections, we review the risk factors (see Table 12.1) for gynaecological cancers throughout the life course, identifying opportunities for prevention. We focus mainly on endometrial, epithelial ovarian (although the most common histotype probably starts in the fallopian tube), and cervical cancers as these are most common. We also highlight variation between different histological subtypes of cancer at the same anatomical site where there is strong supporting evidence for this.

Unsurprisingly, reproductive factors play a key role in the development of gynaecological cancers, and, accordingly, we have structured the chapter by reproductive life phase, noting the potential importance of timing of reproductive and other events in cancer development.

12.2 Early Life to Menarche

Early life exposures reflect a combination of genetics and maternal and childhood factors such as obstetric history, illnesses, nutrition, and lifestyle. Many of these are, in turn, influenced by upstream socioeconomic factors,[2] and they also influence women's experience later in life.

Susan J. Jordan and Penelope M. Webb, *Gynaecological Cancers* In: *A Life Course Approach to Women's Health*. Second Edition. Edited by: Gita D Mishra, Rebecca Hardy, and Diana Kuh, Oxford University Press. © Oxford University Press 2023. DOI: 10.1093/oso/9780192864642.003.0012

Table 12.1 Summary of risk factors across life-stages for endometrial, ovarian, and cervical cancers.

	Endometrial Cancer	Ovarian Cancer	Cervical Cancer
Genetic			
High-risk genes	MMR ↑↑	*BRCA1, BRCA2* ↑↑	–
Moderate-risk genes	*PTEN* ↑	MMR, *BRIP1, RAD51* ↑	–
Hormonal & Reproductive			
Diethylstilboestrol in utero	–	–	↑ Clear cell cancers
Older age at menarche	↓↓	↓	–
HPV infection	–	–	↑↑↑ Likely necessary
Younger sexual activity	–	–	↑↑
Pregnancy:			
Full-term	↓↓↓	↓↓↓	↑
Incomplete	↓	↓	–
Younger age at first	–	–	↑
Older age at last	↓	↓	–
Breastfeeding	↓↓	↓↓	–
Contraception:			
Contraceptive pill	↓↓↓	↓↓↓	↑ Current & recent use
Long-acting reversible	↓?	↓?	–
Infertility treatment	–?	–?	–
Older age at menopause	↑	↑	–
Menopausal hormones:			
Oestrogen only	↑↑	↑	–
+Cyclic progestogen	–	–	–
+Continuous progestogen	↓	–	–
Tamoxifen	↑↑	–	–
Anthropometric			
Greater height:			
Childhood	–	–	–
Adult	↑	↑	↑?
Greater adiposity:			
Childhood & adolescence	↑?	↑?	–
Adult	↑↑↑	↑ Non-HGSC	–?
Weight loss	↓↓	↓? Non-HGSC	–
Medical Exposures:			
Procedures:			
Tubal ligation	?	↓↓	–
Hysterectomy	↓↓↓	–	↓↓↓

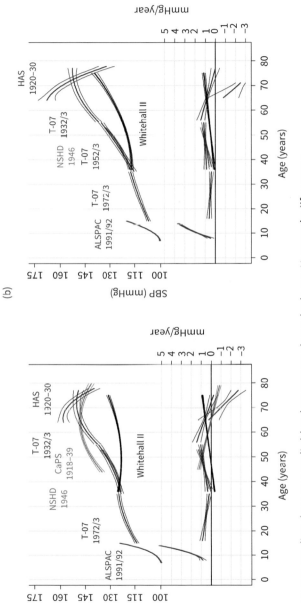

Figure 5.2 Predicted mean systolic blood pressure trajectories in mmHg over the life course.

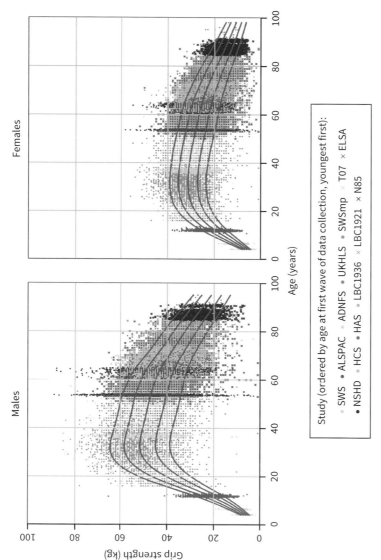

Figure 7.2 Cross-cohort centile curves for grip strength using data from 12 British studies. Centiles shown 10th, 25th, 50th, 75th, and 90th percentiles are shown. The studies include ADNFS Allied Dunbar National Fitness Survey, ALSPAC Avon Longitudinal Study of Parents and Children, ELSA English Longitudinal Study of Ageing, HAS Hertfordshire Ageing Study, HCS Hertfordshire Cohort Study, LBC1921 and LBC1936 Lothian Birth Cohorts of 1921 and 1936, N85 Newcastle 85+ Study, NSHD Medical Research Council National Survey of Health and Development, SWS Southampton Women's Survey, SWSmp Mothers and Their Partners from the SWS, T-07 West of Scotland Twenty-07 Study, UKHLS Understanding Society: the UK Household Panel Study.

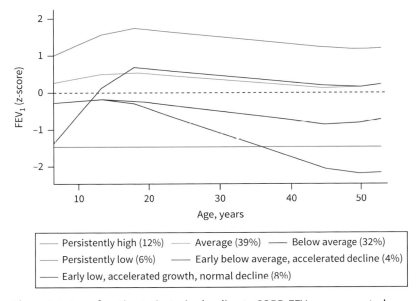

Figure 8.1 Lung function trajectories leading to COPD. FEV_1 was presented in z-scores (standardised for age, height, and sex), with a z-score of zero representing the population average. Individuals in the 'average' trajectory had lung function levels around the population average (z-score around 0) at any time. Individuals in the 'persistently low' trajectory had low childhood lung function, which then grew and declined at the population average rate. Individuals in the 'persistently high' trajectory had high childhood lung function, which then grew and declined at the population average rate. Individuals in the 'early low, accelerated growth, normal decline' trajectory had low childhood lung function, which then grew at a greater rate than the population average rate, but declined at the population average rate. Individuals in the 'early below average, accelerated decline' trajectory had childhood lung function below the population average and lung function declined at a greater rate than the population average rate. Individuals in the 'below average' trajectory had childhood lung function below the population average, which then grew and declined at the population average rate. Three trajectories, namely 'persistently low', 'early below average, accelerated decline', and 'below average', had increased risk of developing COPD by age 53 years.

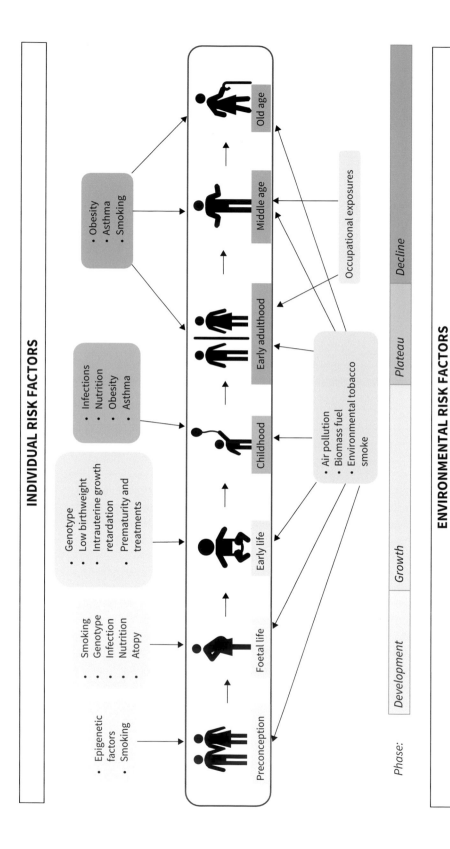

Figure 8.3 Life course risk factors for lung function deficits and COPD.

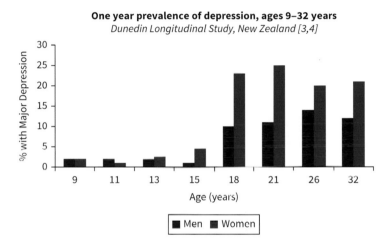

One year prevalence of depression, ages 9–32 years
Dunedin Longitudinal Study, New Zealand [3,4]

Men   Women

Figure 9.1 One-year prevalence of depression in males and females aged 9–32 years in the Dunedin Multidisciplinary Study of Health and Development.

Chain of Risk Model of Body Size and Breast Cancer Risk

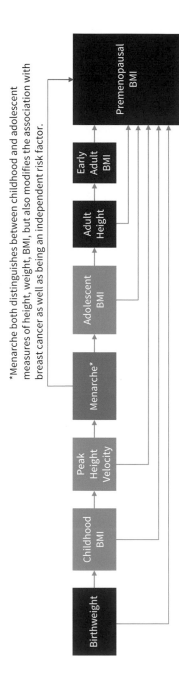

Figure 11.1 Chain of risk model of body size over the life course and premenopausal breast cancer risk.

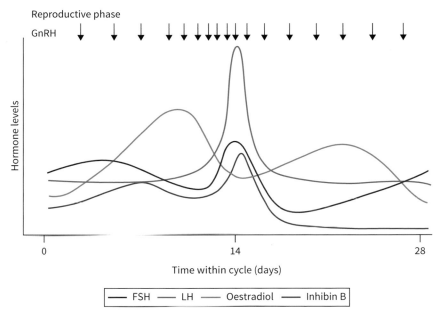

Figure 14.1 Changes in female hormone levels regulated by the pulsatile actions of gonadotropin-releasing hormone in the pituitary gland throughout the menstrual cycle.

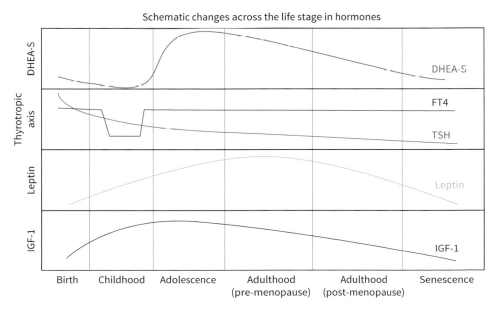

Figure 14.5 Schematic changes across the life course in the main hormones.

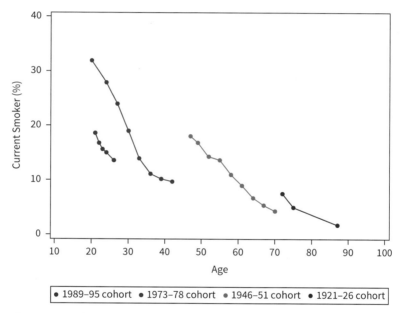

Figure 15.1 The prevalence of current smokers by age across four birth cohorts in the Australian Longitudinal Study on Women's Health.

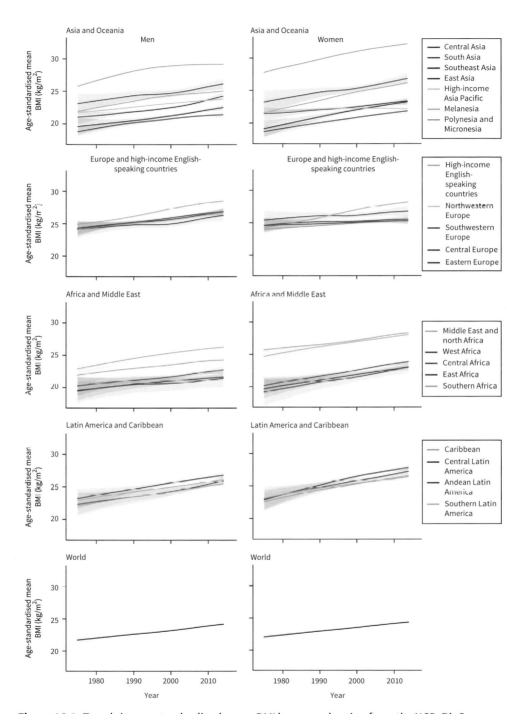

Figure 16.1 Trends in age-standardised mean BMI by sex and region from the NCD-RisC.

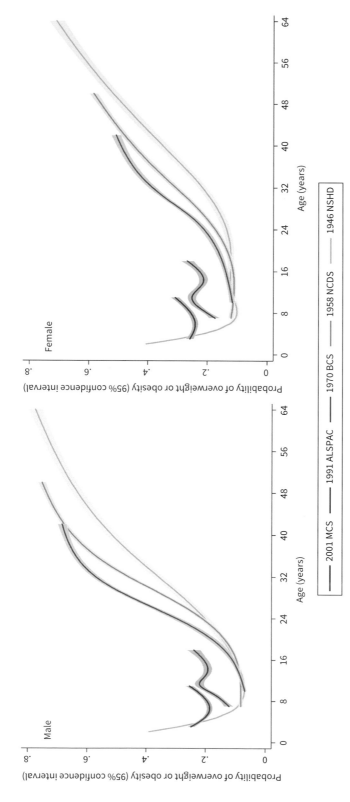

Figure 16.2 Trajectories of the probability of overweight or obesity across the life course from sex- and study-stratified multilevel logistic regression models.

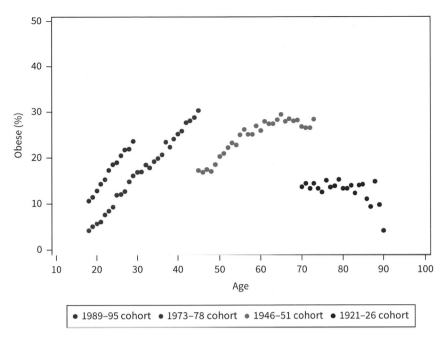

Figure 16.3 Percentage of obese women in each cohort of the Australian Longitudinal Study on Women's Health.

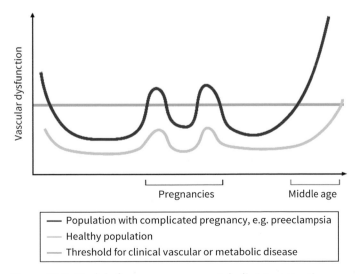

Figure 21.2 Model of pregnancy as a metabolic 'stress test'.

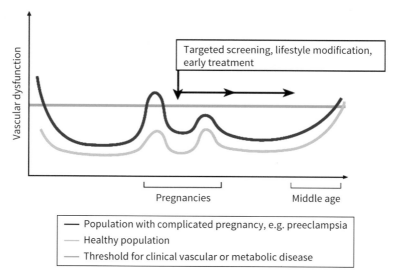

Figure 21.4 Conceptual model of intervention during critical periods in the reproductive life course to reduce disease risk and improve health in adulthood.

Table 12.1 Continued

	Endometrial Cancer	Ovarian Cancer	Cervical Cancer
Medical Conditions:			
Endometriosis	–	↑↑ END & CCC	–
Polycystic ovary syndrome	↑	↓	–
Fibroids	↑?	–	–
Diabetes	↑	–	–
Metabolic syndrome	↑	–	↑?
Medications:			
Aspirin	↓ (Obese women only?)	↓	–
Metformin	–	–	–
Bisphosphonates	↓?	↓?	–
Lifestyle			
Physical activity	↓	↓?	–
Diet:			
Glycaemic load	↑	–	–
Coffee	↓	–	–
Vitamin D	–	↓?	–
Smoking	↓	↓ END/CCC; ↑↑MUC	↑↑
Alcohol	–	–	–

Abbreviations: CCC, clear cell ovarian cancer; END, endometrioid ovarian cancer; HGSC, high-grade serous ovarian cancer; MUC, mucinous ovarian cancer; HPV, human papillomavirus; MMR, mismatch repair genes (*MLH1, MSH2, MSH6,* and *PMS2*).

– = No evidence for an association or insufficient evidence to assess this; ↑/↓ = weak increase/reduction in risk; ↑↑/↓↓ = moderate increase/reduction in risk; ↑↑↑/↓↓↓= strong evidence and/or large increase/reduction in risk; ? = Uncertain if effect is causal.

12.2.1 Genetic Risks

A woman's genetic background plays an important role in determining her subsequent cancer risk. Women with a pathogenic *BRCA1/BRCA2* gene mutation have a 35%–55% and 11%–25% risk, respectively, of developing ovarian cancer by age 80 years[3] versus about 1% in the general population. Women with a mismatch repair gene mutation (*MLH1, MSH2, MSH6,* or *PMS2*) have a 16%–50% risk of developing endometrial cancer by age 70 years, and a modestly increased risk of ovarian cancer.[4] Mutations in other genes including *BRIP1, RAD51, PTEN,* and *STK11* also confer a moderately increased risk of ovarian and/or endometrial cancer,[5] and genome-wide association studies have identified multiple low-risk susceptibility loci associated with ovarian, endometrial, and/or cervical cancer. Identifying high-risk mutations and offering carriers preventive measures (e.g. prophylactic surgery) is an important strategy to reduce incidence.

12.2.2 Exposures in Utero and Birthweight

There is little evidence that exposures in utero have a major influence on a woman's risk of most gynaecological cancers; however, it is well established that daughters of women who used diethylstilboestrol (previously prescribed for morning sickness) have an increased risk of developing rare clear cell adenocarcinomas of the cervix and vagina in adulthood.[6]

Birthweight has been linked to subsequent risk of several cancers,[7] but evidence for gynaecological cancers is conflicting. While a large data-linkage study found both lower and higher-than-average birthweight were associated with subsequent ovarian cancer risk, cohort studies do not support this.[7] There is no evidence for a relation with endometrial cancer and little data for other gynaecological cancers.

12.2.3 Age at Menarche

Observational and Mendelian randomization (MR) studies show the risks of endometrial and ovarian cancer decrease with older age at menarche.[8-10] The association is particularly strong for endometrial cancer, with each additional year decreasing risk by ~9%.[9] Menarcheal age does not appear to affect risk of cervical cancer.[11]

12.2.4 Height and Weight in Childhood

In a large historical cohort study, greater measured height and body mass index (BMI) in childhood (age 7 years) and around menarche (age 13 years) were both associated with increased risk of endometrial and ovarian cancer in later life, although increased growth rate between these two ages did not seem to play a role.[7] Notably, childhood BMI was not strongly correlated with BMI at older ages,[7] suggesting the associations might not simply reflect tracking of overweight/obesity from childhood into adulthood, although others have found childhood BMI is no longer associated with endometrial cancer after adjusting for recent BMI.[12,13]

12.3 From Menarche to Menopause

12.3.1 Sexual Activity and HPV Infection

The primary, and probably necessary, cause of cervical cancer is infection with a carcinogenic strain of the human papillomavirus (HPV);[14] however, other factors such as smoking and oral contraceptive use modify risk among those carrying a high-risk HPV.[15] HPV infection also plays a role in vulval and vaginal cancer development but has not been implicated in either ovarian or endometrial cancer. Genital HPV infections are sexually transmitted, thus the prevalence of infection increases rapidly as girls become sexually active, peaking among women between 20 and 30 years,[16] and it is strongly associated with number of sexual partners.[15] The introduction of HPV vaccination in 2006, coupled with enhanced HPV DNA screening for cervical precancers, has the potential to almost eliminate cervical cancer in the future.[17] UK data show almost a 90% reduction in risk of cervical cancer among girls vaccinated before age 14,[18,19] but benefits were lower for girls vaccinated at older ages, highlighting the importance of vaccination before girls become sexually active. If current vaccination and screening rates are maintained, it has been estimated that cervical cancer will be almost eliminated in girls born in the UK after September 1995,[18] and in countries like Australia that started vaccination early, it could cease to be a public health problem within 20 years.[20]

12.3.2 Pregnancy and Breastfeeding

There is overwhelming evidence that a full-term or incomplete pregnancy reduces the risk of both ovarian[10,21,22] and endometrial[23] cancer, and that risk reduces further with subsequent pregnancies. The timing of pregnancy is also likely to be important such that, after accounting for birth number, the older a woman is at last birth, the lower her risk of developing these cancers.[24,25] This pregnancy-associated risk reduction persists for several decades. For ovarian cancer, the relationship may vary by histotype with the strongest inverse associations seen for the endometrioid and clear cell histotypes.[10,21] In contrast, higher parity is associated with an increased risk of cervical cancer and the younger a woman is at first birth, the higher her risk.[26] This appears to be independent of age at first sexual intercourse and number of sexual partners.[26]

Breastfeeding, independent of parity, also appears to reduce risk of ovarian[23] and endometrial cancers,[27] and risk decreases with increasing breastfeeding duration. For ovarian cancer, individual episodes of breastfeeding that lasted 12 or more months were associated with a 34% lower risk;[23] the equivalent estimate for endometrial cancer was around 13%.[27] Supporting women to breastfeed may be one avenue to help prevent these cancers. Data for other gynaecological cancers are lacking.

12.3.3 Contraception

Use of the combined oral contraceptive (COC) pill substantially reduces the risk of endometrial and ovarian cancer. Risk decreases with increasing duration of use,[28,29] and the protective effect persists for at least 30 years after cessation.[29,30] Further, the risk-reducing benefits of COCs are apparent for newer lower-dose formulations as well as older forms.[29,31] There is less evidence for other hormonal contraceptives, although some studies report reduced risks associated with the progestin-releasing intrauterine device (IUD)[32] and injected progestins.[33,34] Given the increasing use of these long-acting reversible contraceptives, understanding their relationship with cancer is a research priority.

Use of COCs appears to increase cervical cancer risk in a duration-dependent fashion, but risk declines after cessation, returning to background after ~10 years.[35] In contrast, IUD users may have lower cervical cancer risk,[36] but this may reflect greater cervical surveillance rather than a direct causal effect.

Notwithstanding the small increase in risk of cervical cancer and the established short-term increase in breast cancer, estimates show the long-lasting benefits of COCs for ovarian and endometrial cancer equate to an overall reduction in women's cancer risk.[37]

12.3.4   Benign Gynaecological Conditions

Gynaecological conditions, such as endometriosis, polycystic ovary syndrome (PCOS), and fibroids, are associated with ovulatory and/or menstrual abnormalities, aberrations in reproductive hormone levels, and infertility. Endometriosis is also associated with pervasive local inflammation (see Chapter 3). These factors may also affect gynaecological cancer risk.

Endometriosis is associated with a two- to threefold increased risk of clear cell and endometrioid ovarian cancer, but not endometrial cancer.[38] Reduced risks observed for cervical cancer have been attributed to increased surveillance in women with endometriosis.[38]

A large pooled analysis[39] and a MR study suggested women with PCOS have a lower risk of ovarian cancer.[38] While, a data linkage study reported a twofold increase in ovarian cancer risk associated with a PCOS diagnosis, these results were based on relatively few women with PCOS and could not adjust for important covariates such as BMI and oral contraceptive use.[40] That study found no link between PCOS and cervical cancer but, in keeping with most studies,[41] an increased risk of endometrial cancer. There is little information available on whether treatment (including timing) of either PCOS or endometriosis modifies associations with endometrial or ovarian cancer.

Women with a history of fibroids may have an elevated risk of endometrial cancer, perhaps reflecting the role of oestrogen exposure in both conditions.[42]

12.3.5   Infertility and Fertility Treatment

As described above, some common causes of infertility may increase risk of ovarian and endometrial cancer. Whether specific infertility treatments independently affect cancer risk is less clear. A recent meta-analysis indicated that, overall, fertility treatment was not associated with increased risk of endometrial or ovarian cancer.[43] However, the risk may be slightly higher for borderline ovarian tumours (abnormal cells in the tissue covering the ovary that are slow-growing and not considered cancerous) and/or may vary by treatment type (possible 30%–40% increased risks with IVF and clomiphene citrate), although the latter analyses did not consider histotype.[43] A reduction in cervical cancer risk was attributed to frequent screening in women undergoing infertility treatment.[43]

12.3.6   Height, Weight, and Weight Change

Evidence from observational [44] and MR studies[45] indicates that greater adult height is associated with increased risk of ovarian, endometrial, and possibly cervical cancers. Height is determined by a combination of genetics and early life exposures, including nutrition and exposure to insulin, sex steroids, and growth hormones, which likely explain the association rather than height itself.

Obesity may promote carcinogenesis via a number of pathways including increased inflammation, effects on glucose metabolism, and via increased production of a wide range of cytokines and hormones such as oestrogen in adipose tissue.[46] Obesity is a major risk factor for endometrial cancer with risk increasing by approximately 50% for every five-unit increase in BMI.[47] Although obesity is most strongly associated with the more common low-grade type 1 endometrial cancers, it also increases risk of the more aggressive nonendometrioid type 2 cancers, albeit to a lesser extent.[48] Importantly, greater central adiposity has also been associated with increased risk among women within a healthy weight range.[49] While body size in childhood and adolescence may be important (see Section 12.2.4),[7] the strongest associations are with adult weight gain and recent weight,[12,13] with adult overweight and/or obesity accounting for about one third of all endometrial cancers.[50] Encouragingly, a prospective cohort analysis suggests that intentional weight-loss may reduce risk of endometrial cancer,[13] and benefits have also been reported for those who undergo bariatric surgery.[51]

Observational and genetic data suggest obesity also plays a role in the development of non-high-grade serous ovarian cancers[52,53]; however, there is little evidence that it affects the risk of cervical cancer.[35]

12.3.7 Physical Activity

Separating effects of physical activity from those of obesity can be challenging, but several cohort studies have reported that increased physical activity is associated with a lower risk of endometrial cancer independent of obesity. Accordingly, the 2018 WCRF/AICR report concluded that physical activity probably reduces risk of endometrial cancer, and sedentary behaviour might increase risk.[47] Additional support for this being a causal relationship comes from a preliminary MR analysis using genetic markers of objectively measured activity which also reported significantly reduced risk among women predicted to be more active.[54] Data for ovarian cancer are more limited; however, recent large-scale analyses reported a 30% increased risk among women who were inactive[55] or sedentary[56] prior to diagnosis.

12.3.8 Diet

Diet has an indirect effect on risk of gynaecological cancers through its effects on body weight, but although diet affects a wide range of metabolic processes and foods contain both pro- and anti-inflammatory compounds, as well as a wide range of antioxidants, evidence of a direct effect on risk is limited. Prospective data, which are less prone to recall bias than retrospective studies, suggest increased glycaemic load increases endometrial cancer risk and an inverse association with coffee drinking, but little evidence for other dietary components.[47] There is no good evidence that diet plays a role in ovarian or cervical cancer development.[47] While it has been suggested the polyphenols in tea, particularly green tea, might reduce cancer risk, the data are insufficient to draw definitive conclusions.

The role of vitamin D in disease has received much attention, but there is little good evidence that it plays a role in cancer development although one exception may be ovarian cancer, with MR studies suggesting lower risk among women with higher genetically predicted circulating levels of 25-hydroxy vitamin D.[57]

12.3.9 Smoking and Alcohol Consumption

Current smokers have an almost twofold increased risk of developing squamous cell cancers of the cervix, with similar associations seen overall and among women who carry a high-risk HPV infection.[58] The risk is greater for women who start smoking younger, increases with the number of cigarettes smoked per day, and falls again after smoking cessation. Smokers also have a 30%–80% increased risk of mucinous ovarian cancers;[59,60] that increases with increasing duration of smoking and persists for up to 20 years after cessation, but age at initiation appears to be less important.[60] In contrast, smoking has not been associated with adenocarcinomas of the cervix[58] and smokers appear to be at lower risk of developing endometrioid or clear cell ovarian cancers[59] and endometrial cancer,[48] perhaps because smoking lowers endogenous oestrogen levels. There is currently little evidence (observational[47] or genetic[61]) that alcohol consumption increases risk of gynaecological cancer.

12.3.10 Tubal Ligation

Tubal ligation reduces the risk of ovarian cancer,[10,62] particularly the endometrioid and clear cell histotypes. It might act by blocking the passage of preneoplastic cells or carcinogens from the vagina, uterus, or fallopian tube to the ovary; thus, its timing might be expected to affect the relationship (earlier procedures reducing opportunity for exposure). However, there is little evidence of this, as procedures undertaken before and after 40 years of age have been associated with similar risk reductions.[62]

Evidence for a link with endometrial cancer is less convincing. Cohort studies found no association,[63] but a Danish linkage study showed an ~25% reduction in risk among those who had a tubal ligation compared to those without, although they could not adjust for either oral contraceptive use or BMI.[64] Risk of cervical cancer is not associated with tubal ligation.[63]

12.3.11 Hysterectomy

Surgical removal of the uterus (hysterectomy) prevents endometrial and cervical cancer (if the cervix is not left in situ). For ovarian cancer, the relationship is more complex. Earlier studies suggested hysterectomy without oophorectomy reduced ovarian cancer risk; however, more recent studies suggested no overall association,[10,65] possibly reflecting changes in menopausal hormone therapy (MHT) use or misclassification of oophorectomy status. Risk may vary by histotype with inverse associations observed for clear cell cancers in particular.[10] Further, evidence suggests that risk might vary in the presence of underlying heath conditions, with profound risk reductions seen for hysterectomy among women with endometriosis.[66] Whether the association varies by age or menopausal status at the time of surgery requires clarification.[66,67]

12.3.12 Age at Natural Menopause

Older age at natural menopause is associated with increased risk of endometrial[28] and ovarian cancer[10] but not cervical cancer. Menopausal age is influenced by a range of genetic, lifestyle (smoking, BMI),[68] and medical factors that operate across the life course, and some (but not all, see Chapter 4) evidence suggests higher childhood socioeconomic status is associated with later menopausal age even after controlling for adult socioeconomic status, smoking, BMI, and parity.[69] Later menopause means the reproductive organs are, on average, exposed to more ovulatory cycles and the accompanying peaks of reproductive hormones. It is likely these ovulatory and hormonal exposures explain the observed increased risk of endometrial and ovarian cancer.

12.4 After Menopause

12.4.1 Menopausal Hormone Therapy

The relationship between use of menopausal hormone therapy (MHT) and gynaecological cancers appears to vary by formulation. Women with an intact uterus treated with oestrogen-only MHT are at increased risk of developing endometrial cancer.[70] However, cyclic addition of a progestin negates that risk, and continuous progestin use is associated with decreased risk.[71] Pooled analyses indicate MHT use also increases risk of ovarian cancer,[10,72] and while some data suggest that progestin-containing formulations mitigate this increase,[73] this has not been found consistently.[72] Risk appears to increase with increasing duration of use,[10,73] and may vary by ovarian cancer histotype, with stronger positive associations observed for serous and endometrioid cancers, but an inverse association with clear cell cancers.[10,72] Data for cervical cancer are limited; one large cohort study reported an inverse association,[74] but the possibility that this reflected increased screening among MHT users could not be excluded.

The selective oestrogen receptor modulator tamoxifen, which is used as an adjuvant treatment in oestrogen-receptor positive breast cancer, is also known to increase endometrial cancer risk,[75] but there is little evidence that it influences risk of either ovarian or cervical cancer.

12.4.2 Body Size, Diet, Physical Activity and Smoking

As discussed in Sections 12.3.6 and 12.3.9, longer and more recent exposure is likely to be most relevant, at least for the obesity–endometrial cancer and smoking–cervical cancer associations. This suggests that, although obesity and smoking across the life course increase a woman's risk of these cancers, behaviour change even after menopause may still result in some risk reduction. After menopause, adipose tissue is the primary source of endogenous oestrogen while progesterone production has ceased. The association between obesity and endometrial cancer is thus strongest for postmenopausal women who do not take exogenous hormones (MHT),[12,76] while use of MHT, particularly formulations that provide regular progesterone in addition to oestrogen, appears to mitigate some of this obesity-associated risk.[71]

12.4.3 Diabetes, Metabolic Syndrome, and Medications

The prevalence of comorbidity such as metabolic syndrome (the presence of three or more of abdominal obesity, high blood pressure, impaired fasting glucose, high serum triglycerides, and low high-density lipoprotein (LDL) levels), increases with age. As discussed above, obesity is strongly associated with endometrial cancer, but diabetes also increases risk about twofold,[77] with evidence that this is a causal association also coming from MR studies.[78,79] Other components of metabolic syndrome including hypertension may increase risk by an additional 20%–40%; these associations appear independent of obesity but residual confounding is always a possibility.[77] Metabolic syndrome may also increase risk of cervical cancer, but there is little evidence of an association with ovarian cancer.[80]

Given the association between diabetes and endometrial cancer, it is plausible that the antidiabetes medicine metformin might reduce endometrial cancer risk, but current data do not support this.[81] Further, while in some women metformin has reversed endometrial hyperplasia, the precursor of type 1 endometrial cancer, the data are very heterogeneous.[82] There is also little evidence that statins, which inhibit 3-hydroxy-3-methylglutaryl coenzyme A (HMG-CoA) reductase and lower LDL cholesterol, reduce risk of endometrial or ovarian cancer,[83] although a MR study found genetic variants associated with lower LDL cholesterol were associated with lower ovarian cancer risk.[84]

Regular use of aspirin, particularly daily low-dose aspirin, and, potentially, other nonsteroidal anti-inflammatory drugs has been associated with a reduced risks of ovarian[85] and endometrial cancer, although the latter association may be restricted to women who are overweight or obese.[86] However, these studies are potentially subject to confounding by indication because those who take specific medications do so for a reason and thus differ from non-users. An effect is plausible as these medicines inhibit cyclooxygenase (COX) activity, reducing prostaglandin levels, and COX inhibitors down-regulate aromatase activity (and thus oestrogen synthesis) in some cancer cell lines, but randomised controlled trials are required to provide definitive evidence. There is no evidence for an association with cervical cancer. Bisphosphonates, which are used to treat osteoporosis, have been associated with reduced risk of endometrial[87] and possibly ovarian cancer.

12.5 Conclusions

A good understanding of the natural history of cervical cancer and identification of HPV as a necessary cause has enabled successful screening and vaccine development. Squamous cell cervical cancer could, therefore, be eliminated if we can influence the socioeconomic and health system factors necessary to enable universal access to appropriately timed HPV vaccination (before sexual activity commences) and screening.

For endometrial and particularly ovarian cancer, prevention pathways are less clear, as the underlying carcinogenic mechanisms are not well understood. Genetic influences are important for both; thus, early identification of carriers of high-risk mutations will enable informed decision-making around reproductive events and prophylactic surgery. However, most women who develop these cancers do not have high-risk mutations; thus, other approaches need to be considered.

For endometrial cancer, proliferation of endometrial cells caused by exposure to exogenous or endogenous oestrogen unopposed by a progestin is a likely underlying mechanism. While much remains unknown about the drivers of relative oestrogen excess, obesity is one key contributing factor, and recent weight gain or loss appears to influence risk, suggesting that efforts to reduce obesity at all stages throughout the life course would also reduce endometrial cancer rates. In contrast, protective factors (e.g. the oral contraceptive pill, full-term pregnancy, and prolonged breastfeeding) may limit endometrial proliferation or strip away neoplastic or preneoplastic cells and thus slow or halt carcinogenic processes. Timing of these factors is thus likely to be important in determining whether a woman goes on to develop cancer.

For ovarian cancer, it has been posited that recurrent exposure of the ovaries and/or fallopian tubes to the mechanical, hormonal, and/or local inflammatory effects of ovulation lead to neoplastic changes and cancer development; factors that influence lifetime number of ovulations thus affect risk.

For both endometrial and ovarian cancers, the reproductive period of a woman's life is critical in determining her future risk. However, apart from breastfeeding, where multilevel interventions to support initiation and continuation might contribute to prevention, and obesity, where successful intervention is challenging but would deliver benefits in many areas of health and not just gynaecological cancer, most risk factors acting during this period are not readily modifiable. Women should be informed of the potential cancer-preventing benefits of COC use and pregnancy (including timing), but potential prevention of endometrial or ovarian cancer later in life is unlikely to have a major influence on women's decisions about these reproductive issues.

A better understanding of the magnitude of the effects and the implications of the timing of different risk factors could facilitate prevention. For example, downward secular trends in age at menarche and upward trends in height over time point to the potential importance of infant and childhood nutritional habits, physical activity, and socioeconomic factors.[88,89] A life course approach could help tease apart the relative contributions to risk, and the relationships of these factors to exposures later in life and thus give additional insights to the potential for prevention, but, to date, this approach has rarely, if ever, been applied to gynaecological cancer.

Key messages and implications

- Eradication of squamous cell cervical cancer this century is achievable though prioritising appropriately timed universal access to HPV vaccination and adequate screening. This will also likely contribute to a reduction in vulval and vaginal cancers.
- Reducing incidence of endometrial and ovarian cancers presents a greater challenge. While much is known about their aetiology, many of the most important risk factors relate to reproductive factors, which, apart from insufficient breastfeeding, and are not readily modifiable for the purpose of preventing cancers that may occur many years later. However, one important exception is obesity. Lifelong maintenance of a healthy weight, particularly as a woman gets older, would likely reverse increasing incidence trends in endometrial cancer.
- A life course approach to gynaecological cancer has rarely, if ever, been taken in assessing risk factors and their relationships with each other. Such an approach could provide new insights into the life course development of these important female cancers.

References

1. Ferlay J, Ervik M, Lam F, Colombet M, Mery L, Piñeros M, et al. *Global cancer observatory: cancer today* [Data visualisation tool]. Lyon: International Agency for Research on Cancer; 2020 [cited 30 April 2021]. Available from: https://gco.iarc.fr/today/online-analysis-table.

2. Thornburg KL, Boone-Heinonen J, Valent AM. Social determinants of placental health and future disease risks for babies. *Obstetrics and Gynecoly Clinics of North America.* 2020;47(1):1–15.

3. Kuchenbaecker KB, Hopper JL, Barnes DR, Phillips KA, Mooij TM, Roos-Blom MJ, et al. Risks of breast, ovarian, and contralateral breast cancer for BRCA1 and BRCA2 mutation carriers. *Journal of the American Medical Association.* 2017;317(23):2402–16.

4. Bonadona V, Bonaiti B, Olschwang S, Grandjouan S, Huiart L, Longy M, et al. Cancer risks associated with germline mutations in MLH1, MSH2, and MSH6 genes in Lynch syndrome. *Journal of the American Medical Association.* 2011;305(22):2304–10.

5. Ring KL, Modesitt SC. Hereditary cancers in gynecology: what physicians should know about genetic testing, screening, and risk reduction. *Obstetrics and Gynecology Clinics of North America.* 2018;45(1):155–73.

6. Huo D, Anderson D, Palmer JR, Herbst AL. Incidence rates and risks of diethylstilbestrol-related clear-cell adenocarcinoma of the vagina and cervix: update after 40-year follow-up. *Gynecolic Oncology.* 2017;146(3):566–71.

7. Aarestrup J, Bjerregaard LG, Meyle KD, Pedersen DC, Gjaerde LK, Jensen BW, et al. Birthweight, childhood overweight, height and growth and adult cancer risks: a review of studies using the Copenhagen School Health Records Register. *International Journal of Obesity (Lond).* 2020;44(7):1546–60.

8. Day FR, Thompson DJ, Helgason H, Chasman DI, Finucane H, Sulem P, et al. Genomic analyses identify hundreds of variants associated with age at menarche and support a role for puberty timing in cancer risk. *Nature Genetics.* 2017;49(6):834–41.

9. Fuhrman BJ, Moore SC, Byrne C, Makhoul I, Kitahara CM, de Gonzalez AB, et al. Association of the age at menarche with site-specific cancer risks in pooled data from nine cohorts. *Cancer Research.* 2021;81(8):2246–55.

10. Wentzensen N, Poole EM, Trabert B, White E, Arslan AA, Patel AV, et al. Ovarian cancer risk factors by histologic subtype: an analysis from the Ovarian Cancer Cohort Consortium. *Journal of Clinical Oncology.* 2016;34(24):2888–98.

11. Syrjanen K, Shabalova I, Petrovichev N, Kozachenko V, Zakharova T, Pajanidi J, et al. Age at menarche is not an independent risk factor for high-risk human papillomavirus infections and cervical intraepithelial neoplasia. *International Journal of STD and AIDS.* 2008;19(1):16–25.

12. Dougan MM, Hankinson SE, Vivo ID, Tworoger SS, Glynn RJ, Michels KB. Prospective study of body size throughout the life-course and the incidence of endometrial cancer among premenopausal and postmenopausal women. *International Journal of Cancer.* 2015;137(3):625–37.

13. Luo J, Chlebowski R, Hendryx M, Rohan T, Wactawski-Wende J, Thomson C, et al. Intentional weight loss and endometrial cancer risk. *Journal of Clinical Oncology.* 2017;35(11):1189–993.

14. IARC Working Group on the Evaluation of Carcinogenic Risks to Humans. *IARC monographs on the evaluation of carcinogenic risks to humans volume 90. Human papillomaviruses.* Lyon: IARC; 2007.

15. Chelimo C, Wouldes TA, Cameron LD, Elwood JM. Risk factors for and prevention of human papillomaviruses (HPV), genital warts and cervical cancer. *Journal of Infection.* 2013;66(3):207–17.

16. Dunne EF, Unger ER, Sternberg M, McQuillan G, Swan DC, Patel SS, et al. Prevalence of HPV infection among females in the United States. *Journal of the American Medical Association.* 2007;297(8):813–9.

17. Brisson M, Kim JJ, Canfell K, Drolet M, Gingras G, Burger EA, et al. Impact of HPV vaccination and cervical screening on cervical cancer elimination: a comparative modelling analysis in 78 low-income and lower-middle-income countries. *The Lancet.* 2020;395(10224):575–90.

18. Falcaro M, Castanon A, Ndlela B, Checchi M, Soldan K, Lopez-Bernal J, et al. The effects of the national HPV vaccination programme in England, UK, on cervical cancer and grade 3 cervical intraepithelial neoplasia incidence: a register-based observational study. *The Lancet.* 2021;398:2084–92.

19. Lei J, Ploner A, Elfstrom KM, Wang J, Roth A, Fang F, et al. HPV vaccination and the risk of invasive cervical cancer. *New England Journal of Medicine*. 2020;383(14):1340–8.

20. Hall MT, Simms KT, Lew JB, Smith MA, Brotherton JM, Saville M, et al. The projected timeframe until cervical cancer elimination in Australia: a modelling study. *The Lancet Public Health*. 2019;4(1):e19–e27.

21. Lee AW, Rosenzweig S, Wiensch A, Australian Ovarian Cancer Study G, Ramus SJ, Menon U, et al. Expanding our understanding of ovarian cancer risk: the role of incomplete pregnancies. *Journal of the National Cancer Institute*. 2021;113 (3):301–8.

22. Jordan SJ, Na R, Weiderpass E, Adami HO, Anderson KE, van den Brandt PA, et al. Pregnancy outcomes and risk of endometrial cancer: a pooled analysis of individual participant data in the Epidemiology of Endometrial Cancer Consortium. *International Journal of Cancer*. 2021;148(9):2068–78.

23. Babic A, Sasamoto N, Rosner BA, Tworoger SS, Jordan SJ, Risch HA, et al. Association between breastfeeding and ovarian cancer risk. *JAMA Oncology*. 2020;6(6):e200421.

24. Setiawan VW, Pike MC, Karageorgi S, Deming SL, Anderson K, Bernstein L, et al. Age at last birth in relation to risk of endometrial cancer: pooled analysis in the epidemiology of endometrial cancer consortium. *American Journal of Epidemiology*. 2012;176(4):269–78.

25. Wu Y, Sun W, Xin X, Wang W, Zhang D. Age at last birth and risk of developing epithelial ovarian cancer: a meta-analysis. *Bioscience Reports*. 2019;39(9):BSR20182035

26. International Collaboration of Epidemiological Studies of Cervical Cancer. Cervical carcinoma and reproductive factors: collaborative reanalysis of individual data on 16,563 women with cervical carcinoma and 33,542 women without cervical carcinoma from 25 epidemiological studies. *International Journal of Cancer*. 2006;119(5):1108–24.

27. Jordan SJ, Na R, Johnatty SE, Wise LA, Adami HO, Brinton LA, et al. Breastfeeding and endometrial cancer risk: an analysis from the epidemiology of Endometrial Cancer Consortium. *Obstetrics and Gynecology*. 2017;129(6):1059–67.

28. Dossus L, Allen N, Kaaks R, Bakken K, Lund E, Tjonneland A, et al. Reproductive risk factors and endometrial cancer: the European Prospective Investigation into Cancer and Nutrition. *International Journal of Cancer*. 2010;127(2):442–51.

29. Collaborative Group on Epidemiological Studies of Ovarian Cancer, Beral V, Doll R, Hermon C, Peto R, Reeves G. Ovarian cancer and oral contraceptives: collaborative reanalysis of data from 45 epidemiological studies including 23,257 women with ovarian cancer and 87,303 controls. *The Lancet*. 2008;371(9609):303–14.

30. Iversen L, Sivasubramaniam S, Lee AJ, Fielding S, Hannaford PC. Lifetime cancer risk and combined oral contraceptives: the Royal College of General Practitioners' Oral Contraception Study. *American Journal of Obstetrics and Gynecology*. 2017;216(6):580 e1– e9.

31. Burchardt NA, Shafrir AL, Kaaks R, Tworoger SS, Fortner RT. Oral contraceptive use by formulation and endometrial cancer risk among women born in 1947–1964: The Nurses' Health Study II, a prospective cohort study. *European Journal of Epidemiology*. 2021;36(8):827–39.

32. Jareid M, Thalabard JC, Aarflot M, Bovelstad HM, Lund E, Braaten T. Levonorgestrel-releasing intrauterine system use is associated with a decreased risk of ovarian and endometrial cancer, without increased risk of breast cancer: results from the NOWAC Study. *Gynecologic Oncology*. 2018;149(1):127–32.

33. Depot-medroxyprogesterone acetate (DMPA) and risk of endometrial cancer. The WHO Collaborative Study of Neoplasia and Steroid Contraceptives. *International Journal of Cancer*. 1991;49(2):186–90.

34. Phung MT, Lee AW, Wu AH, Berchuck A, Cho KR, Cramer DW, et al. Depot-medroxyprogesterone acetate use is associated with decreased risk of ovarian cancer: the mounting evidence of a protective role of progestins. *Cancer Epidemiology Biomarkers and Prevention*. 2021;30(5):927–35.

35. International Collaboration of Epidemiological Studies of Cervical Cancer, Appleby P, Beral V, Berrington de Gonzalez A, Colin D, Franceschi S, et al. Cervical cancer and hormonal contraceptives: collaborative reanalysis of individual data for 16,573 women with cervical cancer and 35,509 women without cervical cancer from 24 epidemiological studies. *The Lancet*. 2007;370(9599):1609–21.

36. Castellsague X, Diaz M, Vaccarella S, de Sanjose S, Munoz N, Herrero R, et al. Intrauterine device use, cervical infection with human papillomavirus, and risk of cervical cancer: a pooled analysis of 26 epidemiological studies. *The Lancet Oncology*. 2011;12(11):1023–31.

37. Jordan SJ, Wilson LF, Nagle CM, Green AC, Olsen CM, Bain CJ, et al. Cancers in Australia in 2010 attributable to and prevented by the use of combined oral contraceptives. *Australian New Zealand Journal of Public Health*. 2015;39(5):441–5.

38. Kvaskoff M, Mahamat-Saleh Y, Farland LV, Shigesi N, Terry KL, Harris HR, et al. Endometriosis and cancer: a systematic review and meta-analysis. *Human Reproduction Update*. 2021;27(2):393–420.

39. Harris HR, Babic A, Webb PM, Nagle CM, Jordan SJ, Risch HA, et al. Polycystic ovary syndrome, oligomenorrhea, and risk of ovarian cancer histotypes: evidence from the Ovarian Cancer Association Consortium. *Cancer Epidemiology Biomarkers and Prevention*. 2018;27(2):174–82.

40. Yin W, Falconer H, Yin L, Xu L, Ye W. Association between polycystic ovary syndrome and cancer risk. *JAMA Oncology*. 2019;5(1):106–7.

41. Harris HR, Terry KL. Polycystic ovary syndrome and risk of endometrial, ovarian, and breast cancer: a systematic review. *Fertility Research and Practice*. 2016;2:14.

42. Rowlands IJ, Nagle CM, Spurdle AB, Webb PM, ANECS Group, AOCS Group. Gynecological conditions and the risk of endometrial cancer. *Gynecologic Oncology*. 2011;123(3):537–41.

43. Barcroft JF, Galazis N, Jones BP, Getreu N, Bracewell-Milnes T, Grewal KJ, et al. Fertility treatment and cancers-the eternal conundrum: a systematic review and meta-analysis. *Human Reproduction*. 2021;36(4):1093–1107.

44. Choi YJ, Lee DH, Han KD, Yoon H, Shin CM, Park YS, et al. Adult height in relation to risk of cancer in a cohort of 22,809,722 Korean adults. *British Journal of Cancer*. 2019;120(6):668–74.

45. Ong JS, An J, Law MH, Whiteman DC, Neale RE, Gharahkhani P, et al. Height and overall cancer risk and mortality: evidence from a Mendelian randomisation study on 310,000 UK Biobank participants. *British Journal of Cancer*. 2018;118(9):1262–7.

46. Calle EE, Kaaks R. Overweight, obesity and cancer: epidemiological evidence and proposed mechanisms. *Nature Reviews Cancer*. 2004;4(8):579–91.

47. World Cancer Research Fund, American Institute for Cancer Research. *Diet, nutrition, physical activity and cancer: a global perspective: a summary of the Third Expert Report*. London: WCRF International; 2018.

48. Setiawan VW, Yang HP, Pike MC, McCann SE, Yu H, Xiang YB, et al. Type I and II endometrial cancers: have they different risk factors? *Journal of Clinical Oncology*. 2013;31(20):2607–18.

49. Arthur RS, Dannenberg AJ, Kim M, Rohan TE. The association of body fat composition with risk of breast, endometrial, ovarian and colorectal cancers among normal weight participants in the UK Biobank. *British Journal of Cancer*. 2021;124(9):1592–1605.

50. Arnold M, Pandeya N, Byrnes G, Renehan PAG, Stevens GA, Ezzati PM, et al. Global burden of cancer attributable to high body-mass index in 2012: a population-based study. *The Lancet Oncology*. 2015;16(1):36–46.

51. Bruno DS, Berger NA. Impact of bariatric surgery on cancer risk reduction. *Annals of Translational Medicine*. 2020;8(Suppl 1):S13.

52. Dixon SC, Nagle CM, Thrift AP, Pharoah PD, Pearce CL, Zheng W, et al. Adult body mass index and risk of ovarian cancer by subtype: a Mendelian randomization study. *International Journal of Epidemiology*. 2016;45(3):884–95.

53. Olsen CM, Nagle C, Whiteman DC, Ness R, Pearce CL, Pike MC, et al. Obesity and risk of ovarian cancer subtypes: evidence from the Ovarian Cancer Association Consortium. *Endocrine Related Cancer*. 2013;20(2):251–62.

54. Baurecht H, Leitzmann M, O'Mara T, Thompson D, the collaborators of the Endometrial Cancer Association Consortium, Teumer A, et al. Physical activity and risk of breast and endometrial cancers: a Mendelian randomization study. *MedRxiv*. 2019. https://doi.org/10.1101/19005892

55. Cannioto R, LaMonte MJ, Risch HA, Hong CC, Sucheston-Campbell LE, Eng KH, et al. Chronic recreational physical inactivity and epithelial ovarian cancer risk: evidence from the Ovarian Cancer Association Consortium. *Cancer Epidemiology Biomarkers and Prevention*. 2016;25(7):1114–24.

56. Biller VS, Leitzmann MF, Sedlmeier AM, Berger FF, Ortmann O, Jochem C. Sedentary behaviour in relation to ovarian cancer risk: a systematic review and meta-analysis. *European Journal of Epidemiology*. 2021;36(8):769–80.

57. Ong JS, Dixon-Suen SC, Han X, An J, Esophageal Cancer C, Me Research T, et al. A comprehensive re-assessment of the association between vitamin D and cancer susceptibility using Mendelian randomization. *Nature Communications.* 2021;12(1):246.

58. International Collaboration of Epidemiological Studies of Cervical Cancer, Appleby P, Beral V, Berrington de Gonzalez A, Colin D, Franceschi S, et al. Carcinoma of the cervix and tobacco smoking: collaborative reanalysis of individual data on 13,541 women with carcinoma of the cervix and 23,017 women without carcinoma of the cervix from 23 epidemiological studies. *International Journal of Cancer.* 2006;118(6):1481–95.

59. Collaborative Group on Epidemiological Studies of Ovarian Cancer, Beral V, Gaitskell K, Hermon C, Moser K, Reeves G, et al. Ovarian cancer and smoking: individual participant meta-analysis including 28,114 women with ovarian cancer from 51 epidemiological studies. *The Lancet Oncology.* 2012;13(9):946–56.

60. Faber MT, Kjaer SK, Dehlendorff C, Chang-Claude J, Andersen KK, Hogdall E, et al. Cigarette smoking and risk of ovarian cancer: a pooled analysis of 21 case-control studies. *Cancer Causes and Control.* 2013;24(5):989–1004.

61. Larsson SC, Carter P, Kar S, Vithayathil M, Mason AM, Michaelsson K, et al. Smoking, alcohol consumption, and cancer: A mendelian randomisation study in UK Biobank and international genetic consortia participants. *PLoS Medicine.* 2020;17(7):e1003178.

62. Sieh W, Salvador S, McGuire V, Weber RP, Terry KL, Rossing MA, et al. Tubal ligation and risk of ovarian cancer subtypes: a pooled analysis of case-control studies. *International Journal of Epidemiology.* 2013;42(2):579–89.

63. Gaitskell K, Coffey K, Green J, Pirie K, Reeves GK, Ahmed AA, et al. Tubal ligation and incidence of 26 site-specific cancers in the Million Women Study. *British Journal of Cancer.* 2016;114(9):1033–7.

64. Falconer H, Yin L, Altman D. Association between tubal ligation and endometrial cancer risk: a Swedish population-based cohort study. *International Journal of Cancer.* 2018;143(1):16–21.

65. Jordan SJ, Nagle CM, Coory MD, Maresco D, Protani MM, Pandeya NA, et al. Has the association between hysterectomy and ovarian cancer changed over time? A systematic review and meta-analysis. *European Journal of Cancer.* 2013;49(17):3638–47.

66. Dixon-Suen SC, Webb PM, Wilson LF, Tuesley K, Stewart LM, Jordan SJ. The association between hysterectomy and ovarian cancer risk: a population-based record-linkage study. *Journal* of the *National Cancer Institute.* 2019;111(10):1097–103.

67. Rice MS, Hankinson SE, Tworoger SS. Tubal ligation, hysterectomy, unilateral oophorectomy, and risk of ovarian cancer in the Nurses' Health Studies. *Fertility and Sterility.* 2014;102(1):192–8e3.

68. Schoenaker DA, Jackson CA, Rowlands JV, Mishra GD. Socioeconomic position, lifestyle factors and age at natural menopause: a systematic review and meta-analyses of studies across six continents. *International Journal of Epidemiology.* 2014;43(5):1542–62.

69. Hardy R, Kuh D. Social and environmental conditions across the life course and age at menopause in a British birth cohort study. *British Journal of Obstetrics and Gynaecology.* 2005;112(3):346–54.

70. International Agency for Research on Cancer. *IARC monographs on the evaluation of carcinogenic risks to humans volume 72. Hormonal contraception and post-menopausal hormonal therapy.* Lyon: IARC; 1999.

71. Beral V, Bull D, Reeves G, Million Women Study C. Endometrial cancer and hormone-replacement therapy in the Million Women Study. *The Lancet.* 2005;365(9470):1543–51.

72. Collaborative Group on Epidemiological Studies of Ovarian C, Beral V, Gaitskell K, Hermon C, Moser K, Reeves G, et al. Menopausal hormone use and ovarian cancer risk: individual participant meta-analysis of 52 epidemiological studies. *The Lancet.* 2015;385(9980):1835–42.

73. Pearce CL, Chung K, Pike MC, Wu AH. Increased ovarian cancer risk associated with menopausal estrogen therapy is reduced by adding a progestin. *Cancer.* 2009;115(3):531–9.

74. Roura E, Travier N, Waterboer T, de Sanjose S, Bosch FX, Pawlita M, et al. The Influence of hormonal factors on the risk of developing cervical cancer and pre-cancer: results from the EPIC Cohort. *PLoS ONE.* 2016;11(1):e0147029.

75. Fleming CA, Heneghan HM, O'Brien D, McCartan DP, McDermott EW, Prichard RS. Meta-analysis of the cumulative risk of endometrial malignancy and systematic review of endometrial surveillance in extended tamoxifen therapy. *British Journal of Surgery.* 2018;105(9):1098–106.

76. Aune D, Navarro Rosenblatt DA, Chan DS, Vingeliene S, Abar L, Vieira AR, et al. Anthropometric factors and endometrial cancer risk: a systematic review and dose-response meta-analysis of prospective studies. *Annals of Oncology*. 2015;26(8):1635–48.

77. Trabert B, Wentzensen N, Felix AS, Yang HP, Sherman ME, Brinton LA. Metabolic syndrome and risk of endometrial cancer in the United States: a study in the SEER-Medicare linked database. *Cancer Epidemiology Biomarkers and Prevention*. 2015;24(1):261–7.

78. Nead KT, Sharp SJ, Thompson DJ, Painter JN, Savage DB, Semple RK, et al. Evidence of a causal association between insulinemia and endometrial cancer: a Mendelian randomization analysis. *Journal of the National Cancer Institute*. 2015;107(9):djv178.

79. Yuan S, Kar S, Carter P, Vithayathil M, Mason AM, Burgess S, et al. Is Type 2 diabetes causally associated with cancer risk? evidence from a two-sample Mendelian randomization study. *Diabetes*. 2020;69(7):1588–96.

80. Stocks T, Bjorge T, Ulmer H, Manjer J, Haggstrom C, Nagel G, et al. Metabolic risk score and cancer risk: pooled analysis of seven cohorts. *International Journal of Epidemiology*. 2015;44(4):1353–63.

81. Chu D, Wu J, Wang K, Zhao M, Wang C, Li L, et al. Effect of metformin use on the risk and prognosis of endometrial cancer: a systematic review and meta-analysis. *BMC Cancer*. 2018;18(1):438.

82. Meireles CG, Pereira SA, Valadares LP, Rego DF, Simeoni LA, Guerra ENS, et al. Effects of metformin on endometrial cancer: systematic review and meta-analysis. *Gynecologic Oncology*. 2017;147(1):167–80.

83. Desai P, Wallace R, Anderson ML, Howard BV, Ray RM, Wu C, et al. An analysis of the association between statin use and risk of endometrial and ovarian cancers in the Women's Health Initiative. *Gynecologic Oncology*. 2018;148(3):540–6.

84. Yarmolinsky J, Bull CJ, Vincent EE, Robinson J, Walther A, Smith GD, et al. Association between genetically proxied inhibition of HMG-CoA reductase and epithelial ovarian cancer. *Journal* of the *American Medical Association*. 2020;323(7):646–55.

85. Trabert B, Ness RB, Lo-Ciganic WH, Murphy MA, Goode EL, Poole EM, et al. Aspirin, nonaspirin nonsteroidal anti-inflammatory drug, and acetaminophen use and risk of invasive epithelial ovarian cancer: a pooled analysis in the Ovarian Cancer Association Consortium. *Journal of the National Cancer Institute*. 2014;106(2):djt431.

86. Webb PM, Na R, Weiderpass E, Adami HO, Anderson KE, Bertrand KA, et al. Use of aspirin, other nonsteroidal anti-inflammatory drugs and acetaminophen and risk of endometrial cancer: the Epidemiology of Endometrial Cancer Consortium. *Annals of Oncology*. 2019;30(2):310–16.

87. Newcomb PA, Passarelli MN, Phipps AI, Anderson GL, Wactawski-Wende J, Ho GY, et al. Oral bisphosphonate use and risk of postmenopausal endometrial cancer. *Journal of Clinical Oncology*. 2015;33(10):1186–90.

88. Karapanou O, Papadimitriou A. Determinants of menarche. *Reproductive Biology and Endocrinology*. 2010;8:115.

89. Perkins JM, Subramanian SV, Davey Smith G, Ozaltin E. Adult height, nutrition, and population health. *Nutrition Reviews*. 2016;74(3):149–65.

PART IV

BIOLOGICAL AND BEHAVIOURAL PATHWAYS

13

Integrative Omics for Women's Health

Anna Murray and Katherine S. Ruth

13.1 Introduction

Our understanding of the role of genes and environment in diseases and traits has progressed from investigating single candidate genes (e.g. *FSHR* in primary ovarian insufficiency[1]) to uncovering genetic associations with nearly 600 regions of the genome involved in reproductive lifespan.[2,3] Timing of menarche and menopause are multifactorial traits, combining genetic predisposition with environmental influences to determine overall reproductive lifespan. The genetic component results from variation in many genes, often with each variant having a very small effect on the trait. Many female-specific diseases are also multifactorial, including polycystic ovary syndrome (PCOS), endometriosis, and hormone-responsive cancer.

The field of genomics has been facilitated by substantial improvements in technology resulting in enormous reductions in cost and time. Sequencing a whole human genome can now be done in a matter of hours for less than US$1000.[4] Alongside these improved efficiencies in technology, funders have recognised the value of large biobanks, extensive health record data are now available, and researchers have formed large consortia to generate studies with sample sizes large enough to enable associations with only small effects to be detected or to collect enough individuals with rare disorders to enable meaningful insights. The latest study of variation in human height is the largest to date; it included data from 5.5 million individuals and discovered >12,000 genetic variants.[5] This progress is phenomenal, as although Ronald Fisher hypothesised that height was polygenic in 1918,[6] the first genomic variants associated with normal variation in human height were not described until 2007.[7] In the field of rare disease, initiatives such as the Deciphering Developmental Disorders[8] and 100,000 Genomes[9] projects have led the way in finding genetic causes for rare diseases, often resulting in treatment or management changes for patients. A major benefit of investigating the whole genome is that no prior hypothesis is necessary, providing opportunity to discover new biological pathways and mechanisms.

Alongside the field of genomics, similar advances have been made in studying modifications to the structure of DNA (epigenomics); the full complement of proteins in a cell, tissue, or organism (proteomics); the range and abundance of all RNA transcripts (transcriptomics); and the metabolites present in a tissue type (metabolomics). The integration of omics data is a powerful tool to understand and treat disease and traits and has been used extensively in women's health research (Figure 13.1).

Anna Murray and Katherine S. Ruth, *Integrative Omics for Women's Health* In: *A Life Course Approach to Women's Health*. Second Edition. Edited by: Gita D Mishra, Rebecca Hardy, and Diana Kuh, Oxford University Press. © Oxford University Press 2023. DOI: 10.1093/oso/9780192864642.003.0013

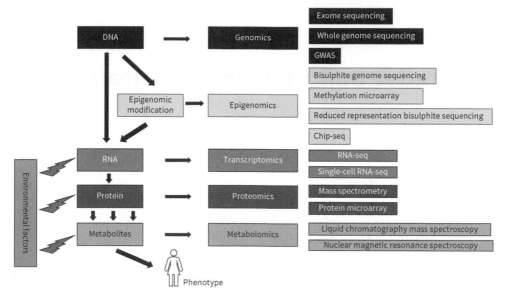

Figure 13.1 Overview of omics discussed in the chapter, how they relate to the central assumption of DNA > RNA > protein, the influence of environmental factors and some of the technologies used in these fields.

13.2 Genomic Variation

13.2.1 Types of Genetic Differences

There are around 20,000 protein-coding genes in the human genome,[10,11] but the protein-coding sequence (or exome) accounts for only between 1% to 2% of the 3 billion bases in the genome. The most common type of variants in the genome are single nucleotide polymorphisms (SNPs), occurring every 100–200 bases. Larger variants occur less frequently and include deletions, insertions, inversions, or variation in repetitive sequences (copy number variants). Many of these variants are benign, having no functional impact on gene function, RNA expression, or protein structure. Variation in the coding sequence can result in loss of protein product (stop-gain, frameshift, splice site variants) or a change in an amino acid (missense). The consequence of alteration to the coding sequence is relatively easy to predict, but it is more challenging to predict the impact of variation in the noncoding genome, which contains important regulatory sequences as well as many repetitive elements and redundant genes. The noncoding genome is no longer considered 'junk DNA'. International efforts, such as the Genome Aggregation Database (gnomAD), have collated exome and genome sequence data from tens of thousands of individuals to inform the wider scientific community about the extent of variation in the genome.[12]

In addition to genomic variation at the DNA sequence level (genomics), there is variation in chemical modifications of DNA that affects gene regulation and expression (epigenomics). Epigenomic modifications can be part of normal cell regulation processes, but can also be caused by environmental factors, such as diet, smoking, and medications, and are altered during ageing and disease.[13]

13.2.2 Role of Genomics in Women's Health

The contribution of genomic variation to a disease or trait is measured by assessing heritability and is best calculated from twin and family study data, for instance measuring the degree of concordance of a trait in dizygous versus monozygous twins. Heritability for female traits across the lifespan varies, but timing of menarche[14,15] and menopause[16,17] have heritability estimates of about 50%. The genetic component of a disease or trait results from variation in many genes, often each variant has a very small effect on the trait, but in combination can explain a larger proportion of the variation in reproductive lifespan. Genetic variants have also been identified for many female-specific diseases, including PCOS,[18] endometriosis,[19] and hormone-responsive cancer.[20] In addition to the common genomic variants with small effects, many traits and diseases have rarer variants with larger effects. In breast cancer, for example, there are a few genes in which coding variants present in < 1% of the population that incur a relatively large risk of breast cancer (e.g. *BRCA1, BRCA2, PTEN*, and *CHEK2*), with carriers of these variants having a >25% lifetime risk of developing breast cancer,[21] compared to the 13% lifetime risk in the general population.[22] However, even in these carriers, the common genomic variation contributes to risk as well, and by combining the common variant risk with the more penetrant rarer variant risk, it is possible to stratify lifetime risk of breast cancer more precisely.[23] Our understanding of the genetic architecture of female-specific traits has been significantly advanced by the omics technologies now available and has the potential to provide women with information that could enable them to take preventative measures, such as increased screening or prophylactic surgery.

13.3 Omics Technologies

13.3.1 Genome Sequencing

Rare variants are best analysed with genomic sequencing. Genome sequencing has been available for over 10 years, since the first exome sequencing for a monogenic disease was reported in 2010.[24] The ability to capture DNA fragments from all exons in a single experiment, followed by high-depth sequencing has enabled the cost of analysing the coding sequence of the entire genome to be reduced substantially. Initial experiments were restricted to small family-based studies of rare disease, but as costs have further plummeted, large-scale exome sequencing at the population level has become a reality. Sequencing the exome has become standard practice in human diagnostic genetics and has resulted in the identification of many new causative variants and genes. Studies of whole genomes including the noncoding genome are less common, in part because of the cost of sequencing, the time taken, storage of data, and difficulties with interpreting functional consequences of variants. However, now that costs are relatively modest and more reference panels are available to assess variation, whole genome sequencing offers the promise of capturing much more of the variation in the genome, with more even coverage enabling variants such as copy number variants to be reliably assessed.

Single gene causes of disorders of reproductive health are rare. Initial candidate gene studies were not very fruitful, although there are a few exceptions (e.g. mutation in the *FSHR* gene in Finnish families has been robustly associated with premature ovarian insufficiency (POI)).[1] The advent of gene-agnostic exome sequencing experiments has identified many new genes. In POI, there are more than 10 examples in the literature of single gene causes identified through whole exome sequencing, including *STAG3*, *MCM8*, *MCM9*, *HFM1*, *SPIDR*, *SOHLH1*, and *SYCE1*.[25] Delayed puberty or idiopathic hypogonadotropic hypogonadism (IHH) also has examples of single gene causes identified through whole exome sequencing, and around 30%–40% of IHH cases can be explained by single gene causes: variants in *KISS1/KISS1R* and *TAC3/TAC3R* have been robustly associated with IHH, but many other genes have also been implicated.[26] In the majority of cases of POI and IHH, the cause is autosomal recessive (i.e. loss of functional variants in both copies of the gene are required).[27,28] The majority of exome sequencing studies have been carried out in families with more than one affected individual or in consanguineous pedigrees where homozygous rare variants are more commonly seen and have phenotypic consequences. Studies in cohorts of cases have found similar variants in the heterozygous state, but many may be coincidental findings as the evidence for them being causal is often limited. Large exome sequencing studies are underway to estimate the penetrance of variants in the general population. Single gene disease-causing variants for which there is robust evidence are curated in repositories including the Human Genome Mutation Database (http://www.hgmd.cf.ac.uk/ac/index.php) and ClinVar (https://www.ncbi.nlm.nih.gov/clinvar/).

13.3.2 Genome-Wide Association Studies

Genome-wide association studies (GWAS) are now the workhorse of common genomic variant discovery. The technique relies on genotyping SNPs. Because SNPs occur so frequently in the genome, neighbouring SNPS often get inherited together and variation at SNPs can be correlated, when they are said to be in linkage disequilibrium.[29] GWAS uses linkage disequilibrium to reduce the number of tests required and to facilitate meta-analyses. Genotyping 500,000–750,000 SNPs on a single microarray enables variation across the majority of the whole genome to be captured. The genotyped SNPs tag un-genotyped SNPs and, by comparison to a reference genome, enable nearly 20 million SNP genotypes to be imputed. Imputation not only increases the number of SNP genotypes, but also enables meta-analysis of samples genotyped on different SNP arrays, which has transformed the success of GWAS consortia. Imputation reference panels have improved substantially since the first GWAS in the late 2000s; from the HapMap of more than 1 million SNPs in four ancestry populations,[30] to the 1000 Genomes Project with around 85 million SNPs from 26 populations,[31] and the Haplotype Reference Consortium (HRC)[32] which has combined multiple panels to provide one of the most comprehensive imputation tools currently available.

GWAS can be used for quantitative, categorical, or binary traits and tests the association of each SNP with the trait of interest. For a quantitative trait such as timing of menarche, the test simply compares the mean menarche age for the three genotypes (homozygous for major allele, heterozygous, and homozygous for minor allele). For a binary trait such as PCOS, the allele frequency in cases is compared to controls. One of the strengths of GWAS has been the high degree of statistical rigour applied to the analyses. Because of the large number of variants tested in a single experiment, correction for multiple testing is essential. The field has used a Bonferroni corrected p-value threshold of $p < 5 \times 10^{-8}$ as standard, as it is estimated that a GWAS includes 1 million independent tests ($P = 0.05/1{,}000{,}000$).[33] However as more variants are discovered and used in GWAS, some studies are using even more stringent thresholds. In addition to stringent p-value thresholds, replication of top signals is commonplace and provides confidence in the validity of the findings. Because of the large number of correlated SNPs in the genome, often at a single position or locus, multiple SNP associations pass the p-value threshold. These correlated SNPs (in linkage disequilibrium) are collapsed into a single signal at each locus, and independent signals are reported and catalogued in public repositories such as the GWAS Catalog (https://www.ebi.ac.uk/gwas/).

While GWAS captures common variants with allele frequencies >0.1% well, SNP arrays do not accurately genotype rare variants. The array method relies on clustering the readout into the three genotype categories: each of the homozygote genotypes, plus the heterozygotes. When the allele frequency is very low, there may only be two clusters, with no rare homozygote group and few heterozygous individuals. The algorithms to detect clusters behave poorly with output that does not fall into the three genotype clusters, and, therefore, miscalling occurs.

13.3.3 Epigenomics

In addition to variation in the coding sequence of the genome, DNA can be chemically modified, which can affect the structure and function of that DNA. These modifications are 'epigenomic' and are involved in chromosome packaging and gene regulation.[34] A key epigenomic modification is methylation of a CG dinucleotide in the genomic sequence, by the addition of a methyl group to the cytosine residue of the DNA. Other modifications include acetylation of histone proteins, which can affect chromatin structure and, thus, accessibility of the genomic sequence to transcription factors. Epigenomic marks are made as a result of a variety of processes, including ageing, diseases, medications, exposure to environmental stimuli, and regulation of gene expression. Ageing can be mapped with 353 CpG sites where methylation levels change with age and together form an 'ageing clock'.[35] The clock is correlated with cell division and, therefore, varies between cell types. There is no evidence of a biological clock in oocytes, with epigenomic age younger in oocytes than in blood.[36] Methylation levels were lower in oocytes compared to blood as women aged. One of the DNA methylation changes in oocytes was near the *DENND1A* gene. Genetic variants in *DENND1A* have been suggested to play a role in susceptibility to PCOS.[37] Differences in the methylome from women with PCOS have been reported in several studies.[38–40] *SIRT1* plays a role in oocyte function in older ages, partly by regulating epigenomic changes that affect oocyte quality.[41] The association of hypertension in pregnancy and low birth weight may be mediated via differential methylation.[42] Smoking can also have a significant effect on the epigenome, including smoking in pregnancy. Differential methylation of three CpGs in *GFI1* explained 12%–19% of the 202g-lower birthweight in the offspring of mothers who smoked. Functional enrichment analysis pointed towards activation of cell-mediated immunity as the underlying mechanism.[43]

13.3.4 Transcriptomics

SNPs that are associated with variation in RNA levels are called eQTLs. Unlike sequence variation, transcript variation will be tissue specific, and, therefore, eQTL analyses rely on appropriate tissues from the relevant developmental stage to be available. A great many transcriptome data are freely available to researchers: for example, in the Genotype-Tissue Expression (GTEx) resource from the Broad Institute, there are eQTL data for >15,000 samples from 49 tissues (Figure 13.2).[44] There are, however, limited female-specific tissue samples available: for example, in GTEx, only 167 samples are from the ovary, and these are not categorised into functional cell types such as follicles and granulosa cells. In the GTEx resource, 67% of tissues are from males; 68% are from people over 50 years of age; and 85% are from people of white European ancestry. Bespoke in-house transcriptome studies are, therefore, often used in reproductive genomics.

The methodologies used to analyse transcriptomics have improved substantially alongside the transformation in genomic technology. Microarrays were the first method used and were able to analyse expression from all known genes, through hybridisation to probes attached to a single array or chip. However, arrays have been superseded by sequence-based technology, known as RNA-seq,[45] which has the advantage of being able to analyse transcripts that were not previous known, thereby identifying novel genes, transcripts, and mechanisms. RNA-seq starts with reverse transcription of the RNA sample, followed by fragmentation of the cDNA and next generation sequencing. The number of sequence reads allows quantification of the amount of target RNA, making RNA-seq both qualitative and quantitative. A further advance has been the introduction of single cell transcriptomics (scRNA-seq),[46] where individual cells can be isolated from complex tissues, by techniques such as laser microdissection, fluorescent activated cell sorting, or microfluidics. Isolation of individual cells can be low- or high-throughput making the technology scalable for large multiomics projects. scRNA-seq has been used in female reproductive biology to determine expression profiles in specific cell types.[47–49] It has also been used to investigate the presence of germline stem cells in the adult ovary,[50] and in female-specific diseases, such as endometriosis, where scRNA-seq showed differential gene expression profiles in oocytes from patients with endometriosis compared to controls.[51]

1.3.5 Proteomics and Metabolomics

Genomics can also be integrated with protein expression data or metabolite level data in order to assess the impact of genomic variation. These directly measured variables are a good intermediary phenotype between the DNA sequence and the clinical phenotype, which may be influenced by various biological pathways and environmental factors. There are often strong associations between genomic variants and their gene products (i.e. proteins, known as pQTLs). For example, variants in the *SHBG* gene are strongly associated with SHBG protein levels in blood.[52] Other pQTLs are far less easy to predict and are, therefore, more likely to identify novel mechanisms. There are now several high-throughput methodologies for assessing large numbers of proteins or metabolites in a single experiment, including microarray-based technologies, mass spectroscopy, and nuclear magnetic resonance imaging. As with the other omics, step changes in technology have facilitated a shift in the

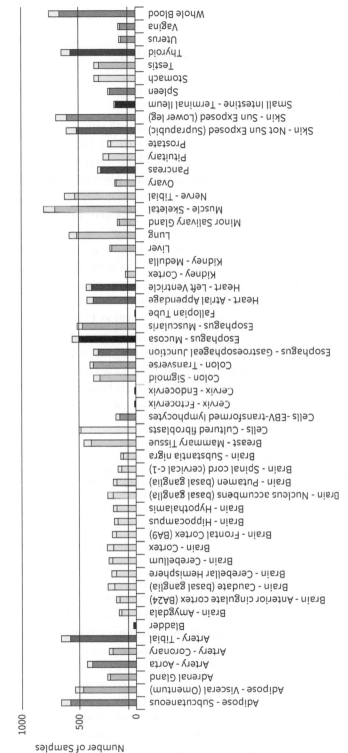

Figure 13.2 Sample counts by tissue in the GTEx portal (https://gtexportal.org/home/, 31/01/2022) with transcriptome data available. The Genotype-Tissue Expression (GTEx) Project was supported by the Common Fund of the Office of the Director of the National Institutes of Health, and by NCI, NHGRI, NHLBI, NIDA, NIMH, and NINDS.

availability of datasets of proteomic and metabolomic data from various tissues and large numbers of individuals.

13.4 Benefits of Omics Studies for Health

13.4.1 Biological Insights

A whole exome study of 119,992 women from the UK Biobank found rare deleterious variants in three genes associated with menopause timing: *CHEK2* and *DCLRE1A* with later menopause and *TOP3A* with earlier menopause.[53] *CHEK2* was a gene highlighted previously by GWAS, and all three are DNA damage repair genes, thus providing further evidence for the role of this pathway in ovarian ageing.

Exome sequencing has recently been used to discover a key gene involved in the sensing of nutrients to trigger puberty onset.[54] In a study of ~200,000 individuals from the UK Biobank, loss-of-function variants in *MC3R* delayed puberty and reduced linear growth, lean mass, and IGF1 levels in the blood, suggesting a role for this gene in sensing calorie levels and influencing growth and reproduction. The value of exome sequencing over GWAS is the ability to more readily get to the causal mechanism involved in the trait with a coding variant and to test it experimentally more easily. In a population-based study, rare variants will only be detected if they have a relatively large effect size. For example, the *MC3R* deleterious variant carried by 0.82% of participants in the UK Biobank, delayed menarche by an average of 4.7 months,[54] which is approximately three times larger than the largest common variant effect from GWAS at the *LIN28B* locus.[55,56] Extremely large sample sizes will be required to detect moderate/small effect alleles, as we have seen in GWAS.

13.4.1.1 Deriving Biological Insights from GWAS

GWAS has identified thousands of genetic signals associated with human traits and disease, but proving which is the causative gene and variant is more challenging. The association signals are more often found within noncoding areas of the genome, making it more difficult to infer mechanism. With genome reference panels including rarer coding variants in addition to the common variants used in GWAS,[57] it is possible to identify coding variants that are correlated with GWAS signals because of linkage disequilibrium. Evidence that a GWAS signal tags a coding variant can prioritise that gene as being potentially causative.

Transcriptomic data can be used to narrow down the potential causative gene at a GWAS locus by assessing variation in gene expression levels depending on SNP genotype. Tissue-specific regulation of gene expression varies throughout development and lifespan and occurs via various genomic elements that lie outside the coding sequence. For example, enhancers can lie several hundred kilobases from the exonic sequence of the gene, and other genes can lie within the intervening region.[58] Other regulatory elements include promoters, insulators, and silencers, and variation at these sites can affect gene expression. There are, therefore, often several potential causative genes that lie under a positive association signal from GWAS, and there are various approaches that have been adopted to infer or demonstrate the causal mechanisms. One of the benefits of GWAS is that it is a hypothesis-free approach to gene discovery, but previous evidence of involvement in related traits can aid gene prioritisation for further follow-up. For example, it is now well established that DNA damage repair is the predominant mechanism that determines timing of menopause.[59] Thus, genes at a GWAS locus known to be involved in DNA damage repair may be more likely to be causative. Evidence from other multifactorial traits has illustrated that the gene closest to the GWAS signal is more likely to be causative than other genes in the region.[60]

GWAS has made a substantial contribution to our understanding of the biology of female-specific traits across the life course (Table 13.1). There are various software packages available that can be used to reveal common biological pathways from the association signals from GWAS. One of the most striking examples of the power of this approach comes from the menopause timing GWAS, where over 60% of the loci are in or near genes involved in DNA damage repair.[59] As sample sizes have increased in GWAS, the number of loci associated has increased and for many traits, no plateau has yet been observed. Even for relatively poorly measured traits, such as timing of menopause, which often occurs over several years and age rounding is apparent, because there is no systematic variability, and robust associations can be detected with sufficiently large studies.

13.4.1.2 Confirming Biological Causation

Despite the various *in silico* methods for prioritising genes identified by omics technologies, functional studies are required to prove causation. The exact functional study will depend on the trait being studied but include in vitro cellular assays and model organisms. In a GWAS of menopause timing, variants near *CHEK2* were identified as strongly associated, with each allele increasing menopause age by 1.3 years.[3] Experimental studies in mice demonstrated that by knocking out *chek2*, reproductive lifespan could be extended in the mice, recapitulating the effect seen in humans and providing evidence that *CHEK2* is the causative gene.[3]

13.4.1.3 Overlaps Between Diseases

Genetic correlations between traits can be used to ascertain shared biology, and although this reflects observational correlation, it does not imply causality. For example in the GWAS of 'number of children',[62] there was correlation between both menarche and menopause timing, indicating that both traits contribute to the number of children a woman has. Additionally, the genetic correlation between menarche timing and menopause timing is not particularly strong; many of the genes associated with menarche timing are expressed in the brain and are related to nutrient sensing or BMI,[2] while menopause-associated genes are more likely to be expressed in the ovary.[3] The most commonly used method for estimating genetic correlation is LD score regression, which can use summary statistics from GWAS rather than individual-level data.[68] The benefit of this method over traditional epidemiological approaches is that correlations between traits that are not measured in the same individuals can be investigated. For example, menopause timing and male pattern balding are traits that are each present in a different sex, so it would be impossible to determine the correlation between the two via traditional epidemiology, but by using LD score regression, we can test the genetic correlation.

13.4.2 Drug Discovery and Repurposing

One of the most promising areas for the application of integrated omics is in the development and repurposing of drugs.[69] The treatment of endometrial cancer, for example, has been guided by the discovery of a GWAS association with the aromatase gene *CYP19A1*, resulting

Table 13.1 Comparison of GWAS for female reproductive traits.

	Phenotype	Number of GWAS Signals	Sample Size	Variance Explained by Top Signals	Effect Size Range per Allele	Publications	Biological Pathways/Insights
Quantitative traits	Menarche timing	389	370,000	7.40%	1 week–5 months	Day FR, et al. 2017[2]	hypothalamic–pituitary-gonadal axis, nutrient sensing
	Cycle length	5	44,871	5.4% (overall SNPs)	<1 day	Laisk T, et al. 2018[61]	hypothalamic–pituitary-gonadal axis
	Number of children	34	478,624	na	0.012–0.025 children	Mathieson I, et al. 2020[62]	overlap with menarche and menopause
	Menopause timing	290	201,323	10.10%	3.5–74 weeks	Ruth KS, et al. 2021[3]	DNA damage response
Diseases/ conditions	Endometriosis	19	17,045 patients; 191,596 controls	5.19%	OR = 1.06–1.46	Sapkota Y, et al. 2017[63]	Sex steroid hormones
	PCOS	19	10,074 patients; 103,164 controls	na	OR = 1.10–1.22	Day F, et al. 2018[64]	BMI, fasting insulin, depression
	Uterine fibroids	22	15,453 patients; 392,628 controls	na	OR = 1.07–1.53	Valimaki N, et al. 2018[65]	Genitourinary development + Genome instability
	Breast cancer	210	133,384 patients; 113,789 controls	18.3% of familial RR		Zhang H, et al. 2020[66]	Cell cycle/apoptosis/ metabolism
	Ovarian cancer	9	8,174 patients; 26,134 controls	4% of familial risk	OR = 1.12–1.44	Pharoah PD, et al. 2013[67]	Ovarian cancer initiation and development/overlap with other cancer susceptibility loci

in promising results for the treatment of endometrial cancer with aromatase inhibitors.[70] GWAS of menopausal symptoms found a single genetic association in the *TACR3* gene, and phase 2 randomised controlled trials of an antagonist to its protein product (Neurokinin 3 receptor) have shown effective amelioration of vasomotor symptoms, such as hot flushes.[71] As more genome sequencing data are generated, causal genes and pathways will be identified, but also the effect of targeting particular genes or proteins can be monitored. By assessing the broader phenotypic consequences of loss of function of a particular gene, off-target effects of a potential antagonist to that protein can be predicted. Also, the identification of slow/fast metabolisers of certain drugs and ethnic differences in drug response can be predicted.

13.4.3 Prediction of Personal and Population Risk

Combining genomic variants into a genetic risk score is becoming a powerful tool for predicting outcomes and is starting to be introduced into clinical settings. Single variants, particularly those that are common and present in >1% of the population, have relatively small effects on disease outcome. However, by combining variants, a much more powerful predictive tool can be generated. This can either be limited to just the GWAS-significant loci (e.g. to distinguish between type 1 and type 2 diabetes) or can use all SNPs in the genome (e.g. in the prediction of heart disease). In both approaches, SNPs are weighted by the size of their effect on the trait and combined for each individual depending on which allele they carry at each locus. When using all variants in the genome, sophisticated statistical methods have been developed to take account of issues, such as linkage disequilibrium. The genetic score can be combined with traditional risk factors to improve the prediction power. A good example of where this has been implemented in female health is in breast cancer; carriers of *BRCA1* and *BRCA2*, with high genetic predisposition to cancer, can have their risk modified substantially by testing their genetic risk profile.[72] For women with the lowest genetic risk score for breast cancer, those who are *BRCA1* carriers can have a risk of breast cancer similar to that in the general population.[73] The power of a genetic risk score will be determined by the variance in the trait of interest that is explained by the variants included in the score. One of the limitations of this technique is that the scores do not perform as well in different ethnic groups.[74] GWAS has currently focused on individuals of European ancestry, and more multiethnic studies are required to improve the method and make it more generally applicable. Recent debate about the potential to use genetic risk scores to select healthy embryos has received considerable attention, but there are significant concerns about the feasibility of the approach, aside from the obvious ethical issues.[75]

13.4.4 Causal Inference for Epidemiology

Genomics can be used to make inferences about the causal relationships between traits using a method known as Mendelian randomization.[76] The basis of the method is that because genomes are present from birth and are not influenced by exposures throughout life, associations with genomic variants not being affected by confounding and reverse causation in the way that epidemiology studies can be. By combining associated genetic variants into an instrument for a trait, you can investigate whether that trait causally influences an outcome. The method is, therefore, analogous to a randomised controlled trial, and similarly to the use in prediction, the variance explained by the genetic instrument will influence the ability to detect causal associations. It is important to note that absence of an association with Mendelian randomization does not mean the exposure is not causally related to the outcome.

13.5 Unmet Needs

Omics studies are generally reliant on large sample sizes to be able to detect the relatively small effects for individual variation, and, therefore, increases in sample size will invariably increase the number of signals detected. A more diverse ancestry background in omics studies is also needed to enable the applications of genomics to benefit a wider proportion of the population. Allele frequencies can vary substantially between ethnic groups, with some variants being population specific. These variations can be leveraged to fine map genomic associations, making identification of causal genes and variants easier. Transcriptomics and proteomics are currently limited by the tissues available, and this is particularly true for female-specific tissue types, such as ovaries. For non-sex-specific tissues, there is also a bias in publicly available transcriptomics datasets for samples from males. Finally, while there is a substantially push from the research community to make omics datasets freely available, most of those resources are combined for males and females. It will be important to make more sex-specific data available, particularly for studies such as Mendelian randomization, where causal pathways may differ between sexes. If testing a sex-specific exposure, such as oestrogen level, it is essential that the outcome is restricted to females.

13.6 Future of Omics Studies

Genomic data are accumulating at an astounding rate, and in the near future, there will be whole exome and whole genome data available on hundreds of thousands of individuals. Whole genome data from different technologies also provides different information. Long-read sequencing is able to detect novel transcripts of a gene, for example, much more efficiently than previous methods, and will provide important insights. Improved sequencing techniques will also improve our ability to analyse the more complex areas of the genome that are not well-captured by techniques such as GWAS (e.g. repetitive regions, telomeres, and larger deletions and insertions). Alongside the increase in genomic datasets, there will be increases in availability of epigenomic data at the population level. One of the limitations of the large population-based cohorts with omic data has been the depth of phenotyping available. This will be improved by moves to include linkage to health care records, including primary care, plus more in-depth measured phenotyping, such as imaging and wearable devices. The COVID-19 pandemic has highlighted the benefits of integrating omics with health care records. The availability of more intermediate phenotypes from metabolomics and proteomics will also facilitate future discoveries. As studies with more diverse ancestry backgrounds become available, omics will become more mainstream. Direct-to-consumer genotyping companies such as 23&Me and Ancestry DNA are already popular, offering information about ancestry and disease risk to the general public. These companies are set to increase as we become more able to make more translational discoveries from omics that have direct impact on lifestyle choices and disease prediction. Genomics is becoming a nonspecialist area of medicine, and in the future, it will become a routine part of women's health care, providing insights for treatment and prevention across the life course.

Key messages and implications

- Many women's health conditions and traits are multifactorial, arising from a combination of genetic and environmental factors.
- Because of advancements in omics technology in the last few decades, we have a better understanding of the genetic factors associated with female-specific conditions and traits.
- As gene sequencing is now quicker and cheaper to perform than before, women will be able to access individualised and targeted treatment.
- Diversity in genomics research needs to be prioritised to enable all populations to benefit from new treatments arising from omics technology.

References

1. Aittomaki K, Lucena JL, Pakarinen P, Sistonen P, Tapanainen J, Gromoll J, et al. Mutation in the follicle-stimulating hormone receptor gene causes hereditary hypergonadotropic ovarian failure. *Cell*. 1995;82(6):959–68.
2. Day FR, Thompson DJ, Helgason H, Chasman DI, Finucane H, Sulem P, et al. Genomic analyses identify hundreds of variants associated with age at menarche and support a role for puberty timing in cancer risk. *Nature Genetics* 2017;49(6):834–41.
3. Ruth KS, Day FR, Hussain J, Martinez-Marchal A, Aiken CE, Azad A, et al. Genetic insights into biological mechanisms governing human ovarian ageing. *Nature*. 2021;596(7872):393–7.
4. Zhao S, Cheng X, Wen W, Qiu G, Zhang TJ, Wu Z, et al. Advances in clinical genetics and genomics. *Intelligent Medicine*. 2021;1(3):128–33.
5. Yengo L, Vedantam S, Marouli E, Sidorenko J, Bartell E, Sakaue S, et al. A saturated map of common genetic variants associated with human height. *Nature*. 2022;610:704–12.
6. Fisher RA. The correlation between relatives on the supposition of Mendelian inheritance. *Transactions of the Royal Society of Edinburgh*. 1918;52:399–433.
7. Weedon MN, Lettre G, Freathy RM, Lindgren CM, Voight BF, Perry JR, et al. A common variant of HMGA2 is associated with adult and childhood height in the general population. *Nature Genetics*. 2007;39(10):1245–50.
8. Firth HV, Wright CF. The Deciphering Developmental Disorders (DDD) study. *Developmental Medicine & Child Neurology*. 2011;53(8):702–3.
9. Turnbull C, Scott RH, Thomas E, Jones L, Murugaesu N, Pretty FB, et al. The 100 000 Genomes Project: bringing whole genome sequencing to the NHS. *British Medical Journal*. 2018;361:k1687.
10. Lander ES, Linton LM, Birren B, Nusbaum C, Zody MC, Baldwin J, et al. Initial sequencing and analysis of the human genome. *Nature*. 2001;409(6822):860–921.
11. Venter JC, Adams MD, Myers EW, Li PW, Mural RJ, Sutton GG, et al. The sequence of the human genome. *Science*. 2001;291(5507):1304–51.
12. Gudmundsson S, Singer-Berk M, Watts NA, Phu W, Goodrich JK, Solomonson M, et al. Variant interpretation using population databases: lessons from gnomAD. *Human Mutation*. 2022;43(8):1012–30.

13. Tiffon C. The impact of nutrition and environmental epigenetics on human health and disease. *International Journal of Molecular Sciences.* 2018;19(11):3425–44.

14. Anderson CA, Zhu G, Falchi M, van den Berg SM, Treloar SA, Spector TD, et al. A genome-wide linkage scan for age at menarche in three populations of European descent. *Journal of Clinical Endocrinology and Metabolism.* 2008;93(10):3965–70.

15. Morris DH, Jones ME, Schoemaker MJ, Ashworth A, Swerdlow AJ. Familial concordance for age at menarche: analyses from the Breakthrough Generations Study. *Paediatric Perinatal Epidemiology.* 2011;25(3):306–11.

16. Murabito JM, Yang Q, Fox C, Wilson PW, Cupples LA. Heritability of age at natural menopause in the Framingham Heart Study. *Journal of Clinical Endocrinology and Metabolism.* 2005;90(6):3427–30.

17. Snieder H, MacGregor AJ, Spector TD. Genes control the cessation of a woman's reproductive life: a twin study of hysterectomy and age at menopause. *Journal of Clinical Endocrinology and Metabolism.* 1998;83(6):1875–80.

18. Dapas M, Lin FTJ, Nadkarni GN, Sisk R, Legro RS, Urbanek M, et al. Distinct subtypes of polycystic ovary syndrome with novel genetic associations: an unsupervised, phenotypic clustering analysis. *PLoS Medicine.* 2020;17(6):e1003132.

19. Mortlock S, Corona RI, Kho PF, Pharoah P, Seo JH, Freedman ML, et al. A multi-level investigation of the genetic relationship between endometriosis and ovarian cancer histotypes. *Cell Reports Medicine.* 2022;3(3):100542.

20. Easton DF, Pooley KA, Dunning AM, Pharoah PD, Thompson D, Ballinger DG, et al. Genome-wide association study identifies novel breast cancer susceptibility loci. *Nature.* 2007;447(7148):1087–93.

21. Shiovitz S, Korde LA. Genetics of breast cancer: a topic in evolution. *Annals of Oncology.* 2015;26(7):1291–9.

22. DeSantis CE, Ma J, Goding Sauer A, Newman LA, Jemal A. Breast cancer statistics, 2017, racial disparity in mortality by state. *CA: A Cancer Journal for Clinicians.* 2017;67(6):439–48.

23. Ho PJ, Ho WK, Khng AJ, Yeoh YS, Tan BK, Tan EY, et al. Overlap of high-risk individuals predicted by family history, and genetic and non-genetic breast cancer risk prediction models: implications for risk stratification. *BMC Medicine.* 2022;20(1):150.

24. Ng SB, Buckingham KJ, Lee C, Bigham AW, Tabor HK, Dent KM, et al. Exome sequencing identifies the cause of a mendelian disorder. *Nature Genetics.* 2010;42(1):30–5.

25. Jiao X, Ke H, Qin Y, Chen ZJ. Molecular genetics of premature ovarian insufficiency. *Trends in Endocrinology and Metabolism.* 2018;29(11):795–807.

26. Perry JR, Murray A, Day FR, Ong KK. Molecular insights into the aetiology of female reproductive ageing. *Nature Reviews Endocrinology.* 2015;11(12):725–34.

27. Franca MM, Mendonca BB. Genetics of primary ovarian insufficiency in the next-generation sequencing era. *J Endocr Soc.* 2020;4(2):bvz037.

28. Louden ED, Poch A, Kim HG, Ben-Mahmoud A, Kim SH, Layman LC. Genetics of hypogonadotropic hypogonadism-human and mouse genes, inheritance, oligogenicity, and genetic counseling. *Mol Cell Endocrinol.* 2021;534:111334.

29. Bush WS, Moore JH. Chapter 11: genome-wide association studies. *PLoS Computational Biology.* 2012;8(12):e1002822.

30. International HapMap Consortium. A haplotype map of the human genome. *Nature.* 2005;437(7063):1299–320.

31. Genomes Project Consortium, Auton A, Brooks LD, Durbin RM, Garrison EP, Kang HM, Korbel JO, Marchini JL, et al. A global reference for human genetic variation. *Nature.* 2015;526:68–74.

32. McCarthy S, Das S, Kretzschmar W, Delaneau O, Wood AR, Teumer A, et al. A reference panel of 64,976 haplotypes for genotype imputation. *Nature Genetics.* 2016;48(10):1279–83.

33. Risch N, Merikangas K. The future of genetic studies of complex human diseases. *Science.* 1996;273(5281):1516–17.

34. Holtzman L, Gersbach CA. Editing the epigenome: reshaping the genomic landscape. *Annual Review of Genomics and Human Genetics.* 2018;19:43–71.

35. Horvath S. DNA methylation age of human tissues and cell types. *Genome Biology.* 2013;14(10):R115.

36. Kordowitzki P, Haghani A, Zoller JA, Li CZ, Raj K, Spangler ML, et al. Epigenetic clock and methylation study of oocytes from a bovine model of reproductive aging. *Aging Cell*. 2021;20(5):e13349.

37. McAllister JM, Modi B, Miller BA, Biegler J, Bruggeman R, Legro RS, et al. Overexpression of a DENND1A isoform produces a polycystic ovary syndrome theca phenotype. *Proceedings of the National Acadamy of Science U S A*. 2014;111(15):E1519–E1527.

38. Pan JX, Tan YJ, Wang FF, Hou NN, Xiang YQ, Zhang JY, et al. Aberrant expression and DNA methylation of lipid metabolism genes in PCOS: a new insight into its pathogenesis. *Clinical Epigenetics*. 2018;10:6.

39. Qu F, Wang FF, Yin R, Ding GL, El-Prince M, Gao Q, et al. A molecular mechanism underlying ovarian dysfunction of polycystic ovary syndrome: hyperandrogenism induces epigenetic alterations in the granulosa cells. *Journal of Molecular Medicine*. 2012;90(8):911–23.

40. Sagvekar P, Kumar P, Mangoli V, Desai S, Mukherjee S. DNA methylome profiling of granulosa cells reveals altered methylation in genes regulating vital ovarian functions in polycystic ovary syndrome. *Clinical Epigenetics*. 2019;11(1):61.

41. Iljas JD, Wei Z, Homer HA. Sirt1 sustains female fertility by slowing age-related decline in oocyte quality required for post-fertilization embryo development. *Aging Cell*. 2020;19(9):e13204.

42. Kazmi N, Sharp GC, Reese SE, Vehmeijer FO, Lahti J, Page CM, et al. Hypertensive disorders of pregnancy and DNA methylation in newborns. *Hypertension*. 2019;74(2):375–83.

43. Kupers LK, Xu X, Jankipersadsing SA, Vaez A, la Bastide-van Gemert S, Scholtens S, et al. DNA methylation mediates the effect of maternal smoking during pregnancy on birthweight of the offspring. *International Journal of Epidemiol*. 2015;44(4):1224–37.

44. GTEx Consortium. The GTEx Consortium atlas of genetic regulatory effects across human tissues. *Science*. 2020;369(6509):1318–30.

45. Wang Z, Gerstein M, Snyder M. RNA-Seq: a revolutionary tool for transcriptomics. *Nature Reviews Genetics*. 2009;10(1):57–63.

46. Hedlund E, Deng Q. Single-cell RNA sequencing: technical advancements and biological applications. *Molecular Aspects Medicine*. 2018;59:36–46.

47. Barrozo ER, Aagaard KM. Human placental biology at single-cell resolution: a contemporaneous review. *British Journal of Obstetrics and Gynecology*. 2022;129(2):208–20.

48. Fan X, Bialecka M, Moustakas I, Lam E, Torrens-Juaneda V, Borggreven NV, et al. Single-cell reconstruction of follicular remodeling in the human adult ovary. *Nature Communications*. 2019;10(1):3164.

49. Zhang Y, Yan Z, Qin Q, Nisenblat V, Chang HM, Yu Y, et al. Transcriptome landscape of human folliculogenesis reveals oocyte and granulosa cell interactions. *Molecular Cell*. 2018;72(6):1021–34e4.

50. Wagner M, Yoshihara M, Douagi I, Damdimopoulos A, Panula S, Petropoulos S, et al. Single-cell analysis of human ovarian cortex identifies distinct cell populations but no oogonial stem cells. *Nature Communications*. 2020;11(1):1147.

51. Ferrero H, Corachan A, Aguilar A, Quinonero A, Carbajo-Garcia MC, Alama P, et al. Single-cell RNA sequencing of oocytes from ovarian endometriosis patients reveals a differential transcriptomic profile associated with lower quality. *Human Reproduction*. 2019;34(7):1302–12.

52. Xita N, Tsatsoulis A. Genetic variants of sex hormone-binding globulin and their biological consequences. *Molecular* and *Cellular Endocrinology*. 2010;316(1):60–5.

53. Ward LD, Parker MM, Deaton AM, Tu HC, Flynn-Carroll AO, Hinkle G, et al. Rare coding variants in DNA damage repair genes associated with timing of natural menopause. *Human Genetics and Genomics Advances*. 2022;3(2):100079.

54. Lam BYH, Williamson A, Finer S, Day FR, Tadross JA, Goncalves Soares A, et al. MC3R links nutritional state to childhood growth and the timing of puberty. *Nature*. 2021;599(7885):436–41.

55. Ong KK, Elks CE, Li S, Zhao JH, Luan J, Andersen LB, et al. Genetic variation in LIN28B is associated with the timing of puberty. *Nature Genetics*. 2009;41(6):729–33.

56. Perry JR, Stolk L, Franceschini N, Lunetta KL, Zhai G, McArdle PF, et al. Meta-analysis of genome-wide association data identifies two loci influencing age at menarche. *Nature Genetics*. 2009;41(6):648–50.

57. The International HapMap Consortium. Integrating common and rare genetic variation in diverse human populations. *Nature.* 2010;467(7311):52–8.

58. Schoenfelder S, Fraser P. Long-range enhancer-promoter contacts in gene expression control. *Nature Reviews Genetics.* 2019;20(8):437–55.

59. Day FR, Ruth KS, Thompson DJ, Lunetta KL, Pervjakova N, Chasman DI, et al. Large-scale genomic analyses link reproductive aging to hypothalamic signaling, breast cancer susceptibility and BRCA1-mediated DNA repair. *Nature Genetics.* 2015;47(11):1294–303.

60. Sun BB, Chiou J, Traylor M, Benner C, Hsu Y-H, Richardson TG, et al. Genetic regulation of the human plasma proteome in 54,306 UK Biobank participants. *bioRxiv.* 2022:2022.06.17.496443.

61. Laisk T, Kukuskina V, Palmer D, Laber S, Chen CY, Ferreira T, et al. Large-scale meta-analysis highlights the hypothalamic-pituitary-gonadal axis in the genetic regulation of menstrual cycle length. *Human Molecular Genetics.* 2018;27(24):4323–32.

62. Mathieson I, Day FR, Barban N, Tropf FC, Brazel DM, Consortium e, et al. Genome-wide analysis identifies genetic effects on reproductive success and ongoing natural selection at the FADS locus. *bioRxiv.* 2020:2020.05.19.104455.

63. Sapkota Y, Steinthorsdottir V, Morris AP, Fassbender A, Rahmioglu N, De Vivo I, et al. Meta-analysis identifies five novel loci associated with endometriosis highlighting key genes involved in hormone metabolism. *Nature Communications.* 2017;8:15539.

64. Day F, Karaderi T, Jones MR, Meun C, He C, Drong A, et al. Large-scale genome-wide meta-analysis of polycystic ovary syndrome suggests shared genetic architecture for different diagnosis criteria. *PLoS Genetics.* 2018;14(12):e1007813.

65. Valimaki N, Kuisma H, Pasanen A, Heikinheimo O, Sjoberg J, Butzow R, et al. Genetic predisposition to uterine leiomyoma is determined by loci for genitourinary development and genome stability. *Elife.* 2018;7:e37110.

66. Zhang H, Ahearn TU, Lecarpentier J, Barnes D, Beesley J, Qi G, et al. Genome-wide association study identifies 32 novel breast cancer susceptibility loci from overall and subtype-specific analyses. *Nature Genetics.* 2020;52(6):572–81.

67. Pharoah PD, Tsai YY, Ramus SJ, Phelan CM, Goode EL, Lawrenson K, et al. GWAS meta-analysis and replication identifies three new susceptibility loci for ovarian cancer. *Nature Genetics.* 2013;45(4):362–70, 70e1–e2.

68. Bulik-Sullivan B, Finucane HK, Anttila V, Gusev A, Day FR, Loh PR, et al. An atlas of genetic correlations across human diseases and traits. *Nature Genetics.* 2015;47(11):1236–41.

69. Reay WR, Cairns MJ. Advancing the use of genome-wide association studies for drug repurposing. *Nature Reviews Genetics.* 2021;22(10):658–71.

70. Paleari L, Rutigliani M, Siri G, Provinciali N, Colombo N, Decensi A. Aromatase inhibitors as adjuvant treatment for ER/PgR positive stage I endometrial carcinoma: a retrospective cohort study. *International Journal of Molecular Sciences.* 2020;21(6):2227.

71. Prague JK, Roberts RE, Comninos AN, Clarke S, Jayasena CN, Nash Z, et al. Neurokinin 3 receptor antagonism as a novel treatment for menopausal hot flushes: a phase 2, randomised, double-blind, placebo-controlled trial. *Lancet.* 2017;389(10081):1809–20.

72. Barnes DR, Rookus MA, McGuffog L, Leslie G, Mooij TM, Dennis J, et al. Polygenic risk scores and breast and epithelial ovarian cancer risks for carriers of BRCA1 and BRCA2 pathogenic variants. *Genetics in Medicine.* 2020;22(10):1653–66.

73. Couch FJ, Wang X, McGuffog L, Lee A, Olswold C, Kuchenbaecker KB, et al. Genome-wide association study in BRCA1 mutation carriers identifies novel loci associated with breast and ovarian cancer risk. *PLoS Genetics.* 2013;9(3):e1003212.

74. Evans DG, van Veen EM, Byers H, Roberts E, Howell A, Howell SJ, et al. The importance of ethnicity: are breast cancer polygenic risk scores ready for women who are not of white European origin? *International Journal of Cancer.* 2022;150(1):73–9.

75. Turley P, Meyer MN, Wang N, Cesarini D, Hammonds E, Martin AR, et al. Problems with using polygenic scores to select embryos. *New England Journal of Medicine.* 2021;385(1):78–86.

76. Smith GD, Ebrahim S. 'Mendelian randomization': can genetic epidemiology contribute to understanding environmental determinants of disease? *International Journal of Epidemiology.* 2003;32(1):1–22.

14
Endocrine Pathways Across the Life Course

Marta Bianchini, Alfonsina Chiefari, Rosa Lauretta,
Marilda Mormando, Giulia Puliani, and Marialuisa Appetecchia

14.1 Introduction

This chapter analyses the physiology of the main endocrine axes throughout life, with the aim of clarifying the role of the endocrine system in women's health. Hormones are key factors in the path to differential well-being. They regulate almost all aspects of female physiology, from gestation to senescence. The fine regulation to which hormones are subjected is controlled by the hypothalamus–pituitary axis, which can be considered as a sort of conductor. Hormones of both maternal and fetal origin act from the development of the fetus and can influence physiological events long after birth, as demonstrated by the correlation between birth weight on the age at the menarche.[1] Further, hormones manage the interaction between people and the environment by organising responses to stimuli, such as stress or workload. Endocrine regulation of metabolism also affects energy use in competing life needs, which ranges from immediate needs for survival to lifetime plans of growth, reproduction, production, and being social, all of which are crucial to well-being.[2]

In this chapter, we provide a summary of the characterisation, regulation, and relationships with health outcomes of the main hormonal systems: hypothalamus–pituitary–gonadal (HPG), hypothalamus–pituitary–adrenal (HPA), and thyrotropic axes, as well as central metabolic regulation and the growth hormone-insulin-like growth factor (IGF-1) axis.

14.2 Hypothalamus–Pituitary–Gonadal (HPG) Axis

Ovarian function is under the control of the central nervous system through HPG axis. Gonadotropin-releasing hormone (GnRH) is secreted from hypothalamic GnRH neurons into the pituitary portal circulation in the median eminence, where it regulates the synthesis and secretion of gonadotropins, luteinising hormone (LH), and follicle-stimulating hormone (FSH), in an intermittent way.[3] The generation of GnRH impulses is regulated by a hypothalamic timing mechanism that begins in the neuronal network of the arcuate nucleus through stimulatory and inhibitory mechanisms mediated by neurokinin B and dynorphin, respectively.[4,5]

Marta Bianchini, Alfonsina Chiefari, Rosa Lauretta, Marilda Mormando, Giulia Puliani, and Marialuisa Appetecchia, *Endocrine Pathways Across the Life Course* In: *A Life Course Approach to Women's Health*. Second Edition. Edited by: Gita D Mishra, Rebecca Hardy, and Diana Kuh, Oxford University Press. © Oxford University Press 2023. DOI: 10.1093/oso/9780192864642.003.0014

14.2.1 Changes in the HPG Axis Across the Life Course

14.2.1.1 HPG Axis During Development

The HPG axis is active in the fetus until the middle of the gestational period and is sub-sequently silenced until the end of gestation. This silencing is removed at birth, leading to axis reactivation and increased gonadotropin concentrations.[6] The LH concentration grad-ually decreases towards 6 months of age, while the FSH concentration in girls remains high until the age of 3–4 years when the active inhibition of GnRH secretion starts and persists throughout childhood. Prenatal and postnatal activation of the HPG axis is associated with maturation of ovarian follicles and an increase in oestradiol (E2) concentrations. This period of activity of the HPG axis in the early stages of life is called 'mini puberty' and is prepara-tory to the subsequent pituitary response of LH and FSH to GnRH during the reproductive phase of adulthood.[6] During childhood, the hypogonadotropic state is a consequence of the suppression of pulsatile GnRH release. Puberty is the transition period between childhood and adulthood, characterised by the development of secondary sexual characteristics (i.e. gonadal maturation) and the achievement of reproductive capacity,[7] and is due to the pulsa-tile release of GnRH from the hypothalamus. The exact mechanism that triggers the onset of puberty remains not fully understood.[8] However, changes in body composition are essential for achieving fertility,[9] linking peripheral hormones and the reproductive axis. Insulin,[10,11] leptin,[12,13] and ghrelin[14,15] are required for the HPG axis maturation, normal pubertal progression, and maintenance of fertility through direct or indirect modulation of GnRH secretion.

The first sign of the onset of puberty in females is typically the development of the breast budding (thelarche). Pubarche is defined as the development of axillary and pubic hair as a result of adrenal androgens production,[16] and happens several years before activation of the HPG axis (gonadarche).[17] Age at menarche (the first menstrual period) varies greatly between individuals and different ethnic populations (see Chapter 2 for more detail).[18] Generally, girls experience the onset of puberty at younger ages than boys; the physiological changes of puberty typically occur between the ages of 8 and 12 years in girls.[19]

14.2.1.2 Regulation of the Menstrual Cycle

The ovarian cycle is characterised by the secretion of relatively low basal levels of LH and FSH, which are interrupted approximately once every 28 days by an upsurge of gonadotropins that triggers ovulation (see Figure 14.1).[20,21] Serum E2 levels start to rise approximately 1 week before ovulation and reach the maximum 1 day before ovulation. Concomitant with the increasing secretion of E2 from the developing follicles is the pro-liferation of the endometrium (follicular phase). Following ovulation, there is a drop in E2 levels before a second (albeit smaller) peak is seen midway through the luteal phase, co-inciding with the peak for progesterone. E2 and progesterone exerts negative feedback on the hypothalamus and pituitary gland to suppress LH and/or FSH secretion (Figure 14.2). Additionally, both progesterone and E2 cause modifications of the endometrium to prepare for potential implantation of an embryo (luteal phase). In the absence of pregnancy, the function of the corpus luteum decreases; E2 and progesterone return to baseline levels; and menstruation occurs.[20]

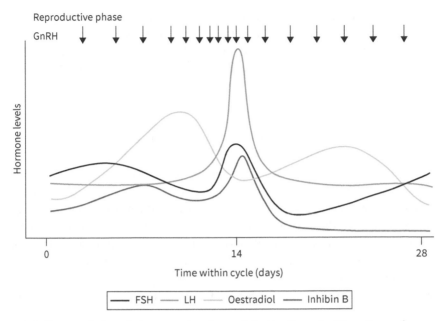

Figure 14.1 Changes in female hormone levels regulated by the pulsatile actions of gonadotropin-releasing hormone in the pituitary gland throughout the menstrual cycle (Davis et al., 2015).[21] See plate section.

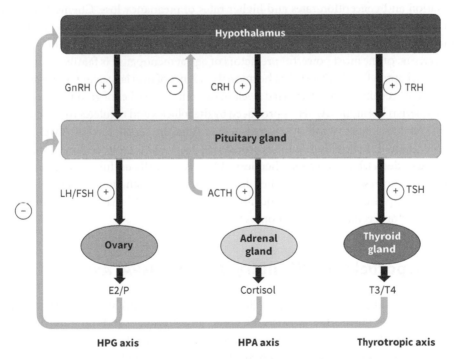

Figure 14.2 The hypothalamic-pituitary axes (hypothalamic-pituitary-gonadal axis, hypothalamic-pituitary-adrenal axis, and thyrotropic axis (HPT)). Gonadotropin-releasing hormone, GnRH. Luteinising hormone, LH. Follicle-stimulating hormone, FSH. Oestrogen, E2. Progesterone, P. Corticotropin-releasing hormone, CRH. Adrenocorticotropic hormone, ACTH. '+' indicates positive feedback loop. '-' indicates negative feedback loop.

In the event of fertilisation, the LH released by the corpus luteum, and human chorionic gonadotropin (hCG) secreted from the embryo stimulates progesterone secretion from the corpus luteum until 6–7-weeks gestation[22] when the developing placenta becomes a key endocrine organ and the primary production site for progesterone, hCG, E2, and other hormones.[23,24]

14.2.1.3 Regulation of Follicular Maturation

As described in Chapter 2, the finite pool of resting follicles in the ovary reaches its maximum in neonatal life. Thereafter, there is a steady decline because of atresia, and, at birth, only one million follicles remain, with a further reduction to a quarter of that by the time of puberty.[25] Between the ages of 30 and 35 years, the percentage of growing follicles increase, and the trajectory of follicle loss is accelerated.[26] Each follicle within the ovary is like a single group of cells that move through the ovarian stroma with two possible fates: dying from apoptosis or ovulating and releasing an egg for fertilisation. Inside the follicle, granulosa cells bind FSH, increasing proliferation and inducing the production of E2 through the conversion of androgens into oestrogens. E2, in turn, through its receptor, plays critical roles in the proliferation of granulosa cells, regulation of FSH receptor activation, and promotion of LH receptor expression.

14.2.1.4 Age-Related Changes in the HPG Axis

Age-related changes in oocyte quality accompany decreased follicle number, with decreased fertilisation and conception rates and higher rates of pregnancy loss. Chemotherapy, radiation, and smoking are all factors that accelerate follicle loss through damage to the oocyte and/or dividing granulosa cells that provide the nutrients and metabolites for the oocyte.[27–30] However, one of the most powerful predictors of age at menopause is family history (as discussed in Chapter 4).[31–33] The earliest hormonal evidence of ovarian ageing is the selective increase in FSH resulting from decreased levels of inhibin B, a marker of granulosa cell number. Anti-Müllerian hormone (AMH) is produced by the follicles and regulates the follicular maturation. As the number of follicles decreases over time, the serum level of AMH in women follows a gradual decline during the reproductive years and a rapid decline at menopause, becoming undetectable soon after. Therefore, AMH is clinically useful as a screening tool for reduced ovarian reserve.[34] With further decrease in ovarian function and loss of ovulatory cycles, GnRH pulses occur more frequently[35] while falling E2 levels allow for increases in both GnRH[36] and gonadotropin responses to GnRH.[36]

14.3 Hypothalamic–Pituitary–Adrenal (HPA) Axis

The adult adrenal gland is made up of the cortex (outer region) and medulla, a stem-like inner structure. The cortex consists of three histologically and functionally distinct zones: glomerulosa, responsible for production of mineralocorticoids (aldosterone); fasciculata, site of glucocorticoids synthesis (mainly cortisol); and reticularis, where adrenal androgens are produced and whose formation is completed with adrenarche.[37] Under stress and other stimuli, the hypothalamic paraventricular nucleus in the hypothalamus secretes corticotropin-releasing hormone (CRH), which induces the anterior pituitary gland to re-lease adrenocorticotropic hormone (ACTH). This stimulates the synthesis and secretion of cortisol and androgen and, to a lesser extent, aldosterone in the adrenal cortex. This endo-crine circuit, commonly referred to as HPA axis, is regulated by feedback mechanisms (see Figure 14.2). Cortisol can limit its own secretion through negative feedback on both the pituitary gland and the hypothalamus. ACTH also provides negative feedback on CRH production.[38]

Cortisol exerts many functions in the human body, both under resting and stressful con-ditions, regulating metabolism, immune response, and the cardiovascular system.[39] Under basal conditions, cortisol production varies throughout the day, following a circadian rhythm, peaking in the morning after waking[40] and then gradually decreasing to its nadir at night.[41,42] These variations show differences based on sex and age, with lower daytime cor-tisol concentration in premenopausal women than men and an age-related increase in cor-tisol levels during late evening and early night in both sexes.[43,44]

14.3.1 Changes in HPA Axis Across the Life Course

14.3.1.1 Adrenarche
The main androgens secreted by the adrenals are androstenedione, dehydroepiandrosterone (DHEA) and its sulphate (DHEAS), and, to a lesser extent, testosterone.[45] They have only weak androgenic activity but provide precursors for conversion to more potent androgens and oestrogens in peripheral tissue. Low concentrations of DHEAS are present up to 5 years of age in both males and females. Then, at 6–8 years of age in girls and 7–9 years of age in boys, a marked rise in DHEAS concentration is observed (another feature of adrenarche in addition to the maturation of the adrenal gland) and is characterised by the appearance of pubic and axillary hair.

14.3.1.2 Pregnancy
Pregnancy represents a condition of relative physiological and temporary hypercortisolism to satisfy the metabolic demands of pregnancy and to contribute to the growth and matur-ation of the fetal organs.[46,47] Increased circulating oestrogens stimulate the hepatic produc-tion of corticosteroid-binding globulin,[48] elevating plasma cortisol values;[47] however, free cortisol also increases, as evidenced by the high urinary free cortisol concentration, which is threefold higher in the third trimester than nonpregnant levels.[49] Hypercortisolism can be explained by several mechanisms: production of CRH and ACTH from the placenta, stimu-lated by the positive feedback of maternal cortisol;[47,50,51] increased responsiveness of the maternal adrenal gland to ACTH; and restoration of maternal HPA feedback mechanisms to higher levels because of resistance to cortisol action.[50,52] The fetus is protected in early gestation from the maternal hypercortisolism by the action of placental 11-hydroxysteroid-dehydrogenase2, which converts active glucocorticoids to inert 11-keto steroids.[53] In the postpartum period, the HPA axis gradually returns to its prepregnant state.[54] Breastfeeding is also a condition of HPA axis hypo-responsiveness; however, unlike pregnancy, it is stimu-lated by suckling.[55] Overall, in pregnancy, parturition, and lactation, the circadian variation in the HPA axis activity is dampened, whereas responses to stressors are attenuated.

14.3.1.3 Ageing
During healthy ageing, cortisol secretion in response to ACTH infusion is increased,[56] and the reduced hypothalamic–pituitary sensitivity to glucocorticoid feedback inhibition is more evident in women than in men.[57] However, the main age-related change in the human adrenal gland is in regards to DHEAS synthesis.[58] Circulating DHEAS concentration reaches its maximum concentration at 25–30 years of age, with levels being higher in males than in females.[59] After this peak, the serum concentration of DHEAS begins to decline until the seventh decade.[60] This age-related decrease is known by the term *adrenopause*, and it morphologically corresponds to a reduction in the size of the adrenal reticular zone,[61] potentially related to some physiological and pathological conditions of ageing.

14.4 Thyrotropic Axis

In the thyrotropic axis (also known as the hypothalamic–pituitary–thyroid axis), thyroid hormone production by the thyroid gland is stimulated by pituitary thyroid-stimulating hormone (TSH), which, in turn, is dependent on thyrotropin-releasing hormone (TRH) that is synthesised in the paraventricular nucleus of the hypothalamus (see Figure 14.2).[62] Thyroid hormones, triiodothyronine (T3) and thyroxine (T4), are synthesised from dietary sources of iodine. Once they are released into the circulation, T3 and T4 are transported by binding to plasma proteins (thyroxin-binding globulin, transthyretin, and albumin) to peripheral tissues, such as the liver, kidney, and adipose tissue.[62] T3 and T4 are released by their transport proteins to allow their uptake by target cells; only the free thyroid hormones (FT3 and FT4) are metabolically active. The thyroid gland produces and secretes mainly T4, while the more active T3 is 20% thyroid origin, with the remaining 80% produced in peripheral tissues through the conversion of T4 to T3 by local deiodinases.[63] T3 and T4 exert inhibitory actions on the hypothalamus and the pituitary gland.

Thyroid hormones play a key role in carbohydrate, lipids, and protein metabolism, cell growth and differentiation, thermoregulation, cardiac function, and bone growth and development.[62,64] Their actions are primarily exerted through regulation of gene expression; however, some nongenomic mechanism have been identified for blood vessel formation[65] and control of cancer cell growth.[66] The thyrotropic axis is regulated by the circadian clock; specifically, TSH levels are lowest in the afternoon, rising throughout the evening and peaking in the first part of night, until the onset of sleep, before gradually decreasing throughout the night and into the morning.[67] The diurnal rhythm of TSH does not differ by sex. TSH secretion is also modulated by neurotransmitters (dopamine and somatostatin) and leptin (a marker of nutritional state).[68]

14.4.1 Changes in Thyrotropic Axis Across the Life Course

14.4.1.1 The Thyrotropic Axis in Development
Thyroid hormones are necessary for brain development in the fetus, which begins from approximately week 10 of gestation.[69] This hormonal requirement is satisfied exclusively by the transplacental passage of T4 before the end of the first trimester. The synthesis of thyroid

hormones begins from weeks 11–12 of gestation and progressively increases during pregnancy, while the maternal thyroid continues to contribute to hormonal needs until the complete maturation of the fetal thyroid gland.[70]

At the time of birth, there is a spike in plasma concentrations of TSH and, therefore, of FT3 and FT4, which remain elevated in the first days of postnatal life to respond to the increased metabolic demands of babies. TSH, then, declines through childhood, adolescence, and adulthood,[71] reflecting a decrease in the pituitary response to hypothalamic TRH.[72–74] Little or no postnatal change in T4 has been observed.[75,76]

14.4.1.2 Pregnancy

During pregnancy, there is a sharp increase in total maternal T4 concentration in the first trimester before it plateaus around midgestation, whereas the rise in total maternal T3 levels is more gradual before it stabilises also at midgestation.[77] From conception, human chorionic gonadotropin (hCG) secretion increases relative to the growth and development of the placenta, resulting in a surge in maternal FT3 and FT4 and suppression of maternal TSH in the first trimester because of the thyrotropic actions of hCG.[78] The gradual increase in TBG secretion from the liver throughout the first trimester until 20 weeks of gestation is thought to be due to the concomitant rise in E2,[79] thus promoting total thyroid hormone production. Consequently, pregnant women have an increased requirement for iodine due to: i) the transplacental transport of thyroid hormones for fetal development,[80,81] and ii) elevated renal clearance of iodine (although, this observation appears to be controversial).[82] Iodine supplementation is currently recommended for pregnant women, particularly in areas where dietary iodine intake is insufficient.[83]

14.4.1.3 The Thyrotropic Axis in Ageing

Amongst healthy individuals, TSH concentration increases with age; however, women have lower levels than men.[84,85] On the other hand, FT4 decreases with age[86] until the age of 60 years when it plateaus.[87] Similarly, FT3 levels are negatively associated with age,[88] possibly because of the reduced activity of deiodinases.[89] Women are more sensitive than men to changes in the thyrotropic axis. Subclinical Hypothyroidism, characterised by elevated serum TSH and normal FT4 levels, is 7–10 times more prevalent in women compared to men and is associated with age.[90,91] Similarly, women are 10–20 times more likely to be diagnosed with hyperthyroidism (low TSH with high FT4); however, the incidence rate is higher amongst younger than older women.[90,91]

14.5 Central Metabolic Regulation

The brain plays a central role in the regulation of energy balance by receiving metabolic signals from the periphery and initiating a response by transmitting the information to the hypothalamus (Figure 14.3).[94,95] The hypothalamus is an area of the brain that acts as a key regulator of metabolism and food intake via a group of neurons called the arcuate nucleus, which is conveniently situated next to the blood-brain barrier. Its position allows easy access to circulating hormones and nutrients.[94] Here, we will focus on hormones, ghrelin and leptin, which are two of the key hormones involved in the modulation of energy balance.

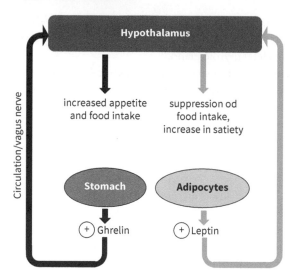

Figure 14.3 The central metabolic pathways for ghrelin and leptin.

14.5.1 Ghrelin

Ghrelin is a peptide secreted by gastrointestinal tract cells to increase food intake. It is a potent stimulator of somatotropic secretion[96] and appetite[97] which reduces fat utilisation and induces hyperglycaemia.[98] Additionally, plasma ghrelin levels rise before meals and decrease after the ingestion of food. The main neuronal targets that mediate ghrelin's orexigenic (appetite-stimulating) action are the arcuate nucleus of hypothalamus and the dorsal vagal brainstem complex (Figure 14.3);[99] however, the exact molecular mechanisms by which this hormone regulates feeding are not completely understood.[94] Ghrelin can be found in two main forms in the circulation: acylated (acyl-ghrelin, the active peptide) and unacylated.[100]

14.5.1.1 The Role of Ghrelin in Development

Ghrelin is strongly expressed in human placenta during the first trimester,[101] and it coincides with a peak in maternal serum levels midgestation.[102] Following this, maternal serum ghrelin levels decreases into the third trimester,[102] and placental expression of ghrelin is undetectable.[103] The role of ghrelin during pregnancy is not clear; however, in vitro experiments and animal models suggest that that it is involved in cell proliferation,[104] uterine contractility,[105] and fetal growth restriction.[106] As ghrelin has inhibitory actions on uterine muscle contraction, its reduction in the third trimester is possibly part of the process for preparing the uterus for delivery.

14.5.1.2 Changes in Ghrelin with Age

One study described the postnatal variations in plasma ghrelin levels from birth to early adulthood.[107] At birth, there was no difference in plasma ghrelin levels between preterm (32–37 weeks gestation) and full-term babies. Then, plasma ghrelin levels almost double within a month after delivery and remain at this level until puberty begins. There is a significant drop in ghrelin (back to the levels observed at birth) in children undergoing Tanner stage II (thelarche in girls and testes enlargement in boys). Circulating ghrelin levels progressively decline as puberty progresses.[107] These observations can be interpreted as a favourable metabolic condition and a permissive signal of HPG axis maturation.[108] There are potentially sex differences in ghrelin secretion as a small Spanish study observed that women had higher plasma ghrelin concentrations than men regardless of age.[109]

There is conflicting evidence regarding the changes in circulating ghrelin levels with age. Some small-scale studies showed no difference between young adults and elderly individuals[109,110] or declining levels with age.[111–113] Other studies demonstrated alterations in ghrelin receptor expression or ghrelin-stimulated signalling in senescent animals.[114] Large-scale studies are needed to determine the relationship between ageing and ghrelin concentration and activity.

14.5.2 Leptin

Leptin is a peptide predominantly secreted by adipocytes,[115] is highly expressed in the mammary epithelium,[116] and is detectable in several other tissues including placenta, ovaries, bone marrow, muscle, brain, endocrine cells of the gastrointestinal system, and lymphoid tissues.[117–120] Circulating leptin levels are directly proportional to body fat mass[121] and fluctuate with acute changes in caloric intake.[122] The main actions of leptin are stimulating pro-opiomelanocortin (POMC) neurons and inhibiting neuropeptide Y/Agouti-related protein (NPY/AGRP) neurons in the arcuate nucleus of the hypothalamus. These neurons have opposing actions: POMC neurons suppress food intake and weight gain,[123,124] while NPY/AGRP neurons induce the sensation of hunger[125] and stimulate feeding.[126]

Plasma leptin concentration also shows significant sex differences, regardless of adiposity. In adults, plasma leptin concentrations per unit of fat mass are about threefold higher in females than in males.[127] Sex-related differences result from different body fat distribution between males and females: the subcutaneous adipose tissue, which is more pronounced in women than men, contain larger adipocytes and express higher leptin levels per unit of fat mass than adipocytes from intra-abdominal fat depots.[128]

14.5.2.1 Changes in Circulating Leptin During Development

Umbilical cord blood leptin levels are closely related to the new-born's adiposity and strongly predictive of subsequent rates of weight gain. Leptin is inversely related to weight gain from birth to 4 months of age; this inverse relationship is still evident at 24 months of age.[129] Children who gain weight more quickly enter puberty earlier and leptin levels may be the signal that reflects the amount of fat stores that trigger pubertal activation of the hypothalamus.[130] In a larger longitudinal study of body composition in a population sample of 40 children (20 boys and 20 girls), leptin levels were observed to gradually increase with age in both boys and girls, until the onset of puberty.[131] After the onset of puberty, leptin levels, correlated to oestrogen concentration, rose further in girls but decreased in boys,[132] resulting in three-to-four-times-higher leptin levels in females than in males. This postpubertal sexual dimorphism can also be explained by a pubertal gain of more fat mass in girls and more lean mass in boys. Thus, the increase in fat percentage during puberty may be necessary for preparation of childbearing and breastfeeding. Further, gonadal steroids (both oestrogens and androgens) can influence the action of leptin through their modulation on neuroendocrine pathways such as NPY, POMC, or melanin-concentrating hormone.[133]

14.5.2.2 The Role of Leptin in Pregnancy

Serum leptin levels rises during pregnancy, especially in the second and the third trimesters.[134] This is not only due to gestational weight gain, but also to placenta-derived leptin and the soluble form of its receptor in the maternal circulation,[135] as well as increased levels of hormones that stimulate leptin secretion (insulin, oestrogens, and human chorionic gonadotropin).[136] The dramatic decline in leptin levels observed after delivery might play a role in the reduced fertility observed during the lactation period.[134,137]

14.5.2.3 Age-Related Changes in Leptin

Several studies have investigated the effects of age on leptin levels and body composition but have produced conflicting evidence as age-related fat increase is the main confounding factor.[138,139] Further, leptin secretion is also affected by several metabolic and hormonal factors that change with ageing. Insulin,[140] glucocorticoids,[141] thyroid hormones,[142] and E2[143] have been shown to stimulate leptin, while testosterone inhibits leptin secretion. In an interesting but under-powered cross-sectional study of 150 men and 320 healthy women of different body weight and of a wide age range (18–77 years), serum leptin was found to gradually decline with age. The BMI-adjusted leptin levels were progressively lower with increasing age in obese and nonobese persons, but in men the difference was not statistically significant. Leptin reduction was also independent of other hormones subject to age-related changes, such as GH, insulin-like growth factor, prolactin, and insulin.[144]

14.6 Growth Hormone

The growth hormone/insulin-like growth factor (GH/IGF) axis regulates growth (e.g. bone growth and mass, and skeletal maturation)[145] and metabolism.[146] GH, also known as somatotropin, is secreted from the pituitary gland into the circulation, which is positively and negatively regulated by hypothalamic peptides, GH-releasing hormone (GHRH) and somatostatin (also known as somatotropin releasing-inhibiting factor, SRIF), respectively (Figure 14.4). GH secretion is also regulated by other neuropeptides and hormones[147] as well as the body's nutritional state (i.e. caloric restriction and overnutrition).[148] Circulating GH, then, stimulates IGF-1 production in many tissues, but primarily the liver. The elevated blood GH and IGF-1 concentration have an inhibitory effect on GH release from the pituitary. GH blocks insulin action, promotes lipolysis, and prevents lipogenesis, whereas IGF-1 has opposite effects.[149,150] The actions of the GH/IGF axis in response to nutrient availability is well-reviewed elsewhere.[146,148]

There are sex differences in the secretion of GH and IGF-1. For pubertal and adult women, spontaneous GH secretion by the pituitary gland is twice that of men, while IGF-1 levels are similar in both sexes, suggesting a lower sensitivity and less peripheral response to GH in females.[151] Oestrogens reduce GH-induced hepatic production of IGF-1; therefore, the increased secretion of GH can be interpreted as a compensatory response of the pituitary gland to counteract this liver resistance mediated by oestrogens. Sex differences in GH secretion begin with puberty, because of the influence of androgens. Jaffe et al. showed that recombinant IGF-1 infusion suppresses GH secretion both in basal and after GHRH stimulation in males but not in females, demonstrating the existence of sexual dimorphism also in the central regulatory mechanisms involved in GH secretion in humans.[152]

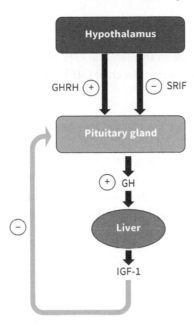

Figure 14.4 The GH/IGF1 axis. GH, growth hormone; IGF-1, insulin-like growth factor; GHRH, growth hormone-releasing hormone; SRIF, somatostatin.

14.5.3 Changes Across the Life Stage in Growth Hormone

14.5.3.1 GH/IGF-1 Axis in Development

The GH/IGF-1 axis is involved in numerous processes during all stages of life, from intra-uterine growth to senescence. During childhood and adolescence, the combined actions of GH and IGF-1 stimulate longitudinal bone growth and somatic maturation.[153] In both sexes, serum concentrations of GH and IGF1 increased during puberty, but earlier in girls than boys[154] and together with sex steroid hormones contribute to adolescent growth spurt.[155] The increase in GH secretion is mainly characterised by an increase in GH pulse amplitude rather than in the frequency and is likely an oestrogen-dependent effect.[156]

14.5.3.2 GH/IGF/1 Axis in Pregnancy

The somatotropic axis during pregnancy undergoes physiological changes with the progressive increase of E2 levels and which at peak increases in concentration by a factor of several hundred, induces a state of liver resistance to GH and, consequently, a reduction of IGF-1 synthesis.[157] From weeks 12–20 of pregnancy, the human placenta begins to produce a form of growth hormone (placental GH), which gradually increases to a peak in the third trimester.[158] Placental GH is not pulsatile secreted, as it is not under hypothalamic control, and has a structure similar to maternal pituitary GH. Therefore, it is able to stimulate the production of IGF-1, which increases two- to threefold in the second half of pregnancy with a peak at about 37 weeks.[159] Meanwhile, because of a negative feedback mechanism, GH secretion by maternal pituitary gland is progressively suppressed.

Placental GH does not appear to have a direct effect on fetal growth, but in the maternal liver and other organs it stimulates gluconeogenesis, lipolysis, and anabolism, thereby increasing nutrient availability for the fetoplacental unit.[160] In summary, placental GH levels progressively increase and exceed resistance to GH during pregnancy; consequently, in the last weeks of pregnancy, both placental GH and IGF-1 reach peak concentrations. Thereafter, a few days after delivery, placental GH becomes undetectable, and IGF-1 drops significantly.[161]

14.5.3.3 Age-Related Changes in the GH/IGF Axis

After reaching adulthood, GH and IGF-1 secretion continuously declines to very low levels in people aged ≥60 years: this phenomenon is known as 'somatopause'.[162] The age-related decline in GH secretion is associated with a general parallel but less-pronounced reduction of IGF-1 levels that is believed to contribute to functional deficits development during ageing. Indeed, recent studies have provided new evidence for the role of IGF-1 in maintaining brain microcirculation in the elderly.[163]

14.6 Conclusions

This chapter provides an overview of the main endocrine axes of women's physiology and their changes throughout their life, as summarised in Figure 14.5. Hormones are primarily involved in all key aspects of female physiology. The responsibility for coordinating the hormonal response to internal and external stimuli rests with the pituitary gland, through the release of stimulating hormones. In particular, information from the surrounding environment and peripherical systems are analysed, mediated by nerve and endocrine pathways, which contribute to the complicated feedback that is the basis of hormonal regulation. These complicated mechanisms clearly vary according to age, both as a consequence of ageing and

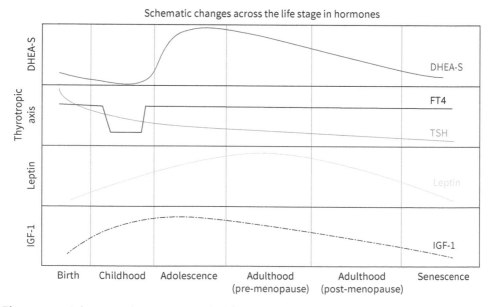

Figure 14.5 Schematic changes across the life course in the main hormones. See plate section.

as regulators of each stage of women's life, such as infancy, puberty, pregnancy, menopause, and senescence.

Key messages and implications

- Hormones are involved in virtually all physiological regulation, including key processes as growth, sexual maturation and fertility, metabolism, and circadian rhythms.
- Hormones secretion is finely regulated by hypothalamus–pituitary axis, which is capable of analysing and integrating information from peripherical organs and external environment.
- This fine regulation constantly adapts and changes throughout a woman's life.
- The regulation of the pituitary axes is responsible for the main changes in women's life, through childhood, puberty, pregnancy, menopause, and senescence.

References

1. Juul F, Chang VW, Brar P, Parekh N. Birth weight, early life weight gain and age at menarche: a systematic review of longitudinal studies. *Obesity Review*. 2017;18(11):1272–88.
2. Krieger N. Commentary: society, biology and the logic of social epidemiology. *International Journal of Epidemiology*. 2001;30(1):44–6.
3. Plant TM. 60 years of neuroendocrinology: the hypothalamo-pituitary-gonadal axis. *Journal of Endocrinology*. 2015;226(2):T41–T54.
4. Rance NE, Krajewski SJ, Smith MA, Cholanian M, Dacks PA. Neurokinin B and the hypothalamic regulation of reproduction. *Brain Research*. 2010;1364:116–28.
5. Wakabayashi Y, Nakada T, Murata K, Ohkura S, Mogi K, Navarro VM, et al. Neurokinin B and dynorphin A in kisspeptin neurons of the arcuate nucleus participate in generation of periodic oscillation of neural activity driving pulsatile gonadotropin-releasing hormone secretion in the goat. *Journal of Neuroscience*. 2010;30(8):3124–32.
6. Kuiri-Hanninen T, Sankilampi U, Dunkel L. Activation of the hypothalamic-pituitary-gonadal axis in infancy: minipuberty. *Hormone Research in Paediatrics*. 2014;82(2):73–80.
7. Terasawa E, Fernandez DL. Neurobiological mechanisms of the onset of puberty in primates. *Endocrine Review*. 2001;22(1):111–51.
8. Abreu AP, Dauber A, Macedo DB, Noel SD, Brito VN, Gill JC, et al. Central precocious puberty caused by mutations in the imprinted gene MKRN3. *New England Journal of Medicine*. 2013;368(26):2467–75.
9. Frisch RE, Revelle R. Height and weight at menarche and a hypothesis of critical body weights and adolescent events. *Science*. 1970;169(3943):397–9.
10. Pralong FP. Insulin and NPY pathways and the control of GnRH function and puberty onset. *Molecular and Cellular Endocrinology*. 2010;324(1-2):82–6.
11. Moret M, Stettler R, Rodieux F, Gaillard RC, Waeber G, Wirthner D, et al. Insulin modulation of luteinizing hormone secretion in normal female volunteers and lean polycystic ovary syndrome patients. *Neuroendocrinology*. 2009;89(2):131–9.
12. Ahima RS, Saper CB, Flier JS, Elmquist JK. Leptin regulation of neuroendocrine systems. *Frontiers in Neuroendocrinology*. 2000;21(3):263–307.
13. Farooqi IS, O'Rahilly S. 20 years of leptin: human disorders of leptin action. *Journal of Neuroendocrinology*. 2014;223(1):T63–T70.
14. Zigman JM, Elmquist JK. Minireview: From anorexia to obesity—the yin and yang of body weight control. *Endocrinology*. 2003;144(9):3749–56.

15. Lanfranco F, Bonelli L, Baldi M, Me E, Broglio F, Ghigo E. Acylated ghrelin inhibits spontaneous luteinizing hormone pulsatility and responsiveness to naloxone but not that to gonadotropin-releasing hormone in young men: evidence for a central inhibitory action of ghrelin on the gonadal axis. *Journal of Clinical Endocrinology and Metabolism*. 2008;93(9):3633–9.

16. Kempna P, Marti N, Udhane S, Fluck CE. Regulation of androgen biosynthesis—a short review and preliminary results from the hyperandrogenic starvation NCI-H295R cell model. *Molecular and Cellular Endocrinology*. 2015;408:124–32.

17. Xing Y, Lerario AM, Rainey W, Hammer GD. Development of adrenal cortex zonation. *Endocrinology and Metabolism Clinics of North America*. 2015;44(2):243–74.

18. Wu T, Mendola P, Buck GM. Ethnic differences in the presence of secondary sex characteristics and menarche among US girls: the Third National Health and Nutrition Examination Survey, 1988–1994. *Pediatrics*. 2002;110(4):752–7.

19. Rosenfield RL, Lipton RB, Drum ML. Thelarche, pubarche, and menarche attainment in children with normal and elevated body mass index. *Pediatrics*. 2009;123(1):84–8.

20. Hall J. Neuroendocrine control of the menstrual cycle In: Strauss JF, Barbieri RL, eds., *Yen and Jaffe's reproductive endocrinology, 7th edition*. Philadelphia: Elsevier. 2013; pp. 141–56.

21. Davis SR, Lambrinoudaki I, Lumsden M, Mishra GD, Pal L, Rees M, et al. Menopause. *Nature Review Disease Primers*. 2015;1:15004.

22. Jarvela IY, Ruokonen A, Tekay A. Effect of rising hCG levels on the human corpus luteum during early pregnancy. *Human Reproduction*. 2008;23(12):2775–81.

23. Roh E, Song DK, Kim MS. Emerging role of the brain in the homeostatic regulation of energy and glucose metabolism. *Experimental & Molecular Medicine*. 2016;48:e216.

24. Malenka RC, Nicoll RA. Long-term potentiation—a decade of progress? *Science*. 1999;285(5435):1870–4.

25. Gougeon A. Regulation of ovarian follicular development in primates: facts and hypotheses. *Endocrine Review*. 1996;17(2):121–55.

26. Gosden RG, Faddy MJ. Ovarian aging, follicular depletion, and steroidogenesis. *Experimetnal Gerontology*. 1994;29(3-4):265–74.

27. Soleimani R, Heytens E, Darzynkiewicz Z, Oktay K. Mechanisms of chemotherapy-induced human ovarian aging: double strand DNA breaks and microvascular compromise. *Aging (Albany NY)*. 2011;3(8):782–93.

28. Mattison DR. The mechanisms of action of reproductive toxins. *American Journal of Industrial Medicine*. 1983;4(1–2):65–79.

29. Cramer DW, Xu H. Predicting age at menopause. *Maturitas*. 1996;23(3):319–26.

30. Gold EB, Bromberger J, Crawford S, Samuels S, Greendale GA, Harlow SD, et al. Factors associated with age at natural menopause in a multiethnic sample of midlife women. *American Journal of Epidemiology*. 2001;153(9):865–74.

31. de Bruin JP, Nikkels PG, Bruinse HW, van Haaften M, Looman CW, te Velde ER. Morphometry of human ovaries in normal and growth-restricted fetuses. *Early Human Development*. 2001;60(3):179–92.

32. Treloar SA, Do KA, Martin NG. Genetic influences on the age at menopause. *Lancet*. 1998;352(9134):1084–5.

33. Snieder H, MacGregor AJ, Spector TD. Genes control the cessation of a woman's reproductive life: a twin study of hysterectomy and age at menopause. *Journal of Clinical Endocrinology and Metabolism*. 1998;83(6):1875–80.

34. Cui L, Qin Y, Gao X, Lu J, Geng L, Ding L, et al. Antimullerian hormone: correlation with age and androgenic and metabolic factors in women from birth to postmenopause. *Fertility and Sterility*. 2016;105(2):481–5e1.

35. Gill S, Lavoie HB, Bo-Abbas Y, Hall JE. Negative feedback effects of gonadal steroids are preserved with aging in postmenopausal women. *Journal of Clinical Endocrinology and Metabolism*. 2002;87(5):2297–302.

36. Gill S, Sharpless JL, Rado K, Hall JE. Evidence that GnRH decreases with gonadal steroid feedback but increases with age in postmenopausal women. *Journal of Clinical Endocrinology and Metabolism*. 2002;87(5):2290–6.

37. Hannah-Shmouni F, Koch C. Adrenal cortex, physiology January 2018. In: *Reference module in biomedical sciences.* Encyclopedia of Endocrine Disease, 2th Edition; 2018. DOI: 10.1016/B978-0-12-801238-3.11098-0.

38. Angelousi A, Margioris AN, Tsatsanis C. ACTH action on the adrenals. In: Feingold KR, Anawalt B, Boyce A, Chrousos G, de Herder WW, Dungan K, et al., eds. *Endotext.* South Dartmouth, MA: MDText.com; 2000.

39. Kadmiel M, Cidlowski JA. Glucocorticoid receptor signaling in health and disease. *Trends in Pharmacological Sciences.* 2013;34(9):518–30.

40. Pruessner JC, Wolf OT, Hellhammer DH, Buske-Kirschbaum A, von Auer K, Jobst S, et al. Free cortisol levels after awakening: a reliable biological marker for the assessment of adrenocortical activity. *Life Sciences.* 1997;61(26):2539–49.

41. Wust S, Wolf J, Hellhammer DH, Federenko I, Schommer N, Kirschbaum C. The cortisol awakening response—normal values and confounds. *Noise & Health.* 2000;2(7):79–88.

42. Edwards S, Clow A, Evans P, Hucklebridge F. Exploration of the awakening cortisol response in relation to diurnal cortisol secretory activity. *Life Sciences.* 2001;68(18):2093–103.

43. Van Cauter E, Leproult R, Kupfer DJ. Effects of gender and age on the levels and circadian rhythmicity of plasma cortisol. *Journal of Clinical Endocrinology and Metabolism.* 1996;81(7):2468–73.

44. Roelfsema F, van Heemst D, Iranmanesh A, Takahashi P, Yang R, Veldhuis JD. Impact of age, sex and body mass index on cortisol secretion in 143 healthy adults. *Endocrine Connections.* 2017;6(7):500–9.

45. Nakamura Y, Gang HX, Suzuki T, Sasano H, Rainey WE. Adrenal changes associated with adrenarche. *Reviews in Endocrine and Metabolic Disorders.* 2009;10(1):19–26.

46. Carr BR, Parker CR, Jr., Madden JD, MacDonald PC, Porter JC. Maternal plasma adrenocorticotropin and cortisol relationships throughout human pregnancy. *American Journal of Obstetrics and Gynecology.* 1981;139(4):416–22.

47. Cousins L, Rigg L, Hollingsworth D, Meis P, Halberg F, Brink G, et al. Qualitative and quantitative assessment of the circadian rhythm of cortisol in pregnancy. *American Journal of Obstetrics and Gynecology.* 1983;145(4):411–16.

48. Wilson EA, Finn AE, Rayburn W, Jawad MJ. Corticosteroid-binding globulin and estrogens in maternal and cord blood. *American Journal of Obstetrics and Gynecology.* 1979;135(2):215–18.

49. Jung C, Ho JT, Torpy DJ, Rogers A, Doogue M, Lewis JG, et al. A longitudinal study of plasma and urinary cortisol in pregnancy and postpartum. *Journal of Clinical Endocrinology and Metabolism.* 2011;96(5):1533–40.

50. Lindsay JR, Nieman LK. The hypothalamic-pituitary-adrenal axis in pregnancy: challenges in disease detection and treatment. *Endocrine Reviews.* 2005;26(6):775–99.

51. Petraglia F, Sawchenko PE, Rivier J, Vale W. Evidence for local stimulation of ACTH secretion by corticotropin-releasing factor in human placenta. *Nature.* 1987;328(6132):717–19.

52. Nolten WE, Rueckert PA. Elevated free cortisol index in pregnancy: possible regulatory mechanisms. *American Journal of Obstetrics and Gynecology.* 1981;139(4):492–8.

53. Seckl JR. Glucocorticoid programming of the fetus: adult phenotypes and molecular mechanisms. *Molecular and Cellular Endocrinology.* 2001;185(1–2):61–71.

54. Magiakou MA, Mastorakos G, Rabin D, Dubbert B, Gold PW, Chrousos GP. Hypothalamic corticotropin-releasing hormone suppression during the postpartum period: implications for the increase in psychiatric manifestations at this time. *Journal of Clinical Endocrinology and Metabolism.* 1996;81(5):1912–17.

55. Brunton PJ, Russell JA, Douglas AJ. Adaptive responses of the maternal hypothalamic-pituitary-adrenal axis during pregnancy and lactation. *Journal of Neuroendocrinology.* 2008;20(6):764–76.

56. Parker CR, Jr., Slayden SM, Azziz R, Crabbe SL, Hines GA, Boots LR, et al. Effects of aging on adrenal function in the human: responsiveness and sensitivity of adrenal androgens and cortisol to adrenocorticotropin in premenopausal and postmenopausal women. *Journal of Clinical Endocrinology and Metabolism.* 2000;85(1):48–54.

57. Wilkinson CW, Peskind ER, Raskind MA. Decreased hypothalamic-pituitary-adrenal axis sensitivity to cortisol feedback inhibition in human aging. *Neuroendocrinology.* 1997;65(1):79–90.

58. Laughlin GA, Barrett-Connor E. Sexual dimorphism in the influence of advanced aging on adrenal hormone levels: the Rancho Bernardo Study. *Journal of Clinical Endocrinology and Metabolism.* 2000;85(10):3561–8.
59. Auchus RJ, Rainey WE. Adrenarche—physiology, biochemistry and human disease. *Clinical Endocrinology (Oxford).* 2004;60(3):288–96.
60. Orentreich N, Brind JL, Rizer RL, Vogelman JH. Age changes and sex differences in serum dehydro-epiandrosterone sulfate concentrations throughout adulthood. *Journal of Clinical Endocrinology and Metabolism.* 1984;59(3):551–5.
61. Parker CR, Jr., Mixon RL, Brissie RM, Grizzle WE. Aging alters zonation in the adrenal cortex of men. *Journal of Clinical Endocrinology and Metabolism.* 1997;82(11):3898–901.
62. Yen PM. Physiological and molecular basis of thyroid hormone action. *Physiological Reviews.* 2001;81(3):1097–142.
63. Larsen PR, Silva JE, Kaplan MM. Relationships between circulating and intracellular thyroid hormones: physiological and clinical implications. *Endocrine Reviews.* 1981;2(1):87–102.
64. Cheng SY, Leonard JL, Davis PJ. Molecular aspects of thyroid hormone actions. *Endocrine Reviews.* 2010;31(2):139–70.
65. Luidens MK, Mousa SA, Davis FB, Lin H-Y, Davis PJ. Thyroid hormone and angiogenesis. *Vascular Pharmacology.* 2010;52(3-4):142–5.
66. Davis PJ, Davis FB, Mousa SA, Luidens MK, Lin H-Y. Membrane receptor for thyroid hormone: physiologic and pharmacologic implications. *Annual Review of Pharmacology and Toxicology.* 2011;51:99–115.
67. Roelfsema F, Boelen A, Kalsbeek A, Fliers E. Regulatory aspects of the human hypothalamus-pituitary-thyroid axis. *Best Practice & Research Clinical Endocrinology & Metabolism.* 2017;31(5):487–503.
68. Mullur R, Liu Y-Y, Brent GA. Thyroid hormone regulation of metabolism. *Physiological Reviews.* 2014;94(2):355–82.
69. Bernal J. Thyroid hormone receptors in brain development and function. *Nature Clinical Practice Endocrinology & Metabolism.* 2007;3(3):249–59.
70. Chan SY, Vasilopoulou E, Kilby MD. The role of the placenta in thyroid hormone delivery to the fetus. *Nature Clinical Practice Endocrinology & Metabolism.* 2009;5(1):45–54.
71. Fisher DA, Nelson JC, Carlton EI, Wilcox RB. Maturation of human hypothalamic-pituitary-thyroid function and control. *Thyroid.* 2000;10(3):229–34.
72. Mariotti S, Barbesino G, Caturegli P, Bartalena L, Sansoni P, Fagnoni F, et al. Complex alteration of thyroid function in healthy centenarians. *Journal of Clinical Endocrinology and Metabolism.* 1993;77(5):1130–4.
73. Runnels BL, Garry PJ, Hunt WC, Standefer JC. Thyroid function in a healthy elderly population: implications for clinical evaluation. *Journal of Gerontology.* 1991;46(1):B39–B44.
74. van Coevorden A, Laurent E, Decoster C, Kerkhofs M, Neve P, van Cauter E, et al. Decreased basal and stimulated thyrotropin secretion in healthy elderly men. *Journal of Clinical Endocrinology and Metabolism.* 1989;69(1):177–85.
75. Knudsen N, Jorgensen T, Rasmussen S, Christiansen E, Perrild H. The prevalence of thyroid dysfunction in a population with borderline iodine deficiency. *Clinical Endocrinology (Oxford).* 1999;51(3):361–7.
76. Wiedemann G, Jonetz-Mentzel L, Panse R. Establishment of reference ranges for thyrotropin, triiodothyronine, thyroxine and free thyroxine in neonates, infants, children and adolescents. *European Journal of Clinical Chemistry and Clinical Biochemistry.* 1993;31(5):277–88.
77. Hotelling DR, Sherwood LM. The effects of pregnancy on circulating triiodothyronine. *Journal of Clinical Endocrinology & Metabolism.* 1971;33(5):783–6.
78. Yoshimura M, Hershman JM. Thyrotropic action of human chorionic gonadotropin. *Thyroid.* 1995;5(5):425–34.
79. Glinoer D. The regulation of thyroid function in pregnancy: pathways of endocrine adaptation from physiology to pathology. *Endocrine Reviews.* 1997;18(3):404–33.
80. Sack J. Thyroid function in pregnancy—maternal-fetal relationship in health and disease. *Pediatric Endocrinology Review.* 2003;1(Suppl 2):170–6; discussion 6.

81. Leung AM. Thyroid function in pregnancy. *Journal of Trace Elements in Medicine and Biology*. 2012;26(2–3):137–40.

82. Andersen SL, Laurberg P. Iodine supplementation in pregnancy and the dilemma of ambiguous recommendations. *European Thyroid Journal*. 2016;5(1):35–43.

83. Gernand AD, Schulze KJ, Stewart CP, West KP, Jr., Christian P. Micronutrient deficiencies in pregnancy worldwide: health effects and prevention. *Nature Reviews Endocrinology*. 2016;12(5):274–89.

84. Surks MI, Boucai L. Age- and race-based serum thyrotropin reference limits. *Journal of Clinical Endocrinology & Metabolism*. 2010;95(2):496–502.

85. Hadlow NC, Rothacker KM, Wardrop R, Brown SJ, Lim EM, Walsh JP. The relationship between TSH and free T4 in a large population is complex and nonlinear and differs by age and sex. *Journal of Clinical Endocrinology & Metabolism*. 2013;98(7):2936–43.

86. Park SY, Kim HI, Oh H-K, Kim TH, Jang HW, Chung JH, et al. Age- and gender-specific reference intervals of TSH and free T4 in an iodine-replete area: data from Korean National Health and Nutrition Examination Survey IV (2013–2015). *PLoS ONE*. 2018;13(2):e0190738.

87. Fontes R, Coeli CR, Aguiar F, Vaisman M. Reference interval of thyroid stimulating hormone and free thyroxine in a reference population over 60 years old and in very old subjects (over 80 years): comparison to young subjects. *Thyroid Research*. 2013;6(1):13.

88. Corsonello A, Montesanto A, Berardelli M, De Rango F, Dato S, Mari V, et al. A cross-section analysis of FT3 age-related changes in a group of old and oldest-old subjects, including centenarians' relatives, shows that a down-regulated thyroid function has a familial component and is related to longevity. *Age and Ageing*. 2010;39(6):723–7.

89. Peeters RP. Thyroid hormones and aging. *Hormones (Athens)*. 2008;7(1):28–35.

90. Vanderpump MPJ, Tunbridge WMG, French JM, Appleton D, Bates D, Clark F, et al. The incidence of thyroid disorders in the community: a twenty-year follow-up of the Whickham Survey. *Clinical Endocrinology*. 1995;43(1):55–68.

91. Turnbridge WMG, Everet DC, Hall R, Appleton D, Brewis M, Clark F, et al. The spectrum of thyroid disease in a community: the Whickham Survey. *Clinical Endocrinology*. 1977;7(6):481–93.

92. Gussekloo J, van Exel E, de Craen AJM, Meinders AE, Frölich M, Westendorp RGJ. Thyroid status, disability and cognitive function, and survival in old age. *Journal of the American Medical Association*. 2004;292(21):2591–9.

93. Jansen SW, Akintola AA, Roelfsema F, van der Spoel E, Cobbaert CM, Ballieux BE, et al. Human longevity is characterised by high thyroid stimulating hormone secretion without altered energy metabolism. *Scientific Reports*. 2015;5(1):11525.

94. Cornejo MP, Hentges ST, Maliqueo M, Coirini H, Becu Villalobos D, Elias CF. Neuroendocrine regulation of metabolism. *Journal of Neuroendocrinology*. 2016;28(7).

95. Roh E, Kim M-S. Brain regulation of energy metabolism. *Endocrinology and Metabolism*. 2016;31(4):519–24.

96. Arvat E, Maccario M, Di Vito L, Broglio F, Benso A, Gottero C, et al. Endocrine activities of ghrelin, a natural growth hormone secretagogue (GHS), in humans: comparison and interactions with hexarelin, a nonnatural peptidyl GHS, and GH-releasing hormone. *Journal of Clinical Endocrinology and Metabolism*. 2001;86(3):1169–74.

97. Wren AM, Seal LJ, Cohen MA, Brynes AE, Frost GS, Murphy KG, et al. Ghrelin enhances appetite and increases food intake in humans. *Journal of Clinical Endocrinology and Metabolism*. 2001;86(12):5992.

98. Broglio F, Arvat E, Benso A, Gottero C, Muccioli G, Papotti M, et al. Ghrelin, a natural GH secretagogue produced by the stomach, induces hyperglycemia and reduces insulin secretion in humans. *Journal of Clinical Endocrinology and Metabolism*. 2001;86(10):5083–6.

99. Mason BL, Wang Q, Zigman JM. The central nervous system sites mediating the orexigenic actions of ghrelin. *Annual Review of Physiology*. 2014;76:519–33.

100. Kojima M, Hosoda H, Date Y, Nakazato M, Matsuo H, Kangawa K. Ghrelin is a growth-hormone-releasing acylated peptide from stomach. *Nature*. 1999;402(6762):656–60.

101. Tanaka K, Minoura H, Isobe T, Yonaha H, Kawato H, Wang DF, et al. Ghrelin is involved in the decidualization of human endometrial stromal cells. *Journal of Clinical Endocrinology and Metabolism*. 2003;88(5):2335–40.

102. Fuglsang J, Skjærbæk C, Espelund U, Frystyk J, Fisker S, Flyvbjerg A, et al. Ghrelin and its relationship to growth hormones during normal pregnancy. *Clinical Endocrinology*. 2005;62(5):554–9.

103. Gualillo O, Caminos JE, Blanco M, Garcìa-Caballero T, Kojima M, Kangawa K, et al. Ghrelin, a novel placental-derived hormone. This work was supported by grants from Xunta de Galicia: PGIDT99PXI20802B, PGIDT99PXI20806B, and Fondo de Investigación Sanitaria, Spanish Ministry of Health, and DGCYT. *Endocrinology*. 2001;142(2):788–94.

104. Nakahara K, Nakagawa M, Baba Y, Sato M, Toshinai K, Date Y, et al. Maternal ghrelin plays an important role in rat fetal development during pregnancy. *Endocrinology*. 2006;147(3):1333–42.

105. Hehir MP, Glavey SV, Morrison JJ. Uterorelaxant effect of ghrelin on human myometrial contractility. *American Journal of Obstetrics and Gynecology*. 2008;198(3):323e1–5.

106. Cortelazzi D, Cappiello V, Morpurgo PS, Ronzoni S, Nobile De Santis MS, Cetin I, et al. Circulating levels of ghrelin in human fetuses. *European Journal of Endocrinology*. 2003;149(2):111–16.

107. Soriano-Guillen L, Barrios V, Chowen JA, Sanchez I, Vila S, Quero J, et al. Ghrelin levels from fetal life through early adulthood: relationship with endocrine and metabolic and anthropometric measures. *Journal of Pediatrics*. 2004;144(1):30–5.

108. Repaci A, Gambineri A, Pagotto U, Pasquali R. Ghrelin and reproductive disorders. *Molecular and Cellular Endocrinology*. 2011;340(1):70–9.

109. Serra-Prat M, Papiol M, Monteis R, Palomera E, Cabré M. Relationship between plasma ghrelin levels and sarcopenia in elderly subjects: a cross-sectional study. *Journal of Nutrition, Health & Aging*. 2015;19(6):669–72.

110. Sturm K, MacIntosh CG, Parker BA, Wishart J, Horowitz M, Chapman IM. Appetite, food intake, and plasma concentrations of cholecystokinin, ghrelin, and other gastrointestinal hormones in undernourished older women and well-nourished young and older women. *Journal of Clinical Endocrinology & Metabolism*. 2003;88(8):3747–55.

111. Rigamonti A, Pincelli A, Corra B, Viarengo R, Bonomo S, Galimberti D, et al. Plasma ghrelin concentrations in elderly subjects: comparison with anorexic and obese patients. *Journal of Endocrinology*. 2002;175(1):R1–R5.

112. Nass R, Farhy LS, Liu J, Pezzoli SS, Johnson ML, Gaylinn BD, et al. Age-dependent decline in acyl-ghrelin concentrations and reduced association of acyl-ghrelin and growth hormone in healthy older adults. *Journal of Clinical Endocrinology & Metabolism*. 2014;99(2):602–8.

113. Amitani M, Amitani H, Cheng KC, Kairupan TS, Sameshima N, Shimoshikiryo I, et al. The role of ghrelin and ghrelin signaling in aging. *International Journal of Molecular Sciences*. 2017;18(7):1511.

114. Yin Y, Zhang W. The role of ghrelin in senescence: a mini-review. *Gerontology*. 2016;62(2):155–62.

115. Cheng-Shine Hwang, Thomas M. Loftus, Mandrup S, Lane MD. Adipocyte differentiation and leptin expression. *Annual Review of Cell and Developmental Biology*. 1997;13(1):231–59.

116. Smith-Kirwin SM, O'Connor DM, Johnston J, de Lancy E, Hassink SG, Funanage VL. Leptin expression in human mammary epithelial cells and breast milk. *Journal of Clinical Endocrinology & Metabolism*. 1998;83(5):1810.

117. Zhang F, Basinski MB, Beals JM, Briggs SL, Churgay LM, Clawson DK, et al. Crystal structure of the obese protein leptin-E100. *Nature*. 1997;387(6629):206–9.

118. Margetic S, Gazzola C, Pegg GG, Hill RA. Leptin: a review of its peripheral actions and interactions. *International Journal of Obesity and Related Metabolic Disorders*. 2002;26(11):1407–33.

119. Cinti S, Matteis RD, Pico C, Ceresi E, Obrador A, Maffeis C, et al. Secretory granules of endocrine and chief cells of human stomach mucosa contain leptin. *International Journal of Obesity and Related Metabolic Disorders*. 2000;24(6):789–93.

120. Jin L, Zhang S, Burguera BG, Couce ME, Osamura RY, Kulig E, et al. Leptin and leptin receptor expression in rat and mouse pituitary cells. *Endocrinology*. 2000;141(1):333–9.

121. Considine RV, Sinha MK, Heiman ML, Kriauciunas A, Stephens TW, Nyce MR, et al. Serum immunoreactive-leptin concentrations in normal-weight and obese humans. *New England Journal of Medicine*. 1996;334(5):292–5.

122. Boden G, Chen X, Mozzoli M, Ryan I. Effect of fasting on serum leptin in normal human subjects. *Journal of Clinical Endocrinology and Metabolism*. 1996;81(9):3419–23.

123. Balthasar N, Coppari R, McMinn J, Liu SM, Lee CE, Tang V, et al. Leptin receptor signaling in POMC neurons is required for normal body weight homeostasis. *Neuron*. 2004;42(6):983–91.

124. Biglari N, Gaziano I, Schumacher J, Radermacher J, Paeger L, Klemm P, et al. Functionally distinct POMC-expressing neuron subpopulations in hypothalamus revealed by intersectional targeting. *Nature Neuroscience*. 2021;24(7):913–29.

125. Betley JN, Xu S, Cao ZFH, Gong R, Magnus CJ, Yu Y, et al. Neurons for hunger and thirst transmit a negative-valence teaching signal. *Nature*. 2015;521(7551):180–5.

126. Clark JT, Kalra PS, Crowley WR, Kalra SP. Neuropeptide Y and human pancreatic polypeptide stimulate feeding behavior in rats. *Endocrinology*. 1984;115(1):427–9.

127. Rosenbaum M, Nicolson M, Hirsch J, Heymsfield SB, Gallagher D, Chu F, et al. Effects of gender, body composition, and menopause on plasma concentrations of leptin. *Journal of Clinical Endocrinology and Metabolism*. 1996;81(9):3424–7.

128. Zhang Y, Zitsman JL, Hou J, Fennoy I, Guo K, Feinberg J, et al. Fat cell size and adipokine expression in relation to gender, depot, and metabolic risk factors in morbidly obese adolescents. *Obesity (Silver Spring)*. 2014;22(3):691–7.

129. Ong KK, Ahmed ML, Sherriff A, Woods KA, Watts A, Golding J, et al. Cord blood leptin is associated with size at birth and predicts infancy weight gain in humans. ALSPAC Study Team. Avon Longitudinal Study of Pregnancy and Childhood. *Journal of Clinical Endocrinology and Metabolism*. 1999;84(3):1145–8.

130. Ong KK, Ahmed ML, Dunger DB. The role of leptin in human growth and puberty. *Acta Paediatrica-Supplement*. 1999;88(433):95–8.

131. Ahmed ML, Ong KK, Morrell DJ, Cox L, Drayer N, Perry L, et al. Longitudinal study of leptin concentrations during puberty: sex differences and relationship to changes in body composition. *Journal of Clinical Endocrinology and Metabolism*. 1999;84(3):899–905.

132. Blum WF, Englaro P, Hanitsch S, Juul A, Hertel NT, Muller J, et al. Plasma leptin levels in healthy children and adolescents: dependence on body mass index, body fat mass, gender, pubertal stage, and testosterone. *Journal of Clinical Endocrinology and Metabolism*. 1997;82(9):2904–10.

133. Mystkowski P, Schwartz MW. Gonadal steroids and energy homeostasis in the leptin era. *Nutrition*. 2000;16(10):937–46.

134. Hardie L, Trayhurn P, Abramovich D, Fowler P. Circulating leptin in women: a longitudinal study in the menstrual cycle and during pregnancy. *Clinical Endocrinology (Oxford)*. 1997;47(1):101–6.

135. Lewandowski K, Horn R, O'Callaghan CJ, Dunlop D, Medley GF, O'Hare P, et al. Free leptin, bound leptin, and soluble leptin receptor in normal and diabetic pregnancies. *Journal of Clinical Endocrinology and Metabolism*. 1999;84(1):300–6.

136. Sivan E, Whittaker PG, Sinha D, Homko CJ, Lin M, Reece EA, et al. Leptin in human pregnancy: the relationship with gestational hormones. *American Journal of Obstetrics & Gynecology*. 1998;179(5):1128–32.

137. Caprio M, Fabbrini E, Isidori AM, Aversa A, Fabbri A. Leptin in reproduction. *Trends in Endocrinology and Metabolism*. 2001;12(2):65–72.

138. Baumgartner RN, Waters DL, Morley JE, Patrick P, Montoya GD, Garry PJ. Age-related changes in sex hormones affect the sex difference in serum leptin independently of changes in body fat. *Metabolism*. 1999;48(3):378–84.

139. Ostlund RE, Jr., Yang JW, Klein S, Gingerich R. Relation between plasma leptin concentration and body fat, gender, diet, age, and metabolic covariates. *Journal of Clinical Endocrinology and Metabolism*. 1996;81(11):3909–13.

140. Ryan AS, Elahi D. The effects of acute hyperglycemia and hyperinsulinemia on plasma leptin levels: its relationships with body fat, visceral adiposity, and age in women. *Journal of Clinical Endocrinology and Metabolism*. 1996;81(12):4433–8.

141. Papaspyrou-Rao S, Schneider SH, Petersen RN, Fried SK. Dexamethasone increases leptin expression in humans in vivo. *Journal of Clinical Endocrinology and Metabolism*. 1997;82(5):1635–7.

142. Diekman MJ, Romijn JA, Endert E, Sauerwein H, Wiersinga WM. Thyroid hormones modulate serum leptin levels: observations in thyrotoxic and hypothyroid women. *Thyroid*. 1998;8(12):1081–6.

143. Licinio J, Negrao AB, Mantzoros C, Kaklamani V, Wong ML, Bongiorno PB, et al. Synchronicity of frequently sampled, 24-h concentrations of circulating leptin, luteinizing hormone, and estradiol in healthy women. *Proceedings of the National Academy of Sciences U S A*. 1998;95(5):2541–6.

144. Isidori AM, Strollo F, More M, Caprio M, Aversa A, Moretti C, et al. Leptin and aging: correlation with endocrine changes in male and female healthy adult populations of different body weights. *Journal of Clinical Endocrinology and Metabolism*. 2000;85(5):1954–62.

145. Mazziotti G, Lania AG, Canalis E. Skeletal disorders associated with the growth hormone-insulin-like growth factor 1 axis. *Nature Reviews Endocrinology*. 2022;18(6):353–65.

146. Møller N, Jørgensen JOL. Effects of growth hormone on glucose, lipid, and protein metabolism in human subjects. *Endocrine Reviews*. 2009;30(2):152–77.

147. Ghigo E, Arvat E, Bellone J, Ramunni J, Camanni F. Neurotransmitter control of growth hormone secretion in humans. *Journal of Pediatric Endocrinology and Metabolism*. 1993;6(3–4):263–6.

148. Caputo M, Pigni S, Agosti E, Daffara T, Ferrero A, Filigheddu N, et al. Regulation of GH and GH signaling by nutrients. *Cells*. 2021;10(6):1376.

149. Moller N, Jorgensen JO. Effects of growth hormone on glucose, lipid, and protein metabolism in human subjects. *Endocrine Reviews*. 2009;30(2):152–77.

150. Junnila RK, List EO, Berryman DE, Murrey JW, Kopchick JJ. The GH/IGF-1 axis in ageing and longevity. *Nature Reviews Endocrinology*. 2013;9(6):366–76.

151. van den Berg G, Veldhuis JD, Frolich M, Roelfsema F. An amplitude-specific divergence in the pulsatile mode of growth hormone (GH) secretion underlies the gender difference in mean GH concentrations in men and premenopausal women. *Journal of Clinical Endocrinology and Metabolism*. 1996;81(7):2460–7.

152. Jaffe CA, Ocampo-Lim B, Guo W, Krueger K, Sugahara I, DeMott-Friberg R, et al. Regulatory mechanisms of growth hormone secretion are sexually dimorphic. *Journal of Clinical Investigation*. 1998;102(1):153–64.

153. Benyi E, Savendahl L. The physiology of childhood growth: hormonal regulation. *Hormone Research in Paediatrics*. 2017;88(1):6–14.

154. Rose SR, Municchi G, Barnes KM, Kamp GA, Uriarte MM, Ross JL, et al. Spontaneous growth hormone secretion increases during puberty in normal girls and boys. *Journal of Clinical Endocrinology and Metabolism*. 1991;73(2):428–35.

155. Kerrigan JR, Rogol AD. The impact of gonadal steroid hormone action on growth hormone secretion during childhood and adolescence. *Endocrine Reviews*. 1992;13(2):281–98.

156. Loche S, Casini MR, Faedda A. The GH/IGF-I axis in puberty. *British Journal of Clinical Practice*. 1996;85:1–4.

157. Abucham J, Bronstein MD, Dias ML. Management of endocrine disease: acromegaly and pregnancy: a contemporary review. *European Journal of Endocrinology*. 2017;177(1):R1–R12.

158. Lacroix MC, Guibourdenche J, Frendo JL, Muller F, Evain-Brion D. Human placental growth hormone—a review. *Placenta*. 2002;23(Suppl A):S87–S94.

159. Muhammad A, Neggers SJ, van der Lely AJ. Pregnancy and acromegaly. *Pituitary*. 2017;20(1):179–84.

160. Alsat E, Guibourdenche J, Couturier A, Evain-Brion D. Physiological role of human placental growth hormone. *Moecular and Cellular Endocrinology*. 1998;140(1–2):121–7.

161. Frankenne F, Closset J, Gomez F, Scippo ML, Smal J, Hennen G. The physiology of growth hormones (GHs) in pregnant women and partial characterization of the placental GH variant. *Journal of Clinical Endocrinology and Metabolism*. 1988;66(6):1171–80.

162. Zadik Z, Chalew SA, McCarter RJ, Jr., Meistas M, Kowarski AA. The influence of age on the 24-hour integrated concentration of growth hormone in normal individuals. *Journal of Clinical Endocrinology and Metabolism*. 1985;60(3):513–6.

163. Sonntag WE, Deak F, Ashpole N, Toth P, Csiszar A, Freeman W, et al. Insulin-like growth factor-1 in CNS and cerebrovascular aging. *Frontiers in Aging Neuroscience*. 2013;5:27.

15

A Life Course Perspective on Women's Health Behaviours

Hsin-Fang Chung and Gita D. Mishra

15.1 Introduction

Observational epidemiological studies have linked a range of health-risk behaviours, such as smoking, alcohol use, unhealthy diet, and physical inactivity, to chronic disease in later life and support the notion that changes in these harmful behaviours can change or mitigate disease risk. However, interventions to change health behaviours and maintain behavioural change over the long term have had limited success.[1] The difficulty of changing adult behaviours has led to studies of young people to better understand the origins and development of individual behaviours and healthy lifestyles, and to recognise possibilities for early interventions.[2,3]

Although women generally engage less in health-risk behaviours than men do, health inequalities are often more pronounced among women, especially in socioeconomically disadvantaged groups. Therefore, it is critical to understand the socioenvironmental effects driving gender differences in health behaviours. This chapter outlines current perspectives on health behaviour research (Section 15.2) and presents a social and temporal context in women's health behaviours (Section 15.3). We set up a developmental life course framework to show the pathways for biological, social, psychological, and environmental factors in the initiation and maintenance of health behaviours through life (Section 15.4). We then discuss health behaviour changes during the COVID-19 pandemic (Section 15.5) and conclude with a brief outline of implications for health policy and future research (Section 15.6).

15.2 Current Perspectives on the Research of Health Behaviours

The role of poor health behaviours, such as smoking, unhealthy diet, and physical inactivity, in the origin of the current epidemic of chronic disease has been the driving factor for research and initiatives to change behaviours,[4] but many such interventions to change health behaviours and achieve long-term behavioural change have had limited success.[1] A recent evaluation of 103 reviews on the effectiveness of health behaviour interventions reported that half of the reviews focused on smoking (either prevention or cessation).[5] Physician advice, individual counselling, and workplace- and school-based activities were judged the most effective interventions across a range of health behaviours, but the evidence mostly related to

Hsin-Fang Chung and Gita D. Mishra, *A Life Course Perspective on Women's Health Behaviours* In: *A Life Course Approach to Women's Health*. Second Edition. Edited by: Gita D Mishra, Rebecca Hardy, and Diana Kuh, Oxford University Press. © Oxford University Press 2023. DOI: 10.1093/oso/9780192864642.003.0015 short-term effects (less than 3 months) rather than long-term impact.[5] Health psychologists previously emphasised the role of individual characteristics (e.g. attitudes, feelings, knowledge, and beliefs) in shaping health behaviours.[3] However, most health behaviours take place in social environments, and, therefore, efforts to change and maintain behaviours must take into account the social context (known as milieu: the social or physical setting in which something occurs or develops) and the political and economic forces that act directly on people's health regardless of individual choices.[4] Despite the importance of social, political, and economic circumstances, the intervention default has traditionally been individual behaviour change. In some ways, this is not surprising because the biggest drivers of the chronic disease epidemic—smoking, alcohol misuse, unhealthy diet, and physical inactivity—are self-evidently behaviours.[4] Thus, if we understand the psychological and socioenvironmental conditions preceding health behaviours, we are better able to support the change to healthier behaviours and their maintenance.

Despite the widely acknowledged link between individual characteristics or socioeconomic position (SEP) and health behaviours, there is still limited evidence addressing social inequalities according to gender, ethnicity, disability, and urban or rural location.[5] There are also challenges for recruitment of 'hard-to-reach' groups, such as ethnic minorities and socially and economically disadvantaged groups.[5] Further, awareness of health disparities among lesbian, gay, bisexual, transgender, intersex, queer, and asexual (LGBTIQA+) populations has increased in recent decades. For example, lesbian and bisexual women were found to have lower levels of engagement in healthy behaviours than were heterosexual women.[6] Continued efforts are needed to engage LGBTIQA + populations for overall well-being, especially in health-related behaviours.

The association between disadvantaged groups and poor health behaviours is well established in HICs, but it is not clear how behavioural risk factors are distributed in LMICs. A recent review of 75 studies from 39 LMICs found that more disadvantaged SEP groups had a significantly higher prevalence of tobacco and alcohol use and consumed less fruit, vegetables, fish, and fibre than advantaged SEP groups, whereas advantaged SEP groups were less physically active and consumed more fats, salt, and processed food than disadvantaged SEP groups.[7] When the studies stratified findings by sex, they mostly showed that inequalities were often more pronounced among women.[7] Compared with HICs, the prevalence of smoking among women is substantially lower in LMICs (3.1% vs 17.2%), while smoking in males is similar (around 30%). However, low rates of smoking among women in low income countries has been linked to high gender inequality and high fertility rate.[8]

15.3 Social and Temporal Context in Women's Health Behaviours

Social and economic development that triggered industrialisation, urbanisation, and globalisation has accelerated the 'epidemiological transition' with its associated changes in lifestyle.[3] Cultural and political forces influence the timing and speed of these lifestyle changes across different countries and social classes.[3] These socioenvironmental factors contribute to gender differences in many aspects, and that is generally greater where there is higher gender inequality.[9] This section presents the global trends in women's health behaviours and inequalities between countries and social classes.

15.3.1 Smoking

Large reductions in the prevalence of daily smoking were observed for both men and women since 1980, but the absolute numbers of smokers have increased because of population growth.[10] Since the adoption of the World Health Organization (WHO) Framework Convention on Tobacco Control in 2003, global smoking rates among women decreased from 8.0% to 5.8% between 2007 and 2017 (from 37.1% to 32.7% among men).[11] However, the prevalence of tobacco use among adolescents aged 13–15 years showed little overall change since 1999; only 20 out of 108 countries reported declining rates in girls and boys.[11] A large Australian study showed that women initiated smoking later than men in earlier cohorts (26.6 vs 19.0 years in the 1910–19 cohort). While both men and women initiated smoking increasingly earlier in the subsequent birth cohorts, this was more pronounced among women, converging in the 1960–69 cohort at 17.8 years for women and 17.6 years for men.[12] Similar patterns and temporal trends for smoking initiation were found in the Asian population, but Asians started smoking later than their Western counterparts.[13] Data from the Australian Longitudinal Study on Women's Health showed a decline in smoking prevalence with increasing age across four birth cohorts. For women in their early 20s, those born in 1989–95 had a much lower smoking prevalence than those born in 1973–78 (Figure 15.1). Girls and boys start smoking for different reasons. Regular smoking among teenage girls is related to low self-esteem, perceived physical development (looking older than their peers), and weight control.[14] Although women smoke less than men overall, women may find it more difficult to maintain long-term abstinence than men.[15] An understanding of the many factors that interact with sex and gender (including biological, psychological, social, environmental, and cultural factors) and how they relate to smoking cessation will help to design better cessation interventions that address these sex/gender differences.[15]

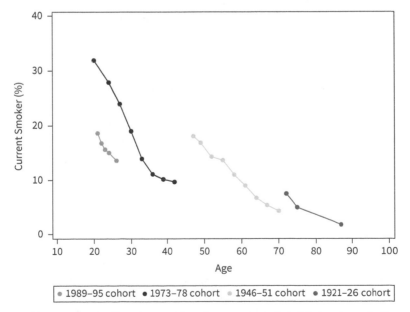

Figure 15.1 The prevalence of current smokers by age across four birth cohorts in the Australian Longitudinal Study on Women's Health. See plate section.

Low income is associated with higher smoking prevalence, particularly among women.[16] Tobacco companies have targeted marketing strategies at socially disadvantaged women in the United States for several decades, including price discounts, developing cheaper brands, and promoting luxury images.[17] Visual appearance and brands of cigarette packets have a strong influence on young women's decisions to take up and continue smoking.[18] In 2012, Australia was the first country to implement plain packaging to reduce the appeal of tobacco products, increase the effectiveness of the health warning, and reduce misperception about the harmfulness of cigarettes.[19] Following the lead of Australia, over 20 countries, including the UK, have adopted plain packaging.[20]

15.3.2 Alcohol and Illicit Drug Use

The global prevalence of current drinking among women decreased from 37.3% to 32.5% between 2000 and 2016 (from 57.9% to 53.6% among men).[21] Youth alcohol consumption and binge drinking are emerging public health issues. Globally, more than a quarter (26.5%) of 15–19 years old adolescents and 40.7% of young adults aged 20–24 are current drinkers.[21] School surveys found that alcohol use starts early in life and before the age of 15 years. There are remarkably small sex differences observed in the prevalence of past-30-days alcohol use between boys and girls aged 15 years in many countries of the Americas and Europe, but the prevalence varies greatly from 20% to 70%.[21] HICs generally have higher alcohol consumption and higher prevalence of current drinkers, while the prevalence of heavy episodic drinking among drinkers is fairly similar between high-income and low-income countries.[21] Frequency of alcohol use, binge drinking, and the type of alcohol consumed tend to vary by country and SEP. In Europe, disadvantaged SEP groups generally consume less alcohol overall, but are more likely to engage in harmful binge drinking and experience more alcohol-related harm.[22] In LMICs, alcohol use is more prevalent in disadvantaged SEP groups in Southeast Asia, but the association is less clear in Africa, and there is an abject paucity of data from other regions.[23]

Conversely, illicit drug use worldwide has been on the rise, increasing from 4.8% of the global population aged 15–64 years in 2009 to 5.3% in 2018, and one in three drug users is a woman.[24] Cannabis is the most used substance globally. Drug use is more widespread in high-income countries than in low-income countries, and it is higher in urban areas than in rural areas.[24] Poverty, low education, and social marginalisation are the major factors that increase the risk of drug use disorder and exacerbate the consequences.[24] Women, youth, vulnerable, and marginalised groups face barriers to receiving treatment services due to discrimination and stigma.[24]

15.3.3 Diet

A suboptimal diet is now one of the leading risk factors for chronic disease. Worldwide, intakes of healthful foods including vegetables, fruit, whole grains, fish, and nuts/seeds are substantially below current recommendations or optimal intakes.[25] Between 1990 and 2010, intakes of fruit, nuts and seeds, and red meat modestly increased; whole grains decreased; and vegetables, seafood, and processed meat remained stable.[25] For the same period, intakes of saturated fat, trans fat, and dietary cholesterol were stable, while omega-6, seafood omega-3, and plant omega-3 fat intakes increased.[26] Generally, energy-adjusted intakes of each food and dietary fats are not substantially different by sex, although women tend to have greater intakes of more healthful foods and consume slightly more saturated fat and plant omega-3 than men.[25,26] Diet quality follows a socioeconomic gradient–advantaged SEP groups consume more whole grains, lean meats, fish, low-fat dairy products, and fresh vegetables and fruit, whereas more disadvantaged groups consume more refined grains, added fats, and fatty meats.[27] The social determinants of food choice are complex and multifactorial and should consider structural factors, such as food prices, ease of access to grocery stores, transportation, inequities in access to healthy foods, as well as education and culture (e.g. social network and cultural traditions).[27]

15.3.4 Insufficient Physical Activity

Insufficient physical activity is defined as not doing at least 150 minutes of moderate-intensity or 75 minutes of vigorous-intensity physical activity per week, including activity at work, at home, for transport, and during leisure time.[28] Globally, more than a quarter (27.5%) of adults were insufficiently active in 2016, and women (31.7%) were less active than men (23.4%).[28] A temporal decrease of insufficient activity between 2001 and 2016 was observed for men (from 25.5% in 2001), but there was no change for women (from 31.5% in 2001), resulting in a widening of an already important gender difference.[28] The same trend was observed among adolescents aged 11–17 years, with a decrease of insufficient activity in boys but no change in girls.[29] With regards to the comparison between countries, the prevalence of insufficient activity among adults has increased over time in HICs (from 31.6% in 2001 to 36.8% in 2016), while it was stable in low-income countries (from 16.0% to 16.2%).[28] In 2016, 42.3% of women in high-income Western countries were insufficiently active, compared with 18.8% of women in low-income countries. Recent reviews reported convincing evidence that disadvantaged SEP is associated with insufficient leisure-time physical activity in both men and women, but is associated with higher levels of occupational physical activity (mainly in men).[30,31]

15.4 Life Course Framework for Health Behaviour

A developmental framework is inherent in the life course approach to health behaviours, showing the pathways from childhood socioeconomic environment to adult health behaviours, influenced by the various factors at different life stages (Figure 15.2).[2] Adolescence is a critical or sensitive period of development that involves biological, social, behavioural, and relationship changes. The changes may lead to special windows of susceptibility and imprint behaviour and have profound influences on health in later life. In this framework, the term *socioeconomic environment* covers any measures of SEP (e.g. education, income, and occupation) or associated dimension of social inequality in relation to social integration, social roles, and other psychosocial factors.[2] The effects of socioeconomic environment in childhood may operate through the development of education, behavioural capital (discussed in more detail in Section 15.4.3), and adult socioeconomic environment. However, the associations

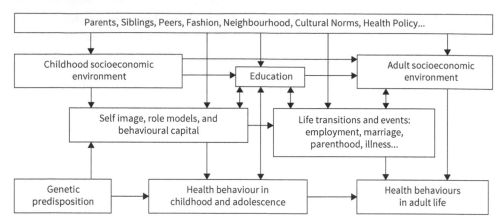

Figure 15.2 Developmental life course framework showing the pathways between childhood socioeconomic environment and adult health behaviours (originally published in Mishra et al., 2010).[2]

with health behaviours and health outcomes in adulthood are population-specific, reflecting social, economic, cultural, and ethnic differences.

15.4.1 Before Birth

Previous research has suggested that maternal age and health behaviours during pregnancy are related to offspring health behaviours. A Swedish study found that young adults who were born to teenage mothers (15–19 years) and older mothers (≥40 years) were more likely to smoke and to consume alcohol regularly, and those born to older mothers were also less likely to exercise regularly.[32] One explanation could be a lasting disadvantage from poor perinatal outcomes.[32] It is known that those born to younger and older mothers are at higher risk of preterm birth, low birthweight, and other pregnancy complications that can have long-term negative consequences.[33] Maternal smoking during pregnancy has been linked with an increased risk of offspring smoking initiation and tobacco dependence.[34–36] Inferring an intrauterine effect from epidemiological studies is difficult because intergenerational transmission of smoking behaviour may be strongly influenced by familial smoking during childhood and sociodemographic characteristics.[36]

A genetic predisposition (also called *genetic susceptibility*) is an increased likelihood of developing a particular disease because of specific genetic variations that are often inherited from a parent. Recent research has shown that genetic variants are also associated with offspring health behaviours. A 38-year longitudinal study of a New Zealand birth cohort found that genetic risk profile was not related to smoking initiation but accelerated the development of smoking behaviour.[37] Among individuals who initiated smoking, those at higher genetic risk were more likely to convert to daily smoking as teenagers, progressed more rapidly to having smoking and nicotine dependence, persisted longer in smoking heavily, and had more difficulty quitting.[37] Critically, the effects of genetic risk seemed to be limited to individuals who initiated smoking during adolescence,[37] yet another reason why adolescence is of crucial importance for preventing smoking initiation and targeting smoking cessation. Recently, a large genome-wide association study (GWAS) identified 18 significant loci associated with heavy drinking and alcohol use disorder,[38] and a systematic review of six GWAS reported up to 10 loci associated with physical activity or sedentary behaviour.[39] However, these genetic findings were not sex specific; there is a lack of sex-stratified GWAS of health behaviours.

15.4.2 Socioeconomic Environment in Childhood and the Initiation and Maintenance of Health Behaviours

The socioeconomic environment in childhood directly constrains that of adulthood through availability of material wealth and social resources or via accessibility to educational opportunities and other learning experiences.[2] Childhood socioeconomic environment also shapes the development of health behaviours during adolescence, primarily through the impact on self-identity and behavioural capital, which can have long-term effects on adult health behaviours.[2] Growing up in a disadvantaged socioeconomic environment (e.g. low parental education and poverty) and having adverse childhood experiences are associated with the initiation of some adverse health behaviours, and girls and boys could be affected differently. The inverse relationship between parental SEP gradients and adolescent substance use was most consistent for cigarette smoking (related to both parental education and income),[40–42] and the inequalities in smoking were more pronounced in girls.[42] However, the association with alcohol and illicit drug use was less consistent, depending on parental education or income.[40,41,43] It was found that alcohol consumption was more common in adolescents with a higher household income, but binge drinking was less common in those with higher maternal education.[41] There was no association between SEP and physical activity in preschool children, while in school-aged children and adolescents, the findings were inconsistent.[30] Many changes with respect to physical development and social interactions (e.g. school environment and peer influences) during the transition from childhood to adolescence might directly influence physical activity levels, making it difficult to accurately identify the impact of SEP.[30]

With respect to the maintenance of health behaviours, evidence has shown that childhood SEP has a long-term impact on adult behaviour, independent of SEP in adulthood. A large British birth cohort found disadvantaged childhood SEP predicted adult smoking for both men and women,[44] but it predicted persistent smoking only among women as the association was not significant among men when adjusted for adulthood SEP.[45] The link between childhood social disadvantage and adult smoking behaviour may be mediated by exposure to parental or peer smoking, adolescent conduct problems, and cognitive and educational factors.[46] Dietary habits have been found to depend partly on food preferences established from early childhood. However, childhood SEP seemed more important for women's adult food intake patterns, whereas adult SEP was more important for men.[47] Recent review studies also showed that lower childhood SEP was associated with less frequent physical activity during adulthood,[48,49] particularly among women.[49] The gender differences are likely explained by social rather than biological pathways given the absence of gender differences in how childhood SEP relates to an adult's capacity to undertake exercise.[49] Adverse childhood experiences, such as abuse and household dysfunction (i.e. separation or divorce, mental illness, substance abuse, violence, and incarceration), have also been related to poorer health behaviours and attributes in adult life, including smoking and drinking behaviour, illicit drug use, sedentary lifestyle, and severe obesity, independent of sex.[50-52] The choice of these harmful behaviours may be the direct result of the stressful experience and associated lifetime psychosocial orientations.

Educational attainment is often a protective factor for adult risk behaviours. Individuals with higher education levels are more likely to engage in health-promoting behaviours, with a particularly pronounced gradient among women.[53] Economic resources (i.e. income, health insurance, and family background), cognitive ability, knowledge, and social networks account for 60%–80% of the education gradient in health behaviours.[53] In turn, the adoption of healthy behaviours in adolescence has been shown to precede educational performance,[54] suggesting that common factors may be behind the better outcomes in both these domains, which we describe as 'behavioural capital'.[2,3]

15.4.3 Behavioural Capital

Behavioural capital is defined as 'the accumulation of positive individual attributes such as social competence, decision making and problem-solving skills, coping strategies, personal efficacy, self-esteem, attitudes and values that help the individual remain resilient in times of adversity or take advantage of talents and opportunities'.[3] It considers the kinds of adverse and protective childhood environments with short- and long-term effects on behavioural choices and the underlying mechanisms through which they may operate.[3] Many of the attributes of behavioural capital are acquired more easily during child and adolescent development, and while they can be acquired later, it is often harder to do so,[55] indicating childhood and adolescence is a sensitive period for initiating beneficial behaviours. Behavioural capital is likely to lead to the choice of healthy behaviours throughout life, either directly or indirectly, by influencing many aspects of adult life (e.g. educational achievements, employment, and social support) that shape adult behaviours.[3] Parental practices may play an important moderating role. It is found that parenting styles may influence child food consumption behaviours[56] and adolescent substance use.[57,58] Positive parenting practices may develop emotional resilience in terms of adversity.

15.4.4 Identity in Adolescence and Role Model

Adolescence is crucial for many aspects of developing self-identity and self-esteem, shaping values, beliefs, and morals. Young adolescents desire autonomy, particularly from parents, along with an increased commitment to social aspects of identity and greater connection with peers.[59] Identity formation during adolescence, together with past experiences in relation to the different health behaviours and characteristics, such as gender, SEP, and personality traits, contribute to the choice of health behaviours.[2] Girls tend to have lower levels of self-esteem, and the gender gap in self-esteem is most prominent in late adolescence, narrowing with increasing age.[60] A large UK study (68% females) showed that low self-esteem appears to be associated with smoking behaviour and excessive alcohol consumption.[61] It is also recognised that an individual's health behaviours are influenced by the behaviour of other people, particularly family member and peers who can act as role models.[2] Parental and sibling smoking is a strong determinant of smoking uptake in childhood and adolescence.[62]

Girls are influenced more by maternal than paternal smoking, while the opposite applies to boys.[62] Peer social networks are also important factors in adolescent behaviour choices.[63]

15.4.5 Tracking from Childhood and Adolescence into Adult Life

Many longitudinal studies of health behaviours from childhood to adulthood have focused on *tracking*, which can be defined as the stability of a health behaviour over time or the maintenance of a behaviour's relative position in a group over time.[64] Identifying trajectories of behaviours across life and examining the factors related to the trajectories is important for planning tailored and well-targeted health behaviour promotion strategies and interventions. Because of the strongly addictive nature of tobacco use, smoking tracks strongly from adolescence into young adult life.[65] Tracking of physical activity, food choice, and alcohol use are also apparent but at low to moderate levels.[66-70] A large US longitudinal study found that healthy behaviours declined dramatically during adolescence to young adulthood.[71] Girls reported fewer healthy behaviours than boys did at age 13 years but had a significantly less rapid decline in healthy behaviours between ages 13 and 24 years. Low psychological distress; high self-efficacy; social support from parents, schools, and peers; and living with nonsmoking parents were associated with higher engagement in healthy behaviours across adolescence and adulthood.[71] Tracking may be due to stable psychological characteristics of the individuals or stable conditions in the social environment. Further, black, Asian, and Hispanic youth were less likely to report risky health behaviours than white youth.[72] More research is needed to characterise tracking of health behaviours further over later adult life and in relation to different ethnic groups.

15.4.6 Adult Transitions

There are many transitions in women's adult life that greatly affect their health behaviours, including workforce (type of employment), marriage and partnership, pregnancy, menopause, and retirement. Pregnancy may be a point in the life course when women are especially amenable to making positive behaviour changes, particularly in smoking cessation.[5] Interventions to promote smoking cessation or smoking reduction among pregnant women are generally effective,[5] but the restarting rate by 6 months postpartum is high. Many women reduce their alcohol consumption when they realise they are pregnant, but alcohol use during pregnancy is still prevalent (20%–80%) and socially pervasive in many countries.[73] These results suggest that effective policy and interventions are required to maintain behaviour change post pregnancy. Menopause is another important change of life as it marks the end of a women's reproductive life. Many women are interested in the potential of lifestyle and behaviour changes (e.g. exercise, weight loss, and intake of soy foods) to manage their menopausal symptoms, although the clinical evidence for the effectiveness of lifestyle changes is mixed and limited.[74] Despite that, midlife is a critical stage in life for adopting healthy behaviours and preventive strategies.[75] The experience of intimate partner violence is also found to influence health behaviours. Victims of intimate partner violence were more likely to engage in smoking and drinking behaviour than non-victims, and SEP did not moderate the relationship.[76,77]

Nicotine and alcohol may serve as coping strategies that aim to reduce negative affect and anxiety related to intimate partner violence.[76]

15.5 Health Behaviour Changes During the COVID-19 Pandemic

Measures which aimed to contain COVID-19, including social distancing, isolation, quarantine, and lockdown, have led to profound changes in health behaviours at a population level. These are likely to include changes in physical activity, alcohol consumption, dietary habits, and sleep patterns, which may have subsequent downstream mental health consequences.[78] Two large UK studies found that during early lockdown, intake of fruit and vegetables decreased; days doing moderate to vigorous physical activity reduced; adverse alcohol use increased; and psychological distress markedly increased;[79,80] surprisingly, current smoking declined.[80] Women and young adults were particularly affected.[79,80] A study of five British birth cohorts provided evidence on the changes to health behaviour linked to lockdown and the differential impacts across generation, gender, socioeconomic circumstances across life, and ethnicity.[81] The Australian Longitudinal Study on Women's Health also found similar behaviour changes during the COVID-19 crisis; younger women (25–31 and 42–47 years) were more likely than older women (69–74 years) to report drinking more alcohol; smoking more; doing less physical activity; gaining weight; consuming less fruit and vegetables but more snacks, fast food or takeaway meals, and sugary drinks; and having multiple sleeping problems and a high levels of stress.[82] The COVID-19 lockdowns and restrictions have disproportionately affected specific population subgroups, with concerns that women, young adults, disadvantaged socioeconomic groups, and ethnic minorities may be at greater risk of health behaviour changes and mental problems. Future research is required to investigate which pandemic-induced behaviour changes are likely to remain and what are the associated characteristics.

15.6 Conclusions

A life course approach considers a temporal and social perspective, highlighting the population changes in smoking, alcohol use, diet, and physical activity over time and investigating inequalities with respect to gender and SEP. The comprehensive nature of life course epidemiology allows researchers to map pathways through life leading to adult health behaviours, which have major implications for developing health intervention policies. First, the time dimension of the life course approach highlights that critical or sensitive time periods, such as childhood and adolescence, can provide an opportunity to initiate beneficial behaviours; for instance, establishing healthy food choices and physical activity in early childhood. Given many adverse behaviours, such as smoking and drinking, are taken up during adolescence and track into adult life, adolescence represents a key period for interventions, both prevention and cessation. Second, a life course perspective identifies vulnerable and disadvantaged groups in their social and environmental context. This facilitates intervention policy not only to engage with at-risk groups but to recognise the social context as an opportunity to change their health behaviours. For instance, providing role models and school connectedness and setting social norms concerning smoking to reduce adolescent smoking, particularly for girls with an adverse childhood socioeconomic environment. In other words, health behaviour policies addressing particular groups at key stages in life and in certain social contexts may be more applicable and effective. The directions for future research on health behaviour should investigate factors influencing the effectiveness and long-term maintenance of behavioural interventions. Large studies or meta-analyses are needed to quantify gender and social inequalities in health behaviours, particularly among ethnic minorities and in LMICs.

Key messages and implications

- Women generally engage less in unhealthy behaviours than men do, but health inequalities are often more pronounced among women, especially in vulnerable and socioeconomically disadvantaged groups.
- A life course approach to women's health behaviours considers a temporal and social perspective, highlighting population changes in health behaviours over time and studying inequalities with respect to gender and socioeconomic position.
- The comprehensive nature of life course epidemiology allows researchers to map pathways through life leading to adult health behaviours, which facilitates intervention policy not only to engage with at-risk groups at key stages in life but to recognise the social context as an opportunity to change their health behaviours.

References

1. Conner M, Norman P. Health behaviour: current issues and challenges. *Psychology & Health*. 2017;32(8):895–906.
2. Mishra GD, Ben-Shlomo Y, Kuh D. A life course approach to health behaviors: theory and methods. In: Steptoe A, ed. *Handbook of behavioural medicine*. New York: Springer; 2010. pp. 525–40.
3. Schooling M, Kuh D, Graham H. A life course perspective on women's health behaviours. In: Kuh D, Hardy R, eds. *A life course approach to women's health*. Oxford: Oxford University Press; 2002. pp. 279–303.
4. Kelly MP, Barker M. Why is changing health-related behaviour so difficult? *Public Health*. 2016;136:109–16.
5. Jepson RG, Harris FM, Platt S, Tannahill C. The effectiveness of interventions to change six health behaviours: a review of reviews. *BMC Public Health*. 2010;10:538.
6. Cunningham TJ, Xu F, Town M. Prevalence of five health-related behaviors for chronic disease prevention among sexual and gender minority adults—25 U.S. States and Guam, 2016. *Morbidity and Mortality Weekly Report*. 2018;67(32):888–93.
7. Allen L, Williams J, Townsend N, Mikkelsen B, Roberts N, Foster C, et al. Socioeconomic status and non-communicable disease behavioural risk factors in low-income and lower-middle-income countries: a systematic review. *Lancet Global Health*. 2017;5(3):e277–e289.
8. Hagen EH, Garfield MJ, Sullivan RJ. The low prevalence of female smoking in the developing world: gender inequality or maternal adaptations for fetal protection? *Evolution, Medicine, and Public Health*. 2016;2016(1):195–211.
9. Wilsnack RW, Wilsnack SC, Kristjanson AF, Vogeltanz-Holm ND, Gmel G. Gender and alcohol consumption: patterns from the multinational GENACIS project. *Addiction*. 2009;104(9):1487–500.
10. Ng M, Freeman MK, Fleming TD, Robinson M, Dwyer-Lindgren L, Thomson B, et al. Smoking prevalence and cigarette consumption in 187 countries, 1980–2012. *JAMA*. 2014;311(2):183–92.

11. World Health Organization. *WHO report on the global tobacco epidemic, 2019.* Geneva: World Health Organization; 2019.

12. Vaneckova P, Wade S, Weber M, Murray JM, Grogan P, Caruana M, et al. Birth-cohort estimates of smoking initiation and prevalence in 20th century Australia: synthesis of data from 33 surveys and 385,810 participants. *PLoS ONE.* 2021;16(5):e0250824.

13. Liu S, Zhang M, Yang L, Li Y, Wang L, Huang Z, et al. Prevalence and patterns of tobacco smoking among Chinese adult men and women: findings of the 2010 national smoking survey. *Journal of Epidemiology and Community Health.* 2017;71(2):154–61.

14. Kaufman AR, Augustson EM. Predictors of regular cigarette smoking among adolescent females: does body image matter? *Nicotine & Tobacco Research.* 2008;10(8):1301–9.

15. Smith PH, Bessette AJ, Weinberger AH, Sheffer CE, McKee SA. Sex/gender differences in smoking cessation: a review. *Preventive Medicine.* 2016;92:135–40.

16. Casetta B, Videla AJ, Bardach A, Morello P, Soto N, Lee K, et al. Association between cigarette smoking prevalence and income level: a systematic review and meta-analysis. *Nicotine & Tobacco Research.* 2017;19(12):1401–7.

17. Brown-Johnson CG, England LJ, Glantz SA, Ling PM. Tobacco industry marketing to low socioeconomic status women in the U.S.A. *Tobacco Control.* 2014;23(e2):e139–e146.

18. Hammond D, Daniel S, White CM. The effect of cigarette branding and plain packaging on female youth in the United Kingdom. *Journal of Adolescent Health.* 2013;52(2):151–7.

19. Wakefield M, Coomber K, Zacher M, Durkin S, Brennan E, Scollo M. Australian adult smokers' responses to plain packaging with larger graphic health warnings 1 year after implementation: results from a national cross-sectional tracking survey. *Tobacco Control.* 2015;24(Suppl 2):ii17–ii25.

20. Cancer Council Victoria. *International developments in plain packaging [Internet].* Victoria: Cancer Council Victoria; 2021 [updated 2021; cited 17 June 2021]. Available from: https://www.cancervic.org.au/plainfacts/timelineandinternationaldevelopments.

21. World Health Organization. *Global status report on alcohol and health 2018.* Geneva: World Health Organization; 2018.

22. Loring B. *Alcohol and inequities: guidance for addressing inequities in alcohol-related harm.* Denmark: World Health Organization. Regional Office for Europe; 2014.

23. Allen LN, Townsend N, Williams J, Mikkelsen B, Roberts N, Wickramasinghe K. Socioeconomic status and alcohol use in low- and lower-middle income countries: a systematic review. *Alcohol.* 2018;70:23–31.

24. United Nations. *UNODC world drug report 2020.* Vienna: UN; 2020.

25. Micha R, Khatibzadeh S, Shi P, Andrews KG, Engell RE, Mozaffarian D, et al. Global, regional and national consumption of major food groups in 1990 and 2010: a systematic analysis including 266 country-specific nutrition surveys worldwide. *BMJ Open.* 2015;5(9):e008705.

26. Micha R, Khatibzadeh S, Shi P, Fahimi S, Lim S, Andrews KG, et al. Global, regional, and national consumption levels of dietary fats and oils in 1990 and 2010: a systematic analysis including 266 country-specific nutrition surveys. *BMJ.* 2014;348:g2272.

27. Darmon N, Drewnowski A. Does social class predict diet quality? *American Journal of Clinical Nutrition.* 2008;87(5):1107–17.

28. Guthold R, Stevens GA, Riley LM, Bull FC. Worldwide trends in insufficient physical activity from 2001 to 2016: a pooled analysis of 358 population-based surveys with 1.9 million participants. *Lancet Global Health.* 2018;6(10):e1077–e1086.

29. Guthold R, Stevens GA, Riley LM, Bull FC. Global trends in insufficient physical activity among adolescents: a pooled analysis of 298 population-based surveys with 1.6 million participants. *Lancet Child & Adolescent Health.* 2020;4(1):23–35.

30. O'Donoghue G, Kennedy A, Puggina A, Aleksovska K, Buck C, Burns C, et al. Socio-economic determinants of physical activity across the life course: a 'Determinants of Diet and Physical Activity'(DEDIPAC) umbrella literature review. *PLoS ONE.* 2018;13(1):e0190737.

31. Stalsberg R, Pedersen AV. Are differences in physical activity across socioeconomic groups associated with choice of physical activity variables to report? *International Journal of Environmental Research and Public Health.* 2018;15(5):922.

32. Barclay K, Myrskyla M. Maternal age and offspring health and health behaviours in late adolescence in Sweden. *SSM - Population Health*. 2016;2:68–76.

33. Goisis A, Remes H, Barclay K, Martikainen P, Myrskyla M. Advanced maternal age and the risk of low birth weight and preterm delivery: a within-family analysis using Finnish population registers. *American Journal of Epidemiology*. 2017;186(11):1219–26.

34. Weden MM, Miles JN. Intergenerational relationships between the smoking patterns of a population-representative sample of US mothers and the smoking trajectories of their children. *American Journal of Public Health*. 2012;102(4):723–31.

35. Lieb R, Schreier A, Pfister H, Wittchen HU. Maternal smoking and smoking in adolescents: a prospective community study of adolescents and their mothers. *European Addiction Research*. 2003;9(3):120–30.

36. Taylor AE, Howe LD, Heron JE, Ware JJ, Hickman M, Munafo MR. Maternal smoking during pregnancy and offspring smoking initiation: assessing the role of intrauterine exposure. *Addiction*. 2014;109(6):1013–21.

37. Belsky DW, Moffitt TE, Baker TB, Biddle AK, Evans JP, Harrington H, et al. Polygenic risk and the developmental progression to heavy, persistent smoking and nicotine dependence: evidence from a 4-decade longitudinal study. *JAMA Psychiatry*. 2013;70(5):534–42.

38. Kranzler HR, Zhou H, Kember RL, Vickers Smith R, Justice AC, Damrauer S, et al. Genome-wide association study of alcohol consumption and use disorder in 274,424 individuals from multiple populations. *Natural Communications*. 2019;10(1):1499.

39. Aasdahl L, Nilsen TIL, Meisingset I, Nordstoga AL, Evensen KAI, Paulsen J, et al. Genetic variants related to physical activity or sedentary behaviour: a systematic review. *International Journal of Behavioral Nutrition and Physical Activity*. 2021;18(1):15.

40. Goodman E, Huang B. Socioeconomic status, depressive symptoms, and adolescent substance use. *Archives of Pediatrics and Adolescent Medicine*. 2002;156(5):448–53.

41. Melotti R, Heron J, Hickman M, Macleod J, Araya R, Lewis G, et al. Adolescent alcohol and tobacco use and early socioeconomic position: the ALSPAC birth cohort. *Pediatrics*. 2011;127(4):e948–e955.

42. Moor I, Rathmann K, Lenzi M, Pfortner TK, Nagelhout GE, de Looze M, et al. Socioeconomic inequalities in adolescent smoking across 35 countries: a multilevel analysis of the role of family, school and peers. *European Journal of Public Health*. 2015;25(3):457–63.

43. Humensky JL. Are adolescents with high socioeconomic status more likely to engage in alcohol and illicit drug use in early adulthood? *Substance Abuse Treatment, Prevention, and Policy*. 2010;5:19.

44. Lacey RE, Cable N, Stafford M, Bartley M, Pikhart H. Childhood socio-economic position and adult smoking: are childhood psychosocial factors important? Evidence from a British birth cohort. *European Journal of Public Health*. 2011;21(6):725–31.

45. Jefferis BJ, Power C, Graham H, Manor O. Effects of childhood socioeconomic circumstances on persistent smoking. *American Journal of Public Health*. 2004;94(2):279–85.

46. Fergusson DM, Horwood LJ, Boden JM, Jenkin G. Childhood social disadvantage and smoking in adulthood: results of a 25-year longitudinal study. *Addiction*. 2007;102(3):475–82.

47. Hare-Bruun H, Togo P, Andersen LB, Heitmann BL. Adult food intake patterns are related to adult and childhood socioeconomic status. *Journal of Nutrition*. 2011;141(5):928–34.

48. Juneau CE, Benmarhnia T, Poulin AA, Cote S, Potvin L. Socioeconomic position during childhood and physical activity during adulthood: a systematic review. *International Journal of Public Health*. 2015;60(7):799–813.

49. Elhakeem A, Cooper R, Bann D, Hardy R. Childhood socioeconomic position and adult leisure-time physical activity: a systematic review. *International Journal of Behavioral Nutrition and Physical Activity*. 2015;12:92.

50. Campbell JA, Walker RJ, Egede LE. Associations between adverse childhood experiences, high-risk behaviors, and morbidity in adulthood. *American Journal of Preventive Medicine*. 2016;50(3):344–52.

51. Lee RD, Chen J. Adverse childhood experiences, mental health, and excessive alcohol use: examination of race/ethnicity and sex differences. *Child Abuse & Neglect*. 2017;69:40–8.

52. Loxton D, Forder PM, Cavenagh D, Townsend N, Holliday E, Chojenta C, et al. The impact of adverse childhood experiences on the health and health behaviors of young Australian women. *Child Abuse & Neglect*. 2021;111:104771.

53. Cutler DM, Lleras-Muney A. Understanding differences in health behaviors by education. *Journal of Health Economics*. 2010;29(1):1–28.

54. Busch V, Loyen A, Lodder M, Schrijvers A, van Yperen T, de Leeuw J. The effects of adolescent health-related behavior on academic performance: a systematic review of the longitudinal evidence. *Review of Educational Research*. 2014;84(2):245–74.

55. Hertzman C, Wiens M. Child development and long-term outcomes: a population health perspective and summary of successful interventions. *Social Science & Medicine*. 1996;43(7):1083–95.

56. Yee AZ, Lwin MO, Ho SS. The influence of parental practices on child promotive and preventive food consumption behaviors: a systematic review and meta-analysis. *International Journal of Behavioral Nutrition and Physical Activity*. 2017;14(1):47.

57. Andersen MR, Leroux BG, Bricker JB, Rajan KB, Peterson AV, Jr. Antismoking parenting practices are associated with reduced rates of adolescent smoking. *Archives of Pediatrics & Adolescent Medicine*. 2004;158(4):348–52.

58. Calafat A, Garcia F, Juan M, Becona E, Fernandez-Hermida JR. Which parenting style is more protective against adolescent substance use? Evidence within the European context. *Drug and Alcohol Dependence*. 2014;138:185–92.

59. Pfeifer JH, Berkman ET. The development of self and identity in adolescence: neural evidence and implications for a value-based choice perspective on motivated behavior. *Child Development Perspectives*. 2018;12(3):158–64.

60. Kiviruusu O, Huurre T, Aro H, Marttunen M, Haukkala A. Self-esteem growth trajectory from adolescence to mid-adulthood and its predictors in adolescence. *Advances in Life Course Research*. 2015;23:29–43.

61. Szinay D, Tombor I, Garnett C, Boyt N, West R. Associations between self-esteem and smoking and excessive alcohol consumption in the UK: a cross-sectional study using the BBC UK Lab database. *Addictive Behaviors Reports*. 2019;10:100229.

62. Leonardi-Bee J, Jere ML, Britton J. Exposure to parental and sibling smoking and the risk of smoking uptake in childhood and adolescence: a systematic review and meta-analysis. *Thorax*. 2011;66(10):847–55.

63. Montgomery SC, Donnelly M, Bhatnagar P, Carlin A, Kee F, Hunter RF. Peer social network processes and adolescent health behaviors: a systematic review. *Preventive Medicine*. 2020;130:105900.

64. Malina RM. Tracking of physical activity and physical fitness across the lifespan. *Research Quarterly for Exercise and Sport*. 1996;67(3 Suppl):S48–S57.

65. Borracci RA, Mulassi AH. Tobacco use during adolescence may predict smoking during adulthood: simulation-based research. *Archivos Argentinos de Pediatria*. 2015;113(2):106–12.

66. Ovesen L. Adolescence: a critical period for long-term tracking of risk for coronary heart disease? *Annuals of Nutrition and Metabolism*. 2006;50(4):317–24.

67. Enstad F, Evans-Whipp T, Kjeldsen A, Toumbourou JW, von Soest T. Predicting hazardous drinking in late adolescence/young adulthood from early and excessive adolescent drinking—a longitudinal cross-national study of Norwegian and Australian adolescents. *BMC Public Health*. 2019;19(1):790.

68. Kelder SH, Perry CL, Klepp KI, Lytle LL. Longitudinal tracking of adolescent smoking, physical activity, and food choice behaviors. *American Journal of Public Health*. 1994;84(7):1121–6.

69. Herman KM, Craig CL, Gauvin L, Katzmarzyk PT. Tracking of obesity and physical activity from childhood to adulthood: the Physical Activity Longitudinal Study. *International Journal of Pediatric Obesity*. 2009;4(4):281–8.

70. Kjonniksen L, Torsheim T, Wold B. Tracking of leisure-time physical activity during adolescence and young adulthood: a 10-year longitudinal study. *International Journal of Behavioral Nutrition and Physical Activity*. 2008;5:69.

71. Frech A. Healthy behavior trajectories between adolescence and young adulthood. *Advances in Life Course Research*. 2012;17(2):59–68.

72. Hoyt LT, Chase-Lansdale PL, McDade TW, Adam EK. Positive youth, healthy adults: does positive well-being in adolescence predict better perceived health and fewer risky health behaviors in young adulthood? *Journal of Adolescent Health*. 2012;50(1):66–73.
73. O'Keeffe LM, Kearney PM, McCarthy FP, Khashan AS, Greene RA, North RA, et al. Prevalence and predictors of alcohol use during pregnancy: findings from international multicentre cohort studies. *BMJ Open*. 2015;5(7):e006323.
74. Nonhormonal management of menopause-associated vasomotor symptoms: 2015 position statement of the North American Menopause Society. *Menopause*. 2015;22(11):1155–72; quiz 73–4.
75. El Khoudary SR, Greendale G, Crawford SL, Avis NE, Brooks MM, Thurston RC, et al. The menopause transition and women's health at midlife: a progress report from the Study of Women's Health Across the Nation (SWAN). *Menopause*. 2019;26(10):1213–27.
76. Crane CA, Hawes SW, Weinberger AH. Intimate partner violence victimization and cigarette smoking: a meta-analytic review. *Trauma, Violence & Abuse*. 2013;14(4):305–15.
77. Devries KM, Child JC, Bacchus LJ, Mak J, Falder G, Graham K, et al. Intimate partner violence victimization and alcohol consumption in women: a systematic review and meta-analysis. *Addiction*. 2014;109(3):379–91.
78. Arora T, Grey I. Health behaviour changes during COVID-19 and the potential consequences: a mini-review. *Journal of Health Psychology*. 2020;25(9):1155–63.
79. Naughton F, Ward E, Khondoker M, Belderson P, Marie Minihane A, Dainty J, et al. Health behaviour change during the UK COVID-19 lockdown: findings from the first wave of the C-19 health behaviour and well-being daily tracker study. *British Journal of Health Psychology*. 2021;26(2):624–43.
80. Niedzwiedz CL, Green MJ, Benzeval M, Campbell D, Craig P, Demou E, et al. Mental health and health behaviours before and during the initial phase of the COVID-19 lockdown: longitudinal analyses of the UK Household Longitudinal Study. *Journal of Epidemiology and Community Health*. 2021;75(3):224–31.
81. Bann D, Villadsen A, Maddock J, Hughes A, Ploubidis GB, Silverwood R, et al. Changes in the behavioural determinants of health during the COVID-19 pandemic: gender, socioeconomic and ethnic inequalities in five British cohort studies. *Journal of Epidemiology and Community Health*. 2021;75(12):1136–42.
82. Australian Longitudinal Study on Women's Health. ALSWH COVID-19 Survey Reports [Internet]. Australia: ALSWH; 2020 [updated September 2021; cited 17 June 2021]. Available from: https://alswh.org.au/outcomes/reports/covid-19-survey-reports/.

16
A Life Course Approach to Body Weight

Rebecca Hardy and Laura D. Howe

16.1 Introduction

Overweight and obesity is acknowledged as a major public health challenge worldwide, as excess adiposity, or fat mass, results in a wide range of negative health outcomes. The rapid rise in the prevalence of obesity, initially in high-income countries (HICs) and, more recently, in low- and middle-income countries (LMICs), suggests that this may be attributable to a Western lifestyle, characterised by high-calorie diets and low levels of physical activity, and an increasingly obesogenic environment—one which encourages such behaviours.

In this chapter, we focus on increased body weight, overweight, and obesity over the life course, but it is acknowledged that being underweight also has important health consequences, as do other components of body composition such as muscle mass. We consider the consequences and causes of high adiposity, highlighting where there are exposures which are specific to women or sex differences in associations.

16.1.1 Defining and Measuring Body Weight Across the Life Course

Weight-for-height indices are the most commonly collected markers of adiposity in longitudinal population-based studies because of the ease with which body weight and height can be obtained. However, fat mass is increasingly being measured directly through dual-energy X-ray absorptiometry, computed tomography (CT), or magnetic resonance imaging scans. BMI(calculated as weight (kg) / (height (m))^2) is by far the most commonly studied weight-for-height measure across the life course. BMI is also used to categorise adult overweight and obesity, as well as underweight, with the most commonly adopted cut-offs defined by the World Health Organization (WHO): < 18.5 kg/m^2 as underweight; ≥18.5 to < 2 5kg/m^2 as normal weight; and ≥25 kg/m^2 to < 30kg/m^2 as overweight; and ≥30 kg/m^2 as obese.[1] These cut-offs represent levels of BMI related to increased risk of mortality and other health outcomes but are based on analysis of observational studies from the United States and Europe in white populations. They are, therefore, not applicable to all ethnic groups where risk of disease is observed at lower levels of BMI.[2] The WHO has subsequently suggested additional action points along the BMI continuum to trigger intervention in Asian populations.[3] Age- and sex-specific cut-offs for children were calculated to represent the same centile as the cut-offs for adulthood by the WHO and are now in widespread use.[4] These cut-offs are lower in girls than boys in childhood until age 9–10 years and then become higher in girls.

Rebecca Hardy and Laura D. Howe, *A Life Course Approach to Body Weight* In: *A Life Course Approach to Women's Health*. Second Edition. Edited by: Gita D Mishra, Rebecca Hardy, and Diana Kuh, Oxford University Press. © Oxford University Press 2023. DOI: 10.1093/oso/9780192864642.003.0016

BMI does have limitations as a measure of adiposity as it does not measure fat mass directly and cannot distinguish heaviness attributable to adiposity from muscularity. It is correlated with fat mass at the population level, but the strength of the correlation is age and sex dependent.[5,6] Further, although division of weight by height^2 is intended to remove the correlation of BMI with height, correlation often remains. The Benn index, the power to which height is raised which ensures the resulting index is uncorrelated with height, has been found to be consistently lower across adulthood, particularly in women. This is due to the higher proportion of weight made up of fat in women, and because fat has a lower correlation with height than do muscle and bone.[7] Indices of weight for height are also unable to measure location of adiposity, with excess adiposity around the abdomen shown to be particularly harmful for health. Many studies deploy measurements of waist circumference or use the ratio of waist-to-hip circumference, to capture central adiposity.

16.1.2 Time Trends in BMI

Average adult BMI has increased worldwide in the last 40 years and is projected to continue increasing. The Non-Communicable Disease Risk Factor Collaboration (NCD-RisC) used 1698 population-based data sources, with more than 19.2 million adult participants in 186 countries to map these changes.[8] Overall, age-standardised mean BMI increased from 22.1 kg/m^2 in 1975 to 24.4 kg/m^2 in 2014 in women, and from 21.7 kg/m^2 to 24.2 kg/m^2 in men (Figure 16.1). In the same time period, age-standardised prevalence of obesity increased from 6.4% to 14.9% in women, and 3.2% to 10.8% in men, while prevalence of underweight decreased. There remain great disparities by region of the world, with HICs having higher mean BMI than LMICs (Figure 16.1). Low BMI was observed in central Africa and South Asia, but extremely high average BMI in Polynesia and Micronesia. Women in English-speaking HICs had substantially higher mean BMI than those in continental Europe in 2014, whereas in 1975, their BMI had been similar or lower. However, rates of increase in BMI were observed to have slowed in HICs and some MICs since the year 2000.

Overweight and obesity in childhood has become an increasing public health challenge as another NCD-RisC paper from 2181 datasets covering 16 million children aged 5–19 years in 200 countries highlights.[9] Highest mean BMI in 2019 for 19 year olds was observed in Pacific Island countries at over 28 kg/m^2, with high levels also seen in Kuwait, Bahrain, The Bahamas, Chile, the United States, and New Zealand; and, for girls, South Africa. Heterogeneity across the globe was apparent with a difference of approximately 9–10 kg/m^2 between the highest and lowest BMI (e.g. in India, Bangladesh, Ethiopia, and Chad). Generally, these global patterns persisted across all ages.

16.2 Changes in Body Size and BMI over the Life Span

In childhood, BMI increases rapidly over the first year of life and then decreases to a nadir around 6–7 years of age before increasing again—the so-called adiposity rebound. Thereafter, BMI increases as height increases and children experience puberty. This average pattern is seen across different populations, although the mean BMI and skewness (length of the right-hand tail) of the BMI distribution may vary. For example, a US study observed

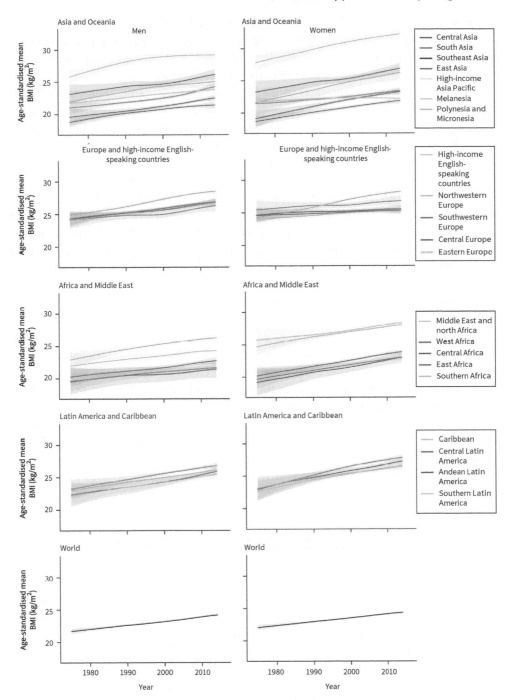

Figure 16.1 Trends in age-standardised mean BMI by sex and region from the NCD-RisC.[8] See plate section.

that children born during the obesity epidemic exhibited lower average BMI before the adiposity rebound but a more rapid subsequent BMI gain.[10] The sex differences in average childhood BMI are relatively small. For example, in the Avon Longitudinal Study of Parents and Children (ALSPAC), mean BMI was similar in boys and girls born in the early 1990s at age

1 year, lower in girls by age 3, but higher in girls from age 7 years onwards.[11] At 18 years, BMI was 2.4% higher in females than males. However, sex differences are considerably greater in height-adjusted fat mass. In ALSPAC, females had higher fat mass at age 9 years, and this difference increased with age such that by18 years, it was 77.8% higher.

In adulthood, mean BMI increases through to older age, where around the eighth decade it levels off and decreases. The decline in BMI observed at older ages is a result of loss of both fat mass and lean mass, with studies suggesting that the decline in lean mass starts considerably earlier in the life course.[12,13] Analysis of data from the British birth cohort studies born in 1946, 1958, and 1970[14] found that each later born cohort exhibited a higher median BMI at all ages, resulting in the age at which the median woman became overweight decreasing from 48 years in those born in 1946 to 41 years in a cohort born in 1970; this is later than for men, where the comparable ages were 41 and 30 years. The impact of an increasingly obesogenic environment in the UK over the period of study is highlighted by the shift towards earlier age at overweight or obesity (Figure 16.2). The same pattern in relation to obesity is observed across birth cohorts in the Australian Longitudinal Study on Women's Health (Figure 16.3). This also implies that more recently born cohorts are experiencing increasing cumulative exposure to overweight and obesity across the life course.

BMI tracks across the life course; a systematic review[15] found that obese children were approximately five times more likely to be obese adults than those not obese, and that 55% of obese children were obese in adolescence, and around 80% of obese adolescents remained obese in adulthood. On the other hand, the majority (70%) of obese adults were not obese children, reflecting the steady increases in BMI across adulthood. Although researchers have investigated early life growth as a predictor of adult BMI, it is difficult to tease out whether associations simply reflect BMI tracking or whether they could be considered causal. Associations with greater risk of adult obesity or adiposity have been observed for higher birthweight,[16–18] early age at adiposity rebound, and rapid early height growth and early puberty, particularly in women.[19,20] However, these characteristics are likely to all be part of the same process of growth.[21–24]

16.3 Social and Health Burden Related to Excess Weight

A J-shaped relationship between BMI and all-cause mortality is generally observed with higher rates at low and high BMI,[23,24] with the nadir of the curve being in the normal weight, or even the overweight category particularly at older ages. The increased rates at low BMI may be a result of confounding by smoking or residual confounding and/or reverse causality, whereby weight loss is a result of underlying disease. A Mendelian randomization (MR) study found similar J-shaped relationships to the observational studies but suggested that the increased risk in the underweight was only observed in smokers.[25]

Higher BMI, overweight, and obesity are associated with cardiovascular disease (CVD),[26,27] type 2 diabetes,[27] specific cancers,[27,28] respiratory diseases,[27] as well as poorer physical capability in later life,[29] and, more recently, with susceptibility to and severity of COVID-19, with a suggestion that this association is stronger in women than in men.[30] MR studies support causal associations for diabetes and coronary artery disease,[31,32] chronic obstructive pulmonary disease (COPD),[32] lung cancer,[32] and endometrial cancer,[33] but for breast cancer, higher BMI has been found to be associated with lower risk,[34] and evidence is

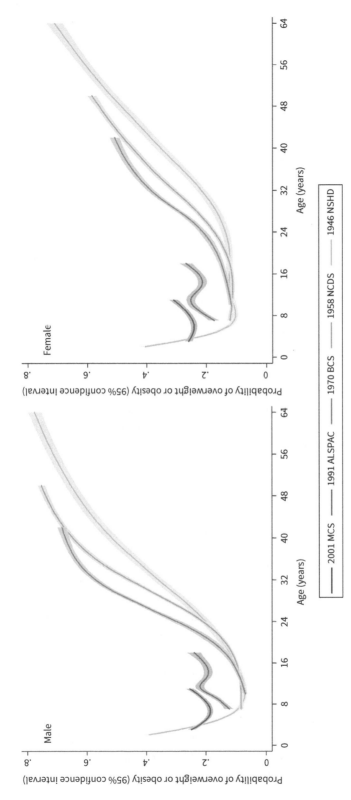

Figure 16.2 Trajectories of the probability of overweight or obesity across the life course from sex- and study-stratified multilevel logistic regression models.[14] See plate section.

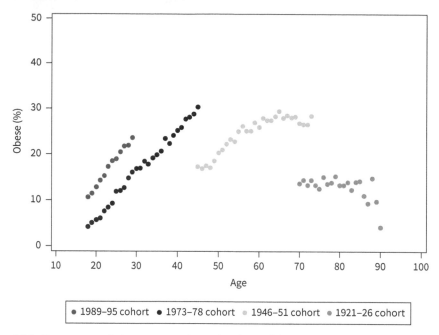

Figure 16.3 Percentage of obese women in each cohort of the Australian Longitudinal Study on Women's Health. See plate section.

inconsistent for cerebrovascular disease.[32,35] The risk of type 2 diabetes associated with a high BMI has been found to be greater in women than in men in observational and MR studies.[27,32] A greater accumulation of time across the life course exposed to high BMI has been shown to be associated with increasing risk of multiple adverse health outcomes. Evidence for accumulation of BMI from childhood have been observed, especially for cardiometabolic outcomes and diabetes.[36,37] Whether there is a long-term effect of early life obesity, if resolved in later life, remains less clear. Cohort studies investigating children who have a high BMI, but normalise their weight trajectory, show little evidence of a lasting detriment to cardiovascular health.[38,39]

Adiposity creates health risks during women's reproductive years, as prepregnancy obesity and higher gestational weight gain are associated with fertility problems[40] and multiple adverse pregnancy outcomes such as gestational hypertensive disorders, gestational diabetes, and large for gestational age at birth.[41,42] Maternal adiposity may also have longer-term impacts on offspring, particularly in terms of cognitive development,[43] asthma, coronary heart disease, stroke, and type 2 diabetes,[44] as well as with higher BMI (see Section 16.4.2), although some evidence suggests associations may, at least in some cases, be driven by shared genetic or shared familial, social, and lifestyle characteristics rather than the intra-uterine environment.[45] Raised BMI is also associated with adverse pregnancy outcomes in women undergoing assisted reproduction technologies such as in vitro fertilisation (IVF) or intracytoplasmic sperm injection (ICSI), including lower live birth rates.[46]

High BMI in adolescence in women, through social stigma and discrimination, for example, or through increased disease burden, may also result in poorer social outcomes in women, such as lower educational attainment and income.[47] However, social causation of BMI means it is challenging to tease out the causal direction. There are also implications for mental health from childhood onwards, [48] and overweight girls have lower self-esteem than others.[49] Detailed analysis from a UK birth cohort found that obesity and internalising symptoms increasingly co-occurred with age, and that weak reciprocal associations emerged between 7 and 14 years of age, with a suggestion that some of the associations could be explained by socioeconomic factors.[50] MR evidence suggests that BMI has a causal effect on depression,[51,52] but studying the reverse direction using MR is challenging because of the genetic variants for depression being relatively weak.

16.4 Causes of Obesity

16.4.1 Genetics

Twin studies suggest that the heritability of BMI is between 0.47 and 0.90, with some evidence that heritability varies across the life course, being higher during childhood than adulthood.[53] Genome-wide association studies (GWAS) of adults have identified numerous genetic variants that affect BMI. Analysis of approximately 700,000 participants of European ethnicity identified 941 single nucleotide polymorphisms (SNPs) that together explain 6% of the variance of BMI.[54] GWAS have also been conducted for other adiposity-related traits, for example measures of fat distribution.[55–57] Whilst the vast majority of GWAS have been performed in people of European ethnicity, there is growing recognition that the genetic determinants of body size may partially differ between populations with different ancestry,[58] and several genetic studies have been conducted in different ethnic groups.[59–62]

Longitudinal analyses have examined how the effects of genetic variants for BMI vary across the life course. In data from 9328 children from England and Australia, Warrington et al. demonstrated that a higher polygenetic risk for BMI was associated with higher BMI at the adiposity peak in infancy, and earlier age and higher BMI at the adiposity rebound during childhood.[63] This demonstrates that the known adult genetic determinants of BMI act from early childhood. In analysis of the MRC National Survey of Health and Development cohort, Hardy et al. observed that the effect of FTO (the SNP with the greatest effect on BMI) on BMI strengthened during childhood and adolescence, reached a peak strength at age 20 years, and then weakened during adulthood.[64]

Attempts have been made to identify genetic variants that affect body weight during specific periods of the life course. Earlier studies were hampered by a lack of power and identified only a few genetic variants that appeared to affect childhood BMI.[65,66] More recently, however, data from the UK Biobank has enabled the identification of a larger set of genetic variants for childhood body size. Adult participants in UK Biobank (mean age 56.5 years) were asked 'When you were 10 years old, compared to average would you describe yourself as thinner, plumper, or about average?' A GWAS of this measure detected 295 independent SNPs for early life body size.[67] In data from the ALSPAC and Norwegian HUNT study, a polygenic score of these early life body size SNPs was shown to be more strongly related to childhood BMI than to adult BMI. Further, the early life body size polygenic score was more strongly related to child BMI than a polygenic score based on SNPs identified in GWAS of adult BMI.[68]

16.4.2 Parental Body Weight and Diabetes

Parental and offspring body size typically display considerable correlations; for example, a study of over 11,000 participants from three European birth cohort studies showed a correlation of 0.29 between maternal prepregnancy BMI and offspring BMI at age 15.[69] Observational studies have also suggested a link between maternal diabetes during pregnancy and greater offspring adiposity.[70–75] The developmental overnutrition hypothesis proposes that mothers with higher levels of adiposity and/or higher glucose levels during pregnancy may 'overfeed' developing infants during gestation, and hence, programme the infant towards a greater tendency to adiposity.[76] However, alternative explanations for the observed intergenerational associations could be shared environmental factors or shared genetic factors.

To attempt to unpick the causality of the relationship between maternal diabetes during pregnancy and offspring adiposity, sibling and maternal-paternal comparison studies have been carried out. Sibling studies in both Sweden and in the Pima Indians of Arizona (a population with very high levels of obesity and type 2 diabetes) have found evidence that children born before a woman is diagnosed with type 2 diabetes are on average lighter than their siblings born after a diagnosis of type 2 diabetes in the mother.[74,77] The study in Pima Indians also found no association between paternal type 2 diabetes and offspring BMI, further supporting the notion of an intrauterine effect of maternal diabetes on offspring BMI.

There is also some evidence from sibling studies suggesting an effect of extreme maternal obesity on offspring BMI; two studies found that children born before their mother underwent bariatric surgery were more adipose than children born after their mother underwent bariatric surgery.[78,79] However, there is much less evidence from studies designed to test causality that greater levels of adiposity outside the case of extreme obesity have a causal effect on offspring BMI. A large Swedish study found that associations between maternal BMI and offspring BMI seen in the total population were not present in between-sibling analysis.[74] Additionally, a MR study using a genetic risk score of 32 BMI-increasing SNPs as an instrumental variable for maternal BMI found little evidence of an effect on offspring adiposity.[80] Further, a study of three European birth cohorts found that genetic confounding is likely to be an important driver of the correlation between maternal and offspring BMI; in these studies, common imputed SNPs explained 43% of the correlation between maternal prepregnancy BMI and offspring BMI at age 15 years.[69]

16.4.3 Social Factors

Socioeconomic inequalities in adiposity are consistently observed in HICs in contemporary cohorts, with disadvantaged socioeconomic position (SEP) being a risk factor for greater adiposity in both children[81] and adults.[82] Historically, this was not always the case. This social patterning has emerged during the course of economic development. In a comparative analysis of four British birth cohorts, in the earlier born cohorts (1946 Medical Research Council National Survey of Health and Development, 1958 National Child Development Study, and 1970 British Cohort Study), a more disadvantaged childhood SEP was associated with lower weight and shorter height during childhood, whereas in the 2001 Millennium Cohort Study (2001 MCS), a more disadvantaged childhood SEP was associated with higher weight and BMI during childhood.[83] In both the 2001 MCS and the ALSPAC cohort (born in 1991/1992), longitudinal analyses have shown that SEP differences in BMI have widened during childhood and adolescence,[83,84] with evidence from the ALSPAC cohort that SEP inequalities in adiposity are contributing to SEP inequalities in cardiovascular risk, even from as young as age 9 years.[85] Despite there being no association between more SEP and BMI during childhood in the 1946 Medical Research Council National Survey of Health and Development, 1958 National Child Development Study, and 1970 British Cohort Study, a more disadvantaged childhood SEP was associated with higher BMI during adulthood in all of these cohorts, with SEP differences typically being greater at older ages.[86] In many LMICs, disadvantaged SEP continues to be associated with lower BMI across the life course from childhood to adulthood,[87,88] although this is likely to change over time, with some evidence that women change to a pattern of higher adiposity with more disadvantaged SEP before men do.[89] Despite the predominant association in the general population being between disadvantaged SEP and higher adiposity in HICs, there is some evidence that the most disadvantaged people are also at increased risk of underweight.[90,91]

In addition to SEP, other social factors have been shown to be associated with higher adiposity, including adverse childhood experiences (ACEs)[92-94] such as abuse, neglect, and parental substance misuse. In a pooled meta-analysis of 10 observational studies with a total of 118,691 participants, exposure to multiple ACEs was associated with a 46% increase in the risk of obesity.[95] However, some studies have shown that the associations between ACEs and BMI/obesity attenuate considerably after adjustment for SEP and other potential confounding factors,[92,96] and associations between ACEs and adiposity were not observed in a Brazilian cohort,[97] where SEP shows either a positive or a null association with BMI.

16.4.4 Infant Feeding

The role of infant feeding in the development of obesity remains controversial. Numerous studies demonstrate associations of formula feeding with more rapid infant weight gain and a higher risk of childhood obesity.[98] However, these studies are potentially highly confounded. Women with obesity before pregnancy are less likely to initiate and continue breastfeeding,[99] breastfeeding initiation and continuation is highly socially patterned in HICs,[100] and maternal perceptions of a 'hungry' baby or being unable to make enough milk to satisfy a baby's demands can lead to women stopping breastfeeding.[101] Evaluating the causality of the relationship between infant feeding and subsequent risk of obesity is challenging. One study compared the relationship in two settings—the UK, where breastfeeding is more common in affluent groups of society, and Brazil, where there is little social patterning of breastfeeding. Breastfeeding was associated with lower BMI in the UK, but not in Brazil, suggesting that confounding by SEP and other factors is driving the association seen in the UK and other high-income settings.[102] Similarly, a randomised controlled trial of breastfeeding promotion in Belarus has shown no evidence of a causal effect of breastfeeding on BMI or other cardiovascular risk factors.[103] The intervention in this RCT led to a substantial increase in breastfeeding duration and exclusivity, but all mothers in both the intervention and control arm initiated breastfeeding, so the results cannot be generalised to breastfeeding initiation.

Current recommendations are that infants should be breastfed exclusively for 6 months, with no complementary food and beverages (CFB) introduced before this age. A systematic review assessed the associations of the timing of introduction of CFB on growth and body size. The authors concluded that there was no strong evidence of an effect of introducing CFB between ages 4 and 5 months (compared with 6 months) on weight status, body composition, weight, or length, but that some limited evidence suggests that introducing CFB before age 4 months may be associated with higher odds of obesity or overweight.[104] As with breast-feeding, the evaluation of causality in these relationships is very challenging, with significant potential for confounding and reverse causality.

16.4.5 Diet and Physical (In)Activity

Whilst a link between energy imbalance and body size must exist, studying the influence of diet and physical (in)activity on body size is fraught with challenges. Both diet and physical activity are extremely difficult to measure, with substantial potential for reporting biases. Isolating the effects of any specific food or component of diet is particularly challenging, given the complex and dynamic nature of diet. Further, observational studies of diet and physical (in)activity in relation to body size are likely to be highly confounded.

MR studies have attempted to assess the causal effects of diet and physical activity on body weight, but these studies are hampered by a lack of strong genetic variants. Nonetheless, a recent MR study in UK Biobank used 14 loci related to physical activity to demonstrate that each standard deviation increase in physical activity was related to a 0.14 standard deviation lower BMI.[105] MR results also suggest that relationships of diet and physical (in)activity may be bidirectional.[105–108]

16.4.6 Behavioural Factors

Numerous behavioural factors are associated with higher body weight and adiposity in observational studies, including short sleep duration, smoking, and alcohol consumption.[109–112] Supporting a causal effect of sleep on BMI, there is some evidence of effectiveness of sleep interventions in reducing BMI in children.[113] MR studies have also provided some evidence of causal effects of sleep duration and insomnia on BMI.[105,114,115]

Smoking has a complex relationship with BMI. Observationally, current smoking tends to have a negative relationship with BMI,[116] but some studies have shown associations between heavy smoking and higher BMI.[116,117] MR studies suggest that heavier smoking leads to a lower BMI, potentially explained by nicotine increasing the metabolic rate and/or lowering appetite.[118–120] There is also evidence from MR that the relationship is bidirectional, with higher BMI affecting smoking initiation and smoking heaviness.[121]

A systematic review of observational studies found that, in general, light to moderate alcohol use is not associated with weight gain, whereas heavy alcohol consumption is associated with weight gain.[122] MR studies support a causal effect of higher alcohol consumption on higher BMI.[123,124]

16.4.7 Reproductive Factors

Earlier puberty is associated with higher BMI and greater risk of cardiovascular disease.[125] However, disentangling the causality of this association is complex because higher adiposity in childhood may induce puberty at an earlier age.[126] Using data from ALSPAC, Bell et al.[127] found that associations between age at menarche or voice breaking and BMI at age 18 years attenuated ten-fold after adjustment for BMI at age 8 years, suggesting that the primary direction of causation may be from higher early life BMI to earlier puberty. Further, in negative control MR analyses, later age at menarche was associated with lower BMI measured at age 8 years, indicating that the genetic variants influencing menarche also influence prepubertal BMI.[127] Similarly, in the same cohort, O'Keeffe et al. used longitudinal data to show evidence of an association of prepubertal fat mass with puberty timing, but little evidence of an association of puberty timing with postpubertal change in fat mass.[128]

Pregnancy is an important period of the life course for women's adiposity. Women who experience high levels of weight gain during pregnancy are approximately three times more likely to be overweight in midlife.[129]

Women undergo the menopause transition at a median age of around age 52 years, and disaggregating the effects of chronological ageing and ovarian ageing is challenging. In a US study tracking the body composition of women through the menopausal transition (Study of Women's Health Across the Nation) and using menopausal age as the time metric, change in body composition accelerated during the transition, showing a two-to-fourfold increase in fat mass.[130] Postmenopause, the trajectories of fat and lean mass decelerated to a zero slope. However, these accelerated premenopausal changes were not observed in Japanese and Chinese women.

16.5 Policy Implications

Given the rising prevalence of obesity, the known health consequences, and the stark social inequalities, there is a pressing need for action. The high prevalence of obesity during childhood suggests a need for early life intervention, but the fact that the majority of adults with obesity were not obese during childhood highlights the need for continued action across the whole life course. In women, there may be opportunities to intervene in the reproductive years, when they are interacting with the health care system, which could be of benefit to both mother and offspring in terms of obesity.[131] Whilst much of the evidence base on the determinants of body size across the life course focuses on individual-level risk factors, there is growing recognition of the importance of commercial factors as targets for both research and policy.[132] Policy responses, particularly focused on individual or family agency, have often been assessed as being ineffective, and this is backed up by continuing rising levels of obesity during periods where policies have been implemented.[131,133] There is increasing understanding of the potential for higher-level interventions, such as taxes, to have a greater impact and to be more equitable than interventions focussed on individuals' diet and physical activity.[134,135]

16.6 Conclusions

The prevalence of obesity has increased dramatically in recent decades as environments become increasingly obesogenic. There are numerous influences on body size across the life course, including social factors, behavioural and psychological factors, and genetics. The evidence in this chapter highlights the potential for intervention to reduce obesity at all stages of the life course. Going forward, more detailed measurement of body composition in longitudinal studies, in addition to BMI, along with increasing use of methods to elucidate causality, should provide additional insights.

Key messages and implications

- The prevalence of obesity has risen in recent decades for both children and adolescents in HICs. As countries move through the epidemiological transition, a similar trend is occurring in LMICs.
- More recent cohorts are, on average, living for greater periods of their life course with overweight and obesity, which will have a detrimental impact on subsequent health.
- Life course research has identified a wide range of social, behavioural, and psychological factors operating at all life stages that are associated with body size across the life course.
- Given the stark socioeconomic inequalities in obesity seen in HICs and the diverse adverse health consequences of obesity, urgent policy action is required at all stages of the life course.
- 'Upstream' interventions which require a low level of individual agency, as well as the more common policies targeted at individuals, will be required to reduce obesity and the social inequalities in obesity.

References

1. WHO Consultation on Obesity. *Obesity: preventing and managing the global epidemic: report of a WHO consultation*. WHO Technical Report Series 894. Geneva: World Health Organization; 1999.
2. Caleyachetty R, Barber TM, Mohammed NI, Cappuccio FP, Hardy R, Mathur R, et al. Ethnicity-specific BMI cutoffs for obesity based on type 2 diabetes risk in England: a population-based cohort study. *Lancet Diabetes & Endocrinology*. 2021;9(7):419–26.
3. WHO expert consultation. Appropriate body-mass index for Asian populations and its implications for policy and intervention strategies. *Lancet (London, England)*. 2004;363(9403):157–63.
4. Cole TJ, Bellizzi MC, Flegal KM, Dietz WH. Establishing a standard definition for child overweight and obesity worldwide: international survey. *BMJ (Clinical Research Ed)*. 2000;320(7244):1240–3.
5. Gallagher D, Visser M, Sepúlveda D, Pierson RN, Harris T, Heymsfield SB. How useful is body mass index for comparison of body fatness across age, sex, and ethnic groups? *American Journal of Epidemiology*. 1996;143(3):228–39.
6. Flegal KM, Shepherd JA, Looker AC, Graubard BI, Borrud LG, Ogden CL, et al. Comparisons of percentage body fat, body mass index, waist circumference, and waist-stature ratio in adults. *American Journal of Clinical Nutrition*. 2009;89(2):500–8.
7. Johnson W, Norris T, Bann D, Cameron N, Wells JK, Cole TJ, et al. Differences in the relationship of weight to height, and thus the meaning of BMI, according to age, sex, and birth year cohort. *Annals of Human Biology*. 2020;47(2):199–207.
8. NCD Risk Factor Collaboration (NCD-RisC). Trends in adult body-mass index in 200 countries from 1975 to 2014: a pooled analysis of 1698 population-based measurement studies with 19.2 million participants. *Lancet (London, England)*. 2016;387(10026):1377–96.

9. NCD Risk Factor Collaboration (NCD-RisC). Height and body-mass index trajectories of school-aged children and adolescents from 1985 to 2019 in 200 countries and territories: a pooled analysis of 2181 population-based studies with 65 million participants. *Lancet (London, England)*. 2020;396(10261):1511–24.

10. Johnson W, Soloway LE, Erickson D, Choh AC, Lee M, Chumlea WC, et al. A changing pattern of childhood BMI growth during the 20th century: 70 y of data from the Fels Longitudinal Study. *American Journal of Clinical Nutrition*. 2012;95(5):1136–43.

11. O'Keeffe LM, Simpkin AJ, Tilling K, Anderson EL, Hughes AD, Lawlor DA, et al. Sex-specific trajectories of measures of cardiovascular health during childhood and adolescence: a prospective cohort study. *Atherosclerosis*. 2018;278:190–6.

12. Westbury LD, Syddall HE, Fuggle NR, Dennison EM, Harvey NC, Cauley JA, et al. Relationships between level and change in sarcopenia and other body composition components and adverse health outcomes: findings from the Health, Aging, and Body Composition Study. *Calcified Tissue International*. 2021;108(3):302–13.

13. Newman AB, Lee JS, Visser M, Goodpaster BH, Kritchevsky SB, Tylavsky FA, et al. Weight change and the conservation of lean mass in old age: the Health, Aging and Body Composition Study. *American Journal of Clinical Nutrition*. 2005;82(4):872–8; quiz 915–16.

14. Johnson W, Li L, Kuh D, Hardy R. How has the age-related process of overweight or obesity development changed over time? Co-ordinated analyses of individual participant data from five United Kingdom birth cohorts. *PLoS Medicine*. 2015;12(5):e1001828; discussion e.

15. Simmonds M, Llewellyn A, Owen CG, Woolacott N. Predicting adult obesity from childhood obesity: a systematic review and meta-analysis. *Obesity Reviews: An Official Journal of the International Association for the Study of Obesity*. 2016;17(2):95–107.

16. Zhao Y, Wang SF, Mu M, Sheng J. Birth weight and overweight/obesity in adults: a meta-analysis. *European Journal of Pediatrics*. 2012;171(12):1737–46.

17. Yu ZB, Han SP, Zhu GZ, Zhu C, Wang XJ, Cao XG, et al. Birth weight and subsequent risk of obesity: a systematic review and meta-analysis. *Obesity Reviews: An Official Journal of the International Association for the Study of Obesity*. 2011;12(7):525–42.

18. Araújo de França GV, Restrepo-Méndez MC, Loret de Mola C, Victora CG. Size at birth and abdominal adiposity in adults: a systematic review and meta-analysis. *Obesity Reviews: An Official Journal of the International Association for the Study of Obesity*. 2014;15(2):77–91.

19. Rolland-Cachera MF, Deheeger M, Bellisle F, Sempé M, Guilloud-Bataille M, Patois E. Adiposity rebound in children: a simple indicator for predicting obesity. *American Journal of Clinical Nutrition*. 1984;39(1):129–35.

20. Prentice P, Viner RM. Pubertal timing and adult obesity and cardiometabolic risk in women and men: a systematic review and meta-analysis. *International Journal of Obesity (2005)*. 2013;37(8):1036–43.

21. Williams S, Davie G, Lam F. Predicting BMI in young adults from childhood data using two approaches to modelling adiposity rebound. *International Journal of Obesity and Related Metabolic Disorders: Journal of the International Association for the Study of Obesity*. 1999;23(4):348–54.

22. Cole TJ. Children grow and horses race: is the adiposity rebound a critical period for later obesity? *BMC Pediatrics*. 2004;4:6.

23. Bhaskaran K, Dos-Santos-Silva I, Leon DA, Douglas IJ, Smeeth L. Association of BMI with overall and cause-specific mortality: a population-based cohort study of 3.6 million adults in the UK. *Lancet Diabetes & Endocrinology*. 2018;6(12):944–53.

24. Global BMI Mortality Collaboration, Di Angelantonio E, Bhupathiraju Sh N, Wormser D, Gao P, Kaptoge S, et al. Body-mass index and all-cause mortality: individual-participant-data meta-analysis of 239 prospective studies in four continents. *Lancet (London, England)*. 2016;388(10046):776–86.

25. Sun YQ, Burgess S, Staley JR, Wood AM, Bell S, Kaptoge SK, et al. Body mass index and all-cause mortality in HUNT and UK Biobank studies: linear and non-linear mendelian randomisation analyses. *BMJ (Clinical Research Ed)*. 2019;364:l1042.

26. Mongraw-Chaffin ML, Peters SAE, Huxley RR, Woodward M. The sex-specific association between BMI and coronary heart disease: a systematic review and meta-analysis of 95 cohorts with 1.2 million participants. *Lancet Diabetes & Endocrinology.* 2015;3(6):437–49.

27. Guh DP, Zhang W, Bansback N, Amarsi Z, Birmingham CL, Anis AH. The incidence of comorbidities related to obesity and overweight: a systematic review and meta-analysis. *BMC Public Health.* 2009;9:88.

28. Renehan AG, Tyson M, Egger M, Heller RF, Zwahlen M. Body-mass index and incidence of cancer: a systematic review and meta-analysis of prospective observational studies. *Lancet (London, England).* 2008;371(9612):569–78.

29. Hardy R, Cooper R, Aihie Sayer A, Ben-Shlomo Y, Cooper C, Deary IJ, et al. Body mass index, muscle strength and physical performance in older adults from eight cohort studies: the HALCyon programme. *PLoS ONE.* 2013;8(2):e56483.

30. Peters SAE, MacMahon S, Woodward M. Obesity as a risk factor for COVID-19 mortality in women and men in the UK biobank: comparisons with influenza/pneumonia and coronary heart disease. *Diabetes, Obesity & Metabolism.* 2021;23(1):258–62.

31. Riaz H, Khan MS, Siddiqi TJ, Usman MS, Shah N, Goyal A, et al. Association between obesity and cardiovascular outcomes: a systematic review and meta-analysis of Mendelian randomization studies. *JAMA Network Open.* 2018;1(7):e183788.

32. Censin JC, Peters SAE, Bovijn J, Ferreira T, Pulit SL, Mägi R, et al. Causal relationships between obesity and the leading causes of death in women and men. *PLoS Genetics.* 2019;15(10):e1008405.

33. Painter JN, O'Mara TA, Marquart L, Webb PM, Attia J, Medland SE, et al. Genetic risk score Mendelian randomization shows that obesity measured as body mass index, but not waist:hip ratio, is causal for endometrial cancer. *Cancer Epidemiology, Biomarkers & Prevention: A Publication of the American Association for Cancer Research, Cosponsored by the American Society of Preventive Oncology.* 2016;25(11):1503–10.

34. Shu X, Wu L, Khankari NK, Shu XO, Wang TJ, Michailidou K, et al. Associations of obesity and circulating insulin and glucose with breast cancer risk: a Mendelian randomization analysis. *International Journal of Epidemiology.* 2019;48(3):795–806.

35. Marini S, Merino J, Montgomery BE, Malik R, Sudlow CL, Dichgans M, et al. Mendelian randomization study of obesity and cerebrovascular disease. *Annals of Neurology.* 2020;87(4):516–24.

36. Norris T, Cole TJ, Bann D, Hamer M, Hardy R, Li L, et al. Duration of obesity exposure between ages 10 and 40 years and its relationship with cardiometabolic disease risk factors: a cohort study. *PLoS Medicine.* 2020;17(12):e1003387.

37. Park MH, Sovio U, Viner RM, Hardy RJ, Kinra S. Overweight in childhood, adolescence and adulthood and cardiovascular risk in later life: pooled analysis of three British birth cohorts. *PloS ONE.* 2013;8(7):e70684.

38. Lawlor DA, Benfield L, Logue J, Tilling K, Howe LD, Fraser A, et al. Association between general and central adiposity in childhood, and change in these, with cardiovascular risk factors in adolescence: prospective cohort study. *BMJ (Clinical Research Ed).* 2010;341:c6224.

39. Juonala M, Magnussen CG, Berenson GS, Venn A, Burns TL, Sabin MA, et al. Childhood adiposity, adult adiposity, and cardiovascular risk factors. *New England Journal of Medicine.* 2011;365(20):1876–85.

40. Brower MA, Hai Y, Jones MR, Guo X, Chen YI, Rotter JI, et al. Bidirectional Mendelian randomization to explore the causal relationships between body mass index and polycystic ovary syndrome. *Human Reproduction.* 2019;34(1):127–36.

41. Santos S, Voerman E, Amiano P, Barros H, Beilin LJ, Bergström A, et al. Impact of maternal body mass index and gestational weight gain on pregnancy complications: an individual participant data meta-analysis of European, North American and Australian cohorts. *International Journal of Obstetrics & Gynaecology.* 2019;126(8):984–95.

42. Tyrrell J, Richmond RC, Palmer TM, Feenstra B, Rangarajan J, Metrustry S, et al. Genetic evidence for causal relationships between maternal obesity-related traits and birth weight. *Journal of the American Medical Association.* 2016;315(11):1129–40.

43. Adane AA, Mishra GD, Tooth LR. Maternal pre-pregnancy obesity and childhood physical and cognitive development of children: a systematic review. *International Journal of Obesity (2005).* 2016;40(11):1608–18.

44. Godfrey KM, Reynolds RM, Prescott SL, Nyirenda M, Jaddoe VW, Eriksson JG, et al. Influence of maternal obesity on the long-term health of offspring. *Lancet Diabetes & Endocrinology.* 2017;5(1):53–64.

45. Bond TA, Richmond RC, Karhunen V, Cuellar-Partida G, Borges MC, Zuber V, et al. Exploring the causal effect of maternal pregnancy adiposity on offspring adiposity: Mendelian randomisation using polygenic risk scores. *BMC Medicine.* 2022;20(1):34.

46. Rittenberg V, Seshadri S, Sunkara SK, Sobaleva S, Oteng-Ntim E, El-Toukhy T. Effect of body mass index on IVF treatment outcome: an updated systematic review and meta-analysis. *Reproductive BioMedicine Online.* 2011;23(4):421–39.

47. Gortmaker SL, Must A, Perrin JM, Sobol AM, Dietz WH. Social and economic consequences of overweight in adolescence and young adulthood. *New England Journal of Medicine.* 1993;329(14):1008–12.

48. Sutaria S, Devakumar D, Yasuda SS, Das S, Saxena S. Is obesity associated with depression in children? Systematic review and meta-analysis. *Archives of Disease in Childhood.* 2019;104(1):64–74.

49. Moradi M, Mozaffari H, Askari M, Azadbakht L. Association between overweight/obesity with depression, anxiety, low self-esteem, and body dissatisfaction in children and adolescents: a systematic review and meta-analysis of observational studies. *Critical Reviews in Food Science and Nutrition.* 2022;62(2):555–70.

50. Patalay P, Hardman CA. Comorbidity, codevelopment, and temporal associations between body mass index and internalizing symptoms from early childhood to adolescence. *Journal of the American Medical Association Psychiatry.* 2019;76(7):721–9.

51. Luppino FS, de Wit LM, Bouvy PF, Stijnen T, Cuijpers P, Penninx BW, et al. Overweight, obesity, and depression: a systematic review and meta-analysis of longitudinal studies. *Archives of General Psychiatry.* 2010;67(3):220–9.

52. Tyrrell J, Mulugeta A, Wood AR, Zhou A, Beaumont RN, Tuke MA, et al. Using genetics to understand the causal influence of higher BMI on depression. *International Journal of Epidemiology.* 2019;48(3):834–48.

53. Elks CE, den Hoed M, Zhao JH, Sharp SJ, Wareham NJ, Loos RJ, et al. Variability in the heritability of body mass index: a systematic review and meta-regression. *Frontiers in Endocrinology (Lausanne).* 2012;3:29.

54. Yengo L, Sidorenko J, Kemper KE, Zheng Z, Wood AR, Weedon MN, et al. Meta-analysis of genome-wide association studies for height and body mass index in ~700,000 individuals of European ancestry. *Human Molecular Genetics.* 2018;27(20):3641–9.

55. Rask-Andersen M, Karlsson T, Ek WE, Johansson Å. Genome-wide association study of body fat distribution identifies adiposity loci and sex-specific genetic effects. *Nature Communications.* 2019;10(1):339.

56. Pulit SL, Stoneman C, Morris AP, Wood AR, Glastonbury CA, Tyrrell J, et al. Meta-analysis of genome-wide association studies for body fat distribution in 694,649 individuals of European ancestry. *Human Molecular Genetics.* 2019;28(1):166–74.

57. Emdin CA, Khera AV, Natarajan P, Klarin D, Zekavat SM, Hsiao AJ, et al. Genetic association of waist-to-hip ratio with cardiometabolic traits, type 2 diabetes, and coronary heart disease. *Journal of the American Medical Association.* 2017;317(6):626–34.

58. Peprah E, Xu H, Tekola-Ayele F, Royal CD. Genome-wide association studies in Africans and African Americans: expanding the framework of the genomics of human traits and disease. *Public Health Genomics.* 2015;18(1):40–51.

59. Liu CT, Monda KL, Taylor KC, Lange L, Demerath EW, Palmas W, et al. Genome-wide association of body fat distribution in African ancestry populations suggests new loci. *PLoS Genetics.* 2013;9(8):e1003681.

60. Wen W, Kato N, Hwang JY, Guo X, Tabara Y, Li H, et al. Genome-wide association studies in East Asians identify new loci for waist-hip ratio and waist circumference. *Scientific Reports.* 2016;6:17958.

61. Liu CT, Buchkovich ML, Winkler TW, Heid IM, Borecki IB, Fox CS, et al. Multi-ethnic fine-mapping of 14 central adiposity loci. *Human Molecular Genetics.* 2014;23(17):4738–44.

62. Hoffmann TJ, Choquet H, Yin J, Banda Y, Kvale MN, Glymour M, et al. A large multiethnic genome-wide association study of adult body mass index identifies novel loci. *Genetics.* 2018;210(2):499–515.

63. Warrington NM, Howe LD, Wu YY, Timpson NJ, Tilling K, Pennell CE, et al. Association of a body mass index genetic risk score with growth throughout childhood and adolescence. *PloS ONE.* 2013;8(11):e79547.

64. Hardy R, Wills AK, Wong A, Elks CE, Wareham NJ, Loos RJ, et al. Life course variations in the associations between FTO and MC4R gene variants and body size. *Human Molecular Genetics.* 2010;19(3):545–52.

65. Warrington NM, Howe LD, Paternoster L, Kaakinen M, Herrala S, Huikari V, et al. A genome-wide association study of body mass index across early life and childhood. *International Journal of Epidemiology.* 2015;44(2):700–12.

66. Felix JF, Bradfield JP, Monnereau C, van der Valk RJ, Stergiakouli E, Chesi A, et al. Genome-wide association analysis identifies three new susceptibility loci for childhood body mass index. *Human Molecular Genetics.* 2016;25(2):389–403.

67. Richardson TG, Sanderson E, Elsworth B, Tilling K, Davey Smith G. Use of genetic variation to separate the effects of early and later life adiposity on disease risk: Mendelian randomisation study. *BMJ (Clinical Research Ed).* 2020;369:m1203.

68. Brandkvist M, Bjørngaard JH, Ødegård RA, Åsvold BO, Smith GD, Brumpton B, et al. Separating the genetics of childhood and adult obesity: a validation study of genetic scores for body mass index in adolescence and adulthood in the HUNT Study. *Human Molecular Genetics.* 2021;29(24):3966–73.

69. Bond TA, Karhunen V, Wielscher M, Auvinen J, Männikkö M, Keinänen-Kiukaanniemi S, et al. Exploring the role of genetic confounding in the association between maternal and offspring body mass index: evidence from three birth cohorts. *International Journal of Epidemiology.* 2020;49(1):233–43.

70. Pettitt DJ, Bennett PH, Saad MF, Charles MA, Nelson RG, Knowler WC. Abnormal glucose tolerance during pregnancy in Pima Indian women: long-term effects on offspring. *Diabetes.* 1991;40(Suppl 2):126–30.

71. Pettitt DJ, Nelson RG, Saad MF, Bennett PH, Knowler WC. Diabetes and obesity in the offspring of Pima Indian women with diabetes during pregnancy. *Diabetes Care.* 1993;16(1):310–4.

72. Lawlor DA, Fraser A, Lindsay RS, Ness A, Dabelea D, Catalano P, et al. Association of existing diabetes, gestational diabetes and glycosuria in pregnancy with macrosomia and offspring body mass index, waist and fat mass in later childhood: findings from a prospective pregnancy cohort. *Diabetologia.* 2010;53(1):89–97.

73. Philipps LH, Santhakumaran S, Gale C, Prior E, Logan KM, Hyde MJ, et al. The diabetic pregnancy and offspring BMI in childhood: a systematic review and meta-analysis. *Diabetologia.* 2011;54(8):1957–66.

74. Lawlor DA, Lichtenstein P, Långström N. Association of maternal diabetes mellitus in pregnancy with offspring adiposity into early adulthood: sibling study in a prospective cohort of 280,866 men from 248,293 families. *Circulation.* 2011;123(3):258–65.

75. Patel S, Fraser A, Davey Smith G, Lindsay RS, Sattar N, Nelson SM, et al. Associations of gestational diabetes, existing diabetes, and glycosuria with offspring obesity and cardiometabolic outcomes. *Diabetes Care.* 2012;35(1):63–71.

76. Lawlor DA. The Society for Social Medicine John Pemberton Lecture 2011. Developmental overnutrition—an old hypothesis with new importance? *International Journal of Epidemiology.* 2013;42(1):7–29.

77. Dabelea D, Hanson RL, Lindsay RS, Pettitt DJ, Imperatore G, Gabir MM, et al. Intrauterine exposure to diabetes conveys risks for type 2 diabetes and obesity: a study of discordant sibships. *Diabetes.* 2000;49(12):2208–11.

78. Kral JG, Biron S, Simard S, Hould FS, Lebel S, Marceau S, et al. Large maternal weight loss from obesity surgery prevents transmission of obesity to children who were followed for 2 to 18 years. *Pediatrics*. 2006;118(6):e1644–e1649.

79. Smith J, Cianflone K, Biron S, Hould FS, Lebel S, Marceau S, et al. Effects of maternal surgical weight loss in mothers on intergenerational transmission of obesity. *The Journal of Clinical Endocrinology & Metabolism*. 2009;94(11):4275–83.

80. Richmond RC, Timpson NJ, Felix JF, Palmer T, Gaillard R, McMahon G, et al. Using genetic variation to explore the causal effect of maternal pregnancy adiposity on future offspring adiposity: a Mendelian randomisation study. *PLoS Medicine*. 2017;14(1):e1002221.

81. Shrewsbury V, Wardle J. Socioeconomic status and adiposity in childhood: a systematic review of cross-sectional studies 1990–2005. *Obesity*. 2008;16:275–84.

82. McClaren L. Socioeconomic status and obesity. *Epidemiologic Reviews*. 2007;29:29–48.

83. Bann D, Johnson W, Li L, Kuh D, Hardy R. Socioeconomic inequalities in childhood and adolescent body-mass index, weight, and height from 1953 to 2015: an analysis of four longitudinal, observational, British birth cohort studies. *Lancet Public Health*. 2018;3(4):e194–e203.

84. Howe LD, Tilling K, Galobardes B, Smith GD, Ness AR, Lawlor DA. Socioeconomic disparities in trajectories of adiposity across childhood. *International Journal of Pediatric Obesity*. 2011;6(2–2):e144–e153.

85. Howe LD, Galobardes B, Sattar N, Hingorani AD, Deanfield J, Ness AR, et al. Are there socioeconomic inequalities in cardiovascular risk factors in childhood, and are they mediated by adiposity? Findings from a prospective cohort study. *International Journal of Obesity (2005)*. 2010;34(7):1149–59.

86. Bann D, Johnson W, Li L, Kuh D, Hardy R. Socioeconomic inequalities in body mass index across adulthood: coordinated analyses of individual participant data from three British birth cohort studies initiated in 1946, 1958 and 1970. *PLoS Medicine*. 2017;14(1):e1002214.

87. Reyes Matos U, Mesenburg MA, Victora CG. Socioeconomic inequalities in the prevalence of underweight, overweight, and obesity among women aged 20-49 in low- and middle-income countries. *International Journal of Obesity (2005)*. 2020;44(3):609–16.

88. Patel R, Tilling K, Lawlor DA, Howe LD, Hughes RA, Bogdanovich N, et al. Socioeconomic differences in childhood BMI trajectories in Belarus. *International Journal of Obesity (2005)*. 2018;42(9):1651–60.

89. Gigante DP, Victora CG, Matijasevich A, Horta BL, Barros FC. Association of family income with BMI from childhood to adult life: a birth cohort study. *Public Health Nutrition*. 2013;16(2):233–9.

90. Pearce A, Rougeaux E, Law C. Disadvantaged children at greater relative risk of thinness (as well as obesity): a secondary data analysis of the England National Child Measurement Programme and the UK Millennium Cohort Study. *International Journal for Equity in Health*. 2015;14:61.

91. Hughes A, Kumari M. Unemployment, underweight, and obesity: findings from Understanding Society (UKHLS). *Preventive Medicine*. 2017;97:19–25.

92. Houtepen LC, Heron J, Suderman MJ, Fraser A, Chittleborough CR, Howe LD. Associations of adverse childhood experiences with educational attainment and adolescent health and the role of family and socioeconomic factors: a prospective cohort study in the UK. *PLoS Medicine*. 2020;17(3):e1003031.

93. Anderson EL, Fraser A, Caleyachetty R, Hardy R, Lawlor DA, Howe LD. Associations of adversity in childhood and risk factors for cardiovascular disease in mid-adulthood. *Child Abuse & Neglect*. 2018;76:138–48.

94. Caleyachetty R, Stafford M, Cooper R, Anderson EL, Howe LD, Cosco TD, et al. Exposure to multiple childhood social risk factors and adult body mass index trajectories from ages 20 to 64 years. *European Journal of Public Health*. 2021;31(2):385–90.

95. Wiss DA, Brewerton TD. Adverse childhood experiences and adult obesity: a systematic review of plausible mechanisms and meta-analysis of cross-sectional studies. *Physiology & Behavior*. 2020;223:112964.

96. Purswani P, Marsicek SM, Amankwah EK. Association between cumulative exposure to adverse childhood experiences and childhood obesity. *PLoS One*. 2020;15(9):e0239940.

97. Soares ALG, Matijasevich A, Menezes AMB, Assunção MC, Wehrmeister FC, Howe LD, et al. Adverse childhood experiences (ACEs) and adiposity in adolescents: a cross-cohort comparison. *Obesity (Silver Spring)*. 2018;26(1):150–9.

98. Appleton J, Russell CG, Laws R, Fowler C, Campbell K, Denney-Wilson E. Infant formula feeding practices associated with rapid weight gain: a systematic review. *Maternal & Child Nutrition*. 2018;14(3):e12602.

99. Huang Y, Ouyang YQ, Redding SR. Maternal prepregnancy body mass index, gestational weight gain, and cessation of breastfeeding: a systematic review and meta-analysis. *Breastfeeding Medicine*. 2019;14(6):366–74.

100. Bærug A, Laake P, Løland BF, Tylleskär T, Tufte E, Fretheim A. Explaining socioeconomic inequalities in exclusive breast feeding in Norway. *Archives of Disease in Childhood*. 2017;102(8):708–14.

101. Ahluwalia IB, Morrow B, Hsia J. Why do women stop breastfeeding? Findings from the Pregnancy Risk Assessment and Monitoring System. *Pediatrics*. 2005;116(6):1408–12.

102. Brion MJ, Lawlor DA, Matijasevich A, Horta B, Anselmi L, Araújo CL, et al. What are the causal effects of breastfeeding on IQ, obesity and blood pressure? Evidence from comparing high-income with middle-income cohorts. *International Journal of Epidemiology*. 2011;40(3):670–80.

103. Martin RM, Kramer MS, Patel R, Rifas-Shiman SL, Thompson J, Yang S, et al. Effects of promoting long-term, exclusive breastfeeding on adolescent adiposity, blood pressure, and growth trajectories: a secondary analysis of a randomized clinical trial. *Journal of the American Medical Association Pediatr*. 2017;171(7):e170698.

104. English LK, Obbagy JE, Wong YP, Butte NF, Dewey KG, Fox MK, et al. Timing of introduction of complementary foods and beverages and growth, size, and body composition: a systematic review. *American Journal of Clinical Nutrition*. 2019;109(Suppl 7):935s–55s.

105. Doherty A, Smith-Byrne K, Ferreira T, Holmes MV, Holmes C, Pulit SL, et al. GWAS identifies 14 loci for device-measured physical activity and sleep duration. *Nature Communications*. 2018;9(1):5257.

106. Freuer D, Meisinger C, Linseisen J. Causal relationship between dietary macronutrient composition and anthropometric measures: a bidirectional two-sample Mendelian randomization analysis. *Clinical Nutrition*. 2021;40(6):4120-4131.

107. Schnurr TM, Viitasalo A, Eloranta AM, Damsgaard CT, Mahendran Y, Have CT, et al. Genetic predisposition to adiposity is associated with increased objectively assessed sedentary time in young children. *International Journal of Obesity (2005)*. 2018;42(1):111–14.

108. Richmond RC, Davey Smith G, Ness AR, den Hoed M, McMahon G, Timpson NJ. Assessing causality in the association between child adiposity and physical activity levels: a Mendelian randomization analysis. *PLoS Medicine*. 2014;11(3):e1001618.

109. Poorolajal J, Sahraei F, Mohamdadi Y, Doosti-Irani A, Moradi L. Behavioral factors influencing childhood obesity: a systematic review and meta-analysis. *Obesity Research & Clinical Practice*. 2020;14(2):109–18.

110. Morrissey B, Taveras E, Allender S, Strugnell C. Sleep and obesity among children: A systematic review of multiple sleep dimensions. *Pediatric Obesity*. 2020;15(4):e12619.

111. Cooper CB, Neufeld EV, Dolezal BA, Martin JL. Sleep deprivation and obesity in adults: a brief narrative review. *BMJ Open Sport & Exercise Medicine*. 2018;4(1):e000392.

112. Garfield V. The association between body mass index (BMI) and sleep duration: where are we after nearly two decades of epidemiological research? *International Journal of Environmental Research and Public Health*. 2019;16(22) 4327.

113. Miller MA, Bates S, Ji C, Cappuccio FP. Systematic review and meta-analyses of the relationship between short sleep and incidence of obesity and effectiveness of sleep interventions on weight gain in preschool children. *Obesity Reviews: An Official Journal of the International Association for the Study of Obesity*. 2021;22(2):e13113.

114. Jansen PR, Watanabe K, Stringer S, Skene N, Bryois J, Hammerschlag AR, et al. Genome-wide analysis of insomnia in 1,331,010 individuals identifies new risk loci and functional pathways. *Nature Genetics*. 2019;51(3):394–403.

115. Lane JM, Jones SE, Dashti HS, Wood AR, Aragam KG, van Hees VT, et al. Biological and clinical insights from genetics of insomnia symptoms. *Nature Genetics*. 2019;51(3):387–93.

116. Audrain-McGovern J, Benowitz NL. Cigarette smoking, nicotine, and body weight. *Clinical Pharmacology & Therapeutics.* 2011;90(1):164–8.

117. Dare S, Mackay DF, Pell JP. Relationship between smoking and obesity: a cross-sectional study of 499,504 middle-aged adults in the UK general population. *PloS ONE.* 2015;10(4):e0123579.

118. Freathy RM, Kazeem GR, Morris RW, Johnson PC, Paternoster L, Ebrahim S, et al. Genetic variation at CHRNA5-CHRNA3-CHRNB4 interacts with smoking status to influence body mass index. *International Journal of Epidemiology.* 2011;40(6):1617–28.

119. Åsvold BO, Bjørngaard JH, Carslake D, Gabrielsen ME, Skorpen F, Smith GD, et al. Causal associations of tobacco smoking with cardiovascular risk factors: a Mendelian randomization analysis of the HUNT Study in Norway. *International Journal of Epidemiology.* 2014;43(5):1458–70.

120. Morris RW, Taylor AE, Fluharty ME, Bjørngaard JH, Åsvold BO, Elvestad Gabrielsen M, et al. Heavier smoking may lead to a relative increase in waist circumference: evidence for a causal relationship from a Mendelian randomisation meta-analysis: the CARTA Consortium. *BMJ Open.* 2015;5(8):e008808.

121. Taylor AE, Richmond RC, Palviainen T, Loukola A, Wootton RE, Kaprio J, et al. The effect of body mass index on smoking behaviour and nicotine metabolism: a Mendelian randomization study. *Human Molecular Genetics.* 2019;28(8):1322–30.

122. Traversy G, Chaput JP. Alcohol consumption and obesity: an update. *Current Obesity Reports.* 2015;4(1):122–30.

123. Lawlor DA, Nordestgaard BG, Benn M, Zuccolo L, Tybjaerg-Hansen A, Davey Smith G. Exploring causal associations between alcohol and coronary heart disease risk factors: findings from a Mendelian randomization study in the Copenhagen General Population Study. *European Heart Journal.* 2013;34(32):2519–28.

124. Holmes MV, Dale CE, Zuccolo L, Silverwood RJ, Guo Y, Ye Z, et al. Association between alcohol and cardiovascular disease: Mendelian randomisation analysis based on individual participant data. *BMJ (Clinical Research Ed).* 2014;349:g4164.

125. Charalampopoulos D, McLoughlin A, Elks CE, Ong KK. Age at menarche and risks of all-cause and cardiovascular death: a systematic review and meta-analysis. *American Journal of Epidemiology.* 2014;180(1):29–40.

126. Ahmed ML, Ong KK, Dunger DB. Childhood obesity and the timing of puberty. *Trends in Endocrinology & Metabolism.* 2009;20(5):237–42.

127. Bell JA, Carslake D, Wade KH, Richmond RC, Langdon RJ, Vincent EE, et al. Influence of puberty timing on adiposity and cardiometabolic traits: a Mendelian randomisation study. *PLoS Medicine.* 2018;15(8):e1002641.

128. O'Keeffe LM, Frysz M, Bell JA, Howe LD, Fraser A. Puberty timing and adiposity change across childhood and adolescence: disentangling cause and consequence. *Human Reproduction.* 2020;35(12):2784–92.

129. Fraser A, Tilling K, Macdonald-Wallis C, Hughes R, Sattar N, Nelson SM, et al. Associations of gestational weight gain with maternal body mass index, waist circumference, and blood pressure measured 16 y after pregnancy: the Avon Longitudinal Study of Parents and Children (ALSPAC). *American Journal of Clinical Nutrition.* 2011;93(6):1285–92.

130. Greendale GA, Sternfeld B, Huang M, Han W, Karvonen-Gutierrez C, Ruppert K, et al. Changes in body composition and weight during the menopause transition. *Journal of Clinical Investigation Insight.* 2019;4(5).e124865.

131. Hanson M, Barker M, Dodd JM, Kumanyika S, Norris S, Steegers E, et al. Interventions to prevent maternal obesity before conception, during pregnancy, and post partum. *Lancet Diabetes & Endocrinology.* 2017;5(1):65–76.

132. Lobstein T, Jackson-Leach R, Moodie ML, Hall KD, Gortmaker SL, Swinburn BA, et al. Child and adolescent obesity: part of a bigger picture. *Lancet (London, England).* 2015;385(9986):2510–20.

133. Adams J, Mytton O, White M, Monsivais P. Why are some population interventions for diet and obesity more equitable and effective than others? The role of individual agency. *PLoS Medicine.* 2016;13(4):e1001990.

292 Biological and Behavioural Pathways

134. Teng AM, Jones AC, Mizdrak A, Signal L, Genç M, Wilson N. Impact of sugar-sweetened beverage taxes on purchases and dietary intake: systematic review and meta-analysis. *Obesity Reviews: An Official Journal of the International Association for the Study of Obesity.* 2019;20(9):1187–204.
135. Pell D, Mytton O, Penney TL, Briggs A, Cummins S, Penn-Jones C, et al. Changes in soft drinks purchased by British households associated with the UK soft drinks industry levy: controlled interrupted time series analysis. *BMJ (Clinical Research Ed).* 2021;372:n254.

PART V
SOCIAL ISSUES IMPACTING WOMEN'S HEALTH

17
Life Course Socioeconomic Trajectories and Health

Rebecca Hardy

17.1 Introduction

There is extensive research highlighting substantial socioeconomic inequalities in a wide range of health outcomes and, of particular relevance to life course epidemiology, inequalities in adult health according to childhood socioeconomic position. These inequalities in health have persisted in many countries, and the global COVID-19 pandemic—which began in 2020—served to further highlight them. To understand how adult socioeconomic inequalities in health develop, an understanding of the social patterning of life course risk factors is required. Indeed, many early life exposures which are risks for later health, and discussed in the previous chapters of this book, are socially patterned. The interdependencies between socioeconomic, reproductive, and health trajectories in women over the life course also need to be understood to tackle inequalities in health.

In this chapter, after consideration of the definitions and measurement of socioeconomic position (SEP), we discuss intergenerational social mobility and the changing nature of childbearing and employment trajectories in women. We then focus on life course social inequalities in health, describing secular changes in these inequalities and the impact of the COVID-19 pandemic. We finish by discussing the pathways through which SEP and health are related across the life course. While it is acknowledged that there are inequalities between countries, this chapter primarily focuses on inequalities according to socioeconomic position within countries, particularly within the UK.

17.2 Socioeconomic Position Across Life

17.2.1 Defining and Measuring Socioeconomic Position

SEP has been defined as the 'social and economic factors that influence what positions individuals or groups hold within the structure of a society'.[1] Galobardes et al.[1] provided an overview of the different measures of SEP including education, housing, income, and occupation. Each measure has its own theoretical basis, measurement, and strengths and weaknesses. For example, social class based on occupation reflects social standing, income, and intellect and can characterise working relations between employers and employees, while

Rebecca Hardy, *Life Course Socioeconomic Trajectories and Health* In: *A Life Course Approach to Women's Health*. Second Edition. Edited by: Gita D Mishra, Rebecca Hardy, and Diana Kuh, Oxford University Press. © Oxford University Press 2023.
DOI: 10.1093/oso/9780192864642.003.0017

income reflects material resources. Although classifications based on occupation have widely been used in studies of inequality, such an approach suffers the disadvantage of not being able to categorise people who are not in employment, including homemakers who are more likely to be women. Therefore, historically, it has often been partner's occupation or income that has been used to represent women's SEP. In life course epidemiology, SEP in childhood, which must be based on measures of parental SEP or household conditions, is of particular interest. Education is often used in research as a common marker of SEP, and while it reflects the knowledge and 'capital' built up through schooling, it is not considered a direct measure of location within the class structure or the status hierarchy.[2]

Societal trends and policy differences over time and place can make comparison of findings on inequalities challenging.[3] For example, declining industrialisation in high-income countries (HICs) has led to a reduction in the overall numbers employed in manual occupations,[4] and changes in education policy have increased years of schooling and higher education participation, particularly for women.[5] Consequently, the distributions in different categories of these SEP measures have changed over time. The process of social stratification in low- and middle-income countries (LMICs) differs from that in HICs, meaning that different measurement tools are required. Howe et al.[6] evaluated the use of education, occupation, and income, noting differences in LMICs, such as the rarity of formal employment and seasonal fluctuations in employment and income. Measures more specific to LMICs include an asset-based measure often called a wealth index, consumption expenditure capturing the extent to which households can meet material needs, and participatory wealth rankings where community members rank the wealth of households within their communities.

17.2.2 Intergenerational Social Mobility

Social mobility can occur across the adult life course (intragenerational mobility), but here we concentrate on mobility between generations. Such intergenerational social mobility can be defined in absolute (the extent to which offspring SEP is different from their parents) or relative (the chance of offspring being in a certain category given that of their parents) terms. Studies have consistently shown continuity in occupational social class and income between fathers and sons.[7-9] Similar patterns have been seen for daughters, but the evidence is far less extensive as women were historically excluded from relevant research because of their lower levels of workforce participation.[7-9] The reason for this continuity in SEP remains debated but could act through transmission of wealth and social norms such as work ethic or social network, while education is widely considered as a mediator of social mobility and is discussed below.

Despite this documented continuity, absolute intergenerational social mobility has increased and remains high across most OECD countries, with upward mobility being greater than downward mobility (except in Australia).[10] However, there is evidence that downward mobility has recently increased compared to earlier findings.[5] Social mobility is particularly high in most Nordic countries, but low in Southern and Central European countries, suggesting differing policies exert an influence. Absolute social mobility is slightly higher between fathers and sons than between mothers and daughters.[10] Time trends in absolute social mobility depend on the changes in class structure within a country over time, such that where countries now have a greater proportion of the population in professional and nonmanual occupations, prospects of upward mobility are less for younger generations. In terms of relative mobility, there is persisting continuity at the very top and very bottom of the SEP distribution, with a more mixed picture for those in the middle.[10] This suggests that those at the very top are particularly good at ensuring assets and advantages are passed onto their children, while the most disadvantaged struggled to move up the social ladder.

In the first edition of this book, Bartley et al.[11] demonstrated how upward intergenerational social mobility of women born in Britain in 1970 was greater than that for women born in 1958. An analysis including these two cohorts, along with an earlier born (1946) and a later born (1980–84) generation, has since provided evidence of increasing social mobility (upward or downward) in absolute and relative terms among men and women across all four generations.[12] However, while total mobility increased, the experience of absolute upward mobility became less common and that of absolute downward mobility more common. Upward mobility was similar in the 1980–84 cohort to that in the 1970 cohort for women, unlike for men where a decrease was observed. There was a divergence in the trends in relative mobility between genders when considering offspring social class at age 38 years. Relative mobility remained constant among men but increased among women, suggesting greater social fluidity among women. Similar trends have been reported using the UK Office of National Statistics Longitudinal Study.[13] The extent to which these differences are due to the more rapidly increasing levels of education in women, women returning to work at lower levels after periods of motherhood—termed *perverse fluidity*,[14] or to policies which have been beneficial to women remains unclear.[12] The role of part-time work in relation to the perverse fluidity hypothesis has been investigated. Although eventual full-time and part-time workers were not found to differ in terms of parental social class nor in educational qualifications, there was a difference in the levels of employment at which they entered the labour market. Women who eventually worked part-time were more likely to start in a working-class position than those who eventually worked full-time, after accounting for family social class and education.[15]

More educated and affluent parents can provide their children with better education, and a higher level of education is associated with higher status jobs and greater earnings. However, analysis using data from the UK Labour Force Survey 2014–18[16] found that higher levels of educational attainment were associated with greater chances of upward mobility and lower risks of downward mobility, and this was not just the result of more privileged children attaining higher levels of education. Men generally gain more social and economic advantage from the same level of educational achievement than women do.[17-19] For example, men are less likely to experience downward and more likely to experience upward mobility with greater education levels, compared with women.[16]

It has been repeatedly demonstrated that in countries with greater income inequality, as indicated by the Gini coefficient, there is less intergenerational income elasticity, a measure of social mobility[20,21]—a relationship dubbed the 'Great Gatsby Curve'.[22] However, despite widespread interest in the relationship, there has been relatively little research examining the mechanisms behind it. The role of education was examined in a cross-national dataset, finding that greater country-level income inequality was associated with less access to higher education, lower financial returns on education, and greater residual effect of parental education upon labour market earnings.[23] The authors, therefore, concluded that educational attainment is an important driver of the relationship between intergenerational mobility and income inequality. High-inequality countries also have greater private, and less public, investment in education and the type of education gained can impact SEP. For example, around 6% attend private schools in Britain once foreign pupils are removed;[24,25] these pupils are from the very top of the family income distribution,[25] and are subsequently over-represented in higher status occupations[26] and earn substantially more in adulthood.[24] Type of schooling may thus play a role in why social mobility remains lower in the very highest end of the distribution.

17.2.3 Family and Work Trajectories

There have been considerable secular changes in family formation, childbearing, and employment among women over the past 70 years. Divorce rates have increased, whilst marriage decreased; the global fertility rate has decreased, likely explained in large part by the secular trend of delayed childbearing,[27] and employment rates for women have increased. For women, family and work trajectories across life are highly interlinked as balancing family and career remains a challenge. Analysis of the British birth cohort studies, using multi-channel sequence analysis, found that women's and men's work and family life courses are becoming increasingly similar as more women engage in continuous full-time employment; however, part-time employment or career breaks remain common for women.[28]

A cross-country comparison, which accounted for the selection of family-oriented women into motherhood, found that having more children had a negative effect on the probability of working and the number of working hours in all country groups, except in the Nordic countries.[29] The timing of childbearing also appears to impact social outcomes, as younger maternal age (in particular teenage motherhood) and having more children have been associated with less schooling and poorer educational attainment, and decreased labour market participation.[30-36] However, background characteristics which select into early pregnancy make it difficult to disentangle the causal impact on subsequent social outcomes. Some analyses have suggested that accounting for differences between pregnant and childless teenagers' backgrounds reduces the observed education gap but does not explain it completely.[37] Therefore, the reduced time in education, time out of the labour force, and discrimination because of early pregnancy may also contribute to worse outcomes.[38] In addition to the well-researched area of pregnancy, menstrual cycles and menopause may also have socio-economic implications, demonstrating the interlinked nature of women's life course reproductive health and social trajectories.[39,40] For example, research using the 1958 British Birth Cohort study[40] found that early menopause (< 45 years), 'bothersome' menopausal symptoms, and psychological problems attributable to menopause were associated with a lower employment rate.

Despite the secular changes in women's participation in the workforce and the slow convergence of the pay of men and women across multiple countries,[41] there remains a gender earnings gap. The average gap between mean male and female hourly earnings in the countries in the European Union in 2020 was 13.0%, with the highest gap in Latvia (22.3%) and Estonia (21.1%), and the lowest in Luxembourg (0.7%) and Romania (2.4%). The UK was the fourth highest at 20.8%.[42] The wage gap tends to vary across the life course, with analysis from cohorts born in 1958 and 1970 in the UK demonstrating the initial gap in early adulthood widens during the childbearing years and then declines.[43,44] Much, but not all, of the gender wage gap has been attributed to divergent work experience primarily due to family formation.[44,45] Further, while family composition is similar for male and female workers, it was detrimental to women's wages but beneficial for men. However, the wage difference is not confined to parents, given the gap existed on entry to the labour market, highlighting the differences cannot just be due to family responsibilities.[44,46] Thus, the lower level of earnings over the life course illustrates how women are more likely to suffer social and economic disadvantage after divorce or widowhood. The implications of changes in partnership status are further discussed in Chapters 18 and 19.

17.3 Life Course Social Inequalities in Health

The UK Office for National Statistics reported that in 2018–20, females living in the most deprived areas in the UK could expect to live 78.33 years compared with 86.3 years in the most advantaged areas.[47] This was smaller than the absolute difference in men, which was 73.5 compared with 83.2 years. As well as having shorter lives, those in the most deprived areas can also expect to live less time in good health. Disability-free life expectancy at birth was 50.3 years in women in the most deprived areas compared with 66.4 years in the least deprived. The comparable figures from men were 51.4 and 69.0 years. These inequalities are replicated across countries and according to multiple individual adult markers of SEP. For example, an EU report in 2020 found that, from 2007 to 2016, the difference in average life expectancy at birth between people with high and low education levels was up to 10 years and more in Estonia, Bulgaria, and Slovakia.[48] There is also evidence of persisting social inequalities across a range of health outcomes and, for adult high body mass index (BMI) and fat mass, there is evidence that such inequalities are greater in women than men.[49–52]

   While most existing research considers social inequalities in the general population, it is increasingly acknowledged that marginalised and highly disadvantaged groups are not represented in most research datasets. Studies of children who spent some of their childhood in out-of-home care,[53–55] homeless people,[56] and refugees[57] highlight the poor physical and mental health outcomes in such groups. It is acknowledged that these are important groups who need to be included in future research; they are not discussed further in this chapter. Neither do we discuss ethnic inequalities in health which are distinct, although related to social inequalities.[58]

17.3.1 Secular Trends in Social Inequalities in Health

Even prior to the COVID-19 pandemic, declining life expectancy in the most disadvantaged areas of both the United States and UK was evident. The Marmot Review 10 Years On report[59] found that, in England, improvements in life expectancy since 2010 had stalled for the first time since 1900. It also reported that the inequalities in life expectancy have increased so that among women in the most deprived 10% of areas, life expectancy fell between 2010–12 and 2016–18. However, this contrasts with findings of narrowing inequalities in mortality by educational attainment over the same period,[60] and persisting inequalities according to multiple SEP indicators from early and adult life across the British birth cohort studies,[61] suggesting trends may be dependent on the measure of SEP and health outcome.

Secular changes in mortality according to education have been extensively studied, particularly in the United States. One study of age, period, and cohort effects of education on mortality risk from 1986 to 2006 found widening educational differences, which were similar in women and men.[62] Cohort changes in the educational gap are more modest among black women and men than among white women and men. Other studies from the same time period, similarly, reported that for some subpopulations in the United States, mortality rates had increased and life expectancy decreased.[63–66] For example, in the period 1986 to 2002, a growing gradient for all-cause mortality in white women was reported, reflecting increasing mortality among low-educated women and decreasing mortality among college-educated women.[66] It has, however, been suggested that these findings do not necessarily represent 'real' trends, but rather are a result of differences in selection into education over time, termed 'lagged selection bias'.[67]

17.3.2 Childhood Socioeconomic Position and Adult Health

Of particular interest to life course epidemiology is the extent to which earlier life SEP is associated with adult health and/or whether accumulation of exposure to disadvantage across life is associated with greater health risks. In HICs, childhood SEP has been found to be associated with mortality[68] and a wide range of disease and health-related outcomes such as CVD,[69] diabetes,[70] respiratory function,[71] physical capability,[72] inflammation,[73] BMI,[49] and body composition,[74] many of which have been discussed in previous chapters. It is generally agreed that this association is not simply due to the continuity of SEP from childhood to adulthood described in Section 17.2.2. While childhood SEP has been extensively studied, there has been less, although increasing, interest in the impact of early adulthood SEP and the transition to adulthood as an important life stage. Analysis of the British Cohort Study 1970 suggested an independent contribution to cardiovascular risk factor inequalities of early adulthood socioeconomic trajectories.[75] The influence of social disadvantage on health is often hypothesised to take a cumulative effect because of the long-term gradual damage to health from harmful exposures and behaviours related to disadvantage across life, and indeed studies have tended to support this idea.[76] Allostatic load also uses the concept of a gradual accumulation of damage and was introduced as a measure of multisystem dysregulation caused by chronic stress.[77] Disentangling the effects of sensitive periods of exposure to disadvantage from accumulation is complex, although multiple advances in statistical approaches have been proposed.[78–80] Applying one such approach to data from Sweden on all-cause mortality, a sensitive period model best described the influence of SEP with a heightened effect in later adult life for both men and women.[81] However, for mortality from circulatory diseases, findings differed between men and women, where for women midlife SEP was most important, while the effect was cumulative among men. This contrasts with the sex differences in models found in the 1946 British Birth Cohort Study, where SEP was generally associated with CVD risk factors in a cumulative manner for women, but the childhood sensitive period was the most common model for men.[82] While replication is therefore needed, it may be that the effects of life course SEP vary by time and place.

17.3.3 The COVID-19 Pandemic

The global COVID-19 pandemic has exposed the stark social inequalities in health. Greater SARS-CoV-2 exposure and COVID-19 severity and mortality have occurred in the most disadvantaged groups,[83–86] and lockdown policies may have amplified these inequalities.[87] Vaccination uptake is less in more disadvantaged areas in the UK[88] and United States.[89] Mental health symptoms have also been exacerbated by the COVID-19 pandemic, and living in crowded households or living alone may be particularly important in contributing to poor mental health during lockdown.[90] Women's mental health appears to have been impacted to a greater extent than men's.[91] This may be partly because women had a larger share of the unpaid tasks, including housework, home-schooling, and caring responsibilities,[92,93] and rates of domestic and gender-based violence have been reported to have increased during lockdowns.[94] As well as health impacts, detrimental social changes, including loss of employment, disruption of food programs, and the subsequent economic recession, have occurred. There are likely to be far-reaching consequences of the inequalities in educational disruption among children. During the first lockdown in the UK in 2020, those in disadvantaged circumstances had approximately 1.5 hours less home schooling per day, and fewer had home computers compared with more advantaged peers.[95]

The pandemic also highlighted the importance of the environment to health. As well as disadvantaged areas having greater rates of COVID-19, mental health was worse among people who lacked access to outdoor facilities during lockdown,[90] consistent with an increasing body of evidence suggesting that access to green space is beneficial for aspects of mental health.[96] Further, other area-level factors, including the food environment and walkability and safety, may influence health outcomes,[97,98] with obesity being perhaps the most commonly studied outcome given the interest in the impact of an increasingly 'obesogenic environment'. It may be that air pollution is a risk factor for greater COVID-19 severity,[99] as well as an exposure related to a range of other negative outcomes.[100–103] All of these neighbourhood risk factors tend to cluster in more disadvantaged areas.[104]

17.4 Explanations for Socioeconomic Inequalities in Health

Life course epidemiology attempts to explain adult health inequalities through socially distributed exposures through the life course. Health behaviours, which are key risk factors for multiple conditions, play a role in explaining social inequalities in health since risky behaviours tend to be socially patterned. When specifically tested as mediators of social inequalities in health, health behaviours generally have not explained all of the inequality, and the extent of mediation may vary by population.[105] A study in the UK found that most of the relationship of education and area deprivation with coronary heart disease risk was accounted for by health-related behaviours, in particular smoking.[106] The difficulty in measuring health behaviours, particularly over the life course, however, may mean that the contribution of lifelong behaviours is underestimated.[107] Further, as the initial uptake of risky behaviours is socially patterned, lifelong health behaviour patterns may explain inequalities in health according to childhood SEP, and Chapter 15 outlines how factors from early life such as adverse childhood experiences and lower parental education influence behaviour development (see Section 15.4.2 for more detail).

We now consider some of the socially distributed childhood exposures that might play a role in adult health inequalities, along with the biological pathways through which early disadvantage might 'get under the skin'. As highlighted in Section 17.3.2, biological measures which are risk factors for subsequent disease, such as lung function, body composition, and inflammation, vary according to childhood SEP. There is also accumulating evidence that biomarkers based on new omics measures and more intense phenotypic information are also socially distributed, although further research is needed. Childhood SEP has been associated with, for example, changes in the epigenome,[108] and early life social disadvantage related to faster rates of ageing marked by epigenetic age,[109-111] telomere length,[112] allostatic load,[113] and a measure termed 'pace of ageing' derived from multiple biomarkers across the body systems.[114]

17.4.1 Health and Physical Development

Disadvantaged SEP in childhood is linked to a range of detrimental early life health outcomes, such as increased respiratory infections and asthma[115] (potentially owing to poor and crowded housing), mental health problems, and poorer physical, cognitive, and socioemotional development.[116] Childhood mental health symptoms and cognition track over the life course, while respiratory infections are associated with lower lung function in later life,[117] and may act to prevent maximum development of the lungs.[117] Clearly, given the COVID-19 pandemic, there has been a renewed interest in the impact of infectious diseases in childhood, which are likely to be more common in crowded and disadvantaged households, on later health. This was initially of interest in the first part of the twentieth century and, then again, stimulated by the discovery that helicobacter-pylori infection contributed to the development of peptic ulcer disease.[118,119]

In most HICs, early life disadvantage is also associated with shorter height and greater childhood BMI,[120] assumed to act through poorer maternal and infant nutrition. However, an analysis across the British birth cohorts demonstrated that although the height inequality was observed in the 1946 cohort, there was little evidence of such height inequalities by the 2000 cohort.[121] In contrast, inequalities in childhood BMI have emerged in more recent cohorts, which were not observed in cohorts born prior to the 1990s in the UK—inequalities are also greatest in the upper tails of the BMI distribution, suggesting greater skewing of the BMI distribution in the most disadvantaged.

As previous chapters have documented, these socially patterned early life exposures may be important for later life health, but there is little direct evidence to explain much of the effect of early life SEP on health. Pathways appear complex and understanding may be enhanced through further examination with modern mediation approaches. Alternatively, poor health in childhood, and indeed throughout the life course, may influence subsequent socioeconomic trajectories. Good health in childhood is associated with better education attainment,[122,123] while the impacts of specific health conditions such as depression[124-127] and asthma[128] is varied, as is the potential mediating role of school absence. There is more consistent evidence linking attention-deficit hyperactivity disorder (ADHD) to educational achievement.[129-131] However, the fact that children who are less advantaged have poorer health means that such associations may be confounded by childhood SEP. Triangulation across observational and genetic approaches has supported a causal influence of ADHD on lower educational attainment, but not of autism spectrum disorder, depression, asthma, or migraine.[132] Similar to health, while advantaged SEP is generally thought to be associated with taller height and lower BMI, owing to better nutrition in childhood, taller stature and lower BMI may have beneficial effects on subsequent SEP,[133-136] through, for example, discrimination against those who are shorter and of greater adiposity. High BMI is associated with weight-related stigma and poorer physical and mental health.[137-139] An MR study in UK Biobank supported prior observational evidence that height and BMI play a causal role in determining SEP.[140] Low BMI in women was related to higher income and lower social deprivation, and taller height in men was beneficial for income and occupation, as well as education. Interestingly, a nonlinear MR analysis suggested both low, as well as high BMI, increased deprivation and reduced income.[141]

17.4.2 Psychosocial Exposures

A comparison of data from the Millennium Cohort study (participants born in 2000–01), the Study of Early Education and Development (participants born in 2010–12), and the 1970 Birth Cohort Study found that inequalities in early cognitive, social, and emotional development have changed little between those born in 2000–01 and those born in the 2010–12.[142] Childhood psychosocial development is influenced by the home environment, which includes the input of parents to educational development, 'emotional' support (such as parent–child relationships and interactions), and parents' mental well-being. Socioeconomic inequalities need to be addressed to allow parents the material, cultural, and social capital to buy books, cook healthy meals, and spend time with their children.[143] The Deaton Review, comparing three cohorts, found improvements in some aspects of early home environments, such as the frequency with which parents read to their children, but deteriorations in others, such as an increase in the prevalence of maternal mental health problems.[144] Further, the differences in these exposures according to family income remained high.

There has been substantial increased interest in the role of adverse childhood experiences (ACEs), and while there is debate in regards of what constitutes an ACE, they have been defined as an 'exposure during childhood or adolescence to environmental circumstances that are likely to require significant psychological, social, or neurobiological adaptation by an average child and that represent a deviation from the expectable environment'.[145] Poverty is strongly related to ACEs, particularly parental separation, sexual abuse, and maternal mental health problems.[146] Further, the transition into poverty has been shown to be an important risk factor for maternal mental health problems in the UK Millennium Cohort Study.[147] Girls are more likely to report maltreatment, particularly sexual abuse, but males are more likely to report physical abuse.[146,148-150] ACEs have also been found to cluster such that those who experience one adversity are much more likely to report another, but no gender differences were found in the way in which ACEs cluster in a UK study.[146] Associations between ACEs and health outcomes are discussed throughout this book, with clearer evidence of a relationship with mental than physical health (see Chapters 5, 9, 15, 16, 19, and 20). It has been suggested that the associations vary between men and women, with possibly stronger effects on mental health in women.[151] However, there is currently a lack of clear evidence as a meta-analysis of gender differences in associations between child maltreatment and adult mental health found only five studies which had stratified analyses by gender,[152] and these showed no gender differences. In the US Fragile Families and Child Wellbeing Study, ACEs by age 5 years were related to both internalised and externalised psychological distress for boys and were mainly related to externalised distress for girls.[153]

Mental health could explain any pathway between ACEs and poorer physical health, while a systematic review of research on ACEs and biomarkers in early life found an effect of ACEs on markers of the immune system such as C-reactive protein, and interleukin-6 (IL-6).[154] Studies have also provided some evidence of changes in DNA methylation by ACE exposure,[155] and that exposure to ACEs might be related to increased epigenetic age in children[156] and adults[157] and elevated allostatic load.[158] In addition, as for childhood health, ACEs likely impact subsequent social trajectories, potentially via lower educatinal attainment, drug use and smoking.[159]

17.5 Conclusions

Social inequalities in health are perhaps the biggest current public health challenge. A life course approach to tackle these inequalities which starts in childhood is required, acknowledging the highly interlinked nature of work, family, and health trajectories across the life course in women, and the differences in social context according to birth cohort. Inequalities have been further highlighted and exacerbated by the COVID-19 pandemic, and effective policies are required to mitigate the worst impacts of the pandemic and the subsequent economic recession. Follow-up of longitudinal studies of women who have experienced the pandemic at different ages will be needed to monitor the progress made.

Key messages and implications

- Intergenerational social mobility in women has increased over subsequent generations, but there remains substantial continuity particularly at the top and bottom of the social distribution.
- Women's family and work trajectories are highly interrelated across the life course, have implications for health, and change according to the social context.
- There are wide and persistent inequalities in mortality and health according to adult and childhood socioeconomic position.
- Health-related behaviours play a major role in explaining the social inequalities in health, but potential socially patterned early life factors may also contribute.
- Childhood health, and physical, cognitive, and socioemotional development impact subsequent social trajectories in women.

References

1. Galobardes B, Shaw M, Lawlor DA, Lynch JW, Davey Smith G. Indicators of socioeconomic position (part 1). *Journal of Epidemiology and Community Health*. 2006;60(1):7–12.
2. Blane D. Commentary: the place in life course research of validated measures of socioeconomic position. *International Journal of Epidemiology*. 2006;35(1):139–40.

3. Bann D, Wright L, Goisis A, Hardy R, Johnson W, Maddock J, et al. Investigating change across time in prevalence or association using observational data: guidance on utility, methodology, and interpretation. *OSF Preprints*. 27 August 2021.

4. Tregenna F. Characterising deindustrialisation: an analysis of changes in manufacturing employment and output internationally. *Cambridge Journal of Economics*. 2008;33(3):433–66.

5. Gakidou E, Cowling K, Lozano R, Murray CJ. Increased educational attainment and its effect on child mortality in 175 countries between 1970 and 2009: a systematic analysis. *Lancet*. 2010;376(9745):959–74.

6. Howe LD, Galobardes B, Matijasevich A, Gordon D, Johnston D, Onwujekwe O, et al. Measuring socio-economic position for epidemiological studies in low- and middle-income countries: a methods of measurement in epidemiology paper. *International Journal of Epidemiology*. 2012;41(3):871–86.

7. Erikson R, Goldthorpe JH. *The constant flux: a study of class mobility in industrial societies*. Oxford: Clarendon Press; 1992.

8. Kuh D, Head J, Hardy R, Wadsworth M. The influence of education and family background on women's earnings in midlife: evidence from a British national birth cohort study. *British Journal of Sociology of Education*. 1997;18(3):21.

9. Causa O, Johansson A. Intergenerational social mobility in OECD countries. *OECD Journal: Economic Studies*. 2010;2010(1):44.

10. OECD. *A broken social elevator? How to promote social mobility*. Paris: OECD Publishing; 2018.

11. Bartley M, Sacker A, Schoon I. Social and economic trajectories and women's health. In: Kuh D, Hardy R, eds. *A life course approach to women's health, 1st edition*. Oxford: Oxford University Press; 2002. pp. 233–54.

12. Bukodi E, Goldthorpe JH, Waller L, Kuha J. The mobility problem in Britain: new findings from the analysis of birth cohort data. *British Journal of Sociology*. 2015;66(1):93–117.

13. Buscha F, Sturgis P. Declining social mobility? Evidence from five linked censuses in England and Wales 1971–2011. *British Journal of Sociology*. 2018;69(1):154–82.

14. Goldthorpe JH, Mills C. Trends in intergenerational class mobility in Britain in the late twentieth century. In: Breen R, ed. *Social mobility in Europe*. Oxford: Oxford University Press; 2004. pp. 195–224.

15. Bukodi E, Goldthorpe JH, Joshi H, Waller L. Why have relative rates of class mobility become more equal among women in Britain? *British Journal of Sociology*. 2017;68(3):512–32.

16. Macmillan L, McKnight A. *Understanding recent patterns in intergenerational social mobility: differences by gender, ethnicity, education, and their intersections*. London: London School of Economics and Political Science; May 2022. SPDORP11.

17. Subotnik RF, Arnold K, ed. *Beyond Terman: longitudinal studies in contemporary gifted education*. Norwood, NJ: Ablex; 1993.

18. OECD. *Education at a glance 2020: OECD indicators*. Paris: OECD Publishing; 2020.

19. Fan X, Sturman M. Has higher education solved the problem? Examining the gender wage gap of recent college graduates entering the workplace. *Compensation & Benefits Review*. 2019;51(1):5–12.

20. World Economic Forum. *The global social mobility report 2020: equality, opportunity and a new economic imperative*. Geneva: World Economic Forum; 2020.

21. Hertel FR, Groh-Samberg O. The relation between inequality and intergenerational class mobility in 39 countries. *American Sociological Review*. 2019;84(6):34.

22. Krueger AB. *The rise and consequences of inequality in the United States, speech, presented at the Center for American Progress*, Washington, DC; 12 January 2012.

23. Jerrim J, Macmillan L. Income inequality, intergenerational mobility, and the Great Gatsby curve: is education the key? *Social Forces*. 2015;94(2):29.

24. Green F, Machin S, Murphy R, Zhu Y. The changing economic advantage from private schools. *Economica*. 2011;79(316):12.

25. Green F, Anders J, Henderson M, Henseke G. *Who chooses private schooling in Britain and why?* London: Centre for Learning and Life Chances in Knowledge Economies and Societies; LLAKES Research Paper 62. 2017

26. The Cabinet Office. *Fair access to professional careers: a progress report by the Independent Reviewer on Social Mobility and Child Poverty*. London: The Cabinet Office; 2012.

27. Global Burden of Disease Population Fertility Collaborators. Population and fertility by age and sex for 195 countries and territories, 1950–2017: a systematic analysis for the Global Burden of Disease Study 2017. *Lancet*. 2018;392(10159):1995–2051.

28. McMunn A, Lacey RE, Worts D, McDonough P, Stafford M, Booker C, et al. De-standardization and gender convergence in work–family life courses in Great Britain: a multi-channel sequence analysis. *Advances in life Course Research*. 2015;26:60–75.

29. Baranowska-Rataj A, Matysiak A. The causal effects of the number of children on female employment—do European institutional and gender conditions matter? *Journal of Labor Research*. 2016;37:343–67.

30. Finlay JE, Lee MA. Identifying causal effects of reproductive health improvements on women's economic empowerment through the Population Poverty Research Initiative. *Milbank Quarterly*. 2018;96(2):300–22.

31. Ermisch J. *Does a 'teen-birth' have longer-term impacts on the mother? Suggestive evidence from the British Household Panel Study*. Colchester: Institute for Social and Economic Research; Nov. 2003. ISER Working paper Series 2003-32.

32. Pevalin DJ. *Outcomes in childhood and adulthood by mother's age: evidence from the 1970 British Cohort Study*. Colchester: Institute for Social and Economic Research; Oct. 2003. ISER Working Paper Series 2003-31.

33. Hobcraft J, Kiernan K. Childhood poverty, early motherhood and adult social exclusion. *British Journal of Sociology*. 2001;52(3):495–517.

34. Klein JD, and the Committee on Adolescence. Adolescent pregnancy: current trends and issues. *Pediatrics*. 2005;116(1):281–6.

35. Levine D, Painter G. The schooling costs of teenage out-of-wedlock childbearing: analysis with a within-school propensity-score-matching estimator. *Review of Economics and Statistics*. 2003;85:884–900.

36. Taniguchi H, Rosenfeld RA. Women's employment exit and reentry: differences among whites, blacks, and Hispanics. *Social Science Research*. 2002;31(3):432–71.

37. Hoffman SD. Teen childbearing and economics: a short history of a 25-year research love affair. *Societies*. 2015;5(3):646–63.

38. Gorry D. Heterogeneous consequences of teenage childbearing. *Demography*. 2019;56(6):2147–68.

39. Ichino A, Moretti E. Biological gender differences, absenteeism, and the earnings gap. *American Economic Journal: Applied Economics*. 2009;1(1):183–218.

40. Bryson A, Conti G, Hardy R, Peycheva D, Sullivan A. The consequences of early menopause and menopause symptoms for labour market participation. *Social Science & Medicine*. 2022;293:114676.

41. Kunze A. The *gender wage gap in developed countries*. Bonn: Institute of Labor Economics; June 2017. IZA Discussion Paper No. 10826.

42. Eurostat: Statistics Explained. *Gender pay gap statistics [Internet]*. Brussel: Eurostat; 2022 [updated March 2022; cited 29 July 2022]. Available from: https://ec.europa.eu/eurostat/statistics-explained/index.php?title=Gender_pay_gap_statistics.

43. Bryson A, Joshi H, Wielgoszewska B, Wilkinson D. *A short history of the gender wage gap in Britain*. Bonn: Institute of Labor Economics; May 2020. IZA DP No. 13289.

44. Joshi H, Bryson A, Wilkinson D, Ward K. The gender gap in wages over the life course: evidence from a British cohort born in 1958. *Gender, Work & Organization*. 2021;28(1):397–415.

45. Costa Dias M, Joyce R, Parodi F. *The gender pay gap in the UK: children and experience in work*. London: Institute for Fiscal Studies; Feb. 2018. IFS Working Paper 18/02.

46. Manning A, Swaffield J. The gender gap in early-career wage growth. *Economic Journal*. 2008;118(530):983–1024.

47. Office of National Statistics. *Health state life expectancies by national deprivation deciles, England: 2018 to 2020*. London: Office of National Statistics; 2022.

48. European Core Health Indicators. *Data from: European Core Health Indicators (ECHI) Data Tool, Version 3.1.0*. Brussel: European Core Health Indicators; 2021 [cited 5 July 2022]. Available from: https://webgate.ec.europa.eu/dyna/echi/.

49. Newton S, Braithwaite D, Akinyemiju TF. Socio-economic status over the life course and obesity: systematic review and meta-analysis. *PLoS ONE*. 2017;12(5):e0177151.
50. McLaren L. Socioeconomic status and obesity. *Epidemiologic Reviews*. 2007;29:29–48.
51. Bridger Staatz C, Kelly Y, Lacey RE, Blodgett JM, George A, Arnot M, et al. Socioeconomic position and body composition in childhood in high- and middle-income countries: a systematic review and narrative synthesis. *International Journal of Obesity (London)*. 2021;45(11):2316–34.
52. Bann D, Johnson W, Li L, Kuh D, Hardy R. Socioeconomic inequalities in body mass index across adulthood: coordinated analyses of individual participant data from three British birth cohort studies initiated in 1946, 1958 and 1970. *PLoS Medicine*. 2017;14(1):e1002214.
53. Murray ET, Lacey R, Maughan B, Sacker A. Non-parental care in childhood and health up to 30 years later: ONS Longitudinal Study 1971–2011. *European Journal of Public Health*. 2020;30(6):1121–7.
54. Botchway SK, Quigley MA, Gray R. Pregnancy-associated outcomes in women who spent some of their childhood looked after by local authorities: findings from the UK Millennium Cohort Study. *BMJ Open*. 2014;4(12):e005468.
55. Akister J, Owens M, Goodyer IM. Leaving care and mental health: outcomes for children in out-of-home care during the transition to adulthood. *Health Research Policy and Systems*. 2010;8:10.
56. Fazel S, Geddes JR, Kushel M. The health of homeless people in high-income countries: descriptive epidemiology, health consequences, and clinical and policy recommendations. *Lancet*. 2014;384(9953):1529–40.
57. Müller M, Khamis D, Srivastava D, Exadaktylos AK, Pfortmueller CA. Understanding refugees' health. *Seminars in Neurology*. 2018;38(02):152–62.
58. Bhopal RS. *Ethnicity, race, and health in multicultural societies: foundations for better epidemiology, public health, and health care*. Oxford: Oxford University Press; 2007.
59. Marmot M, Allen J, Boyce T, Goldblatt P, Morrison J. *Health equity in England: the Marmot Review 10 years on*. London: Institute of Health Equity; 2020.
60. McCartney G, Popham F, Katikireddi SV, Walsh D, Schofield L. How do trends in mortality inequalities by deprivation and education in Scotland and England & Wales compare? A repeat cross-sectional study. *BMJ Open*. 2017;7(7):e017590.
61. Fluharty ME, Hardy R, Ploubidis G, Pongiglione B, Bann D. Socioeconomic inequalities across life and premature mortality from 1971 to 2016: findings from three British birth cohorts born in 1946, 1958 and 1970. *Journal of Epidemiology and Community Health*. 2021;75(2):193–6.
62. Masters RK, Hummer RA, Powers DA. Educational differences in U.S. adult mortality: a cohort perspective. *American Sociological Review*. 2012;77(4):548–72.
63. Olshansky SJ, Antonucci T, Berkman L, Binstock R, Boersch-Supan A, Cacioppo JT, et al. differences in life expectancy due to race and educational differences are widening, and many may not catch up. *Health Affairs*. 2012;31(8):1803–13.
64. Montez JK, Hummer RA, Hayward MD, Woo H, Rogers RG. Trends in the educational gradient of U.S. adult mortality from 1986 through 2006 by race, gender, and age group. *Research on Aging*. 2011;33(2):145–71.
65. Kindig DA, Cheng ER. Even as mortality fell in most US counties, female mortality nonetheless rose in 42.8 percent of counties from 1992 to 2006. *Health Affairs*. 2013;32(3):451–8.
66. Montez JK, Zajacova A. Trends in mortality risk by education level and cause of death among US white women from 1986 to 2006. *American Journal of Public Health*. 2013;103(3):473–9.
67. Dowd JB, Hamoudi A. Is life expectancy really falling for groups of low socio-economic status? Lagged selection bias and artefactual trends in mortality. *International Journal of Epidemiology*. 2014;43(4):983–8.
68. Galobardes B, Lynch JW, Smith GD. Is the association between childhood socioeconomic circumstances and cause-specific mortality established? Update of a systematic review. *Journal of Epidemiology and Community Health*. 2008;62(5):387–90.
69. Galobardes B, Smith GD, Lynch JW. Systematic review of the influence of childhood socioeconomic circumstances on risk for cardiovascular disease in adulthood. *Annals of Epidemiology*. 2006;16(2):91–104.
70. Agardh E, Allebeck P, Hallqvist J, Moradi T, Sidorchuk A. Type 2 diabetes incidence and socio-economic position: a systematic review and meta-analysis. *International Journal of Epidemiology*. 2011;40(3):804–18.

71. Rocha V, Soares S, Stringhini S, Fraga S. Socioeconomic circumstances and respiratory function from childhood to early adulthood: a systematic review and meta-analysis. *BMJ Open*. 2019;9(6):e027528.

72. Birnie K, Cooper R, Martin RM, Kuh D, Sayer AA, Alvarado BE, et al. Childhood socioeconomic position and objectively measured physical capability levels in adulthood: a systematic review and meta-analysis. *PLoS ONE*. 2011;6(1):e15564.

73. Milaniak I, Jaffee SR. Childhood socioeconomic status and inflammation: a systematic review and meta-analysis. *Brain, Behavior, and Immunity*. 2019;78:161–76.

74. Bridger Staatz C, Kelly Y, Lacey RE, Blodgett JM, George A, Arnot M, et al. Life course socioeconomic position and body composition in adulthood: a systematic review and narrative synthesis. *International Journal of Obesity*. 2021;45(11):2300–15.

75. Winpenny EM, Howe LD, van Sluijs EMF, Hardy R, Tilling K. Early adulthood socioeconomic trajectories contribute to inequalities in adult cardiovascular health, independently of childhood and adulthood socioeconomic position. *Journal of Epidemiology and Community Health*. 2021;75(12):1172–80.

76. Pollitt RA, Rose KM, Kaufman JS. Evaluating the evidence for models of life course socioeconomic factors and cardiovascular outcomes: a systematic review. *BMC Public Health*. 2005;5(1):7.

77. McEwen BS, Stellar E. Stress and the individual: mechanisms leading to disease. *Archives of Internal Medicine*. 1993;153(18):2093–101.

78. Mishra G, Nitsch D, Black S, De Stavola B, Kuh D, Hardy R. A structured approach to modelling the effects of binary exposure variables over the life course. *International Journal of Epidemiology*. 2008;38(2):528–37.

79. Smith ADAC, Heron J, Mishra G, Gilthorpe MS, Ben-Shlomo Y, Tilling K. Model selection of the effect of binary exposures over the life course. *Epidemiology*. 2015;26(5).719–26.

80. Madathil S, Joseph L, Hardy R, Rousseau M-C, Nicolau B. A Bayesian approach to investigate life course hypotheses involving continuous exposures. *International Journal of Epidemiology*. 2018;47(5):1623–35.

81. Mishra GD, Chiesa F, Goodman A, De Stavola B, Koupil I. Socio-economic position over the life course and all-cause, and circulatory diseases mortality at age 50–87 years: results from a Swedish birth cohort. *European Journal of Epidemiology*. 2013;28(2):139–47.

82. Murray ET, Mishra GD, Kuh D, Guralnik J, Black S, Hardy R. Life course models of socioeconomic position and cardiovascular risk factors: 1946 birth cohort. *Annals of Epidemiology*. 2011;21(8):589–97.

83. Hawkins RB, Charles EJ, Mehaffey JH. Socio-economic status and COVID-19–related cases and fatalities. *Public Health*. 2020;189:129–34.

84. Niedzwiedz CL, O'Donnell CA, Jani BD, Demou E, Ho FK, Celis-Morales C, et al. Ethnic and socioeconomic differences in SARS-CoV-2 infection: prospective cohort study using UK Biobank. *BMC Medicine*. 2020;18(1):160.

85. Marmot M, Allen J, Goldblatt P, Herd E, Morrison J. *Build back fairer: the COVID-19 Marmot Review: the pandemic, socioeconomic and health inequalities in England*. London: Institute of Health Equity; 2020.

86. Williamson EJ, Walker AJ, Bhaskaran K, Bacon S, Bates C, Morton CE, et al. Factors associated with COVID-19-related death using OpenSAFELY. *Nature*. 2020;584(7821):430–6.

87. Bajos N, Jusot F, Pailhé A, Spire A, Martin C, Meyer L, et al. When lockdown policies amplify social inequalities in COVID-19 infections: evidence from a cross-sectional population-based survey in France. *BMC Public Health*. 2021;21(1):705.

88. Glampson B, Brittain J, Kaura A, Mulla A, Mercuri L, Brett SJ, et al. Assessing COVID-19 vaccine uptake and effectiveness through the North West London Vaccination Program: retrospective cohort study. *JMIR Public Health Surveillance*. 2021;7(9):e30010.

89. Curtis AF, Rodgers M, Miller MB, McCrae CS. Impact of sex on COVID-19 media exposure, anxiety, perceived risk, and severity in middle-aged and older adults. *Journal of Aging and Health*. 2022;34(1):51–9.

90. Keller A, Groot J, Matta J, Bu F, El Aarbaoui T, Melchior M, et al. Housing environment and mental health of Europeans during the COVID-19 pandemic: a cross-country comparison. *Scientific Reports*. 2022;12(1):5612.

91. Moreno-Agostino D, Fisher HL, Hatch SL, Morgan C, Ploubidis GB, Das-Munshi J. Inequalities in mental and social wellbeing during the COVID-19 pandemic: prospective longitudinal observational study of five UK cohorts. *medRxiv*. 2022:2022.02.07.22270588.

92. Xue B, McMunn A. Gender differences in unpaid care work and psychological distress in the UK Covid-19 lockdown. *PLoS ONE*. 2021;16(3):e0247959.

93. Seedat S, Rondon M. Women's wellbeing and the burden of unpaid work. *BMJ*. 2021;374:n1972.

94. Feder G, Lucas d'Oliveira AF, Rishal P, Johnson M. Domestic violence during the pandemic. *BMJ*. 2021;372:n722.

95. Andrew A, Cattan S, Costa Dias M, Farquharson C, Kraftman L, Krutikova S, et al. Inequalities in children's experiences of home learning during the Covid-19 lockdown in England. *Fiscal Studies*. 2020;41(3):653–83.

96. Vanaken G-J, Danckaerts M. Impact of green space exposure on children's and adolescents' mental health: a systematic review. *International Journal of Environmental Research and Public Health*. 2018;15(12):2668.

97. Wilkins E, Radley D, Morris M, Hobbs M, Christensen A, Marwa WL, et al. A systematic review employing the GeoFERN framework to examine methods, reporting quality and associations between the retail food environment and obesity. *Health & Place*. 2019;57:186–99.

98. Gianfredi V, Buffoli M, Rebecchi A, Croci R, Oradini-Alacreu A, Stirparo G, et al. Association between urban greenspace and health: a systematic review of literature. *International Journal of Environmental Research and Public Health*. 2021;18(10):5137.

99. Walton H, Evangelopoulos D, Kasdagli M, Selley L, Dajnak D, Katsouyanni K. *Investigating links between air pollution, COVID-19 and lower respiratory infectious diseases*. London: Imperial College London; 2021.

100. Raaschou-Nielsen O, Andersen ZJ, Beelen R, Samoli E, Stafoggia M, Weinmayr G, et al. Air pollution and lung cancer incidence in 17 European cohorts: prospective analyses from the European Study of Cohorts for Air Pollution Effects (ESCAPE). *Lancet Oncology*. 2013;14(9):813–22.

101. Jacquemin B, Siroux V, Sanchez M, Carsin A-E, Schikowski T, Adam M, et al. Ambient air pollution and adult asthma incidence in six European cohorts (ESCAPE). *Environmental Health Perspectives*. 2015;123(6):613–21.

102. Doiron D, Bourbeau J, de Hoogh K, Hansell AL. Ambient air pollution exposure and chronic bronchitis in the Lifelines cohort. *Thorax*. 2021;76(8):772–9.

103. Doiron D, de Hoogh K, Probst-Hensch N, Fortier I, Cai Y, De Matteis S, et al. Air pollution, lung function and COPD: results from the population-based UK Biobank study. *European Respiratory Journal*. 2019;54(1):1802140.

104. Ferguson L, Taylor J, Zhou K, Shrubsole C, Symonds P, Davies M, et al. Systemic inequalities in indoor air pollution exposure in London, UK. *Build Cities*. 2021;2(1):425–48.

105. Petrovic D, de Mestral C, Bochud M, Bartley M, Kivimäki M, Vineis P, et al. The contribution of health behaviors to socioeconomic inequalities in health: a systematic review. *Preventive Medicine*. 2018;113:15–31.

106. Floud S, Balkwill A, Moser K, Reeves GK, Green J, Beral V, et al. The role of health-related behavioural factors in accounting for inequalities in coronary heart disease risk by education and area deprivation: prospective study of 1.2 million UK women. *BMC Medicine*. 2016;14(1):145.

107. Stringhini S, Sabia S, Shipley M, Brunner E, Nabi H, Kivimaki M, et al. Association of socioeconomic position with health behaviors and mortality. *JAMA*. 2010;303(12):1159–66.

108. Cerutti J, Lussier AA, Zhu Y, Liu J, Dunn EC. Associations between indicators of socioeconomic position and DNA methylation: a scoping review. *Clinical Epigenetics*. 2021;13(1):221.

109. Raffington L, Belsky DW. Integrating DNA methylation measures of biological aging into social determinants of health research. *Current Environmental Health Reports*. 2022;9(2):196–210.

110. George A, Hardy R, Castillo Fernandez J, Kelly Y, Maddock J. Life course socioeconomic position and DNA methylation age acceleration in mid-life. *Journal of Epidemiology and Community Health*. 2021;75(11):1084–90.

111. Hughes A, Smart M, Gorrie-Stone T, Hannon E, Mill J, Bao Y, et al. Socioeconomic position and DNA methylation age acceleration across the life course. *American Journal of Epidemiology*. 2018;187(11):2346–54.

112. Ridout KK, Levandowski M, Ridout SJ, Gantz L, Goonan K, Palermo D, et al. Early life adversity and telomere length: a meta-analysis. *Molecular Psychiatry*. 2018;23(4):858–71.

113. Dowd JB, Simanek AM, Aiello AE. Socio-economic status, cortisol and allostatic load: a review of the literature. *International Journal of Epidemiology*. 2009;38(5):1297–309.

114. Belsky DW, Caspi A, Cohen HJ, Kraus WE, Ramrakha S, Poulton R, et al. Impact of early personal-history characteristics on the pace of aging: implications for clinical trials of therapies to slow aging and extend health span. *Aging Cell*. 2017;16(4):644–51.

115. Uphoff E, Cabieses B, Pinart M, Valdes M, Anto JM, Wright J. A systematic review of socioeconomic position in relation to asthma and allergic diseases. *European Respiratory Journal*. 2015;46(2):364–74.

116. Pillas D, Marmot M, Naicker K, Goldblatt P, Morrison J, Pikhart H. Social inequalities in early childhood health and development: a European-wide systematic review. *Pediatric Research*. 2014;76(5):418–24.

117. Allinson JP, Hardy R, Donaldson GC, Shaheen SO, Kuh D, Wedzicha JA. Combined impact of smoking and early-life exposures on adult lung function trajectories. *American Journal of Respiratory and Critical Care Medicine*. 2017;196(8):1021–30.

118. Kuh D, Ben Shlomo Y, Ezra S. A life course approach to chronic disease epidemiology. In: Kuh D, Ben Shlomo Y, Ezra S, eds. London: Oxford University Press; 2004. pp. 3–14.

119. Marshall BJ, Armstrong JA, McGechie DB, Clancy RJ. Attempt to fulfil Koch's postulates for pyloric Campylobacter. *Medical Journal of Australia*. 1985;142(8):436–9.

120. Wu S, Ding Y, Wu F, Li R, Hu Y, Hou J, et al. Socio-economic position as an intervention against overweight and obesity in children: a systematic review and meta-analysis. *Scientific Reports*. 2015;5:11354.

121. Bann D, Johnson W, Li L, Kuh D, Hardy R. Socioeconomic inequalities in childhood and adolescent body-mass index, weight, and height from 1953 to 2015: an analysis of four longitudinal, observational, British birth cohort studies. *Lancet Public Health*. 2018;3(4):e194–e203.

122. Case A, Fertig A, Paxson C. The lasting impact of childhood health and circumstance. *Journal of Health Economics*. 2005;24(2):365–89.

123. Brekke I. Health and educational success in adolescents: a longitudinal study. *BMC Public Health*. 2015;15(1):619.

124. Fletcher JM. Adolescent depression and educational attainment: results using sibling fixed effects. *Health Economics*. 2010;19(7):855–71.

125. Veldman K, Bültmann U, Stewart RE, Ormel J, Verhulst FC, Reijneveld SA. Mental health problems and educational attainment in adolescence: 9-year follow-up of the TRAILS Study. *PLoS ONE*. 2014;9(7):e101751.

126. McLeod JD, Uemura R, Rohrman S. Adolescent mental health, behavior problems, and academic achievement. *Journal of Health and Social Behavior*. 2012;53(4):482–97.

127. Evensen M, Lyngstad TH, Melkevik O, Mykletun A. The role of internalizing and externalizing problems in adolescence for adult educational attainment: evidence from sibling comparisons using data from the Young HUNT Study. *European Sociological Review*. 2016;32(5):552–66.

128. Milton B, Whitehead M, Holland P, Hamilton V. The social and economic consequences of childhood asthma across the lifecourse: a systematic review. *Child: Care, Health and Development*. 2004;30(6):711–28.

129. Stergiakouli E, Martin J, Hamshere ML, Heron J, St Pourcain B, Timpson NJ, et al. Association between polygenic risk scores for attention-deficit hyperactivity disorder and educational and cognitive outcomes in the general population. *International Journal of Epidemiology*. 2016;46(2):421–8.

130. Fletcher J, Wolfe B. Child mental health and human capital accumulation: the case of ADHD revisited. *Journal of Health Economics*. 2008;27(3):794–800.

131. Currie J, Stabile M. Child mental health and human capital accumulation: the case of ADHD. *Journal of Health Economics*. 2006;25(6):1094–118.

132. Hughes A, Bao Y, Smart M, Kumari M. Body mass index, earnings and partnership: genetic instrumental variable analysis in two nationally representative UK samples. *bioRxiv*. 2019:608588.

133. Anne Case, Christina Paxson. Stature and status: height, ability, and labor market outcomes. *Journal of Political Economy*. 2008;116(3):499–532.

134. Magnusson PKE, Rasmussen F, Gyllensten UB. Height at age 18 years is a strong predictor of attained education later in life: cohort study of over 950 000 Swedish men. *International Journal of Epidemiology*. 2006;35(3):658–63.

135. Gortmaker SL, Must A, Perrin JM, Sobol AM, Dietz WH. Social and economic consequences of overweight in adolescence and young adulthood. *New England Journal of Medicine*. 1993;329(14):1008–12.

136. Lundborg P, Nystedt P, Rooth D-O. Body size, skills, and income: evidence from 150,000 teenage siblings. *Demography*. 2014;51(5):1573–96.

137. Tomiyama AJ, Carr D, Granberg EM, Major B, Robinson E, Sutin AR, et al. How and why weight stigma drives the obesity 'epidemic' and harms health. *BMC Medicine*. 2018;16(1):123.

138. Puhl RM, Liu S. A national survey of public views about the classification of obesity as a disease. *Obesity*. 2015;23(6):1288–95.

139. Spahlholz J, Baer N, König H-H, Riedel-Heller SG, Luck-Sikorski C. Obesity and discrimination—a systematic review and meta-analysis of observational studies. *Obesity Reviews*. 2016;17(1):43–55.

140. Tyrrell J, Jones SE, Beaumont R, Astley CM, Lovell R, Yaghootkar H, et al. Height, body mass index, and socioeconomic status: mendelian randomisation study in UK Biobank. *BMJ*. 2016;352:i582.

141. Howe LD, Kanayalal R, Harrison S, Beaumont RN, Davies AR, Frayling TM, et al. Effects of body mass index on relationship status, social contact and socio-economic position: Mendelian randomization and within-sibling study in UK Biobank. *International Journal of Epidemiology*. 2020;49(4):1173–84.

142. Joyce R, Xu X. *Inequalities in the twenty-first century: introducing the IFS Deaton Review*. London: Institute for Fiscal Studies; 2019.

143. Kamphuis CBM, Jansen T, Mackenbach JP, van Lenthe FJ. Bourdieu's cultural capital in relation to food choices: a systematic review of cultural capital indicators and an empirical proof of concept. *PLoS ONE*. 2015;10(8):e0130695.

144. Cattan S, Fitzsimons E, Goodman A, Phimister A, Ploubidis GB, Wertz J. *Early childhood inequalities*. London: IFS Deaton Review of Inequalities; 2022.

145. McLaughlin KA. Future directions in childhood adversity and youth psychopathology. *Journal of Clinical Child and Adolescent Psychology*. 2016;45(3):361–82.

146. Lacey RE, Howe LD, Kelly-Irving M, Bartley M, Kelly Y. The clustering of adverse childhood experiences in the Avon Longitudinal Study of Parents and Children: are gender and poverty important? *Journal of Interpersonal Violence*. 2022;37(5–6):2218–41.

147. Wickham S, Whitehead M, Taylor-Robinson D, Barr B. The effect of a transition into poverty on child and maternal mental health: a longitudinal analysis of the UK Millennium Cohort Study. *Lancet Public Health*. 2017;2(3):e141–e148.

148. Martin G, Bergen HA, Richardson AS, Roeger L, Allison S. Sexual abuse and suicidality: gender differences in a large community sample of adolescents. *Child Abuse and Neglect*. 2004;28(5):491–503.

149. Dube SR, Anda RF, Whitfield CL, Brown DW, Felitti VJ, Dong M, et al. Long-term consequences of childhood sexual abuse by gender of victim. *American Journal of Preventive Medicine*. 2005;28(5):430–8.

150. Brown GR, Anderson B. Psychiatric morbidity in adult inpatients with childhood histories of sexual and physical abuse. *American Journal of Psychiatry*. 1991;148(1):55–61.

151. Gershon A, Minor K, Hayward C. Gender, victimization, and psychiatric outcomes. *Psychological Medicine*. 2008;38(10):1377–91.

152. Gallo EAG, Munhoz TN, Loret de Mola C, Murray J. Gender differences in the effects of childhood maltreatment on adult depression and anxiety: a systematic review and meta-analysis. *Child Abuse and Neglect*. 2018;79:107–14.

153. Jones MS, Pierce H, Shafer K. Gender differences in early adverse childhood experiences and youth psychological distress. *Journal of Criminal Justice*. 2022;83:101925.

154. Soares S, Rocha V, Kelly-Irving M, Stringhini S, Fraga S. Adverse childhood events and health biomarkers: a systematic review. *Frontiers in Public Health*. 2021;9:649825.

155. Houtepen LC, Hardy R, Maddock J, Kuh D, Anderson EL, Relton CL, et al. Childhood adversity and DNA methylation in two population-based cohorts. *Translational Psychiatry*. 2018;8(1):266.

156. Tang R, Howe LD, Suderman M, Relton CL, Crawford AA, Houtepen LC. Adverse childhood experiences, DNA methylation age acceleration, and cortisol in UK children: a prospective population-based cohort study. *Clinical Epigenetics*. 2020;12(1):55.

157. Lawn RB, Anderson EL, Suderman M, Simpkin AJ, Gaunt TR, Teschendorff AE, et al. Psychosocial adversity and socioeconomic position during childhood and epigenetic age: analysis of two prospective cohort studies. *Human Molecular Genetics*. 2018;27(7):1301–8.

158. Finlay S, Roth C, Zimsen T, Bridson TL, Sarnyai Z, McDermott B. Adverse childhood experiences and allostatic load: a systematic review. *Neuroscience & Biobehavioral Reviews*. 2022;136:104605.

159. Houtepen LC, Heron J, Suderman MJ, Fraser A, Chittleborough CR, Howe LD. Associations of adverse childhood experiences with educational attainment and adolescent health and the role of family and socioeconomic factors: a prospective cohort study in the UK. *PLoS Medicine*. 2020;17(3):e1003031.

18
Women's Social Relationships and Links with Health and Well-being over the Life Course

Anne McMunn

18.1 Introduction

For many years, it has generally been accepted that, with the notable exception of marriage, social relationships are more important for women than for men. Empirical work has often highlighted women's larger social networks, particularly friendship networks, and greater reported levels of providing and receiving social support compared with men in the United States[1] and in the UK.[2] However, while women appear to be more socially integrated and exchange more social support with contacts outside their partnerships than men do, there is some evidence that women may be more likely than men to report loneliness.[3,4] Several hypotheses have been proposed for why social relationships may be particularly important for women. Evolutionary theorists reason that women's historical responsibility for the care of dependent and immature offspring meant they had greater need than men to turn to their social groups for joint protection in times of threat. This resulted in a more developed awareness of the quality of their social relationships, because of their greater need to depend upon them.[5] This model points to neuroendocrine explanations for women's predilection to 'tend and befriend', such as release of oxytocin in response to stress, which may have a calming effect and increase affiliative behaviour.[5] In addition, there is a long history of sociological and social psychological work demonstrating the impact of social norms and institutions in structuring and legitimating gendered life course paths, reinforcing competitiveness and barriers to intimacy for boys, and encouraging intimacy and nurturance among girls.[6] The impact of such imposed gendered roles across life course paths is discussed further in Chapter 19. Given the weakening of traditional gender norms and socialisation processes seen in many countries over the past 40 years,[7] we might expect gendered patterns in social relations and their impact on health to be in flux.[8,9]

A life course perspective allows us to understand how different relationships gain or lose salience as people develop and age, how early life circumstances and life course transitions influence later social relationships, and the pathways through which social relationships influence health and well-being.[10,11] While the link between social relationships and various health outcomes is strong and well-known, the relative importance of particular social relationships at different stages of the life course and the extent to which relationships track

Anne McMunn, *Women's Social Relationships and Links with Health and Well-being over the Life Course* In: *A Life Course Approach to Women's Health*. Second Edition. Edited by: Gita D Mishra, Rebecca Hardy, and Diana Kuh, Oxford University Press.
© Oxford University Press 2023. DOI: 10.1093/oso/9780192864642.003.0018

across life is less clear.[12] Distinct aspects of social relationships—network size or composition, emotional or instrumental support, engagement with organisations or communities—may have different functions at different stages of the life course, and, as described by the Convoy model, social relationships that are longstanding foster exchanges of support at different life stages.[13]

This chapter is structured around the stages of the life course, reviewing current evidence on women's social relationships and their influence on health and well-being. It assesses gender differences in the pattern and meaning of social relationships over the life course, and the notion that social relationships are more central to the lives of women and, therefore, more strongly linked with health, while men continue to rely on their partners for health-enhancing support. Research on the experiences of LBGTIQA + people is still in its infancy; hence, the evidence here reflects on a traditional relationship construct between men and women.

18.2 Women's Relationships in Early Life and Adolescence

18.2.1 Parental Relationships and Early Family Life

The importance of intimate bonds created from secure attachment to a primary caregiver in early life for psychological and social development is now well-accepted.[14] Family attachment and parent-child relationship quality, parenting styles, and, at the extreme end, child maltreatment, have all been linked with a range of behavioural and relationship outcomes,[15-17] including through into mid- and later life,[18,19] with parental conflict and depression particularly detrimental.[17,20,21] Material deprivation and financial strain often drive the parental depression and conflict that have a negative impact on development.[20,22] Indeed, poverty may explain the greater risk of health and well-being problems amongst children in single parent families,[23] as single parent families continue to be much more likely than two-parent families to live in poverty.[24] However, outcomes amongst children are also generally worse in 'reconstituted' families in which parents repartner, despite the increasing diversity of family forms, and this does not appear to be explained by socioeconomic disadvantage.[25] The large majority of studies find early life relationships to be equally important for boys and girls, although a few have shown family conflict or maternal distress to be associated with adiposity and substance use disorders for girls and not boys.[21,26]

18.2.2 Peer Relationships and Adolescent Loneliness

As children reach adolescence, peer relationships become increasingly important, and some of the gendered aspects of social relationships that we see in adulthood begin to appear more strongly in adolescence. For example, there is some evidence to suggest that the wider social networks and higher levels of friend support reported by adult women can already be seen in adolescence, although adolescent boys may be just as satisfied as adolescent girls are with friend support.[27] One study suggested that girls' greater reactivity to interpersonal stressors such as peer events explained the higher prevalence of depressive symptoms in girls aged 13–18 years,[28] although evidence from Sweden has shown friendship networks and mental health to be equally correlated for girls and boys in bidirectional, longitudinal models.[29] Another study found peer relationships to vary more within genders than between them.[30] Much peer relationship exchange is now lived out through social media, particularly for adolescents and young adults. Increased frequency of social media interaction has been associated with declines in well-being for girls, but not boys, aged 10–15, in the UK.[31] Another UK study found links between persistent very frequent social media use and mental health worked through increased cyberbullying, as well as a lack of sleep and physical activity for girls, while the same was not true for boys.[32] And, while much research focuses on social isolation and loneliness in later life (see Section 18.3.2), evidence increasingly points to adolescence as a life course stage in which people are at the greatest risk for loneliness.[3,33] In a study of Dutch adolescents, girls had significantly higher levels of loneliness, depressive symptoms, and neuroticism than did boys, but there was no gender difference in the bidirectional associations between loneliness and depressive symptoms.[34]

18.3 Women's Adult Relationships

Social relationships and their importance for health and well-being in adulthood has been a burgeoning area of study for several decades.[35–37] Social relationships can be thought of in terms of their structural, quantitative aspects, such as the size and characteristics of social networks and frequency of contact with network members, or their functional or qualitative features, such as the support derived from them or the closeness felt.[36,38] The term *social capital* is also used to refer to the resources derived from social relationships at either the individual or community level,[39] although evidence included in this chapter is focused on women's social relationships at the individual level. Structural aspects of social relationships, such as having a large social network, may influence well-being through the higher levels of support and resources (i.e. the functional aspects of social relationships) that larger networks provide.[36] Social support may also buffer the negative impact of social or economic stress on well-being,[40] and socioeconomic advantage may foster large networks with more resources such that social relationships act to mediate inequalities in health.[41]

18.3.1 Social Support and Women's Relational Resources

Since the 1980s, studies from the United States have shown that, relative to men, women tend to have larger social networks, particularly larger friendship networks, and report providing and receiving more support.[1] This has similarly been seen in Spain,[42] Australia,[43] and in the UK.[2] There is evidence to suggest that women perceive, receive, and provide greater emotional social support than do men,[2–4] and these differences are likely to continue in older age.[2] While we might expect gender differences in social relationships to be reducing, given some evidence for the weakening of traditional gender norms and socialisation processes,[7] there is little evidence to support this expectation in the few studies to have included participants born towards the end of the twentieth century.[1,3,7,42] Much of the current evidence is based on participants born much earlier,[2,4,43] and not all studies find gender differences in social contact.[44] We must also be careful not to extrapolate studies from Western cultures to elsewhere.

A variety of structural and functional aspects of social relationships have been investigated in relation to many different health outcomes, the most common of which are mental health or well-being, cardiovascular disease, cognition, and mortality. Based on the notion that social relationships are more central to women's identity than men's, women are thought to be more 'reactive' than men to the quality of their relationships.[5,45] Evidence generally supports this notion in relation to mental health, with the majority of studies showing associations between social support and mental health to be stronger for women than for men,[46] although not always.[43,47] Beyond mental health there appears to be little evidence to support the notion that associations between social relationships and health are stronger for women than for men. When it comes to cardiovascular disease and mortality, greater social integration is associated with greater likelihood of survival for both men and women.[35,37,48,49] Similarly, negative relationships and isolation are equally linked with age-related declines in cognitive function in men and women,[50,51] although many studies in this area have not investigated gender differences. Those that have investigated gender differences have found none,[38,50] with the exception of a study of British civil servants, which found network size to be associated with all-cause and cardiovascular-related mortality in men but not women,[52] and a recent study which found links between the size and quality of social networks and insomnia in men but not women.[53]

Sources of support may be differentially important for women and men, and this may vary across cultures. There is some evidence from both Finland and the UK to suggest that the mental health of women and men benefit equally from contact with friends, while contact with family may largely benefit the mental health of men in the UK.[54] Other evidence from England supports traditional notions of gendered sources of support: men with high levels of positive social support from their spouse or partner had slower cognitive decline over 8 years, while for women, positive support from children and friends was associated with higher levels of cognitive function.[55] In Japan and Finland, contact with relatives was only associated with improved mental health for women,[54] while a recent study of older Mexican Americans found associations between living alone, compared with support from and closeness with children, more strongly associated with depression for men than women.[56]

18.3.2 Isolation and Loneliness

Later life has been a life course period of particular focus for social and family relationships, as retirement, widowhood, and reductions in functioning may serve to increase the risk for social isolation and loneliness.[2,57] The Socioemotional Selectivity theory suggests that network size and frequency of contact may decline with age as people focus on maintaining their closest relationships,[58] and there is evidence to suggest that nonfamily network size decreases with age.[58,59] While women appear to be more socially integrated and exchange more social support with contacts outside their partnerships than men do, some evidence has suggested that women may be more likely than men to report loneliness.[3,4] However, a recent meta-analysis has shown that, while boys and young men are slightly more likely to be lonely than girls or young women, the prevalence of loneliness is similar for men and women in mid- and later life.[60] Meta-analyses of the health and mortality risks associated with social isolation, loneliness, and living alone appear to be similar for men and women,[35,37] although slightly stronger for men (44% increased risk) than women (26% increased risk) in the most recent meta-analysis of loneliness and all-cause mortality.[61]

18.3.3 Partnership

Marriage and partnership have been singled out in the study of social relationships as particularly important close, personal ties. Married people generally have better health than unmarried people do, although often more so for men than women,[8,62,63] and the better health of married people is somewhat explained by healthier people being more likely than their less healthy counterparts to enter into marriage, although certainly not entirely (see discussion in Chapter 19).[64,65] Early studies in older populations suggested that women were less socially dependent on marriage and that mechanisms linking marriage with health differed for men and women, with emotional support and support for positive health behaviours more important for men, and financial advantages for women.[44,66] Traditionally, marriage has also represented caring and domestic responsibilities for women, in particular, and several studies have concluded that women have lower levels of marital satisfaction than do men.[67] There is also some evidence suggesting that widowhood is worse for men's health, while divorce is worse for women's health,[68] and we know that divorce continues to lead to reductions in income for women and not men, at least in the UK.[24]

However, the nature of marriage has changed dramatically over the past 40 years, particularly in relation to gender norms and expectations.[7] Williams[8] and Strohschein[9] have both argued that our current conception that marriage benefits men's health more than women's is based on an outdated version of marriage in which married women were economically dependent on their husbands and subsequently confined to the domestic sphere. Partnership has become more egalitarian as increases in women's occupational attainment has reduced the economic necessity of marriage for many women as well as potentially increasing their power within partnerships.[69] Certainly, evidence from large panel studies and longitudinal studies of ageing in the United States and Australia shows the psychological effects of marital status, marital transitions, and marital quality to be similar for men and women,[9,46,70] as is the marriage premium in mortality,[71] while marital loss has been linked with cardiovascular risk in women and not men in some studies.[72] On the other hand, a recent study in New Zealand found that emotional support mediated more of the association between partnership and well-being for men than for women, suggesting that men continue to be more reliant than women on their partnerships for emotional support, although the study was cross-sectional in design and did not test for cohort and age differences amongst participants who were born across the second half of the twentieth century.[73] Given that most evidence on partnership and women's health is based in Western cultures, it's important to remember there may be cultural differences. Studies in China and India have found worse health amongst unmarried and widowed women across a range of health outcomes, while the same was not found for men, although the association for women was weaker if they were socially active.[74,75]

18.4 Life Course Pathways Linking Social Relationships with Health and Well-being in Women

While the evidence base linking social relationships and mental health, cardiovascular disease, cognitive decline, and premature mortality is fairly substantial, the pathways linking them are less clear. Research has suggested that both behavioural pathways—such as smoking, nutrition, physical activity, alcohol consumption, and sleep[76]—as well as direct biological pathways[77] are likely to play a role.

18.4.1 Behavioural Pathways

Isolation, loneliness, and living alone have each been linked with less healthy behaviour,[78,79] while married people have been shown to have healthier, more varied diets,[80] and to be less likely to smoke[81] and drink heavily.[8,82] Evidence on physical activity is more mixed,[85] and married people tend to have higher BMIs than do single people.[81,83] These associations generally hold true for women and men with some studies showing no gender difference,[4,78,82,84] and some showing stronger associations for men.[79,85] Gendered norms governing health behaviours, such as smoking, alcohol consumption, and physical activity, have weakened since the 1970s,[86,87] so we might expect behavioural pathways linking social relationships and health to be increasingly similar for men and women. Indeed, this reduction in gender differences is thought to explain, at least partly, much of the recent decrease in the gender mortality gap.[87,88] There may be cultural differences as well as the marriage link with reduced alcohol consumption seen in the United States and the UK was not found for French women.[89]

18.4.2 Biological Pathways

Thinking about the potential biological mechanisms that may link social relationships with chronic disease, considerable attention has been paid to blood pressure,[90] heart rate variability,[91] inflammation,[92] and adiposity,[93] each of which has been linked with both biological stress responses and chronic disease risk and so may provide a mechanism through which stressful social environments directly influence health.[94] Studies investigating gender differences in associations between social relationships and biological outcomes have been fairly equally split as to whether men[4,95] or women[96] appear to be more biologically reactive to their social relationships in terms of inflammation, blood pressure, or allostatic load (a measure assessing physiological activity across a range of biological systems pertinent to chronic disease risk[94]); however, some of the most recent studies have found various aspects of social relationships to be equally associated with biomarker risk factors for men and women.[97] Thus far, studies have tended to show functional aspects of social relationships to be more strongly associated with immune responses[98,99] and inflammation[100] in women, while structural aspects are more likely to be associated with inflammatory markers in men.[4,95] However, currently there is inadequate evidence to draw confident conclusions regarding gender differences in social relationships and biological mechanisms. A recent study in Japan showed both structural and functional aspects of social relationships to be associated with raised inflammation in men, but lower inflammation in women,[101] while in Canada, structural aspects were associated with hypertension in women and men.[74] As with studies of other social relationships, studies have investigated inflammation,[100] blood pressure,[102] and markers of adiposity[103] as potential mechanisms linking partnership and health, and gender differences in these associations have not been consistent.[74,102,103]

18.5 Conclusions

Traditional orthodoxy states that women provide and receive more support than men from a wider network of contacts, and that men rely on their partnerships for provision of social support and impetus to adopt healthy behaviours. As a result, men's health benefits more than women's from partnership, while women are more reactive to their social relationships because of the centrality of relationships in women's lives. If we accept that women's greater propensity to develop social relationships is at least partially influenced by the social world around them, to what extent does current evidence show changes in these differences between men and women, given dramatic changes in gender relations and weakening of traditional gender norms in many societies over the past half century? Recent evidence does continue to show that women provide and receive more support from a wider and more diverse social network than men do,[1,2] but there is more evidence to support change in the gendered nature of partnership. Evidence supporting the greater health benefits of partnership for men appears to be diminishing in more recent cohorts in Western contexts.[9,70] This suggests that partnership is one site in which we are beginning to see the result of changing gender relations coming through in the evidence base, perhaps partly because of partnerships being more egalitarian in nature, but possibly also because of the growing ability of women, both financially and legally, to divest themselves of unsatisfying relationships.

Regarding women's greater reactivity to relationships, leading to a greater impact on women's health, evidence supports the idea that women may be more psychologically reactive to negative relationships than men are, but they do not appear to be more reactive physiologically. Many studies show a stronger association between social relationships and mental health outcomes for women than for men,[46] but this is not seen for cardiovascular disease,[38,52] mortality, or cognitive outcomes,[50] although the evidence base for gender differences in these areas remains somewhat thin. In terms of the biological pathways through which social stressors, such as isolation, loneliness, or a lack of support, may impact physical health, the evidence is inconsistent. There is some suggestion, however, that functional or qualitative aspects of relationships may be more strongly linked with stress-related biomarkers in women,[98-100] while structural aspects (e.g. social isolation) are more strongly linked with biomarker outcomes for men.[4,95] Further hypothesis-led research is needed in this area to determine the reasons for these differences.

Increasingly, the availability of longitudinal data has allowed for a life course focus on social relationships. The importance of establishing close personal ties from the beginning of life is clear, and social relationships remain vitally important for well-being and quality of life throughout the life course, perhaps changing in nature[58] but not in importance.[13] Most urgent for future research into women's social relationships is capturing the life courses of the most recent generations as they transition to adulthood and age, as their life courses have been less traditional than those of women who are now old enough for chronic disease and declines in functioning to be prevalent enough for population research.[104]

Key messages and implications

- It is generally accepted that, with the notable exception of marriage, social relationships are more important for women than for men, and recent evidence continues to show that women provide and receive more support from a wider and more diverse social network than men do.
- There is now an extensive body of evidence showing that a variety of aspects of social relationships are crucial for well-being and happiness, and a lack of social integration is strongly linked with poor health and earlier mortality. Women are thought to be more 'reactive' than men are to the quality of their relationships. Evidence reviewed in this chapter suggests that this may be true psychologically, but not in terms of CVD, mortality, or cognitive outcomes, or in terms of biological stress responses which may link social stressors such as isolation with health outcomes.
- There is more evidence to support change in the gendered nature of partnership. Evidence supporting the greater health benefits of partnership for men, compared with women, appears to be diminishing in more recent cohorts in Western contexts, suggesting that partnership is one area in which we are beginning to see the result of changing gender relations.

References

1. McPherson M, Smith-Lovin L, Brashears ME. Social isolation in America: changes in core discussion networks over two decades. *American Sociological Review*. 2006;71(3):353–75.
2. Jivraj S, Nazroo J, Barnes M. Short- and long-term determinants of social detachment in later life. *Ageing & Society*. 2016;36(5):924–45.
3. Lasgaard M, Friis K, Shevlin M. 'Where are all the lonely people?' A population-based study of high-risk groups across the life span. *Social Psychiatry & Psychiatric Epidemiology*. 2016;51(10):1373–84.
4. Shankar A, McMunn A, Banks J, Steptoe A. Loneliness, social isolation, and behavioral and biological health indicators in older adults. *Health Psychology*. 2011;30(4):377–85.
5. Taylor SE, Klein LC, Lewis BP, Gruenewald TL, Gurung RA, Updegraff JA. Biobehavioral responses to stress in females: tend-and-befriend, not fight-or-flight. *Psychological Review*. 2000;107(3):411–29.
6. Scott J, Dex S, Plagnol A, ed. *Gendered lives: gender inequalities in production and reproduction*. Cheltenham: Edward Elgar; 2012.
7. Scott J, Clery E. Gender roles: an incomplete revolution? In: Park A, Bryson C, Clery E, Curtice J, Phillips M, eds. *British social attitudes: the 30th report*. London: National Centre for Social Research; 2013. pp. 115–38.
8. Williams K. Has the future of marriage arrived? A contemporary examination of gender, marriage, and psychological well-being. *Journal of Health & Social Behavior*. 2003;44(4):470–87.
9. Strohschein L. Do men really benefit more from marriage than women? *American Journal of Public Health*. 2016;106(9):E2.
10. Burton-Jeangros C, Cullati S, Sacker A, Blane D, ed. *A life course perspective on health trajectories and transitions*. Cham: Springer; 2015.

11. Kuh D, Ben-Shlomo Y, ed. *A life course approach to chronic disease epidemiology*. Oxford: Oxford University Press; 1997.

12. Ertel KA, Glymour MM, Berkman LF. Social networks and health: a life course perspective integrating observational and experimental evidence. *Journal of Social & Personal Relationships*. 2009;26(1):73–92.

13. Fuller HR, Ajrouch KJ, Antonucci TC. Original voices the Convoy Model and later-life family relationships. *Journal of Family Theory Review*. 2020;12(2):126–46.

14. Bowlby J. *A secure base*. London: Routledge; 1988.

15. Bevilacqua L, Kelly Y, Heilmann A, Priest N, Lacey RE. Adverse childhood experiences and trajectories of internalizing, externalizing, and prosocial behaviors from childhood to adolescence. *Child Abuse & Neglect*. 2021;112.

16. Chiang CJ, Chen YC, Wei HS, Jonson-Reid M. Social bonds and profiles of delinquency among adolescents: differential effects by gender and age. *Child & Youth Services Review*. 2020;110. https://ideas.repec.org/a/eee/cysrev/v110y2020ics0190740919308485.html

17. Lacey RE, Bartley M, Kelly-Irving M, Bevilacqua L, Iob E, Kelly Y, et al. Adverse childhood experiences and early life inflammation in the Avon Longitudinal Study of Parents and Children. *Psychoneuroendocrinology*. 2020;122. https://www.sciencedirect.com/science/article/pii/S0306453020303371?via%3Dihub

18. Chen P, Harris KM. Association of positive family relationships with mental health trajectories from adolescence to midlife. *JAMA Pediatrics*. 2019;173(12).

19. Stafford M, Kuh DL, Gale CR, Mishra G, Richards M. Parent-child relationships and offspring's positive mental wellbeing from adolescence to early older age. *Journal of Positive Psychology*. 2016;11(3):326–37.

20. Acquah D, Sellers R, Stock L, Harold G. *Inter-parental conflict and outcomes for children in the context of poverty and economic pressure*. London: Early Intervention Foundation; 2017.

21. Skeer MR, McCormick MC, Normand SLT, Mimiaga MJ, Buka SL, Gilman SE. Gender differences in the association between family conflict and adolescent substance use disorders. *Journal of Adolescent Health*. 2011;49(2):187–92.

22. Conger RD, Conger KJ, Martin MJ. Socioeconomic status, family processes, and individual development. *Journal of Marriage & Family*. 2010;72(3):685–704.

23. Lacey RE, Kumari M, McMunn A. Parental separation in childhood and adult inflammation: the importance of material and psychosocial pathways. *Psychoneuroendocrinology*. 2013;38(11):2476–84.

24. Brewer M, Nandi A. Partnership dissolution: how does it affect income, employment and well-being? Colchester: University of Essex, Institute of Economic and Social Research; ISER Working Paper Series No. 2014-30; 2014.

25. Pearce A, Lewis H, Law C. The role of poverty in explaining health variations in 7-year-old children from different family structures: findings from the UK Millennium Cohort Study. *Journal of Epidemiology & Community Health*. 2013;67(2):181–9.

26. Tommerup K, Lacey RE. Maternal and paternal distress in early childhood and child adiposity trajectories: evidence from the Millennium Cohort Study. *Obesity*. 2021;29(5):888–99.

27. Colarossi LG. Adolescent gender differences in social support: structure, function, and provider type. *Social Work Research*. 2001;25(4):233–41.

28. Hankin BL, Mermelstein R, Roesch L. Sex differences in adolescent depression: stress exposure and reactivity models. *Child Develoment*. 2007;78(1):279–95.

29. Miething A, Almquist YB, Ostberg V, Rostila M, Edling C, Rydgren J. Friendship networks and psychological well-being from late adolescence to young adulthood: a gender-specific structural equation modeling approach. *BMC Psychology*. 2016;4(1):34.

30. Mjaavatn PE, Frostad P, Pijl SJ. Adolescents: differences in friendship patterns related to gender. *Issues in Educational Research*. 2016;26(1):45–64.

31. Booker CL, Kelly YJ, Sacker A. Gender differences in the associations between age trends of social media interaction and well-being among 10–15 year olds in the UK. *BMC Public Health*.2018;18. https://bmcpublichealth.biomedcentral.com/articles/10.1186/s12889-018-5220-4#citeas

32. Viner RM, Aswothikutty-Gireesh A, Stiglic N, Hudson LD, Goddings AL, Ward JL, et al. Roles of cyberbullying, sleep, and physical activit y in mediating the effects of social media use on mental

health and wellbeing among young people in England: a secondary analysis of longitudinal data. *Lancet Child & Adolescent Health*. 2019;3(10):685–96.

33. Barreto M, Victor C, Hammond C, Eccles A, Richins MT, Qualter P. Loneliness around the world: age, gender, and cultural differences in loneliness. *Personal & Individual Diffferences*. 2021;169:110066.
34. Vanhalst J, Klimstra TA, Luyckx K, Scholte RH, Engels RC, Goossens L. The interplay of loneliness and depressive symptoms across adolescence: exploring the role of personality traits. *Journal of Youth & Adolescence*. 2012;41(6):776–87.
35. Holt-Lunstad J, Smith TB, Layton JB. Social relationships and mortality risk: a meta-analytic review. *PLoS Medicine*. 2010;7(7). https://journals.plos.org/plosmedicine/article?id=10.1371/journal.pmed.1000316
36. Berkman L, Krisha A. Social network epidemiology. In: Berkman LF, Kawachi I, Glymour MM, eds. *Social epidemiology*. Oxford: Oxford University Press; 2014. pp. 234–89.
37. Holt-Lunstad J, Smith TB, Baker M, Harris T, Stephenson D. Loneliness and social isolation as risk factors for mortality: a meta-analytic review. *Perspectives in Psychological Science*. 2015;10(2):227–37.
38. Valtorta NK, Kanaan M, Gilbody S, Ronzi S, Hanratty B. Loneliness and social isolation as risk factors for coronary heart disease and stroke: systematic review and meta-analysis of longitudinal observational studies. *Heart*. 2016;102(13):1009–16.
39. Kawachi I, Berkman L. Social capital, social cohesion, and health. In: Berkman LF, Kawachi I, Glymour MM, eds. *Social epidemiology*. Oxford: Oxford University Press; 2014. pp. 290–319.
40. Veenstra G, Patterson AC. Capital relations and health: mediating and moderating effects of cultural, economic, and social capitals on mortality in Alameda County, California. *International Journal of Health Services*. 2012;42(2):277–91.
41. Vonneilich N, Jockel KH, Erbel R, Klein J, Dragano N, Siegrist J, et al. The mediating effect of social relationships on the association between socioeconomic status and subjective health—results from the Heinz Nixdorf Recall cohort study. *BMC Public Health*. 2012;12.
42. Matud MP, Ibanez I, Bethencourt JM, Marrero R, Carballeira M. Structural gender differences in perceived social support. *Personal & Individual Differences*. 2003;35(8):1919–29.
43. McLaughlin D, Vagenas D, Pachana NA, Begum N, Dobson A. Gender differences in social network size and satisfaction in adults in their 70s. *Journal of Health Psychology*. 2010;15(5):671–9.
44. Rogers RG, Everett BG, Saint Onge JM, Krueger PM. Social, behavioral, and biological factors, and sex differences in mortality. *Demography*. 2010;47(3):555–78.
45. Saphire-Bernstein S, Taylor S. Close relationships and happiness. In: Boniwell I, David S, eds. *Oxford handbook of happiness*. Oxford: Oxford University Press; 2014. pp. 821–33.
46. Milner A, Krnjacki L, LaMontagne AD. Age and gender differences in the influence of social support on mental health: a longitudinal fixed-effects analysis using 13 annual waves of the HILDA cohort. *Public Health*. 2016;140:172–8.
47. Hakulinen C, Pulkki-Raback L, Jokela M, Ferrie JE, Aalto AM, Virtanen M, et al. Structural and functional aspects of social support as predictors of mental and physical health trajectories: Whitehall II Cohort Study. *Journal of Epidemiology & Community Health*. 2016;70(7):710–15.
48. Tabue Teguo M, Simo-Tabue N, Stoykova R, Meillon C, Cogne M, Amieva H, et al. Feelings of loneliness and living alone as predictors of mortality in the elderly: the PAQUID Study. *Psychosomatic Medicine*. 2016;78(8):904–9.
49. Tanskanen J, Anttila T. A Prospective study of social isolation, loneliness, and mortality in Finland. *American Journal of Public Health*. 2016;106(11):2042–8.
50. Liao J, Head J, Kumari M, Stansfeld S, Kivimaki M, Singh-Manoux A, et al. Negative aspects of close relationships as risk factors for cognitive aging. *American Journal of Epidemiology*. 2014;180(11):1118–25.
51. Shankar A, Hamer M, McMunn A, Steptoe A. Social isolation and loneliness: relationships with cognitive function during 4 years of follow-up in the English Longitudinal Study of Ageing. *Psychosomatic Medicine*. 2013;75(2):161–70.

52. Stringhini S, Berkman L, Dugravot A, Ferrie JE, Marmot M, Kivimaki M, et al. Socioeconomic status, structural and functional measures of social support, and mortality the British Whitehall II Cohort Study, 1985–2009. *American Journal of Epidemiology*. 2012;175(12):1275–83.

53. Park K, Cho D, Lee E, Kim J, Shim JS, Youm Y, et al. Sex differences in the association between social relationships and insomnia symptoms. *Journal of Clinical Sleep Medicine*. 2020;16(11):1871–81.

54. Cable N, Chandola T, Lallukka T, Sekine M, Lahelma E, Tatsuse T, et al. Country specific associations between social contact and mental health: evidence from civil servant studies across Great Britain, Japan and Finland. *Public Health*. 2016;137:139–46.

55. Liao J, Scholes S. Association of social support and cognitive aging modified by sex and relationship type: a prospective investigation in the English Longitudinal Study of Ageing. *American Journal of Epidemiology*. 2017;186(7):787–95.

56. Pei YL, Cong Z, Wu B. The impact of living alone and intergenerational support on depressive symptoms among older Mexican Americans: does gender matter? *International Journal of Aging & Human Development*. 2020;90(3):255–80.

57. Yang KM, Victor C. Age and loneliness in 25 European nations. *Ageing & Society*. 2011;31:1368–88.

58. Lang FR, Carstensen LL. Close emotional relationships in late-life—further support for proactive aging in the social domain. *Psychological Aging*. 1994;9(2):315–24.

59. Van Groenou MIB, Van Tilburg T. Network size and support in old age: differentials by socio-economic status in childhood and adulthood. *Ageing and Society*. 2003;23:625–45.

60. Maes M, Qualter P, Vanhalst J, Van den Noortgate W, Goossens L. Gender differences in loneliness across the lifespan: a meta-analysis. *European Journal of Personality*. 2019;33(6):642–54.

61. Rico-Uribe LA, Caballero FF, Martin-Maria N, Cabello M, Ayuso-Mateos JL, Miret M. Association of loneliness with all-cause mortality: a meta-analysis. *PLoS ONE*. 2018;13(1). e0190033. https://doi.org/10.1371/journal.pone.0190033.

62. Clouston SAP, Lawlor A, Verdery AM. The role of partnership status on late-life physical function. *Canadian Journal of Aging*. 2014;33(4):413–25.

63. Pachana NA, McLaughlin D, Leung J, McKenzie SJ, Dobson A. The effect of having a partner on activities of daily living in men and women aged 82–87 years. *Maturitas*. 2011;68(3):286–90.

64. Carr D, Springer KW. Advances in families and health research in the 21st century. *Journal of Marriage & Family*. 2010;72(3):743–61.

65. Wood N, McMunn A, Webb E, Stafford M. Marriage and physical capability at mid to later life in England and the USA. *PLoS ONE*. 2019;14(1).

66. Gurung RAR, Taylor SE, Seeman TE. Accounting for changes in social support among married older adults: insights from the MacArthur studies of successful aging. *Psychology & Aging*. 2003;18(4):487–96.

67. Boerner K, Jopp DS, Carr D, Sosinsky L, Kim SK. 'His' and 'her' marriage? The role of positive and negative marital characteristics in global marital satisfaction among older adults. *Journals of Gerontology Series B: Psychological Sciences & Social Sciences*. 2014;69(4):579–89.

68. Grundy EMD, Tomassini C. Marital history, health and mortality among older men and women in England and Wales. *BMC Public Health*. 2010;10.

69. Folbre N. *The economics of family*. Cheltenham: Edward Elgar; 1996.

70. Guner N, Kulikova Y, Llull J. Marriage and health: selection, protection, and assortative mating. *European Economic Review*. 2018;104:138–66.

71. Bookwala J, Gaugler T. Relationship quality and 5-year mortality risk. *Health Psychology*. 2020;39(8):633–41.

72. McFarland MJ, Hayward MD, Brown D. I've got you under my skin: marital biography and biological risk. *Journal of Marriage & Family*. 2013;75(2):363–80.

73. Stronge S, Overall NC, Sibley CG. Gender differences in the associations between relationship status, social support, and wellbeing. *Journal of Family Psychology*. 2019;33(7):819–29.

74. Hosseini Z, Veenstra G, Khan NA, Conklin AI. Associations between social connections, their interactions, and obesity differ by gender: a population-based, cross-sectional analysis of the Canadian Longitudinal Study on Aging. *PLoS ONE*. 2020;15(7):e0235977.

75. Perkins JM, Lee HY, James KS, Oh J, Krishna A, Heo J, et al. Marital status, widowhood duration, gender and health outcomes: a cross-sectional study among older adults in India. *BMC Public Health*. 2016;16(1):1032.

76. Shiovitz-Ezra S, Litwin H. Social network type and health-related behaviors: evidence from an American national survey. *Social Science & Medicine*. 2012;75(5):901–4.

77. Walker E, Ploubidis G, Fancourt D. Social engagement and loneliness are differentially associated with neuro-immune markers in older age: time-varying associations from the English Longitudinal Study of Ageing. *Brain Behavior & Immunity*. 2019;82:224–9.

78. Schrempft S, Jackowska M, Hamer M, Steptoe A. Associations between social isolation, loneliness, and objective physical activity in older men and women. *BMC Public Health*. 2019;19.

79. Herttua K, Martikainen P, Vahtera J, Kivimaki M. Living alone and alcohol-related mortality: a population-based cohort study from Finland. *PLoS Medicine*. 2011;8(9).

80. Stahl ST, Schulz R. Changes in routine health behaviors following late-life bereavement: a systematic review. *Journal of Behavioral Medicine*. 2014;37(4):736–55.

81. Keenan K, Ploubidis GB, Silverwood RJ, Grundy E. Life-course partnership history and midlife health behaviours in a population-based birth cohort. *Journal of Epidemiology & Community Health*. 2017;71(3):232–8.

82. Watt RG, Heilmann A, Sabbah W, Newton T, Chandola T, Aida J, et al. Social relationships and health related behaviors among older US adults. *BMC Public Health*. 2014;14.533

83. Hanson KL, Sobal J, Vermeylen FM. Social selection and social causation in marriage and health: longitudinal evidence of body weight change. *Marriage & Family Review*. 2014;50(5):373–94.

84. Jones-Johnson G, DeLisi M, Hochstetler A, Johnson W, Frishman N. Gender differences in social relationships, social integration and substance use. *Sociology Mind*. 2013;3(1):103–13.

85. Vinther JL, Conklin AI, Wareham NJ, Monsivais P. Marital transitions and associated changes in fruit and vegetable intake: findings from the population-based prospective EPIC-Norfolk cohort, UK. *Social Science & Medicine*. 2016;157:120–6.

86. National Center for Health Statistics. *Health, United States, 2011: with special feature on socioeconomic status and health*. Hyattsville, MD: US Department of Health and Human Services; May 2012. DHHS Publication No. 2012-1232.

87. Waldron I. Trends in gender differences in morality: relationships to changing gender differences in behaviour and other causal factors. In: Annandale E, Hunt K, eds. *Gender inequalities in health*. Buckingham: Open University Press; 2000. pp. 150–81.

88. Luy M, Wegner-Siegmundt C. The impact of smoking on gender differences in life expectancy: more heterogeneous than often stated. *European Journal of Public Health*. 2015;25(4):706–10.

89. Zins M, Gueguen A, Leclerc A, Goldberg M. Alcohol consumption and marital status of French women in the GAZEL cohort: a longitudinal analysis between 1992 and 1996. *Journal of Studies in Alcohol & Drugs*. 2003;64(6):784–9.

90. Uchino BN, Kent de Grey RG, Cronan S. The quality of social networks predicts age-related changes in cardiovascular reactivity to stress. *Psychological Aging*. 2016;31(4):321–6.

91. Gerteis AKS, Schwerdtfeger AR. When rumination counts: perceived social support and heart rate variability in daily life. *Psychophysiology*. 2016;53(7):1034–43.

92. Uchino BN, Trettevik R, de Grey RGK, Cronan S, Hogan J, Baucom BRW. Social support, social integration, and inflammatory cytokines: a meta-analysis. *Health Psychology*. 2018;37(5):462–71.

93. Pachucki MC, Goodman E. Social relationships and obesity: benefits of incorporating a lifecourse perspective. *Current Obesity Reports*. 2015;4(2):217–23.

94. McEwen BS, Seeman T. Protective and damaging effects of mediators of stress—elaborating and testing the concepts of allostasis and allostatic load. *Annals of the New York Academy of Sciences*. 1999;896:30–47.

95. Loucks EB, Berkman LF, Gruenewald TL, Seeman TE. Relation of social integration to inflammatory marker concentrations in men and women 70 to 79 years. *American Journal of Cardiology*. 2006;97(7):1010–16.

96. Elliot AJ, Heffner KL, Mooney CJ, Moynihan JA, Chapman BP. Social relationships and inflammatory markers in the MIDUS Cohort: the role of age and gender differences. *Journal of Aging Health*. 2018;30(6):904–23.

97. Seeman TE, Gruenewald TL, Cohen S, Williams DR, Matthews KA. Social relationships and their biological correlates: Coronary Artery Risk Development in Young Adults (CARDIA) Study. *Psychoneuroendocrinology*. 2014;43:126–38.

98. Robles TF. Annual research review: social relationships and the immune system during development. *Journal of Child Psychology & Psychiatry*. 2021;62(5):539–59.

99. Woods R, McInnis O, Bedard M, Asokumar A, Santoni S, Anisman H, et al. Social support and unsupportive interactions in relation to depressive symptoms: implication of gender and the BDNF polymorphism. *Social Neuroscience-Uk*. 2020;15(1):64–73.

100. Ford J, Anderson C, Gillespie S, Giurgescu C, Nolan T, Nowak A, et al. Social integration and quality of social relationships as protective factors for inflammation in a nationally representative sample of black women. *Journal of Urban Health*. 2019;96:35–43.

101. Koyama Y, Nawa N, Yamaoka Y, Nishimura H, Sonoda S, Kuramochi J, et al. Interplay between social isolation and loneliness and chronic systemic inflammation during the COVID-19 pandemic in Japan: results from U-CORONA study. *Brain, Behavior and Immunity*. 2021;94:51–9.

102. Birditt KS, Newton NJ, Cranford JA, Ryan LH. Stress and negative relationship quality among older couples: implications for blood pressure. *Journals of Gerontology Series B: Psychological Sciences*. 2016;71(5):775–85.

103. Ploubidis GB, Silverwood RJ, DeStavola B, Grundy E. Life-course partnership status and biomarkers in midlife: evidence from the 1958 British Birth Cohort. *American Journal of Public Health*. 2015;105(8):1596–603.

104. McMunn A, Lacey R, Worts D, McDonough P, Stafford M, Booker C, et al. De-standardization and gender convergence in work family life courses in Great Britain: a multi-channel sequence analysis. *Advances in Life Course Research*. 2015;26:60–75.

19

Structural Sexism Across the Life Course

How Social Inequality Shapes Women's Later-Life Health

Jessica A. Kelley and Marissa Gilbert

19.1 Introduction

A long-standing axiom in public health literature is that despite women's advantage in overall life expectancy, they spend more of their years in poor health and limited functionality compared to men.[1,2] Life course epidemiologists have shown that women are overrepresented at each stage of the disablement process, from pathology to disability. To give just a few examples, lifetime obesity rates are higher in women in the United States, increasing the likelihood of functional problems in older adulthood.[3] Women have higher rates of midlife chronic diseases associated with later-life physical impairment, such as arthritis.[4] Finally, women have, on average, shorter disability-free life expectancies than men do, meaning that women live longer but with more functional impairment compared with their male counterparts.[5]

The impact of chronic diseases on later-life disability varies by sex as well. Figure 19.1, adapted from research by Nusselder and colleagues, shows the relative contribution of types of chronic conditions to disability for men and women.[6] For both genders, musculoskeletal diseases contribute most to long-term disability though markedly more for women. For women, but not men, the next highest contributors to disability are anxiety and depression, followed closely by heart disease. The strength of the linkage between mental health and disability is likely due to substantially higher rates of both episodic and lifetime prevalence of these psychological conditions in women.[7] For men, the contribution of depression and anxiety to disability risk is much lower, tying with accidents.

It is widely acknowledged that women's health profiles are the result of gender (social construction), sex-linked biology, and interactions between them. Krieger provides a useful typology of the differential roles of gender and sex, demonstrating when either could be sufficient or when they may interact to affect health outcomes.[8] For example, onset of perimenopause (sex-linked biology) happens at younger ages among women experiencing lifetime economic deprivation (gender-based exposure).[9] The distinctions and unique contributions of sex and gender to health are reflected in growing efforts among funders and journals to account for sex as a biological variable, rectifying decades of scientific and public health neglect.

To add to this discourse, we explore women's health in midlife and later life from a lens at the nexus of structural sexism and the life course perspective. We focus on gender differences in health that are largely due to environmental, cultural, and social factors that organise the

Jessica A. Kelley and Marissa Gilbert, *Structural Sexism Across the Life Course* In: *A Life Course Approach to Women's Health.*
Second Edition. Edited by: Gita D Mishra, Rebecca Hardy, and Diana Kuh, Oxford University Press. © Oxford University Press 2023.
DOI: 10.1093/oso/9780192864642.003.0019

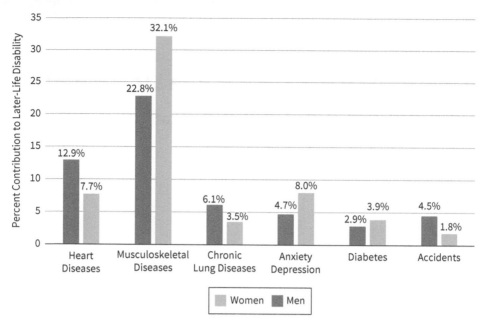

Figure 19.1 Relative contribution of specific health conditions to later-life disability by gender (adapted from Nusselder et al.[6]).

lives of men and women differently, translating into differential health.[8,10,11] By providing specific examples to illustrate this nexus, we are also able to highlight other forms of social inequality, such as low education and race/ethnicity, that stratify health outcomes among women across the life course. After a brief description of our conceptual framework, we turn to three empirical examples of the ways that structural sexism shapes women's mental and physical health in mid-to-late life: i) work history, caregiving expectations, and downward health selection; ii) de-partnering and later-life health; and iii) the hidden impact of stress and trauma on women's health. Although many of our examples are drawn from the US context, the conceptual framework of linking structural sexism to the life course perspective is applicable across societies.

19.2 Structural Sexism and Life Course Dynamics

Research on women's health over the life course generally follows three streams: i) maternal and reproductive health; ii) comparative differences between males and females on specific health outcomes; and iii) impact of social constructions of gender on the health of women. Research in this last category has come under critique for over-emphasising the interactional level of social life (i.e. discrimination, bias, and roles), with much less attention to structural sexism as a fundamental cause of gender health disparities.[8,10,12]

   Applying a structural sexism framework allows for the identification of the scaffolding of discrimination and inequality embedded in the present institutional arrangements of culture, policy, and economics, which are then perpetuated or justified by narratives of a natural—and hierarchical—division between men and women. Parallel with conceptual work on structural racism,[13] gender scholars argue that the '... most obdurate features of our current gender system, such as the household division of labor, the sex segregation of jobs, or gender differences in status and authority are overdetermined ... [in that] ... they are created and maintained by multiple, complementary processes acting simultaneously, often at different levels of analysis, such that the elimination of any single process will not be sufficient to eliminate the phenomenon.'[12] Using such a framework in no way precludes interrogation of gender health disparities at the micro or interactional level. Rather, the structural sexism lens expands the sociological imagination to recognise that while inequality-generating mechanisms are macro and systemic, they operate across all system levels.[10,14]

When framing the ways in which structural inequality influences women's health in mid-to-late life, it is useful to apply the life course perspective. This allows for examination of the roles, transitions, and accumulative processes that interact to shape health as we age and move in, through, and out of life domains. Yet, critical scholars argue that a shortcoming in traditional applications of the life course perspective has been the inherent assumption of 'a' life course. They note that research typically focuses on the privileged life course, or more specifically the male life course, leaving uninterrogated the myriad ways that major life domains are socially arranged by gender.[15,16] Integrating a structural sexism framework centres the inquiry on the powerful gendered forces that shape the life courses of women and their subsequent health, including caregiving expectations,[17] family responsibilities,[18] (re) partnering prospects,[19] and labour force value.[20,21]

We further apply Dannefer's concept of life course reflexivity, which emphasises that the life course is not a 'conveyor belt' set in motion based on early life circumstances but rather a dynamic experience with potential health-changing 'input' at all ages.[14] These can include both purposeful agentic choices, such as returning to school in midlife after raising children, as well as more nuanced gendered forces, such as pressure to retire early in order to care for elderly parents. In the following sections, we provide three extended examples of how women are structurally disadvantaged across the life course relative to men in ways that compromise their mental and physical health. We also focus on intersectional identities that serve to disadvantage some women more than others.

19.3 Work History, Caregiving, and Downward Health Selection

Two prevailing forces intersect to place women at significant risk of adverse health outcomes relative to men when facing familial caregiving needs: i) prevailing cultural preference for female caregivers and ii) devaluation of the caregiving work itself.[22] Economists note that the current caregiving marketplace is able to operate predominantly because of the exploitation of women's labour.[23] Few-to-no policy supports buffer the deleterious effects of lost wages, career stagnation, and compromised health that can result from intensive caregiving, and little political will exists to address this inequality.[24,25] The interrelated health and socioeconomic disadvantages create what Pavalko and Woodbury call the 'vicious cycle' for women: 'Taking on family responsibilities leads to intermittent work history and employment loss, followed by earnings losses, and, eventually, poor economic and health outcomes.'[26] These forms of downward health selection suppress accumulation of later-life resources, which could in turn provide some health protection.[27]

Although an intensive caregiving situation may be temporary, researchers show that even when caregiving responsibilities end, women frequently do not return to the same level of work or pay, further exacerbating their economic disadvantage.[26,28] We offer two key explanations for this, both related to downward health selection. First, among women in the lowest economic strata, they are doubly at risk for: i) needing to leave the labour force to care for a loved one and ii) having poorer health themselves. As such, even when the period of caregiving is over, women's own health problems may preclude return to full-time or high-demand work.[29] Second, caregiving itself can adversely affect physical and mental health of the caregiver. The US Department of Labor reports that female caregivers of older adults tend to provide care for longer hours and for a greater variety of tasks, such as medical care, mobility assistance, and housework, compared with their male caregiving counterparts.[30] The physical stress, coupled with the emotional stress of caring for a loved one, may be why female eldercare givers commonly report depression, anxiety, sleep problems, pain, weakness, low energy, and exhaustion and may neglect management of their own chronic conditions.[31–33]

While caring for a relative can bring personal health and economic costs for women, it is also important to recognise that women are overrepresented in the paid caregiving marketplace, particularly women of colour and immigrant women.[34,35] Home health care has one of the highest risks of musculoskeletal injury, exacerbated by higher average rates of obesity among care workers.[36] Most home health care workers have no sick leave, but the most common reason for lost work time is injuries sustained in the execution of the job.[37] Unlike nurses in regulated workplaces, home health care workers can face additional health risks associated with working in a care recipient's home, such as unfriendly animals, tripping hazards, and lack of cleanliness.[37] Given the extremely low pay, many home health aides work in more than one job, which considerably increases risk of injury because of fatigue.[38]

While caregiving responsibilities may take women out of the labour force prematurely, it can also trap women in the labour force despite their own health challenges.[16] Many older women remain in the labour force as a consequence of either having extended periods out of the labour force at younger ages for caregiving responsibilities or having current caregiving responsibilities that require some level of residential or financial support.[39–41] Meyer's research on grandmothers who work demonstrates intergenerational dependence on not just instrumental care tasks for grandchildren but financial support as well.[42] This is especially true if the grandchild has a disability.[43] Extended working life has been heralded, particularly in European countries with historically mandated retirement ages, as a 'freedom to choose' to continue working, but this obscures the reality that many women in the most disadvantaged socioeconomic positions are simply unable to retire.

The financial need to continue working poses a fresh set of health threats that may stem from the conditions of the work: inflexible schedules, no paid sick time, and physical demands of the job (including sedentary or repetitive motions) that can exacerbate musculoskeletal conditions which are more prevalent in older women than older men, particularly those who worked in physically demanding jobs throughout adulthood.[44,45] Ergonomic considerations and productivity quotas in the workplace have input assumptions that have been largely based on younger workers with regard to energy, capacity, and strength, which leave older workers at risk of injury as they 'keep up' with their younger co-workers.[46] The conditions of work are an important area of consideration, but especially so in the sectors that employ a significant proportion of older women: clerical and sales.[39]

We provide this discussion of women's disrupted and uneven work histories to demonstrate the linkages between economic and health precarity for older women. Critical scholars note that the male life course has been the model for work, pension, and retirement policies, which presumes a steady arc of employment and wages until reaching a logical transition out of the labour force and into a financially secure older adulthood.[16] Women's higher risk of midlife degenerative and autoimmune conditions, plus gendered expectations for raising children or caregiving for an older relative undermine their access to the trajectory-based accumulation model for later-life financial well-being—in turn, placing them at risk of poorer health outcomes.

19.4 De-partnering and Later-Life Health

Marriage has long been understood to provide health-promoting and health-protecting resources including greater household wealth, social and emotional support, and first-line caregiving.[47,48] Early research on gender differences in the benefits of marriage focused largely on the costs to women because of the rigid sex roles in the marriage itself.[49] As gender parity in employment status, education, and parenting responsibilities has risen in recent decades, little evidence remains that women bear greater costs or receive less psychological benefit from marriage.[50] The health effects of marriage are discussed in further detail in Chapter 18.

A long line of inquiry has examined health selection into marriage.[51] The likely mechanisms include positive health selectivity, assortative mating, and stronger likelihood of marriage among those with higher socioeconomic status. No matter how it occurs, these selection patterns account for most of what researchers consider to be the strong linkage between marriage and health.[52] Interestingly, much less attention has been given to the health circumstances that select women out of marriage and the consequences of that dissolution. Mental and physical health can select one out of marriage through either widowhood or divorce. Regardless of how marriages end, women experience social and structural disadvantages that can increase risk of economic precarity and poor health. We trace both pathways out of midlife marriage below and then discuss the consequences for women of becoming de-partnered in later life.

First, women are substantially more likely than men to have marriage end because of death of a spouse. While men have lower life expectancy than women do at all ages, men who are in the lowest economic strata and lower education levels carry the highest risk of premature mortality. Average life expectancy in the United States for white men and for black men with education less than a college degree is 69 and 67, respectively.[53] This means that socioeconomically disadvantaged women face elevated risk of losing their spouse in midlife or early older adulthood. Upon widowhood, these women can face negative financial shocks because of a number of factors, many of which are grounded in policy. For example, widows may face expensive end-of-life bills for the deceased spouse not covered by Medicare (Australia's universal health insurance scheme) and, simultaneously, have reduced Social Security and pension income since widow benefits are substantially lower than recipient benefits. Policy analysts agree that these structural factors significantly disadvantage women, and this inequality represents the primary reason why poverty rates of widows have remained persistently three to four times greater than same-age married men for decades.[54]

Second, poor mental or physical health can select one out of midlife marriage via divorce. Health problems of either spouse increase risk of divorce among adults in midlife and early older adulthood.[55-58] While unexpected health crises are not linked strongly to subsequent divorce, expected health problems are. The onset of chronic health problems in midlife, largely related to lifestyle risk factors, increases risk of divorce relative to couples who have no major health problems.[59]

The evidence is mixed regarding whether the wife's poor health or the husband's poor health are more likely to contribute to dissolution. Some evidence shows that women's poor self-rated health and depression are strongly linked to divorce risk, while men's depression and work-related injuries increase odds of divorce.[60] Severe midlife disablement among women, but not among men, also tends to be a catalyst for divorce.[61] One reason for the increased risk of divorce when wives become ill or disabled has to do with the gendered caregiving reversal within the dyad and renegotiation of roles.[62] Indeed, married women report more unmet needs during recovery from a heart attack than men do, with a likely explanation attributable to an imbalance in caregiving experience in the couple.[63]

The health consequences of midlife divorce, however, are much more substantial for women. In their innovative longitudinal study, Lorenz et al. found that upon entering divorce, women reported significantly more psychological distress than their married counterparts did but no difference in physical health.[64] A decade later, these same divorced women continued to present with higher psychological distress, but now also with more illness and physical health problems. The authors attribute this to the greater number of stressful life events that followed the divorce, which is a consistent conclusion drawn in other work showing that women experience economic aftershocks of divorce for a longer period than men, prolonging the period of stress and psychological distress.[65] This may, in part, explain why divorced women have higher cumulative odds of work-limiting disability in the next 2 decades, despite of selection factors into divorce in the first place.

A key reason for the extended and adverse consequences of divorce for older women is that they are likely to experience what Crowley coined the 'gray divorce economic penalty' relative to men.[66] Despite the fact that 'gray divorce' is more likely among socioeconomically disadvantaged couples, women who experience later-life divorce have higher risk of economic precarity than men.[67-69] Economic risk following divorce is most likely when access to public and private programs in a society are tied to marriage. In the United States, for example, women who experience a later-life divorce are nearly twice as likely to live in poverty than women who experience widowhood.[70] This is largely attributed to the fact that widowed women are eligible to receive benefits based on their male spouse's earnings, buffering the consequence of having a lower earned benefit themselves because of having have spent some earning years out of the labour force or earned lower lifetime pay than their former husbands.[67,71] To qualify for benefits through their ex-spouse, divorced women must meet strict requirements and then still only qualify for half the benefit a widowed spouse receives.[67]

No matter how marital dissolution happens, women are substantially more likely than men to be unpartnered for a longer period in older adulthood.[72] This is for two key reasons. First, women's longer average life expectancy increases the odds of outliving their partner. The gender gap in likelihood of re-partnership increases with age, largely because of the imbalanced sex ratio at upper ages.[73] Second, some gender differences in preference for re-partnership shape who is 'in the market'. Older men tend to re-partner quickly, particularly those with smaller social networks or few close family connections. Widowed women, on the other hand, often express less interest in repartnering, citing their satisfaction with new independence and concern about being roped into more caregiving.[74] That said, women's health plays a substantial role in odds of repartnering, but not so for men.[19,75] Women who have fewer limitations and better self-rated health are more likely to re-partner even in late adulthood.

Taken together, we are better able to see how health and socioeconomic status interact over the life course to influence the likelihood of entering marriage, remaining married, and repartnering following dissolution. Women's disproportionate risk of widowhood throughout midlife and older adulthood shows how the health of the spouse can trigger social and economic vulnerability. While few gender differences appear to exist in terms of whose health problems may spur divorce, the evidence is overwhelming that women experience substantially more adverse psychological distress following dissolution, which can lead to rapid acceleration of physical health problems.

19.5 Hidden Costs of Accumulative Stress and Trauma on Women's Health

Stress and trauma over the life course have been linked to myriad adverse health outcomes.[76,77] Women bear a substantially greater burden of these adverse exposures than men do because of unique vulnerabilities and pressures on females, stressful roles disproportionately occupied by women, and social vulnerabilities that allow stressors and traumas to perpetuate.[8,10] Returning to Dannefer's concept of life course reflexivity, understanding women's health in midlife and older adulthood requires a life course lens to see the accumulative effects of socioenvironmental stressors, as well as new and different stressors that women may experience as they move into and through different roles such as worker, partner, parent, or caregiver.[14] As such, we can understand how patterns in the long-term health of women are shaped by the social organisation of gender in society. To illustrate, we briefly address the gendered impact of both stress and trauma.

19.5.1 Stress

Women are overrepresented in lower-wage occupations, that combines chronic financial strain with low-control and high-demand hourly work.[78] Solo parents are overwhelmingly likely to be women (81% women versus 19% men in the United States), and the proportion is even higher among black women (89% versus 13%).[79] Mothers who work full-time often carry the classically labelled 'second shift' of family responsibilities. The American Time Use survey indicates that, among employed adults, 46% of women report also performing daily household tasks compared to 22% of men, and that women spend, on average, 1.5 more daily hours than their male partners on child-related tasks.[80]

With women facing higher levels, more frequent, and domain-crossing stressors, it is not surprising that they also have disproportionate prevalence of stress-related morbidities. Stress is widely understood to be part of the causal pathway to a number of midlife morbidities for women, including obesity, heart disease (see Chapter 5), and depression (see Chapter 9).[76,81] Sometimes referred to as stress-related accelerated biological ageing, the cumulative impact of metabolic dysregulation, inflammation, and perpetually activated cortisol breaks down major body systems and accelerates disablement.[81] Concomitantly, behavioural response (e.g. inadequate sleep) or adverse coping (e.g. excessive eating or substance abuse) accelerate the breakdown of these systems. Women's substantially higher rates of disablement are linked closely with the downstream effects of stress-related morbidities, including depression and anxiety, which accounted for 8% of the disability (compared to 4.7% in men) in the French Disability Health Survey.[6]

The interaction between biological sex and gender is seen clearly in the prevalence of auto-immune conditions. While these conditions such as lupus, thyroid disease, and rheumatoid arthritis affect about 8% of the population overall, 78%–80% of the diagnoses are in women.[82,83] Evidence is mixed about the balance of contribution from biology and environment to developing autoimmune conditions, but women's heightened sensitivity to these conditions between puberty and menopause suggest that hormones and genes play a non-trivial role.[83,84] That said, stress has been identified as a significant trigger for those who may be predisposed to autoimmune conditions. This suggests an interaction between biology and environment, where the latter represents the structural arrangements and exposures organised by gender. Hence, women's genetic vulnerability to these conditions is actualised at rates fivefold higher than men's equivalent genetic vulnerability.[85]

The long-term health impact of stress-related morbidities can also become exacerbated in the context of stigma. Excess weight in women directly influences risk of chronic metabolic and musculoskeletal conditions, but the social experience of overweight and obesity has its own consequences to health.[86,87] For example, women with obesity are more likely to delay routine health care compared to their normal weight counterparts, including cancer screenings, often because of perceived discrimination in their clinical encounters.[11] Avoidance is even more frequent among women with obesity who have been diagnosed with depression or anxiety. Indeed, research shows that obesity and depression are reciprocally causal and mutually reinforcing in middle-aged women.[88,89] These frequently present together among those with midlife functional or work limitations, indicating more rapid onset of disability.[90] Taken together, we observe the perfect storm of overall increased disease and disablement risk, adverse coping, and delay in care, which translates to later diagnoses and worse long-term prognosis.[11]

19.5.2 Trauma

Women also report higher rates of neglect and psychological abuse in childhood than men, although there appears to be no gender difference in reports of physical abuse.[91] Women also report higher rates of childhood sexual abuse and uninitiated sexual contact by adults.[92] The adult health consequences of childhood abuse and trauma are well documented, with outcomes including depression and anxiety,[93,94] substance abuse, and suicide attempts.[95]

Utilising a life course epidemiology framework, the linkage between early life trauma and adult health can be traced through both direct and indirect mechanisms. First, when acute negative events occur during the critical period of biopsychosocial development, the trauma can imprint damage even if not seen until later. As Nettle argues, repeated physiological stress response and psychosocial investment in mere survival when body systems are growing and developing can limit their ultimate capacity and ability to repair itself in adulthood.[96] The true extent of the damage is not seen until midlife when bodies begin to need that reserve capacity to prevent chronic disease. Other studies demonstrate more direct causal links from the trauma: young adults who experienced adverse childhood experiences present very early with posttraumatic stress disorder, anxiety, depression, and body dysmorphia.[94,97]

However, the robust relationship between childhood trauma and adult health is only partially explained by the direct, sometimes called *latent, causality*.[98,99] Rather, compromised adult health and elevated risk of mortality among those traumatised in their youth most often operates through accumulative and additive risks as they age. These indirect mechanisms include sustained health-risky behaviours such as overeating and substance abuse,[100] work-limiting mental health problems,[101] and repeated exposure to sexual and physical violence in adulthood.[102]

Overwhelming evidence shows that the linkage between adverse childhood experiences and compromised health in adulthood is fundamentally a public health issue for women. Indeed, some research calls for a feminist lens to understand women's differential risk and poorer outcomes following early life trauma.[102] This is for several reasons. First, girls have a disproportionately higher risk of abuse, particularly sexual abuse, than boys (see Chapter 20). Population studies estimate that 25% of women compared with 16% of men report childhood sexual abuse and that women are disproportionately more likely to experience multiple types of abuse or neglect (15.2% versus 9.2%).[92] Second, the impact of childhood trauma on adult mental and physical health may be worse for women. Some research indicates that women have a higher proportion of psychiatric disorder risk attributable to traumatic childhood events than men and a greater number of suicide attempts.[103,104] However, much more work is needed to understand gender differences in processing and coping with trauma into adulthood. This includes interacting with systems that fail to recognise the impact of trauma.[105] Finally, females have unique vulnerabilities in adulthood that increase their risk of repeated or perpetuated trauma. Early sexual trauma, witnessing domestic violence as a child, and other forms of abuse can lead to chaotic and unstable adult relationships with high risk of intimate partner violence.[102,105,106]

19.6 Conclusions

Women's health over the life course is shaped by powerful and obdurate forces related to structural sexism, yet the fact that many of these forces are unseen means that they are continually uninterrogated in the study of health disparities. We propose utilising a conceptual framework at the nexus of structural sexism and the life course perspective to better understand the social origins of gendered health disparities and their consequences as women age. Utilising this framework in no way diminishes inquiry into biological sex differences in health between males and females, but rather complements such work by asking: in what ways does the social organisation of the roles, responsibilities, and treatment of women disadvantage their health relative to men?

In this chapter, we provide three extended examples of the ways in which the social construction of gender has a significant impact on women's midlife and later-life health. First, we demonstrated how the cultural preference for and pressure on women to provide caregiving to elderly relatives can serve to compromise their health and place them at an economic disadvantage in later life that carries its own health risks. Second, we discussed how marriage dissolution—through either widowhood or divorce—disproportionately impacts women's mental and physical health relative to men. Third, we showed how lifetime stress and adverse childhood experiences, including sexual abuse, manifest in significantly compromised health in midlife, through both direct and indirect pathways.

While the majority of our examples draw from the economic and social context in the United States, the framework of combining structural sexism and life course is applicable to any societal context. A starting place is to recognise, as Ridgeway and Correll argue, that structural sexism is overdetermined in any society, and dismantling it would take significant and deliberate action to overhaul its many components.[12] These include—but are certainly not limited to—cultural assumptions about gender roles, male-centred economic policies, and 'gender-blind' practices that do not address particular vulnerabilities of girls and women in society.

Key messages and implications

- An understanding women's health across the life course requires an integrated framework combining knowledge of biological mechanisms and social inequalities stemming from sexism.
- The expectations placed on women to provide familial caregiving and the experience of de-partnering has more health implications at mid-to-later life for women than men.
- The prevalence of stressors, including but not limited to abuse and violence, is greater amongst women, contributing to their risk of adverse physical and mental health.
- Recognising the impact of structural sexism on women's health and driving change in the constructs underpinning this narrative will help reduce the disparities in health outcomes across the life course.

References

1. Freedman VA, Wolf DA, Spillman BC. Disability-free life expectancy over 30 years: a growing female disadvantage in the US population. *American Journal of Public Health*. 2016;106(6):1079–85.
2. Zunzunegui MV, Alvarado BE, Guerra R, Gomez JF, Ylli A, Guralnik JM, et al. The mobility gap between older men and women: the embodiment of gender. *Archives of Gerontology and Geriatrics*. 2015;61(2):140–8.
3. Stokes A, Ni Y, Preston SH. Prevalence and trends in lifetime obesity in the US, 1988–2014. *American Journal of Preventive Medicine*. 2017;53(5):567–75.
4. Sokka T, Toloza S, Cutolo M, Kautiainen H, Makinen H, Gogus F, et al. Women, men, and rheumatoid arthritis: analyses of disease activity, disease characteristics, and treatments in the QUEST-RA Study. *Arthritis Research and Therapy*. 2009;11(1):1–12.
5. Sole-Auro A, Beltran-Sanchez H, Crimmins EM. Are differences in disability-free life expectancy by gender, race, and education widening at older ages? *Population Research and Policy Review*. 2015;34(1):1–18.
6. Nusselder WJ, Wapperom D, Looman CWN, Yokota RTC, van Oyen H, Jagger C, et al. Contribution of chronic conditions to disability in men and women in France. *European Journal of Public Health*. 2019;29(1):99–104.

7. Viana MC, Corass RB. Epidemiology of psychiatric disorders in women. In: Renno Jr J, Valdares G, Cantilano A, Mendes-Ribeiro J, Rocha R, Geraldo da Silva A, eds. *Women's mental health: a clinical and evidence-based guide, 1st edition.* Cham: Springer Publishing; 2020. pp. 17–30.

8. Krieger N. Genders, sexes, and health: what are the connections—and why does it matter? *International Journal of Epidemiology.* 2003;32(4):652–7.

9. Wise LA, Krieger N, Zierler S, Harlow BL. Lifetime socioeconomic position in relation to onset of perimenopause. *Journal of Epidemiology and Community Health.* 2002;56(11):851–60.

10. Homan P. Structural sexism and health in the United States: a new perspective on health inequality and the gender system. *American Sociological Review.* 2019;84(3):486–516.

11. McGuigan RD, Wilkinson JM. Obesity and healthcare avoidance: a systematic review. *Aims Public Health.* 2015;2(1):56–63.

12. Ridgeway CL, Correll SJ. Unpacking the gender system—a theoretical perspective on gender beliefs and social relations. *Gender and Society.* 2004;18(4):510–31.

13. Bailey ZD, Krieger N, Agenor M, Graves J, Linos N, Bassett MT. Structural racism and health inequities in the USA: evidence and interventions. *Lancet.* 2017;389(10077):1453–63.

14. Dannefer D. Systemic and reflexive: foundations of cumulative dis/advantage and life-course processes. *Journal of Gerontology Social Sciences.* 2020;75(6):1249–63.

15. Moen P. The gendered life course. In: Binstock RH, George LK, eds. *Handbook of aging and the social sciences* San Diego, CA: Academic Press; 2001. pp. 179–96.

16. Street D, Ni Leime A. Problems and prospects for current policies to extend working lives. In: Ni Leime A, Ogg J, Rasticova M, Street D, Krekula C, Bediova M, et al., eds. *Extended working life policies: international gender and health perspectives.* Cham: Springer Publishing; 2020. pp. 85–116.

17. Pillemer K, Suitor JJ. Who provides care? A prospective study of caregiving among adult siblings. *Gerontologist.* 2014;54(4):589–98.

18. Craig L. Is there really a second shift, and if so, who does it? A time-diary investigation. *Feminist Review* 2007(86):149–70.

19. Brown SL, Lin IF, Hammersmith AM, Wright MR. Later life marital dissolution and repartnership status: a national portrait. *Journal of Gerontology Social Sciences* 2018;73(6):1032–42.

20. Meyer MH, Herd P. *Market friendly or family friendly? The state and gender inequality in old age.* New York: Russell Sage Foundation; 2007.

21. Ni Leime A, Ogg J, Rasticova M, Street D, Krekula C, Bediova M, et al. *Extended working life policies: international gender and health perspectives.* Cham: Springer Publishing; 2020.

22. Glenn EN. *Forced to care: coercion and caregiving in America.* Cambridge, MA: Harvard University Press; 2010.

23. Gibson MJ, Houser A. Valuing the invaluable: a new look at the economic value of family caregiving. *Issue Brief (Public Policy Institute (American Association of Retired Persons)).* 2007;IB82:1–12.

24. Chattopadhyay J. Political impediments to aging in place: the example of informal caregiving policy. *Public Policy & Aging Report.* 2020;30(2):56–61.

25. Rocco P. Informal caregiving and the politics of policy drift in the United States. *Journal of Aging and Social Policy.* 2017;29(5):413–32.

26. Pavalko EK, Woodbury S. Social roles as process: caregiving careers and women's health. *Journal of Health and Social Behavior.* 2000;41(1):91–105.

27. Wakabayashi C, Donato KM. Does caregiving increase poverty among women in later life? Evidence from the health and retirement survey. *Journal of Health and Social Behavior.* 2006;47(3):258–74.

28. Pavalko EK, Artis JE. Women's caregiving and paid work: causal relationships in late midlife. *Journal of Gerontology Social Sciences.* 1997;52(4):S170–S179.

29. Gonzales E, Lee Y, Brown C. Back to work? Not everyone. Examining the longitudinal relationships between informal caregiving and paid work after formal retirement. *Journal of Gerontology Social Sciences.* 2017;72(3):532–9.

30. US Department of Labor. *Navigating the demands of work and eldercare.* Washington, DC: US Department of Labor; 2011.

31. MetLife Mature Market Institute. *The MetLife study of caregiving costs to working caregivers: double jeopardy for baby boomers caring for their parents.* Westport, CT: MetLife; 2021.

32. Penning MJ, Wu Z. Caregiver stress and mental health: impact of caregiving relationship and gender. *Gerontologist*. 2016;56(6):1102–13.

33. Samuel-Hodge CD, Headen SW, Skelly AH, Ingram AF, Keyserling TC, Jackson EJ, et al. Influences on day-to-day self-management of type 2 diabetes among African-American women—spirituality, the multi-caregiver role, and other social context factors. *Diabetes Care*. 2000;23(7):928–33.

34. Kronenfeld JJ. Health care system issues and race/ethnicity, immigration, SES and gender as sociological issues linking to health and health care. In: Kronenfeld JJ, ed. *Issues in health and health care related to race/ethnicity, immigration, SES and gender*. Bingley: Emerald Group Publishing Limited; 2012. pp. 3–18.

35. Zallman L, Finnegan KE, Himmelstein DU, Touw S, Woolhandler S. Care for America's elderly and disabled people relies on immigrant labor. *Health Affairs*. 2019;38(6):919–26.

36. Hittle B, Agbonifo N, Suarez R, Davis KG, Ballard T. Complexity of occupational exposures for home health-care workers: nurses vs. home health aides. *Journal of Nursing Management*. 2016;24(8):1071–9.

37. Centers for Disease Control and Prevention. *NIOSH hazard review: occupational hazards in home healthcare*. Cincinnati, OH: National Institute for Occupational Safety and Health, Department of Health and Human Services; 5 May 2021. DHHS (NIOSH) Publication No. 2010–125.

38. Houston A, Young Y, Fitzgerald EF. Work-related injuries: an old problem revisited in the first representative US sample of home health aides. *Journal of Aging and Health*. 2013;25(6):1065–81.

39. Hill ET. The labor force participation of older women: retired? Working? Both? *Monthly Labor Review*. 2002;125(9):39–48.

40. Angel J, Settersten RA. What changing American families mean for aging policies: an overview. *Gerontologist*. 2015;55:623.

41. Kreider RM, Ellis R. Living arrangements of children, 2009. Washington, DC: U.S. Census Bureau; Current Population Reports P70-126; 2009.

42. Meyer MH. *Grandmothers at work: juggling families and jobs*. New York: NYU Press; 2014.

43. Meyer MH, Abdul-Malak Y. *Grandparenting children with disabilities*. Cham: Springer Publishing; 2020.

44. Gjesdal S, Bratberg E, Maeland JG. Gender differences in disability after sickness absence with musculoskeletal disorders: five-year prospective study of 37,942 women and 26,307 men. *BMC Musculoskeletal Disorders*. 2011;12:1–9.

45. Cavallari JM, Ahuja M, Dugan AG, Meyer JD, Simcox N, Wakai S, et al. Differences in the prevalence of musculoskeletal symptoms among female and male custodians. *American Journal of Industrial Medicine*. 2016;59(10):841–52.

46. Mital A. Editorial comment—the need to accommodate older workers in the workplace. *Journal of Occupational Rehabilitation*. 1999;9(1):1–2.

47. Waite LJ. Does marriage matter? *Demography*. 1995;32(4):483–507.

48. Waite LJ, Gallagher M. *The case for marriage: why married people are happier, healthier, and better off financially*. New York: Crown Publishing Group; 2001.

49. Aneshensel CS, Frerichs RR, Clark VA. Family roles and sex-differences in depression. *Journal of Health and Social Behavior*. 1981;22(4):379–93.

50. Williams K, Frech A, Carlson DL. Marital status and mental health. In: Scheid TL, Brown TN, eds. *A handbook for the study of mental health: social contexts, theories, and systems, 2nd edition*. Cambridge: Cambridge University Press; 2010. pp. 306–20.

51. Guner N, Kulikova Y, Llull J. Marriage and health: selection, protection, and assortative mating. *European Economic Review*. 2018;109:162–90.

52. Tumin D. Does marriage protect health? A birth cohort comparison. *Social Science Quarterly*. 2018;99(2):626–43.

53. Case A, Deaton A. Life expectancy in adulthood is falling for those without a BA degree, but as educational gaps have widened, racial gaps have narrowed. *Proceedings of the National Academy of Sciences USA*. 2021;118(11):e2024777118.

54. McGarry K, Schoeni RF. Medicare gaps and widow poverty. *Social Security Bulletin*. 2005;66(1):58–74.

55. Blekesaune M, Barrett AE. Marital dissolution and work disability—a longitudinal study of administrative data. *European Sociological Review*. 2005;21(3):259–71.

56. Joung IMA, Van de Mheen HD, Stronks K, Van Poppel FWA, MacKenbach JP. A longitudinal study of health selection in marital transitions. *Social Science and Medicine*. 1998;46(3):425–35.

57. Waldron I, Hughes ME, Brooks TL. Marriage protection and marriage selection—prospective evidence for reciprocal effects of marital status and health. *Social Sciences and Medicine*. 1996;43(1):113–23.

58. Wilson SE, Waddoups SL. Good marriages gone bad: health mismatches as a cause of later-life marital dissolution. *Population Research and Policy Review*. 2002;21(6):505–33.

59. Yu P, Couch KA. Work limiting health and divorce behaviour: a retrospective analysis with SIPP data. *Applied Economics*. 2021;53(25):2799–831.

60. Percheski C, Meyer JM. Health and union dissolution among parenting couples: differences by gender and marital status. *Journal of Health and Social Behavior*. 2018;59(4):569–84.

61. Walsh PN, LeRoy B. *Women with disabilities aging well: a global view*. Baltimore, MD: Paul H Brookes Publishing Company; 2004.

62. Seymour J. Using gendered discourses in negotiations: couples and the onset of disablement in marriage. In: McKie L, Bowlby S, Gregory S, eds. *Gender, power and the household*. London: Palgrave Macmillan; 1999. pp. 76–96.

63. Smith R, Frazer K, Hall P, Hyde A, O'Connor L. 'Betwixt and between health and illness'—women's narratives following acute coronary syndrome. *Journal of Clinical Nursing*. 2017;26(21–22):3457–70.

64. Lorenz FO, Wickrama KAS, Conger RD, Elder GH. The short-term and decade-long effects of divorce on women's midlife health. *Journal of Health and Social Behavior* 2006;47(2):111–25.

65. Leopold T. Gender differences in the consequences of divorce: a study of multiple outcomes. *Demography*. 2018;55(3):769–97.

66. Crowley JE. *Gray divorce: what we lose and gain from mid-life splits*. Oakland: University of California Press; 2018.

67. Carr D. *Golden years? Social inequality in later life*. New York: Russell Sage Foundation; 2019.

68. Lin IF, Brown SL, Wright MR, Hammersmith AM. Antecedents of gray divorce: a life course perspective. *Journal of Gerontology Social Sciences*. 2018;73(6):1022–31.

69. Lin IF, Brown SL. The economic consequences of gray divorce for women and men. *Journal of Gerontology Social Sciences*. 2021;76(10):2073–85.

70. Lin IF, Brown SL, Hammersmith AM. Marital biography, social security receipt, and poverty. *Research on Aging*. 2017;39(1):86–110.

71. Meyer MH, Wolf DA, Himes CL. Linking benefits to marital status: race and social security in the US. *Feminist Economics*. 2005;11(2):145–62.

72. Wu Z, Schimmele CM. Repartnering after first union disruption. *Journal of Marriage and Family*. 2005;67(1):27–36.

73. Schimmele CM, Wu Z. Repartnering after union dissolution in later life. *Journal of Marriage and Family*. 2016;78(4):1013–31.

74. Talbott MM. Older widows' attitudes towards men and remarriage. *Journal of Aging Studies*. 1998;12(4):429–49.

75. Vespa J. Union formation in later life: economic determinants of cohabitation and remarriage among older adults. *Demography*. 2012;49(3):1103–25.

76. Gowey MA, Khodneva Y, Tison SE, Carson AP, Cherrington AL, Howard VJ, et al. Depressive symptoms, perceived stress, and metabolic health: the REGARDS Study. *International Journal of Obesity*. 2019;43(3):615–32.

77. Pearlin LI, Schieman S, Fazio EM, Meersman SC. Stress, health, and the life course: some conceptual perspectives. *Journal of Health and Social Behavior*. 2005;46(2):205–19.

78. Jacobs AW, Padavic I. Hours, scheduling and flexibility for women in the US low-wage labour force. *Gender, Work and Organization*. 2015;22(1):67–86.

79. Livingston G. *The changing profile of unmarried parents*. Washington, DC: Pew Research Center; 2021.

80. Geronimus AT, Hicken MT, Pearson JA, Seashols SJ, Brown KL, Cruz TD. Do US black women experience stress-related accelerated biological aging? *Human Nature.* 2010;21(1):19–38.

81. Raikkonen K, Matthews KA, Kuller LH. The relationship between psychological risk attributes and the metabolic syndrome in healthy women: antecedent or consequence? *Metabolism.* 2002;51(12):1573–7.

82. Fairweather D, Rose NR. Women and autoimmune diseases. *Emerging Infectious Diseases.* 2004;10(11):2005–11.

83. Klein SL, Flanagan KL. Sex differences in immune responses. *Nature Reviews Immunology.* 2016;16(10):626–38.

84. Lockshin MD. Sex differences in autoimmune disease. *Lupus.* 2006;15(11):753–6.

85. Stojanovich L, Marisavljevich D. Stress as a trigger of autoimmune disease. *Autoimmune Review* 2008;7(3):209–13.

86. Abdelaal M, le Roux CW, Docherty NG. Morbidity and mortality associated with obesity. *Annals of Translational Medicine.* 2017;5(7):161–173.

87. Ferraro KF, Kelley-Moore JA. Cumulative disadvantage and health: long-term consequences of obesity? *American Sociological Review.* 2003;68(5):707–29.

88. Simon GE, Ludman EJ, Linde JA, Operskalski BH, Ichikawa L, Rohde P, et al. Association between obesity and depression in middle-aged women. *General Hospital Psychiatry.* 2008;30(1):32–9.

89. Luppino FS, de Wit LM, Bouvy PF, Stijnen T, Cuijpers P, Penninx BW, et al. Overweight, obesity, and depression: a systematic review and meta-analysis of longitudinal studies. *Archives of General Psychiatry.* 2010;67(3):220–9.

90. Arterburn D, Westbrook EO, Ludman EJ, Operskalski B, Linde JA, Rohde P, et al. Relationship between obesity, depression, and disability in middle-aged women. *Obesity Research and Clinical Practice.* 2012;6(3):E197–E206.

91. McDonnell CJ, Garbers SV. Adverse childhood experiences and obesity: systematic review of behavioral interventions for women. *Psychological Trauma.* 2018;10(4):387–95.

92. Dube SR, Anda RF, Whitfield CL, Brown DW, Felitti V, Dong MX, et al. Long-term consequences of childhood sexual abuse by gender of victim. *American Journal of Preventive Medicine.* 2005;28(5):430–8.

93. Cambron C, Gringeri C, Vogel-Ferguson MB. Physical and mental health correlates of adverse childhood experiences among low-income women. *Health Social Work.* 2014;39(4):221–9.

94. Lee H, Kim Y, Terry J. Adverse childhood experiences (ACEs) on mental disorders in young adulthood: latent classes and community violence exposure. *Preventive Medicine.* 2020;134:106039. https://www.sciencedirect.com/science/article/pii/S0091743520300633?casa_token=e3g6yxLbX dwAAAAA:DLgi03xfwhz60jpYlIz6h2z6rsr3Jgjsq58hZIy4qYgNcPW7v31DTcFWnALYEVK rUhXUzzxHvA.

95. Grummitt LR, Kreski NT, Kim SG, Platt J, Keyes KM, McLaughlin KA. Association of childhood adversity with morbidity and mortality in US adults: a systematic review. *Journal of American Medical Association Pediatrics.* 2021;175(12):1269–78.

96. Nettle D. What the future held: childhood psychosocial adversity is associated with health deterioration through adulthood in a cohort of British women. *Evolution and Human Behavior.* 2014;35(6):519–25.

97. Fuemmeler BE, Dedert E, McClernon FJ, Beckham JC. Adverse childhood events are associated with obesity and disordered eating: results from a US Population-based survey of young adults. *Journal of Traumatic Stress.* 2009;22(4):329–33.

98. Kuh D, Ben-Shlomo Y, Lynch J, Hallqvist J, Power C. Life course epidemiology. *Journal of Epidemiology and Community Health.* 2003;57(10):778–83.

99. Dannefer D, Kelley-Moore JA, Huang W. Opening the social: sociological imagination in life course studies. In: Shanahan MJ, Mortimer JT, Johnson MK, eds. *Handbook of life course, 2nd edition.* New York: Springer Publishing; 2015. pp. 87–110.

100. Dube SR, Anda RF, Felitti VJ, Edwards VJ, Croft JB. Adverse childhood experiences and personal alcohol abuse as an adult. *Addictive Behaviors.* 2002;27(5):713–25.

101. Cambron C, Gringeri C, Vogel-Ferguson MB. Adverse childhood experiences, depression and mental health barriers to work among low-income women. *Social Work in Public Health*. 2015;30(6):504–15.

102. Jones MS, Worthen MGF, Sharp SF, McLeod DA. Life as she knows it: the effects of adverse childhood experiences on intimate partner violence among women prisoners. *Child Abuse and Neglect*. 2018;85:68–79.

103. Afifi TO, Enns MW, Cox BJ, Asmundson GJG, Stein MB, Sareen J. Population attributable fractions of psychiatric disorders and suicide ideation and attempts associated with adverse childhood experiences. *American Journal of Public Health*. 2008;98(5):946–52.

104. Ammerman BA, Serang S, Jacobucci R, Burke TA, Alloy LB, McCloskey MS. Exploratory analysis of mediators of the relationship between childhood maltreatment and suicidal behavior. *Journal of Adolescence*. 2018;69:103–12.

105. Erdmans MP, Black T. What they tell you to forget: from child sexual abuse to adolescent motherhood. *Qualitative Health Research*. 2008;18(1):77–89.

106. Whitfield CL, Anda RF, Dube SR, Felitti VJ. Violent childhood experiences and the risk of intimate partner violence in adults—assessment in a large health maintenance organization. *Journal of Interpersonal Violence*. 2003;18(2):166–85.

20

The Influence of Gender-Based Violence Across the Life Course

Elizabeth McLindon, Minerva Kyei-Onanjiri, and Kelsey Hegarty

20.1 Introduction

Violence against women (VAW) includes intimate partner violence (IPV), domestic violence, family violence, and sexual assault. VAW is a leading contributor to poor psychological and physical health as well as premature death for adult women.[1] When VAW is perpetrated by an intimate partner, as is most commonly the case, it is defined as behaviour that, 'results in, or is likely to result in, physical, sexual or psychological harm or suffering to women, including threats of such acts, coercion or arbitrary deprivation of liberty, whether occurring in public or in private life'.[2] Sexual VAW (including rape) is characterised as, 'any sexual act, attempt to obtain a sexual act, unwanted sexual comments or advances, or acts to traffic, or otherwise directed, against a person's sexuality using coercion, by any person regardless of their relationship to the victim, in any setting'.[3] Throughout this chapter, we use the term *victim/survivor* to denote someone who has experienced VAW in recognition of both the harmful impacts of violence and the strength and resilience of people with lived experience.

20.2 VAW Prevalence and Contributing Factors

Data from over 150 countries indicate that 736 million or 31% of all women aged 15 years and older have experienced physical and/or sexual IPV from a current or former intimate partner or sexual violence from someone else at least once in their lifetime.[4] Further, a study of 10 countries reported that the proportion of women who have experienced psychological abuse by a partner in the last year is between 12% to 58%.[5] For Australian women aged 18 years and older, 37% reported an incident of physical and/or sexual violence since the age of 15 years, and 23% had experienced violence by an intimate partner.[6] Moreover, 13% of Australian women witnessed violence toward their mother by a partner when they were children, whereas 4.7% witnessed violence towards their father by a partner.[6] Of women who have experienced violence from a partner, approximately two-thirds identified that their children had also been exposed.[6] Adolescence marks a time of increased risk of sexual violence for young women, with a meta-analysis of the global incidence by continent suggesting that it affects 11.3% of young women in Asia, 13.5% in Europe, 20.1% in the United States

Elizabeth McLindon, Minerva Kyei-Onanjiri, and Kelsey Hegarty, *The Influence of Gender-Based Violence Across the Life Course* In: *A Life Course Approach to Women's Health*. Second Edition. Edited by: Gita D Mishra, Rebecca Hardy, and Diana Kuh, Oxford University Press.

and Canada, and 21.5% in Australia.[7] Sexual assault more commonly occurs within families, perpetrated by a partner, rather than outside intimate relationships.[4,6] Women with disabilities, First Nations women, and women who belong to ethnic, cultural, and religious minorities are consistently over-represented as victim/survivors of VAW.[8] Disability, ethnicity, and transgenerational dispossession and trauma intersect to define the experience of VAW and shape its interpretation.[9]

Violence against women is so called because women and their children account for the majority of victim/survivors, usually offended against by men known to them, across the life course (see Figure 20.1).[8,10] Evidence spotlights the power disparity and unequal access to resources by women compared to men as the largest force underpinning VAW.[11] The gendered power disparity, that is, to varying degrees, confronted by every community around the world, is fuelled by rigid hegemonic gender roles and attitudes linking masculinity with toughness, aggression, and dominance.[12-14] Countries with greater equality between the sexes (assessed using leading international indicators such as life expectancy and workforce participation), generally demonstrate a lower incidence of IPV.[15] Personal, situational, and sociocultural factors all intersect to affect the perpetration of VAW. While a single-factor explanation of male dominance for VAW is inadequate, an ecological framework for violence starts with gender inequality as the foundation.[11,16]

20.3 Ecological Understanding of VAW

Human beings are complex, as are their experiences and relationships, and Heise's (2011) Ecological Framework attempts to identify and synthesise the many distinct factors that contribute to VAW.[11,17] The purpose of the framework is to aid VAW prevention and move towards recovery and healing for victim/survivors. People's lives are layered with different interacting systems, from the micro level (personal experience from birth) to the macro (global health crisis affecting society) (see Figure 20.2).[17,18]

Most of the longitudinal evidence about factors that contribute to VAW has been drawn from studies with victim/survivors, not perpetrators, at the individual level of personal experience. The strength of the evidence about associative factors decreases at each ecological level until the macrosocial (structural) level, where it ceases altogether.[14] Supporting the ecological model, a quantitative multicountry study about VAW perpetration with more than 13,000 people found that stopping one associated factor will not end VAW, because of complex interconnections between individual, relationship, community, and society factors associated with perpetration.[12] The ecological framework will be revisited in Section 20.9 for discussion of how COVID-19 has affected VAW. The next section looks at lifetime impacts of VAW, taking the example of the impacts for children when IPV occurs during pregnancy.

20.4 Exposure to IPV During the Early Childhood Years

Violence can begin in the womb; IPV poses particular risks to women of childbearing age as well as their offspring. The antenatal period may be a time of increased risk that violence will start or escalate,[19-21] and hospital injury data highlights that the pelvis is often a target for physical assaults during pregnancy.[22] A systematic review of all IPV risk and protective

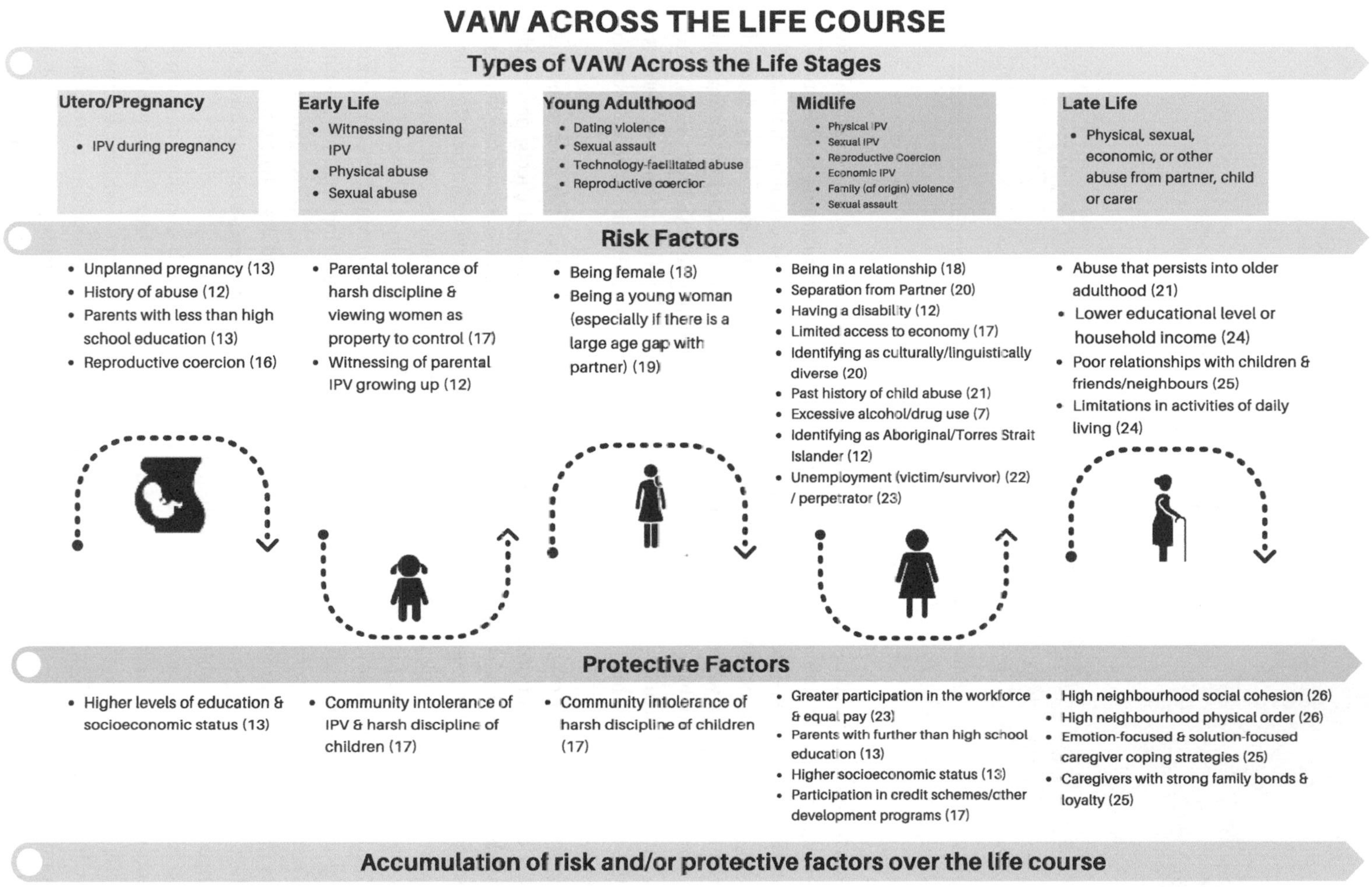

VAW ACROSS THE LIFE COURSE

Types of VAW Across the Life Stages

Utero/Pregnancy	Early Life	Young Adulthood	Midlife	Late Life
• IPV during pregnancy	• Witnessing parental IPV • Physical abuse • Sexual abuse	• Dating violence • Sexual assault • Technology-facilitated abuse • Reproductive coercion	• Physical IPV • Sexual IPV • Reproductive Coercion • Economic IPV • Family (of origin) violence • Sexual assault	• Physical, sexual, economic, or other abuse from partner, child or carer

Risk Factors

• Unplanned pregnancy (13) • History of abuse (12) • Parents with less than high school education (13) • Reproductive coercion (16)	• Parental tolerance of harsh discipline & viewing women as property to control (17) • Witnessing of parental IPV growing up (12)	• Being female (13) • Being a young woman (especially if there is a large age gap with partner) (19)	• Being in a relationship (18) • Separation from Partner (20) • Having a disability (12) • Limited access to economy (17) • Identifying as culturally/linguistically diverse (20) • Past history of child abuse (21) • Excessive alcohol/drug use (7) • Identifying as Aboriginal/Torres Strait Islander (12) • Unemployment (victim/survivor) (22) / perpetrator (23)	• Abuse that persists into older adulthood (21) • Lower educational level or household income (24) • Poor relationships with children & friends/neighbours (25) • Limitations in activities of daily living (24)

Protective Factors

• Higher levels of education & socioeconomic status (13)	• Community intolerance of IPV & harsh discipline of children (17)	• Community intolerance of harsh discipline of children (17)	• Greater participation in the workforce & equal pay (23) • Parents with further than high school education (13) • Higher socioeconomic status (13) • Participation in credit schemes/other development programs (17)	• High neighbourhood social cohesion (26) • High neighbourhood physical order (26) • Emotion-focused & solution-focused caregiver coping strategies (25) • Caregivers with strong family bonds & loyalty (25)

Accumulation of risk and/or protective factors over the life course

Figure 20.1 VAW risk and protective factors across the life course.

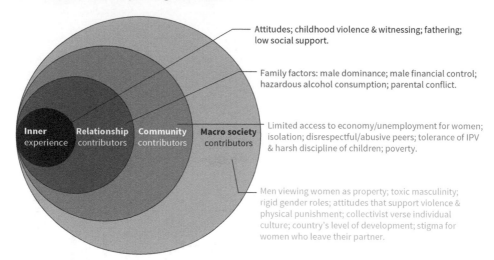

Attitudes; childhood violence & witnessing; fathering; low social support.

Family factors: male dominance; male financial control; hazardous alcohol consumption; parental conflict.

Limited access to economy/unemployment for women; isolation; disrespectful/abusive peers; tolerance of IPV & harsh discipline of children; poverty.

Men viewing women as property; toxic masculinity; rigid gender roles; attitudes that support violence & physical punishment; collectivist verse individual culture; country's level of development; stigma for women who leave their partner.

Figure 20.2 Ecological framework of individual and systemic contributing factors related to VAW (adapted from Heise 2011).[17]

factors found that unplanned pregnancy and having parents with less than high school education were the only known risk factors, although there were limitations to this study.[14] Reproductive coercion—behaviour that sabotages the autonomous decision-making of a woman in relation to becoming pregnant, or continuing or ending a pregnancy—is much more likely to affect a woman whose intimate relationship is already violent.[23] Postpartum impacts for women who experience violence during pregnancy include depression, drug use,[24] infant attachment issues,[25] and social isolation.[26,27] IPV during pregnancy also presents a time point at which to begin an examination of a possible IPV life course effect (see Figure 20.3).

Exposure to IPV during the very earliest stage of life, while in utero, has been associated with a cascade of emotional, developmental, behavioural, and physical effects, observable throughout childhood and into adolescence.[27-31] Following victim/survivor mothers and their children, international longitudinal and birth cohort studies have examined the effects of exposure to IPV during pregnancy. Even after adjusting for potentially confounding factors, varied impacts were present at different time points from birth to late childhood and early adulthood among both boys and girls.[29] Emotional impacts include elevated stress responses like posttraumatic stress disorder (PTSD) and emotional dysregulation that may manifest as lowered mood or hyperactivity in children up to 10 years old.[28,32-34] Developmental impacts span infant sleep problems,[35] underdeveloped language in toddlers,[36] kids unprepared to start school,[28] and aggressive behaviour.[27] Physical impacts encompass low birthweight,[37] a range of respiratory problems,[30,38] and obesity.[39]

Molecular changes that detrimentally affect psychological health may start in utero for infants exposed to IPV and become part of their life course picture. Transgenerational epigenetic changes to the methylation of the glucocorticoid receptor gene—which has a role in growth, immune function, behaviour, and psychology—have been found in a small study of young people aged 10–19 years whose mothers suffered IPV during pregnancy.[40] Cross-sectional studies point to another likely impact of exposure to IPV as a child: increased reporting of IPV in adult relationships.

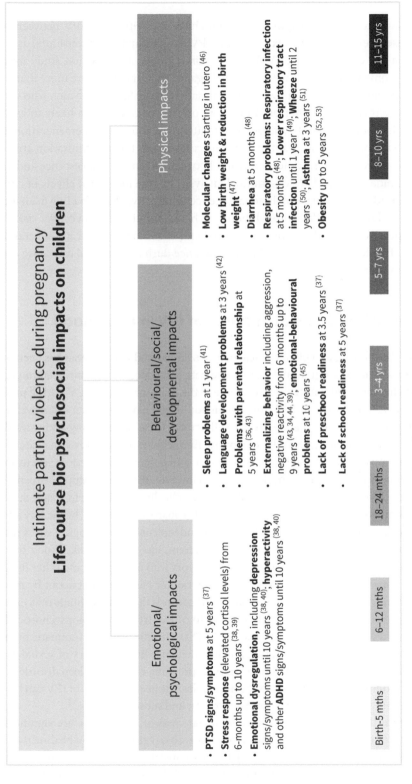

Figure 20.3 Biopsychosocial impacts experienced by children after IPV occurs in pregnancy.

20.5 The Link Between Childhood and Adult Abuse

Evidence suggests that past exposure to child abuse and witnessing IPV between parents, may increase one's likelihood of experiencing IPV in an intimate relationship(s) as an adult, indicating a life course effect of VAW.[13,41,42] For example, a population study found that Australian women who as girls witnessed IPV against their mother, were more than twice as likely to experience IPV in their own adult intimate relationships; while men who witnessed IPV against either their mother or father were up to four times more likely to experience IPV in adulthood.[13] A recent synthesis of the literature about the intergenerational transmission of violence, suggests that the strongest connections for revictimisation are between child abuse and violence in adolescence, and between violence in adolescence and violence in early to midadulthood.[43] A longitudinal analysis into the long-term effects of childhood adversity found that the harms of disadvantage accumulate over time, leading to an increased risk of abuse during late life; although boosting health in midlife reduces that risk.[44] While more prospective-longitudinal studies are needed to better understand and substantiate the repetition of violence, it is indisputable that violence during childhood can cause considerable harm in later life.[14]

20.6 Health and Social Impacts of IPV in Adulthood

Because of the life-long and often cyclical nature of abuse and violence that has been outlined so far in this chapter, longitudinal studies indicate associated biopsychosocial impacts.[45–47] While the chapter has already canvassed some of the many impacts of IPV during pregnancy, health impacts of exposure to IPV throughout adulthood have also been extensively studied and found to be wide-ranging. Figure 20.4 illustrates three of the many pathways through which IPV can lead to adverse health outcomes. Empirical evidence shows an association between cumulative abuse and significantly worse health outcomes, with more severe abuse associated with more concerning health.[45,46,48,49] However, the relationship between violence and health is complex.[3] Adverse health outcomes may be directly caused, for example, through injuries sustained during physical IPV, or indirectly caused, for example, by the way a survivor physiologically or behaviourally responds to fear and violence.[3] Physiological stress responses to prolonged threats may weaken the immune system, increasing the likelihood of viral infections and cancer cell spread.[3] Meanwhile, survivors who use alcohol and other drugs in an attempt to cope with violence risk poor liver function or harm brought about by misadventure.[3] Women whose abusive partner isolates and controls their whereabouts may experience health problems stemming from a lack of access to care or treatment.[3] Biopsychosocial health impacts linked with IPV include depression,[49] PTSD, chronic pain,[42,45] traumatic brain[50] and other injuries,[42] and suicide attempts.[46] Further, evidence links a history of sexual assault at any age to an increased risk of lifetime anxiety, depression, eating and sleep disorders, PTSD, and suicide attempts.[51] Among First Nations peoples, the health impacts of IPV can be exacerbated by racism, transgenerational trauma, poverty, and substance abuse.[52]

Apart from the individual, familial, and social costs of VAW, there are significant economic costs for society.[42] While financial impacts across regions may not be directly comparable because of different inclusion criteria, the costs are substantial. The bill to the Australian economy was $22 billion in 2015–16; in England and Wales, the cost reached £32.96 billion; while in the United States, it was $5.8 billion.[53,54]

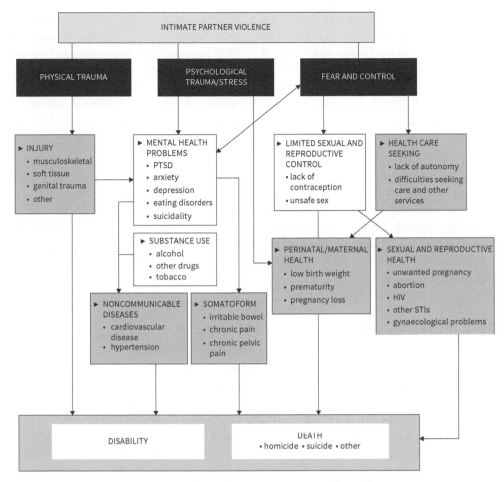

Figure 20.4 Pathways and health effects of intimate partner violence.[4]

20.7 Intervening with Individuals and Communities to Prevent VAW

Against the background of increased risks of further VAW victimisation resulting from previous experience, it is important to take steps that could alter this life course trajectory, preventing violence before it happens.[55] Some literature has identified predictors of VAW that could serve as potential points of intervention. For example, Fulu et al. (2013) studied the motivations, associated factors and outcomes of men who use violence in Asia and the Pacific, found that sexual offending behaviour often began during adolescence, was most commonly motivated by a sense of sexual entitlement, followed by entertainment-seeking, anger, or punishment, and the majority of perpetrators did not face legal consequences.[12] VAW perpetration is linked to societal and attitudinal gender inequality, lived experience of abuse, and witnessing IPV in childhood leading to serious social and health consequences, including depression, low levels of education, under-employment, and the use of violence outside the home.[12] Although, individual factors do not necessarily cause violence and do not exist in isolation, a more meaningful way of preventing violence may be to understand clusters of factors associated with perpetration and how they are interconnected in each context.[12]

Early engagement through the health and community service sectors has the potential to engage individuals and families before a crisis and safety response is required by specialist services.[56] The World Health Organization (WHO) has identified the critical and unique role that an effective health system can play to intervene early with at-risk groups (i.e. young people, pregnant women, and people with mental health issues) to identify warning signs and respond to VAW.[57] A best-practice response towards a victim/survivor who has entered the health system includes: belief and empathy, exploration of the woman's situation with a focus on risk and protective factors, reassurance against blame, offers of practical care that do not intrude upon autonomy, and referral to longer term, specialised support.[58] It has been suggested that early engagement in response to all types of violence should be strongly person centred, considering the context of lived experience, rather than defined subcategories of abuse or violence.[59] For instance, violence-prevention programs focusing on child abuse should strategically address common factors related to dating violence and IPV and elder abuse in later years.[59] Similarly, services targeting people who use violence should link with different organisations and address the fact that perpetrators offend in a variety of contexts and may have experienced victimisation themselves.[59]

20.8 Elder Abuse

Elder abuse can be defined as 'a single or repeated act or lack of appropriate action that causes harm or distress to an older person'.[60] Abuse against an older person (typically defined as people aged 60 years and over) may be psychological, financial, sexual, physical, or take the form of neglect.[61] A meta-analysis has suggested that the global prevalence of elder abuse is 15.7% with little difference by gender.[62] Belonging to a minority culture, suffering from depression, experiencing limitations with activities-of-daily-living, and previous exposure to abuse in childhood, young adulthood, or into late adulthood, are all risk factors for elder abuse (see Figure 20.1).[43,44,63] Protective factors for elder abuse have not been widely studied. A longitudinal investigation conducted in India reported that older people with high neighbourhood social cohesion (perceived support and trust among neighbours) were 38% less likely to experience abuse, and elders who lived in an orderly neighbourhood (i.e. clean) were 48% less likely to experience abuse, compared with those from neighbourhoods with low social cohesion.[64] Other protective factors include acaregivers' own use of emotion and solution focused coping strategiesand caregivers with strong family bonds and sense of loyalty.[65]

20.9 COVID-19 Pandemic and Impact on VAW

On 30 January 2020, the WHO categorised COVID-19 as a public health emergency of international concern.[66] This pandemic has triggered an unprecedented health and social emergency. Diverse policy responses from governments and health organisations around the world presented short- and long-term consequences for the safety of women and children as restrictions on movement forced people to stay at home for protracted time periods.

Dubbed 'the shadow pandemic',[1] because of the insidious and largely hidden nature of VAW during COVID-19, early data indicate worldwide increases in frequency and severity

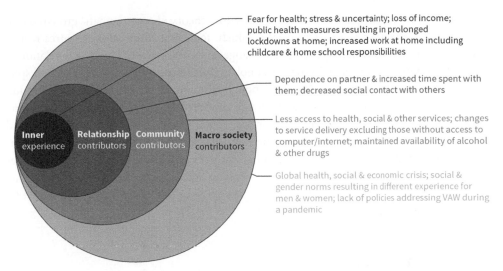

Fear for health; stress & uncertainty; loss of income; public health measures resulting in prolonged lockdowns at home; increased work at home including childcare & home school responsibilities

Dependence on partner & increased time spent with them; decreased social contact with others

Less access to health, social & other services; changes to service delivery excluding those without access to computer/internet; maintained availability of alcohol & other drugs

Global health, social & economic crisis; social & gender norms resulting in different experience for men & women; lack of policies addressing VAW during a pandemic

Inner experience

Relationship contributors

Community contributors

Macro society contributors

Figure 20.5 Ecological model of additional violence risk factors presented by COVID-19 pandemic (inspired by the work of Sánchez et al., 2020).[16]

of all forms of VAW.[16,67] Violence or abuse may be exacerbated by stressors imposed by the pandemic conditions, including income or job loss, increased childcare responsibilities and home-schooling, working remotely, loss of social interactions, boredom and frustration associated with the restrictions, and problematic coping strategies such as substance abuse.[16,68] Compounding these problems are reduced access to resources and disruptions in families' usual sources of support because of lockdown measures. Decreased availability of services, changes to service mode of delivery (i.e. telehealth), increased demand for assistance, overworked and stressed service providers and challenges to help-seeking by women, were further consequences of COVID-19.[16,68] The ecological model for understanding VAW has recently been updated to highlight the additional challenges and risk factors induced by COVID-19 across all systems with which women and children interact (see Figure 20.5).[16]

The full extent to which the pandemic might have worsened both the violence trajectorty and experience of women and children is yet to be determined but is likely to extend beyond the crisis.[68] The pandemic offers an important lesson for health and social policy to prepare for events that disrupt normal social order, however rare. Health systems may benefit from exploring alternative approaches to supporting victim/survivors that allow room to balance competing risks and promote continued learning and action. Any strategy will require input from key stakeholders, including from victim/survivors, to build public trust essential for program implementation.

20.10 Resilience and Posttraumatic Growth

Sitting alongside the harm sequent from VAW, human beings appear to demonstrate enormous capacity for psychological growth after trauma.[69] The term *posttraumatic growth* describes both positive psychological change, and the process of change, that can emerge out of the challenges and struggles of severe adversity, both nature (i.e. COVID-19, bushfire) and human induced, such as VAW.[69] One explanatory theory of posttraumatic growth is that crisis indelibly alters a person's world view, which, following rumination, requires reconstruction.[70] Contemplation may precipitate change and a new sense of meaning in relation to personal strength, coping capacity, one's outlook on life, relationships with others, and spirituality.[71] A systematic review of 16 studies about posttraumatic growth following IPV found that high personal growth is possible, although mediated by a range of factors, including the level of social support a victim/survivor has, ongoing contact with the perpetrator, and self-belief.[72] Posttraumatic growth is not the absence of distress; it does not describe victim/survivors returning to pretrauma functioning, nor does it manufacture a rosy ending after extreme hardship. Rather, posttraumatic growth is an organic process that some victim/survivors experience evolving out of the struggle of surviving IPV and making new sense of a world where old assumptions no longer hold.

20.11 Conclusions

From birth to our later years, women and their children are disproportionally exposed to violence directed towards them within their closest relationships. VAW has a clear life course affect, with exposure in early life setting up a greater likelihood of violence in future partner and familial relationships. This chapter has canvassed the many implications of VAW for emotional, behavioural, physical, and psychological development, health and recovery. Prevention and early intervention guidelines should recognise the interrelations among different forms of violence across the lifespan and current and potential risk factors for further victimisation. Particular groups, such as First Nations women, culturally and linguistically diverse women and women with a disability, bear an even greater violence and abuse burden, which must be considered by service providers, policymakers, and researchers when responding to victim/survivors and devising interventions, strategy, policy, and research. The evidence underscores the importance of an ecological and life course lens to understand a victim/survivor's inner experience and the context of her relationships, community, and society. A long-term commitment to addressing inequality between women and men requires rethinking of, and re-education about, gender roles and attitudes normalised by society. More research, particularly longitudinal studies with both victim/survivors and people who use violence, is required to better understand and inform relevant targeted preventive health strategies. Women and children with lived experience of VAW must be at the centre of all of our efforts to move towards a more desired world in which VAW is prevented and victim/survivors' health, social, and economic needs are better met by professionals, organisations, policy, and research.

Key messages and implications

- VAW affects women and children across the globe at every age and stage, and can profoundly alter the health, relationships, and opportunities of those to whom it is directed.
- VAW imposes significant social and economic costs on women, families, and society.

- There are key time points associated with increased risk of VAW, as well as opportunities for intervention.
- An ecological lens (victim/survivor's inner experience, relationships, community, and society) is critical to the success of VAW prevention programs as well as interventions with women and children after violence has occurred.
- Victim/survivors demonstrate enormous capacity for psychological growth and recovery after the trauma of VAW, but this is mediated by a range of factors, including the social support they receive.
- COVID-19 related restrictions and other events that disrupt normal social order present increased risk for victim/survivors of VAW and available data indicates an increase in intensity of all forms of VAW.
- Health and social policy must consider and make provisions for events that disrupt normal social order, however rare they may be.
- More longitudinal studies with both VAW victim/survivors and perpetrators will enhance prevention and response health and social strategies.

References

1. United Nations Women. *Measuring the shadow pandemic: violence against women during COVID-19*. New York: United Nations; 24 November 2021.
2. United Nations General Assembly. *Declaration on the elimination of violence against women*. New York: United Nations; 20 December 1993.
3. Krug EG, Dahlberg LL, Mercy JA, Zwi AB, Lozano R. *World report on violence and health*. Geneva: World Health Organization; 2002.
4. World Health Organization. *Violence against women prevalence estimates, 2018: global, regional and national prevalence estimates for intimate partner violence against women and global and regional prevalence estimates for non-partner sexual violence against women*. Geneva: World Health Organization; 2021.
5. Heise L, Pallitto C, Garcia-Moreno C, Clark CJ. Measuring psychological abuse by intimate partners: constructing a cross-cultural indicator for the Sustainable Development Goals. *SSM - Population Health*. 2019;9:100377.
6. Australian Bureau of Statistics. *Personal Safety, Australia: statistics for family, domestic, sexual violence, physical assault, partner emotional abuse, child abuse, sexual harassment, stalking and safety [Internet]*. Canberra: Australian Bureau of Statistics; 2017 [updated 8 November 2017; cited 29 June 2022]. Available from: https://www.abs.gov.au/statistics/people/crime-and-justice/personal-safety-australia/latest-release.
7. Stoltenborgh M, van Ijzendoorn MH, Euser EM, Bakermans-Kranenburg MJ. A global perspective on child sexual abuse: meta-analysis of prevalence around the world. *Child Maltreatment*. 2011;16(2):79–101.
8. World Health Organization. *Caring for women subjected to violence: a WHO curriculum for training health-care providers*. Geneva: World Health Organization; 2019.
9. Kelly UA. Theories of intimate partner violence: from blaming the victim to acting against injustice: intersectionality as an analytic framework. *ANS Advances in Nursing Science*. 2011;34(3):E29–E51.
10. Australian Institute of Health and Welfare. *Family, domestic and sexual violence in Australia: continuing the national story 2019*. Canberra: Australian Institute of Health and Welfare; 2019. Cat. No. FDV 3.

11. Heise LL. Violence against women: an integrated, ecological framework. *Violence Against Women.* 1998;4(3):262–90.

12. Fulu E, Warner X, Miedema S, Jewkes R, Roselli T, Lang J. Why do some men use violence against women and how can we prevent it? Quantitative findings from the United Nations multi-country study on men and violence in Asia and the Pacific. Bangkok: UNDP, UNFPA, UN Womens and UNV; 201313. Australian Institute of Health and Welfare. *Family, domestic and sexual violence in Australia 2018.* Canberra: Australian Institute of Health and Welfare; 2018. Cat. No. FDV 2.

14. Yakubovich AR, Stockl H, Murray J, Melendez-Torres GJ, Steinert JI, Glavin CEY, et al. Risk and protective factors for intimate partner violence against women: systematic review and meta-analyses of prospective-longitudinal studies. *American Journal of Public Health.* 2018;108(7):e1–e11.

15. United Nations Development Fund for Women. *Investing in gender equality: ending violence against women and girls.* New York: UN Women; 2010.

16. Sanchez OR, Vale DB, Rodrigues L, Surita FG. Violence against women during the COVID-19 pandemic: an integrative review. *International Journal of Gynecology and Obstetrics.* 2020;151(2):180–7.

17. Heise LL. *What works to prevent partner violence: an evidence review.* London: STRIVE Research Consortium; 2011.

18. Bronfenbrenner U. Ecological systems theory. In: Vasta R, ed. *Six theories of child development: revised formulations and current issues.* London: Jessica Kingsley Publishers; 1992. pp. 187–249.

19. Howell KH, Miller-Graff LE, Hasselle AJ, Scrafford KE. The unique needs of pregnant, violence-exposed women: a systematic review of current interventions and directions for translational research. *Aggression and Violent Behavior.* 2017;34:11.

20. Martin SL, Harris-Britt A, Li Y, Moracco KE, Kupper LL, Campbell JC. Changes in intimate partner violence during pregnancy. *Journal of Family Violence.* 2004;19(4):10.

21. World Health Organization. *Intimate partner violence during pregnancy: information sheet.* Geneva: World Health Organization; 2011. WHO/RHR/11.35.

22. Cassell E, Clapperton A. Hospital-treated assault injury among Victorian women aged 15 years and over due to intimate partner violence (IPV), Victoria 2009–10 to 2013–14. *Hazard.* 2015;Winter 2015:1–24.

23. Tarzia L, Wellington M, Marino J, Hegarty K. 'A huge, hidden problem': Australian health practitioners' views and understandings of reproductive coercion. *Qualitative Health Research.* 2019;29(10):1395–407.

24. Bacchus LJ, Ranganathan M, Watts C, Devries K. Recent intimate partner violence against women and health: a systematic review and meta-analysis of cohort studies. *BMJ Open.* 2018;8(7):e019995.

25. Levendosky AA, Leahy KL, Bogat GA, Davidson WS, von Eye A. Domestic violence, maternal parenting, maternal mental health, and infant externalizing behavior. *Journal of Family Psychology.* 2006;20(4):544–52.

26. Silove D, Mohsin M, Klein L, Tam NJ, Dadds M, Eapen V, et al. Longitudinal path analysis of depressive symptoms and functioning among women of child-rearing age in postconflict Timor-Leste. *BMJ Global Health.* 2020;5(3):e002039.

27. Zvara BJ, Mills-Koonce R, the Family Life Project Key C. Intimate partner violence, parenting, and children's representations of caregivers. *Journal of Interpersonal Violence.* 2021;36(21–22):NP11756–NP11779.

28. Enlow MB, Blood E, Egeland B. Sociodemographic risk, developmental competence, and PTSD symptoms in young children exposed to interpersonal trauma in early life. *Journal of Trauma Stress.* 2013;26(6):686–94.

29. Skinner L, Gavidia-Payne S, Brown S, Giallo R. Mechanisms underlying exposure to partner violence and children's emotional-behavioral difficulties. *Journal of Family Psychology.* 2019;33(6):730–41.

30. MacGinty R, Lesosky M, Barnett W, Nduru PM, Vanker A, Stein DJ, et al. Maternal psychosocial risk factors and lower respiratory tract infection (LRTI) during infancy in a South African birth cohort. *PLoS One.* 2019;14(12):e0226144.

31. Bowen E. The impact of intimate partner violence on preschool children's peer problems: an analysis of risk and protective factors. *Child Abuse and Neglect.* 2015;50:141–50.

32. Isaksson J, Lindblad F, Valladares E, Hogberg U. High maternal cortisol levels during pregnancy are associated with more psychiatric symptoms in offspring at age of nine—a prospective study from Nicaragua. *Journal of Psychiatic Research*. 2015;71:97–102.

33. Martinez-Torteya C, Bogat GA, Levendosky AA, von Eye A. The influence of prenatal intimate partner violence exposure on hypothalamic-pituitary-adrenal axis reactivity and childhood internalizing and externalizing symptoms. *Developmental Psychopathology*. 2016;28(1):55–72.

34. Dejonghe E, von Eye A, Bogat GA, Levedosky A. Does witnessing intimate partner violence contribute to toddlers' internalizing and externalizing behaviors? *Applied Developmental Science*. 2011;15(3):11.

35. Cook F, Conway L, Gartland D, Giallo R, Keys E, Brown S. Profiles and predictors of infant sleep problems across the first year. *Journal of Developmental Behavioral Pediatrics*. 2020;41(2):104–16.

36. Peterson CC, Riggs J, Guyon-Harris K, Harrison L, Huth-Bocks A. Effects of intimate partner violence and home environment on child language development in the first 3 years of life. *Journal of Developmental Behavioral Pediatrics*. 2019;40(2):112–21.

37. McFarlane J, Parker B, Soeken K. Abuse during pregnancy: associations with maternal health and infant birth weight. *NursingResearch*. 1996;45(1):37–42.

38. Suglia SF, Enlow MB, Kullowatz A, Wright RJ. Maternal intimate partner violence and increased asthma incidence in children: buffering effects of supportive caregiving. *Archives of Pediatrics and Adolescent Medicine*. 2009;163(3):244–50.

39. Boynton-Jarrett R, Fargnoli J, Suglia SF, Zuckerman B, Wright RJ. Association between maternal intimate partner violence and incident obesity in preschool-aged children: results from the Fragile Families and Child Well-being Study. *Archives of Pediatrics and Adolescent Medicine*. 2010;164(6):540–6.

40. Radtke KM, Ruf M, Gunter HM, Dohrmann K, Schauer M, Meyer A, et al. Transgenerational impact of intimate partner violence on methylation in the promoter of the glucocorticoid receptor. *Translational Psychiatry*. 2011;1:e21.

41. World Health Organization Prevention of Violence Unit. *Violence info [Internet]*. Geneva: World Health Organization; 2017 [updated unknown date; cited 9 November 2021]. Available from: https://apps.who.int/violence-info/.

42. World Health Organization. *Violence against women [Internet]*. Geneva: WHO; 2021 [updated 9 March 2021; cited 9 November 2021]. Available from: https://www.who.int/news-room/fact-sheets/detail/violence-against-women.

43. Herrenkohl TI, Fedina L, Roberto KA, Raquet KL, Hu RX, Rousson AN, et al. Child maltreatment, youth violence, intimate partner violence, and elder mistreatment: a review and theoretical analysis of research on violence across the life course. *Trauma, Violence, and Abuse*. 2022;23(1):314–28.

44. Easton SD, Kong J. Childhood adversities, midlife health, and elder abuse victimization: a longitudinal analysis based on Cumulative Disadvantage theory. *Journal of Gerontology: Series B*. 2021;76(10):2086–97.

45. Davies L, Ford-Gilboe M, Willson A, Varcoe C, Wuest J, Campbell J, et al. Patterns of cumulative abuse among female survivors of intimate partner violence: links to women's health and socioeconomic status. *Violence Against Women*. 2015;21(1):30–48.

46. Devries KM, Mak JY, Bacchus LJ, Child JC, Falder G, Petzold M, et al. Intimate partner violence and incident depressive symptoms and suicide attempts: a systematic review of longitudinal studies. *PLoS Medicine*. 2013;10(5):e1001439.

47. Kong J, Easton SD. Re-experiencing violence across the life course: histories of childhood maltreatment and elder abuse victimization. *Journal of Gerontology: Series B*. 2019;74(5):853–7.

48. Lagdon S, Armour C, Stringer M. Adult experience of mental health outcomes as a result of intimate partner violence victimisation: a systematic review. *European Journal of Psychotraumatology*. 2014;5: 1–12.49. Rees S, Silove D, Chey T, Ivancic L, Steel Z, Creamer M, et al. Lifetime prevalence of gender-based violence in women and the relationship with mental disorders and psychosocial function. *JAMA*. 2011;306(5):513–21.

50. Campbell JC, Anderson JC, McFadgion A, Gill J, Zink E, Patch M, et al. The effects of intimate partner violence and probable traumatic brain injury on central nervous system symptoms. *Journal of Women's Health*. 2018;27(6):761–7.

51. Chen LP, Murad MH, Paras ML, Colbenson KM, Sattler AL, Goranson EN, et al. Sexual abuse and lifetime diagnosis of psychiatric disorders: systematic review and meta-analysis. *Mayo Clinic Proceedings*. 2010;85(7):618–29.

52. Chmielowska M, Fuhr DC. Intimate partner violence and mental ill health among global populations of Indigenous women: a systematic review. *Social Psychiatry and Psychiatric Epidemiology*. 2017;52(6):689–704.

53. KPMG. *The cost of violence against women and their children in Australia.* Canberra: KPMG; 2016.

54. United Nations Women. *The economic costs of violence against women.* Geneva: UN Women; 2016.

55. Our watch. *Change the story: a shared framework for the primary prevention of violence against women and their children in Australia.* Uploaded 2015. Available from: https://www.ourwatch.org.au/change-the-story/.

56. World Health Organization. *Responding to intimate partner violence and sexual violence against women: WHO clinical and policy guidelines.* Geneva: World Health Organization; 2013.

57. Garcia-Moreno C, Hegarty K, d'Oliveira AF, Koziol-McLain J, Colombini M, Feder G. The health-systems response to violence against women. *Lancet*. 2015;385(9977):1567–79.

58. World Health Organization. *Health care for women subjected to intimate partner violence or sexual violence: a clinical handbook.* Geneva: World Health Organization; 2014.

59. Hamby S, Grych J. Implications for prevention and intervention: a more person-centered approach. In: Hamby S, Grych J, eds. *The web of violence: exploring connections among different forms of interpersonal violence and abuse.* Dordrecht: Springer Netherlands; 2013. pp. 81–103.

60. World Health Organization Regional Office for the Western Pacific. *Elder abuse.* Manila: World Health Organization; 2016. WPR/2016/DNH/010.

61. Yon Y, Mikton C, Gassoumis ZD, Wilber KH. The prevalence of self-reported elder abuse among older women in community settings: a systematic review and meta-analysis. *Trauma, Violence, and Abuse.* 2019;20(2):245–59.

62. Yon Y, Mikton CR, Gassoumis ZD, Wilber KH. Elder abuse prevalence in community settings: a systematic review and meta-analysis. *Lancet Global Health.* 2017;5(2):e147–e156.

63. McDonald L, Thomas C. Elder abuse through a life course lens. *International Psychogeriatrics.* 2013;25(8):1235–43.

64. Chang ES, Levy BR. Protective effects of neighborhood community factors on elder abuse in India. *Journal of Elder Abuse and Neglect.* 2021;33(1):1–16.

65. Fang B, Yan E, Lai DWL. Risk and protective factors associated with domestic abuse among older Chinese in the People's Republic of China. *Archives of Gerontology and Geriatrics.* 2019;82:120–7.

66. World Health Organization. *Listings of WHO's response to COVID-19 2020 [Internet].* Geneva: World Health Organization; 2020 [updated 29 June 2020; cited 9 November 2021]. Available from: https://www.who.int/news/item/29-06-2020-covidtimeline.

67. Boxall H, Morgan A, Brown R. *The prevalence of domestic violence among women during the COVID-19 pandemic.* Canberra: Australian Institute of Criminology; 13 July 2020. Statistical Bulletin no. 28.

68. Humphreys KL, Myint MT, Zeanah CH. Increased risk for family violence during the COVID-19 pandemic. *Pediatrics.* 2020;146(1):1–3. 69. Tedeschi RG, Calhoun LG. The Posttraumatic Growth Inventory: measuring the positive legacy of trauma. *Journal of Traumatic Stress.* 1996;9(3):455–71.

70. Valdez CE, Lilly MM. Posttraumatic growth in survivors of intimate partner violence: an assumptive world process. *Journal of Interpersonal Violence.* 2015;30(2):215–31.

71. Tedeschi RG, Park CL, Calhoun LG. Posttraumatic growth: conceptual issues. In: Tedeschi RG, Park CL, Calhoun LG, eds. *Posttraumatic growth: positive changes in the aftermath of crisis.* Mahwah, NJ: Lawrence Erlbaum Associates Publishers; 1998. pp. 1–22.

72. Elderton A, Berry A, Chan C. A systematic review of posttraumatic growth in survivors of interpersonal violence in adulthood. *Trauma, Violence, and Abuse.* 2017;18(2):223–36.

PART VI
FROM EVIDENCE TO PRACTICE

21

A Life Course Approach to Women's Health Care

Judith Stephenson, Jennifer Hall, and Louise F. Wilson

21.1 Introduction

This chapter outlines the implications of a life course approach for the organisation and delivery of women's health care and considers the evidence for the impact of such an approach in the context of high-income countries (HICs). It expands and updates an earlier publication by Stephenson and others that has now been archived,[1] but has formed the cornerstone of national strategies for women's care in the UK in 2012 and 2019.[2] Earlier chapters in this book have described how a life course perspective investigates the long-term effects of biological, behavioural, and social exposures during gestation, childhood, adolescence, and young adulthood on health and chronic disease in later life and across generations. Here, we consider the intuitive relevance of a life course approach to women's health care and the potential for early intervention to reduce disease risk or severity.

21.2 What Features of Women's Health Care Have Particular Relevance to a Life Course Approach?

Unlike disease episodes that arise sporadically in subgroups of men and women, reproductive and sexual health issues are relevant to almost all women for several decades, prompting a wide range of health care needs that unfold across the life course in a more predictable way. An examination of the rates of consultation in primary care between women and men in the UK in 2010 showed that age-specific rates of consultation were higher for girls and women at all ages from 10 to 80 years, and that reproductive events contribute substantially to consultations in women but not to consultation rates in men.[3]

In Figure 21.1, early vaccination programs, which are relevant to male and female infants, are included because they exemplify the success of early intervention in preventing later disease. Aside from the essential role of sexual and reproductive activity for continuing human existence, the great majority of women want to enjoy sexual relationships while controlling their fertility. This requires timely and accurate education about sexual health with access to, and choice of, effective contraception and safe abortion. In HIC, the midtwentieth century saw a significant trend towards earlier onset of sexual activity that has since plateaued,[4] while the age at which women have their first child has been increasing for over 40 years.[5]

Judith Stephenson, Jennifer Hall, and Louise F. Wilson, *A Life Course Approach to Women's Health Care* In: *A Life Course Approach to Women's Health*. Second Edition. Edited by: Gita D Mishra, Rebecca Hardy, and Diana Kuh, Oxford University Press.

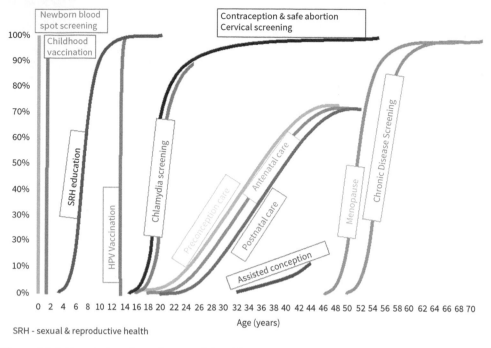

Figure 21.1 Population view of women's health care needs across the life course (adapted from Stephenson et al.[1]).

This means that most women now require effective, reversible contraception for 3 decades or more, while a small but growing number of older women (one in seven in the UK) seek assisted conception as fertility declines with age. The overall picture, which reflects the unfolding of a global demographic transition, is one of declining fertility, with around one in five women remaining childless in the UK.[6] At older ages, the onset of the menopause and increasing incidence of cancer and other chronic diseases become relevant for a very high proportion of the population.

For women who do go through pregnancy, the 'stressor effect' of pregnancy on maternal metabolic and cardiovascular function can act as an 'early warning' by demonstrating a higher risk of health problems in later life (see Figure 21.2). For example, women who develop diabetes in pregnancy (gestational diabetes) are at very high risk of developing type 2 diabetes, particularly between 3 and 6 years after delivery,[7] and they have a significantly increased risk of hypertension and ischaemic heart disease.[8] As obesity has become more common, so has gestational diabetes, which now affects one in every seven pregnancies in Australia[9] and one in twenty-three in the UK[10] (differences in prevalence may reflect diagnostic cut-off criteria).

21.3 What Are the Implications of a Life Course Approach for Delivery of Women's Health Care?

Figure 21.3 presents a comprehensive model of women's healthcare, from puberty to menopause, based on what women seek from health services. It implies integration of primary and

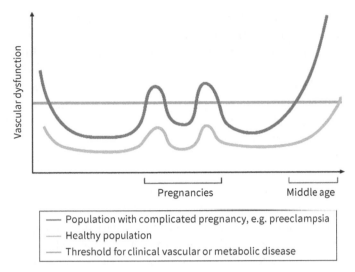

Figure 21.2 Model of pregnancy as a metabolic 'stress test' (adapted from Sattar and Greer[11]). See plate section.

specialist services, whereby core community services for the majority of women link seamlessly into more specialist care for the smaller proportion who need it.

Integrated, woman-centred, holistic care has become something of a mantra in health care policy, but it is often hard to achieve in practice. We will, therefore, consider more specifically the changes that are implied by a life course approach to women's health care. These can relate

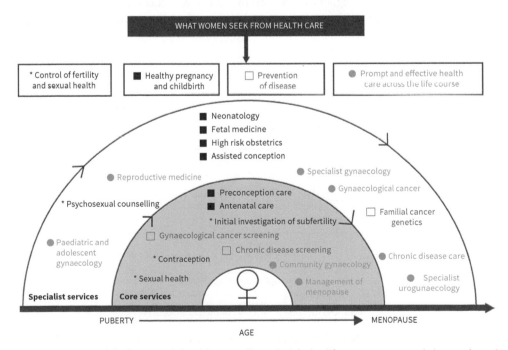

Figure 21.3 A model of women's health care aligned with the life course approach (reproduced with permission from Stephenson et al.[1]).

to the health of the woman herself or, for women who become pregnant, the health of their child or to the health of both generations. HPV vaccination for prevention of cervical cancer provides a clear example of effective early intervention to reduce disease in adulthood and is currently delivered through national vaccination programs in over 100 countries. Screening young women for *Chlamydia trachomatis* to prevent ectopic pregnancy and tubal infertility is included in national prevention strategies in a few HICs, including the UK and Australia (although the extent of implementation differs), but there is little evidence of effectiveness in reducing these adverse health outcomes.

Other aspects of women's health care that focus on maternal and child health—including preconception, antenatal, and postnatal care—impact the health of two or more generations and thus relate more directly to the life course approach expressed by the concept of the Developmental Origins of Health and Disease (DOHaD). Evidence for this concept, accumulated over more than 4 decades, has shown that maternal physiology and nutrition in pregnancy have profound effects on the long-term health of adult offspring. In other words, experience in utero is linked to the risk of cardiovascular disease, obesity, diabetes, respiratory disease, and other diseases of childhood and adulthood. Pregnancy, therefore, becomes an obvious window of opportunity to intervene in accordance with knowledge of DOHaD and life course epidemiology to improve health outcomes for both mother and child. It is also a convenient opportunity for intervention, providing a captive audience for health education and care with pregnant women attending numerous antenatal visits. An example of a life course approach to antenatal care is conceptualised in Figure 21.4. It implies that targeted treatment and lifestyle at critical stages can reverse increasing risk of chronic disease in later life. In support of this hypothesis, a recent meta-analysis of lifestyle interventions in women with gestational diabetes found that intervention implemented within 3 years of delivery (but not during pregnancy) resulted in a marked reduction in the long-term risk of type 2 diabetes.[12] Other systematic reviews have also found that interventions aiming to

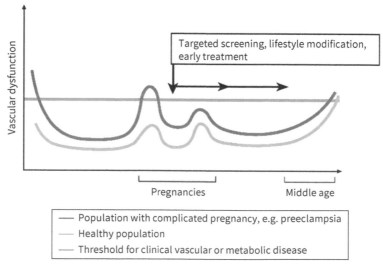

Figure 21.4 Conceptual model of intervention during critical periods in the reproductive life course to reduce disease risk and improve health in adulthood (adapted from Sattar and Greer[11]). See plate section.

reduce gestational diabetes, gestational weight gain, pre-eclampsia, and preterm birth, which started in pregnancy, had little or no impact on pregnancy outcomes.[13]

Owing in part to the disappointing results of lifestyle interventions starting in pregnancy,[13] recent attention has turned to the preconception and postnatal or interconception periods (see Figure 21.1). Indeed, postnatal care has been dubbed the fourth trimester[14] in an attempt to improve care and avoid the usual discontinuity of care associated with transfer from maternity services to primary care. In practical terms, this would mean, for example, ensuring that women who have had gestational diabetes are followed up and supported to reduce their risk of developing type 2 diabetes or their risk of developing gestational diabetes again in a subsequent pregnancy. Evidence-based guidance in the UK recommends annual review of all women who have had gestational diabetes,[10] but this seldom happens in practice,[15] although there are signs of improvement in the proportion of women with gestational diabetes being followed up at 12 weeks after delivery (using a one-off blood test, HbA1c, rather than the less convenient oral glucose tolerance test). Acceptance of the meta-analysis finding that postpartum lifestyle intervention can be highly effective[12] should renew efforts to reduce the number of women with gestational diabetes going on to develop type 2 diabetes.

Broadly speaking, women's reproductive health care is geared towards prevention of pregnancy, through contraception services, or towards antenatal care for women who have become pregnant, while opportunities to reduce risk factors and improve health during the preconception and interconception periods are often missed. For example, a woman seeking removal of a contraceptive device at a sexual health clinic in order to become pregnant may receive little or no advice about taking folic acid, nor support to stop smoking, improve nutrition, or achieve a healthier weight in preparation for a healthy pregnancy. A life course approach implies closing such gaps with a more integrated model of care, such as that shown in Figure 21.5.[16]

In other settings (e.g. general practice) where an intention to become pregnant may not be disclosed, a shift in mindset is required for health care providers to ask women of reproductive age whether they are considering (another) pregnancy.[17] Reorganisation of existing healthcare services is not required, but training of health care practitioners (e.g. nurses, health visitors, and midwives) so that they feel equipped to support women towards having a healthy pregnancy will be important. Experience with the UK NHS Make Every Contact Count program[18,19] shows that this approach is feasible although scaling-up training rapidly would be a challenge.

A life course approach must also include system-wide or public health interventions that recognise the crucial role of the wider determinants of health. These determinants include a diverse range of social, economic, and environmental factors affecting physical and mental health, and their relationship with individual-level factors. A growing appreciation of the interconnectedness of individuals and systems is reflected in recent 'systems approaches' to tackle obesity,[20] and to some extent reproductive health.[21] A systems approach conceptualises poor health and health inequalities as outcomes of many interdependent elements within a connected whole. So, for example, the changing distribution of obesity across a population can be conceptualised as arising out of the interplay of food, transport, employment, economic, and other systems that influence the pattern of energy intake and expenditure of individuals and families. In fact, this kind of thinking 'out of the usual healthcare box' lies at the core of a life course approach to health and is set to develop further over the coming years.[22] Addressing the wider determinants is essential to avoid the problems of individually targeted

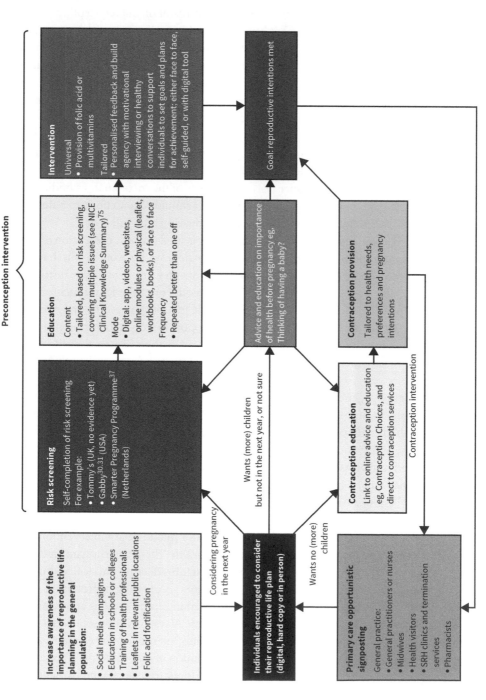

Figure 21.5 Model of integrated care for pregnancy prevention and preparation across the reproductive life course (adapted from Hall et al.[16]).

interventions which include limited impact, widening health inequalities, and engendering feelings of guilt and over-responsibility for health outcomes among individual women.

21.4 Is There Evidence for the Impact of a Life Course Approach to Women's Health Care?

To explore this question, we looked at data on uptake of some key healthcare interventions outlined in Figure 21.1 and compared findings between two high-incomes countries, the UK and Australia. Table 21.1 shows a pattern of near-universal uptake for newborn screening and high uptake levels for childhood intervention, which relate to parental responsibility, but declining rates of participation at older ages when individual (rather than parental) decisions are made about interventions, such as assisted conception or breast cancer screening. Across the life course, uptake of services is related to socioeconomic and cultural factors and influenced by publicity and social media. Adverse publicity about the MMR vaccine led to a substantial fall in uptake, while the death from cervical cancer of a young woman in a popular reality TV show led to a sharp upturn in cervical screening rates in the UK.

Not surprisingly, established public health programs with centrally organised implementation, like vaccination programs, show the highest participation levels. The impact of this is demonstrated in the massive reduction of cases and deaths from childhood illnesses such as whooping cough since the implementation of national vaccination programs.[23] By contrast, uptake of folic acid supplements before conception, which requires awareness and planning for pregnancy, occurred in less than a third of pregnancies, and in only 15% of pregnancies in younger women where social deprivation is greater.[13] The effectiveness of folic acid in preventing neural tube defects is well known; other less well-known benefits include a reduction in fetal growth restriction, increase in birthweight,[24] and a lower risk of severe language delays in childhood.[25] An alternative prevention approach through fortification of food with folic acid has been implemented in 82 countries with impressive effect: a rapid population-wide decline in neural tube defects of around 50%, an achievement that promotion of individual folic acid supplementation cannot expect to match. Flour is the most common food to be fortified: in Australia, for example, all wheat flour used for bread-making must contain folic acid (with the exception of organic flour). However, there is much still to do: the UK, for example, has only recently taken this step, and the lack of fortification worldwide is estimated to be responsible for 5 million pregnancies with preventable neural tube defects since 1991.[26]

Prevention efforts centred on a single cause-and-effect intervention model (e.g. vaccination programs and folic acid fortification) are more likely than prevention initiatives aiming to improve numerous health outcomes by addressing multiple risk factors, such as preconception health care, to achieve rapid, measurable success. This should not discourage such initiatives, but rather point to the importance of adopting a systems-wide approach that conceptualises poor health and health inequalities as outcomes of many interdependent elements within a connected whole.[20] As such, a complex systems approach needs to engage governments, civil society, and practitioners in creating effective movements for change. The rapid rise in obesity among children and adults has triggered this kind of response in many countries. For example, the WHO[27] Commission on Ending Childhood Obesity has six recommendations, framed around critical periods in the life course, including diet and physical activity in childhood, and preconception and pregnancy care, to address the obesogenic

Table 21.1 Uptake of health care interventions relating to population health care needs depicted in Figure 21.1.

Health Care Factor	United Kingdom	Australia
Newborn blood spot screening	Screen for 9 conditions; 97%–99% of babies screened	Screen for 25 conditions; ~99% of babies screened
Childhood vaccination	Vaccination coverage for England at age: 1 year 93% 2 years 91% 5 years 91%	Vaccination coverage at age: 1 year 95% 2 years 92% 5 years 95%
Sexual health education	All secondary schools in the UK required to teach relationships and sex education	National curriculum in place, but each State and Territory implements curriculum to differing extents
Human papillomavirus (HPV) vaccination	84% of year 9 girls completed full of course of vaccine (2 doses)	80% of girls aged 15 years completed full course of vaccine (3 doses)
Contraception	84% of women aged 15–49 used contraception in 2018	43% of women aged 18–39 years reported using hormonal contraceptive
Cervical screening	72% of eligible women screened in England in 2019–20	Over the 2-year period 2016–17, the age-standardised participation rate was 56.0%
Preconception care	28% of women in antenatal care took folic acid supplements before becoming pregnant, and 55% of smokers quit before becoming pregnant, in England in 2017	32% of women took folic acid supplements before becoming pregnant In 2018, 9.2% of pregnant women in Australia smoked during the first 20 weeks of pregnancy
Antenatal care	In 2019–20, 63% who had recorded deliveries in the Hospital Episodes Statistics had their first antenatal visit between 8 and 11 weeks pregnancy	In 2018, 61% of women who gave birth had their first antenatal visit in the first 10 weeks (74% in first trimester); 99.8% of mothers had at least 1 antenatal visit; 94% had 5 or more visits; and 57% had 10 or more visits
Assisted conception	In 2018: 68,724 IVF cycles and 5,651 donor insemination cycles; the average birth rate per embryo transferred to all IVF patients was 23%	In 2017: 74,942 ART treatment cycles, ≈ 14.8 cycles per 1000 women of reproductive age (15–44 years); of all initiated ART treatments in 2017, 22% resulted in a clinical pregnancy, and 18% in a live delivery
Breast cancer screening	2018–19 England: 71% participation rate (women aged 50–70 years); 75% of eligible women (aged 53–70 years) up to date with screening	2017–18: participation rate of 55% (women aged 50–74 years)

environment. The UK[28] response includes a soft drinks levy, a sugar reduction program to remove sugar from the products that children eat most, making school food healthier, better labelling and information about food content, and increasing physical activity in schools. In Australia, the food industry exerts strong influence with the country only adopting a National Obesity Strategy in 2022. National initiatives include a voluntary health star rating system for packaged food and a voluntary program encouraging food companies to reduce fat, sodium, and sugar content of selected foods; all states and territories have policies for healthy eating in schools and most have policies on minimum weekly time spent doing physical activity in schools. However, although many of the causes of obesity are preventable and reversible, no country has yet succeeded in reversing the growth of this epidemic; evidence of impact is, therefore, eagerly awaited.

21.5 Impact of COVID-19

As the UN stated in April 2020, 'the impacts of COVID-19 are exacerbated for women and girls simply by virtue of their sex'.[29] While men are more likely to die of COVID-19, women are at greater risk of infection as they dominate the health and social care workforce, as well as having informal caring responsibilities, which puts them at increased risk of ongoing morbidity from nonacute COVID-19.[30,31] During various 'lockdowns', rates of gender-based violence against women rose[32] (see Chapter 20), and women faced an increased burden of unpaid work as schools were closed and older relatives became isolated, with clear implications for women's mental and physical health.[33] Women in the workforce more often have part-time and short-term or 'zero hours' contracts, are also vulnerable to job losses, and are already more likely to have been earning less and, therefore, have lower savings to fall back on.

Where health care resources are redirected to fight the pandemic, women's sexual and reproductive health care is often a target for resource reallocation. This makes it harder for women to access vital services, such as contraception, termination care, and routine cancer screening. Data from the UK showed that women were 10 times more likely to say that they had difficulty accessing contraception during or after the first national lockdown (from late March 2020), and there was a corresponding increase in the proportion of unplanned pregnancies.[34] Similarly in the United States and Australia,[35] women were more likely to express a desire to avoid pregnancy and to report difficulties accessing contraception.[36]

Against this backdrop of COVID-related difficulty and deprivation, one positive development stands out: analysis of national UK data on over 52,000 early medical abortions before and after the pandemic showed that having abortions at home was safe, effective, and more accessible to women.[37] A change in the law to allow women to access early medical abortions at home was approved in March 2020. Before this time, anyone seeking an abortion had to attend an in-person appointment for an ultrasound scan and take medication to bring about an abortion within the clinic. Under the new guidelines, consultations could take place by phone or video call, and medication could be taken at home, with ultrasound scanning only if needed. As a result of this change, waiting times were reduced from 10.7 to 6.5 days; the duration of pregnancy at the time of abortion was significantly reduced; treatment success (99%) and adverse events were unaffected; and 80% of women reported a preference for this approach in future.

21.6 Conclusions

A life course approach to women's health care is now an established concept, promulgated by a growing number of national and international health policy documents. The COVID-19 pandemic has exacerbated preexisting entrenched health inequalities faced by women in particular and placed them under more intense scrutiny. The integrated, woman-centred, holistic system of care implied by a life course approach to women's health care remains largely aspirational, but important evidence that we need about when and how to intervene to alter unhealthy trajectories, such as the development of gestational diabetes into type 2 diabetes, is now within our sights.

Key messages and implications

- The health care needs of women are distinguished from those of men by more predictable sexual and reproductive events across the life course.
- A life course approach to women's health calls for services to become more aligned around women's predictable healthcare needs with less discontinuity across health care sectors.
- Addressing individual risk factors in health care will not be enough to achieve population-wide impact; public health and system-wide changes that address the wider determinants of health are crucial.
- Raising awareness of a life course approach and the implications for health care requires training and resources. This can enable and equip a wide range of health care practitioners to support women in achieving better health outcomes.

References

1. Stephenson J, Shawe J, Kuh D. *Why should we consider a life course approach to women's health care?* London: Royal College of Obstetricians and Gynaecologists; 1 August 2011. Scientific Advisory Committee opinion paper 27.
2. Royal College of Obstetricians and Gynaecologists. *Better for women. Improving the health and wellbeing of girls and women.* London: RCOG; December 2019.
3. Wang Y, Hunt K, Nazareth I, Freemantle N, Petersen I. Do men consult less than women? An analysis of routinely collected UK general practice data. *BMJ Open.* 2013;3(8):e003320.
4. Rissel C, Heywood W, de Visser RO, Simpson JM, Grulich AE, Badcock PB, et al. First vaginal intercourse and oral sex among a representative sample of Australian adults: the Second Australian Study of Health and Relationships. *Sex Health.* 2014;11(5):406–15.
5. Office for National Statistics. *Childbearing for women born in different years, England and Wales: 2019.* London: UK ONS; 4 December 2020.
6. Office for National Statistics. *Living longer: implications of childlessness among tomorrow's older population.* London: UK ONS; 17 August 2020.
7. Song C, Lyu Y, Li C, Liu P, Li J, Ma RC, et al. Long-term risk of diabetes in women at varying durations after gestational diabetes: a systematic review and meta-analysis with more than 2 million women. *Obesity Reviews.* 2018;19(3):421–9.

8. Daly B, Toulis KA, Thomas N, Gokhale K, Martin J, Webber J, et al. Increased risk of ischemic heart disease, hypertension, and type 2 diabetes in women with previous gestational diabetes mellitus, a target group in general practice for preventive interventions: a population-based cohort study. *PLoS Medicine*. 2018;15(1):e1002488.

9. Australian Institute of Health and Welfare. *Incidence of gestational diabetes in Australia*. Canberra: Australian Institute of Health and Welfare; 2019. Cat. no. CVD 85.

10. National Institute for Health and Care Excellence. *Diabetes in pregnancy: management from pre-conception to the post-natal period [Internet]*. London: National Institute for Health and Care Excellence; 2015 [updated 16 December 2020; cited 15 June 2021]. Available from: https://www.nice.org.uk/guidance/ng3/chapter/Recommendations#postnatal-care.

11. Sattar N, Greer IA. Pregnancy complications and maternal cardiovascular risk: opportunities for intervention and screening? *British Medical Journal*. 2002;325(7356):157–60.

12. Li N, Yang Y, Cui D, Li C, Ma RCW, Li J, et al. Effects of lifestyle intervention on long-term risk of diabetes in women with prior gestational diabetes: a systematic review and meta-analysis of randomized controlled trials. *Obesity Reviews*. 2021;22(1):e13122.

13. Stephenson J, Heslehurst N, Hall J, Schoenaker DA, Hutchinson J, Cade JE, et al. Before the beginning: nutrition and lifestyle in the preconception period and its importance for future health. *The Lancet*. 2018;391(10132):1830–41.

14. ACOG Committee Opinion No. 736. Optimizing postnatal care. ACOG Committee Opinion No 736. *Obstetrics & Gynecology* 2018;131:e140–50.

15. McGovern A, Butler L, Jones S, van Vlymen J, Sadek K, Munro N, et al. Diabetes screening after gestational diabetes in England: a quantitative retrospective cohort study. *British Journal of General Practice*. 2014;64(618):e17.

16. Hall J, Chawla M, Watson D, Jacob CM, Schoenaker D, Connolly A, et al. Addressing reproductive health needs across the life course: An integrated, community-based model combining contraception and preconception care. *The Lancet Public Health*. 2023;8(1):E76–E84. https://doi.org/10.1016/S2468-2667(22)00254-7

17. Stephenson J, Schoenaker DA, Hinton W, Poston L, Barker M, Alwan NA, et al. A wake-up call for preconception health: a clinical review. *British Journal of General Practice*. 2021;71(706):233–6.

18. Nelson A, de Normanville C, Payne K, Kelly MP. Making every contact count: an evaluation. *Public Health*. 2013;127(7):653–60.

19. Lawrence W, Black C, Tinati T, Cradock S, Begum R, Jarman M, et al. 'Making every contact count': evaluation of the impact of an intervention to train health and social care practitioners in skills to support health behaviour change. *Journal of Health Psychology*. 2016;21(2):138–51.

20. Rutter H, Savona N, Glonti K, Bibby J, Cummins S, Finegood DT, et al. The need for a complex systems model of evidence for public health. *The Lancet*. 2017;390(10112):2602–4.

21. Public Health England. *A consensus statement. Reproductive health is public health*. London: Public Health England; June 2018.

22. Academy of Medical Sciences. *Improving the health of the public by 2040*. London: Academy of Medical Sciences; July 2016.

23. Rodrigues CMC, Plotkin SA. Impact of vaccines; health, economic and social perspectives. *Frontiers in Microbiology*. 2020;11:1526.

24. Fekete K, Berti C, Trovato M, Lohner S, Dullemeijer C, Souverein OW, et al. Effect of folate intake on health outcomes in pregnancy: a systematic review and meta-analysis on birth weight, placental weight and length of gestation. *Nutrition Journal*. 2012;11:75.

25. Roth C, Magnus P, Schjølberg S, Stoltenberg C, Surén P, McKeague IW, et al. Folic acid supplements in pregnancy and severe language delay in children. *Journal of the American Medical Association*. 2011;306(14):1566–73.

26. Wald NJ, Morris JK, Blakemore C. Public health failure in the prevention of neural tube defects: time to abandon the tolerable upper intake level of folate. *Public Health Reviews*. 2018;39:2.

27. World Health Organization. *Report of the Commission on Ending Childhood Obesity*. Geneva: WHO; 21 January 2016.

28. UK Government Prime Minister's Office. *Childhood obesity: a plan for action [press release].* London: UK Government Prime Minister's Office; 20 January 2017. Commonwealth of Australia 2022. The National Obesity Strategy 2022–2032. Health Ministers Meeting.

29. United Nations. *Policy brief: the impact of COVID-19 on women.* New York: UN; 9 April 2020.

30. Sudre CH, Murray B, Varsavsky T, Graham MS, Penfold RS, Bowyer RC, et al. Attributes and predictors of long COVID. *Nature Medicine.* 2021;27(4):626–31.

31. UN Women. *Whose time to care? Unpaid care and domestic work during COVID-19.* New York: UN Women; 25 November 2020.

32. Mittal S, Singh T. Gender-based violence during COVID-19 pandemic: a mini-review. *Frontiers in Global Women's Health.* 2020;1:4.

33. Hammarberg K, Tran T, Kirkman M, Fisher J. Sex and age differences in clinically significant symptoms of depression and anxiety among people in Australia in the first month of COVID-19 restrictions: a national survey. *BMJ Open.* 2020;10(11):e042696.

34. Balachandren N, Barrett G, Stephenson J, Yasmin E, Mavrelos D, Davies M, et al. Impact of the SARS-CoV-2 pandemic on access to contraception and pregnancy intentions: a national prospective cohort study of the UK population. *BMJ Sexual & Reproductive Health.* 2022;48(1):60–5.

35. Coombe J, Kong F, Bittleston H, Williams H, Tomnay J, Vaisey A, et al. Contraceptive use and pregnancy plans among women of reproductive age during the first Australian COVID-19 lockdown: findings from an online survey. *European Journal of Contraception and Reproductive Health Care.* 2021;26(4):265–71.

36. Lin TK, Law R, Beaman J, Foster DG. The impact of the COVID-19 pandemic on economic security and pregnancy intentions among people at risk of pregnancy. *Contraception.* 2021;103(6):380–5.

37. Aiken A, Lohr PA, Lord J, Ghosh N, Starling J. Effectiveness, safety and acceptability of no-test medical abortion (termination of pregnancy) provided via telemedicine: a national cohort study. *British Journal of Obstetrics and Gynaecology: An International Journal of Obstetrics and Gynaecology.* 2021;128(9):1464–74.

22

Translating Women's Health Research into Policy and Practice

Helen Brown, Stephanie Best, and Trina Hinkley

'To him who devoted his life to science, nothing can give more happiness than increasing the number of discoveries, but his cup of joy is full when the results of his studies immediately find practical applications.' Louis Pasteur (quoted in René J. Dubos, Louis Pasteur, Free Lance of Science (1960))[1]

22.1 Introduction

Previous chapters highlight the unprecedented growth in the breadth and volume of scientific evidence available and research currently being conducted in women's health. This evidence aims to inform and improve women's health across the life course. Traditionally, the process whereby such scientific evidence has been made available to and accessible by knowledge users has been haphazard and passive, at best, and typical routes have included publications in academic journals or presentations at scientific conferences, where audiences are generally other academics.[2,3] Occasionally, new evidence has been able to trickle down to knowledge users, but it is generally unlikely to reach a level that elicits sufficient change for women to benefit.

Another challenge has been the time it takes to translate evidence into practice, with data showing a 15-to-17-year lag for research evidence to reach practice.[4,5] This evidence is alarming considering the growing evidence in a life course approach to women's health that links early life to adult health outcomes. If we do not reduce this evidence-to-practice gap, we will be missing valuable time to intervene across the lifespan and prevent poor health outcomes.

It is apparent that strong evidence alone is insufficient to change practice, behaviour, or outcomes. It is, therefore, critical to ensure robust processes exist to enable evidence to be adopted and implemented in a timely manner, resulting in increased preventive health policies, leading to fewer adverse events, lower health system costs, and favourable health and well-being outcomes for women.

Multiple barriers exist between knowledge creation, integration into the real lives of women (including prevention efforts), and favourable change.[2,6] These barriers may include:

Helen Brown, Stephanie Best, and Trina Hinkley, *Translating Women's Health Research into Policy and Practice* In: *A Life Course Approach to Women's Health*. Second Edition. Edited by: Gita D Mishra, Rebecca Hardy, and Diana Kuh, Oxford University Press.

- time resources
- competing priorities
- limited capacity for searching, appraising, and applying research evidence
- resistance to change
- unsupportive organisational culture and leadership
- the political context of decision-making.

Life course researchers need to be mindful of these barriers when considering strategies to translate knowledge into practice. The evidence-to-practice, or knowledge-to-action, gap creates an opportunity for the science of Knowledge Translation (KT) to optimise our return on investment in scientific research and ensure best quality care and outcomes for all.

22.2 What Is Knowledge Translation?

There is often misunderstanding surrounding the concepts relating to 'putting evidence into practice'. Many terms are used to describe the knowledge-to-action process, including *knowledge utilisation, diffusion, knowledge transfer, research utilisation,* and *dissemination.*[2,7] However, as a process, KT involves broader constructs than any of these individual terms can support.

Knowledge Translation is defined by the Canadian Institutes of Health Research of Knowledge Translation, an early institutional leader in the field, as 'a dynamic and iterative process that includes the synthesis, dissemination, exchange, and ethically sound application of knowledge to improve health, provide more effective health services and products, and strengthen the healthcare system'.[2,8,9] This definition, adopted by the World Health Organization, outlines the move beyond dissemination to use of knowledge. Additionally, successful KT ensures 'all stakeholders are aware of and use research evidence to inform their health and healthcare decision-making'.[3] A broad range of stakeholders or 'knowledge users' are included in this definition, including policymakers, health professionals, consumers (men, women, and children), and researchers. Key to understanding the true nature of KT is that it is a process.

Major components in the definition of KT are the synthesis, exchange, and application of knowledge.[2,10] The KT process is about a collaborative exchange of information between knowledge creators and knowledge users such that knowledge users can help guide and shape the knowledge that is required and the form in which it is available. This process ensures decision-makers at all levels (e.g. health professionals, policymakers, and women) are aware of, can access, and use research evidence to inform their decision-making.

Past KT projects have typically relied on pushing knowledge to users and have been conducted at the end of a project (e.g. implementing a plan to disseminate knowledge after the knowledge has been created). However, the ideal scenario is to begin the KT process at the commencement of a project, which is often referred to as 'integrated KT'.[11,12] KT fosters a collaborative and participatory approach through engaging knowledge users at each stage of the project to ensure relevance, applicability, and usability in practice. Rather than pushing out information, this bidirectional approach ensures the process will more likely lead to optimal uptake, meet knowledge users' needs, and result in more positive outcomes.[12] Working with knowledge users allows knowledge creators to gain insight into how the key messages of the research can be best used in practice through gaining a better understanding of real-world problems and the contexts in which they occur. This collaborative community approach is particularly useful when working with populations that experience marginalisation, such as women and indigenous populations, as it supports the development of respectful relationships, particularly in sharing control over individual and group health and social conditions.[11,13]

22.3 Knowledge Translation Theories, Models, and Frameworks

Models and frameworks, underpinned by theory, are recommended as a way of considering the multiple, dynamic, and interactive factors that influence the uptake of evidence into practice.[14,15] Use of a KT framework makes the process of KT more systematic, with greater likelihood of uptake and sustainable change in practice.[2,14] A variety of theories, models, and frameworks (TMFs) are available to guide KT; the number available is growing rapidly. A 2020 scoping review by Esmail et al. found 36 KT TMFs for use to guide researchers, including the Ottawa Model of Research Use, the Knowledge-to-Action Process, the Coordinate Implementation Model, the Stetler Model of Research Utilisation, and Conner's conceptual model for research-utilisation evaluation.[14] Despite evidence that using TMFs may improve the likelihood of successful implementation and sustainability and decrease the evidence-to-practice gap, reviews of the field to date suggest that researchers are failing to utilise them appropriately or even at all.[14,16]

One of the most widely adopted and comprehensive frameworks is the Knowledge to Action (K2A) cycle based on planned-action theories, adopted by the World Health Organization and the Canadian Institutes of Health Research. This framework was developed by Graham and colleagues following a review of 31 planned-action theories.[2,5]

The K2A framework presents KT as an iterative and dynamic process, constructed to culminate in the continued application of learned information by knowledge users. It is presented as inner and outer processes (see Figure 22.1) both of which begin with identifying a problem. Ideally, this is done in collaboration with knowledge users or their representatives, such as community organisations that advocate a specific health issue for a particular group of women.

The inner process is focused on tailoring knowledge to address the needs of knowledge users. This process may be applied in isolation (e.g. as an end-of-project KT process) or as part of an integrated KT process. The three steps in this process are:

1. **Knowledge inquiry:** known as first-generation knowledge (knowledge in its raw form directly from evidence); this step explores what knowledge already exists to address the identified problem.
2. **Knowledge synthesis:** the process of creating second-generation knowledge; existing knowledge is synthesised so the most relevant information can be extracted and applied to address the identified problem.
3. **Knowledge tools/products:** this process produces third-generation knowledge, which is more applicable to and accessible by knowledge users.

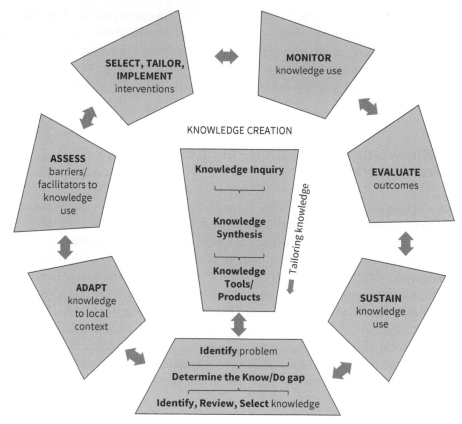

Figure 22.1 The Knowledge to Action Cycle (adapted from Straus, Tetroe, and Graham, 2013).[17]

The outer process is known as the action cycle and is focused on the application of knowledge. It includes seven steps, which are:

1. **Identifying the problem** to be addressed, reviewing, and selecting applicable knowledge.
2. **Adapting knowledge to the local context** to ensure that knowledge is fit for purpose. This step ensures that knowledge can be integrated into the contexts in which it needs to be applied and is accessible by knowledge users who will benefit most.
3. **Assessing barriers/facilitators to knowledge use** to ensure that the necessary supports are incorporated into the KT process to foster the greatest chance of change.
4. **Selecting, tailoring, and implementing interventions and strategies** that adequately address the identified problem.
5. **Monitoring knowledge use** allows knowledge creators to capture how, by whom, and in what contexts the created knowledge is accessed and applied. Information gleaned is essential to inform any project as it moves forward and future projects.
6. **Evaluating outcomes** to determine if change has occurred. While it is necessary to monitor knowledge use (step 5 above), use of knowledge alone does not guarantee change; thus, evaluation is required. Additionally, any knowledge created may have

unintended consequences which cannot be captured in merely monitoring use. For instance, created knowledge may be intended to address a particular problem identified by middle-aged women (intended consequence) but may also address similar problems for younger or older women (unintended consequence).

7. **Sustaining knowledge use** to ensure that any change is sustained.

The K2A framework is frequently used with varying degrees of completion.[18] Its use ranges from simple attribution via a reference, through informal planning, to making a full contribution to science. Inadequate time, funding, and personnel may limit the use of the full framework, support for knowledge creators is required to either use particular stages of the process or fully apply the entire KT process.[6,10] This will ensure the greatest chance of undertaking, translating, and applying robust evidence so that women benefit across all stages of the life course.

22.4 Knowledge Translation in Women's Health

By its very nature, KT as a process is flexible and adaptable and can suit the changing needs of women across the life course. It can be adjusted to meet the needs of adolescents, young, middle-aged, and older women equally well, as it is flexible to accommodate the unique needs, circumstances, and contexts of each group. In the life course approach to women's health, effective KT enables health services to connect with their audience at opportune times to improve outcomes in later life for women at all ages.

Few studies specifically targeting women's health have used an entire KT framework. This may reflect multiple barriers, including coordinating complex initiatives with diverse stakeholders, funding or time constraints, or lack of incentive to engage in longer, more expensive research.[6,10] It may also reflect the aim or purpose of the study. However, evidence of the effectiveness of using a KT framework to guide knowledge use, as well as increased scrutiny on the impact of research by funders, provides a comprehensive rationale for its use.

An important consideration in adopting and implementing new knowledge is the significance of key stages throughout women's lives where the interactive nature of biological and social processes influence disease risk. For example, the knowledge that adopting health-compromising behaviours during early adolescence can adversely affect overall adolescent development, and also track into adult years and even have significant impact on the health of future generations provides rich evidence to support effective KT use.

22.4.1 Applying the K2A Cycle to Menopause

The stage in a woman's life known as menopause will be used as a theoretical example to highlight the use of the K2A cycle. Ideally, these steps are undertaken collaboratively with a variety of stakeholders to provide solutions that meet the user's needs (see Table 22.1).

As can be seen from this example, the application of KT is critical to ensure tailored, accessible information reaches knowledge users (e.g. women) effectively and efficiently at an appropriate time across their life course to prevent health-compromising behaviours developing prior to the onset of the menopause. Ensuring the timely and effective delivery of knowledge around the menopause can also:

- increase women's awareness of the menopause and what may occur during this transition.
- assist in decision-making around factors, such as timing of hysterectomy, use of Menopausal Hormone Therapy, and symptom management.
- inform and support women who may experience early or late menopause.
- support practitioners to deliver messages to patients.

Two recent examples of studies where a comprehensive KT framework has been utilised in women's health to reduce the evidence-to-practice gap are provided here. A 2020 study by Yeganeh et al.[19] used an interdisciplinary co-design research translation model underpinned

Table 22.1 An example of processes involved in the K2A cycle applied to menopause.

Inner Process	Outer Process
Knowledge inquiry	Identifying the problem • Age at natural menopause has been linked to numerous chronic disease risks in later life. • A variety of biological and social factors across the life course can affect the timing of menopause and decisions around factors such as hysterectomy or symptom management. • Interventions or strategies are required to prevent chronic disease risk factors at an early age. • Risk factors for early menopause need to be identified early.
Knowledge synthesis	Adapting knowledge to local context • Work with key stakeholders (e.g. women, medical practitioners, and researchers) • Explore the local context in relation to knowledge use, needs, priorities, policies, and existing resources related to menopause.
Knowledge tools or products	Assessing barriers or facilitators to knowledge use • Work with key stakeholder to identify potential barriers and facilitators to knowledge use. • For example, do resources require translation into other languages? Do women use online resources? Selecting, tailoring, and implementing strategies • Consider all evidence and select, tailor, and implement strategies. These strategies may include online resources, podcasts, or webinars but must be selected according to evidence of use by the stakeholders. Monitoring knowledge use (critical!) • A system is developed to capture how, by whom, and in what contexts the created knowledge is accessed and used. This may be through surveys, interviews, or online statistical data collection but should include a measure of the use of the knowledge. Evaluate outcomes • Determine if change has occurred (e.g. behaviour change towards symptom management). • This phase may uncover unintended consequences to address in the next iteration (e.g. a problem encountered in accessing resources).

by the K2A framework to improve middle-aged women's health. The study highlighted the complex process required to address multiple barriers at the individual, organisational, and political level. Initial research identified early menopause or premature ovarian insufficiency knowledge gaps for both health practitioners and women. Those gaps resulted in delayed diagnosis, suboptimal care, variation in care, and poor outcomes. Using a five-phased KT model, an early menopause digital resource was co-developed, evaluated, and implemented with direct input from both women and health professionals to better inform and support them in timely diagnosis and management.[19]

The five stages included: i) needs analysis with stakeholders to frame the problem, identify priorities, and scope (mixed methods study); ii) evidence synthesis; iii) development of digital resources; iv) evaluation of outcomes; and v) dissemination and implementation. The use of a KT model enabled the research team to maximise the potential for uptake. The study has yet to be evaluated for the impact on women's health; however, it provides a model for successful co-design research translation to improve women's health.

Another study by Hazel et al.[20] used integrative and participatory KT processes to conceptualise their study which aimed to increase women's eye health services in rural Nepal. The research team acknowledged the multiple and interconnected determinants of health, as well as unique barriers to accessing information and services that rural Nepalese women face (e.g. cost, distance, and lack of gender-responsive care). They used a six-step KT process, including: forming an advisory group, collecting and interpreting evidence from formative research, redesign of a program intervention, and implementating/evaluating an action-oriented pragmatic trial. The study reported the importance of building on deep contextual knowledge using a participatory approach, a willingness to challenge stereotypes and 'dive deep into the underlying issues that affect access through a gender lens'.[20]

Other studies on women's health outcomes have used one or more components of a KT framework or model instead of an entire model. Most have focused on knowledge transfer activities or strategies (i.e. pushing out knowledge without engaging women to provide the information they want in a form that they want to receive it). These strategies have been adopted to reduce the 'evidence-to-practice gap'. However, as they are not part of an overall KT process, they do not optimise the potential learnings and related healthcare gains for women.

22.5 Approaching KT Across the Life Course

An important consideration in adopting and implementing new knowledge is the significance of key stages throughout women's lives where the interactive nature of biological and social processes influence disease risk. The life course approach featured in this book acknowledges the relevance of these key stages to provide evidence for a variety of women's health issues during the life course. For example, significant evidence exists relating to a number of adolescent behaviours and risk factors that can influence later health, including sexual health and pregnancy (e.g. condom use, teenage pregnancy especially in indigenous adolescents), mental health (e.g. self-harm, eating behaviours or disorders), and lifestyle behaviours (e.g. alcohol consumption, sun-safe behaviours). However, adolescent women tend to lack concern about how their current behaviours may influence future health risks.[21] Instead, they are often more occupied with current interests, focused on appearance and social interaction and connection. The use of KT, therefore, provides an opportune time to work with adolescent women and co-create strategies tailored to them, providing key messages to prepare and/or intervene in this population in readiness for later health. In comparison, older women are faced with health issues such as cognitive decline (particularly memory and attention), physical function decline (e.g. increased falls, instability), and noncommunicable disease (e.g. stroke, osteoarthritis, and osteoporosis). Older women tend to focus on trying to stay well, though they can find behaviour change challenging.[22] Therefore, there is a need to consider relatable KT strategies that intersect with, or influence, key factors at play in women's different life stages to ensure the greatest chance of successful translation and favourable outcomes.

KT strategies have purposefully aimed to provide preventive messages, such as information about osteoporosis prevention, to specific groups such as young adult women or middle-aged women. In the past, osteoporosis prevention education was heavily tailored to those at-risk, particularly to older women.[23] However, evidence that many osteoporotic bone fractures that occur in older postmenopausal women can be prevented has led to a shift in targeting young adults as they are still at a life stage where they are building bone, and their food choices have the potential to affect their peak bone mass and their future food behaviours.[24] A study by Holland et al.[25] sought to explore how this knowledge can best be translated to younger women for prevention reasons. To gain an understanding of young adult women's needs, interviews with young adults were conducted. The results identified that prevention programs for this age group should make use of traditional sources of knowledge, such as peers, family members, and medical professionals, where the choice of source related to the perceived trust and authority, as well as emerging technologies such as social media. The study also found that messaging should relate directly to the interests of the young adults (e.g. food and fitness) and link to where they are currently seeking information from, rather than delivered as specific osteoporosis information. Messaging needed to be relatable, short, and encourage small behavioural changes.[25]

A study of First Nations women in Alberta, Canada, using a community-based participatory research approach, explored how cultural differences can shape the menopause experience.[26] Researchers worked collaboratively with women to explore, through workshops, their perceptions and experiences of menopause and the impact of menopause on their quality of life. This participatory approach recognised the importance of understanding the context through the eyes of the women themselves, reporting that most women felt they had insufficient information about what to expect prior to the menopause transition before their own transition as it was 'not talked about' by family members or their doctors. They also believed that there was a need to educate spouses, their children, and family members about menopause symptoms so that they were prepared for the impact of the menopause transition. These findings informed the co-development of separate pamphlets for men and women, containing different key messages.[26] Although evaluation of this strategy was not reported in this paper, the results supported the need for tailored KT approaches implemented at a stage in women's lives where knowledge prior to the onset of the menopause transition was useful in preparation for both the families and the women.

Thus, engaging with women at specific life stages is recognised and employed as an appropriate and useful KT strategy to ensure that knowledge creators are able to appropriately reach and influence knowledge users to raise awareness and potentially improve their health-related outcomes. Greater use of the other strategies, namely identifying barriers and facilitators, and selecting appropriate mechanisms and evaluation, may further support effective KT for women.

The majority of existing KT studies report on strategies trialled without appropriate consideration of the mechanisms required to change behaviour. Identifying mechanisms for change and behaviour change techniques used will increase the likelihood of effectiveness. A poorly planned KT program might succeed by chance; however, the success may lead to incorrect conclusions about the effectiveness of the program. Consideration of the life course is integral to this process, as different mechanisms of change and/or behaviour change techniques will be appropriate at different life stages because of differing biological and social influences. If preventive messages or strategies based on appropriate behavioural change techniques can be developed and implemented prior to the onset of chronic disease in women, the likelihood of success will be increased. Linking identified barriers and facilitators for behaviour change to specific KT mechanisms is key to facilitating knowledge use. KT strategies will typically include multiple components to ensure relevant barriers and facilitators are addressed.

An example of a KT study that linked mechanisms for change to behaviour change techniques focused on urinary incontinence in older women. While several behavioural techniques available for use by older women to manage urinary incontinence have been identified, most older women remain untreated, highlighting the need to improve health services for these women. A study by Holroyd-Leduc et al.[27] identified that older women with urinary incontinence often do not seek help from others, preferring to self-manage, but they have low self-efficacy towards managing this condition. Given this, a risk factor modification tool for older women was co-designed as an initial step to manage incontinence, clearly linking the behaviour to change (self-management) to the behaviour change technique (self-management tool). The study evaluation has shown that the tool decreased the number of daily urinary leakage episodes by 50% and improved both self-efficacy and the women's quality of life.[27]

22.6 Conclusions

The aim of this chapter was to highlight the importance of using a robust KT approach in scientific research to enable evidence to be adopted and implemented into practice in a timely manner, to improve care, reduce adverse events, and increase favourable outcomes for women. To optimise the translation of robust evidence into practice for the benefit of women, it is critical to consider the differing biological and social processes at key stages throughout women's lives. The collaborative, participatory nature of KT allows us to gain an understanding of the unique circumstances and contexts of women at these key stages of life, enabling appropriate mechanisms of change to be implemented. Many KT frameworks exist, most commonly with three key stages or processes: understanding the need, selecting and trialling appropriate mechanisms for change, and evaluating effectiveness. Methodological rigour must be balanced with timely, practical, and doable approaches in the real world; however, all knowledge creation projects, however small, should consider their KT plan at the outset of any study to engage women to ensure their needs are understood and met.

Key messages and implications

- A life course approach to women's health highlights phases during a woman's lifetime that can influence health outcomes later in life. Therefore, adopting KT principles becomes critical to ensure key messages are delivered to targeted audiences efficiently and effectively at the most relevant time in women's lives.
- The KT process can be complex, take time and require careful planning. It should be underpinned by strong theoretical models or frameworks to maximise impact.
- KT involves engaging with knowledge users and stakeholders in an appropriate and meaningful way from the beginning of the research process (wherever possible).
- The flexibility of KT is ideally suited to the life course approach to women's health, which addresses the differing needs of women at the various stages of their lives.

References

1. Dubos R. *Louis Pasteur: free lance of science*. New York: Da Capo Press; 1960.
2. Graham ID, Logan J, Harrison MB, Straus SE, Tetroe J, Caswell W, et al. Lost in Knowledge Translation: time for a map? *Journal of ContinuingEducation in the Health Professions* 2006;26(1):13–24.
3. Grimshaw JM, Eccles MP, Lavis JN, Hill SJ, Squires JE. Knowledge Translation of research findings. *Journal of Implementation Science*. 2012;7:Article number: 50.
4. Straus SE, Tetroe JM, Graham ID. Knowledge Translation is the use of knowledge in health care decision making. *Journal of Clinical Epidemiology*. 2011;64(1):6–10.
5. Straus SE, Tetroe J, Graham I. Defining Knowledge Translation. *Canadian Medical Association Journal*. 2009;181(3–4):165–8.
6. Azimi A, Fattahi R, Asadi-Lari M. Knowledge Translation status and barriers. *Journal of Medical Library Association*. 2015;103(2):96–9.
7. McKibbon KA, Lokker C, Wilczynski NL, Ciliska D, Dobbins M, Davis DA, et al. A cross-sectional study of the number and frequency of terms used to refer to Knowledge Translation in a body of health literature in 2006: a Tower of Babel? *Journal Implementation Science*. 2010;5:16.
8. McLean RKD, Graham ID, Bosompra K, Choudhry Y, Coen SE, MacLeod M, et al. Understanding the performance and impact of public Knowledge Translation funding interventions: protocol for an evaluation of Canadian Institutes of Health Research Knowledge Translation funding programs. *Journal of Implementation Science*. 2012;7:Article number: 57.
9. Lavis J, D. R, Woodside JM, McLeod CB, Abelson J, Transfer Study Group K. Understanding the performance and impact of public Knowledge Translation funding interventions? *Milbank Quarterly*. 2003;81(2):221–72.
10. Field B, Booth A, Ilott I, Gerrish K. Using the Knowledge to Action framework in practice: a citation analysis and systematic review. *Journal of Implementation Science*. 2014;9:Article number: 172.
11. Nguyen T, Graham ID, Mrklas KJ, Bowen S, Cargo M, Estabrooks CA, et al. How does integrated Knowledge Translation (IKT) compare to other collaborative research approaches to generating and translating knowledge? Learning from experts in the field. *Journal of Health Research and Policy Systems*. 2020;18:Article number: 35.
12. Wathen CN, MacMillan HL. The role of integrated Knowledge Translation in intervention research. *Journal of Prevention Science*. 2018;19(3):319–27.
13. Esmail R, Hanson HM, Holroyd-Leduc J, Brown S, Strifler L, Straus SE, et al. A scoping review of full-spectrum Knowledge Translation theories, models, and frameworks. *Journal of Implementation Science*. 2020;15:Article number: 11.

14. Davies P, Walker AE, Grimshaw JM. A systematic review of the use of theory in the design of guideline dissemination and implementation strategies and interpretation of the results of rigorous evaluations. *Journal of Implementation Science*. 2010;5:Article number: 14.

15. LaRocca R, Yost J, Dobbins M, Ciliska D, Butt M. The effectiveness of Knowledge Translation strategies used in public health: a systematic review. *BMC Public Health*. 2012;12:Article number: 751.

16. Nilsen P. Making sense of implementation theories, models and frameworks. *Journal of Implementation Science*. 2015;10:Article number: 53.

17. Straus SE, Tetroe J, Graham ID. *Knowledge Translation in health care: moving from evidence to practice*. Chichester, West Sussex: John Wiley & Sons; 2013.

18. Strifler L, Cardoso R, McGowan J, Cogo E, Nincic V, Khan PA, et al. Scoping review identifies significant number of Knowledge Translation theories, models, and frameworks with limited use. *Journal of Clinical Epidemiology*. 2018;100:92–102.

19. Yeganeh L, Johnston-Ataata K, Vincent AJ, Flore J, Kokanovic R, Teede H, et al. Co-designing an early menopause digital resource: model for interdisciplinary Knowledge Translation. *Journal of Seminal Reprodroductive Medicine*. 2020;38(04/05):315–22.

20. Hazel YP, Malla C, Afford A, Hillgrove T, Gurung R, Dahal A, et al. Continuous Knowledge Translation in action: designing a programmatic research trial for equitable eye health for rural Nepalese women. *International Journal of Environmental Research and Public Health*. 2020;17(1):345.

21. Reynen E, Grabell J, Ellis AK, James P. Let's talk period! Preliminary results of an online bleeding awareness Knowledge Translation project and bleeding assessment tool promoted on social media. *Journal of Haemophilia*. 2017;23(4):E282–E286.

22. Carmel S. Health and well-being in late life: gender differences worldwide. *Journal of Frontiers in Medicine-Lausanne*. 2019;6:218.

23. Holland A, Moffat T. Gendered perceptions of osteoporosis: implications for youth prevention programs. *Journal of Global Health Promotion*. 2020;27(2):91–9.

24. Miller PD. Underdiagnoses and undertreatment of osteoporosis: the battle to be won. *Journal of Clinical Endocrinology and Metabolism*. 2016;101(3):852–9.

25. Holland A. Osteoporosis Knowledge Translation for young adults: new directions for prevention programs. *Journal of Health Promotion Chronicles*. 2017;37(8):229–37.

26. Sydora BC, Graham B, Oster RT, Ross S. Menopause experience in First Nations women and initiatives for menopause symptom awareness; a community-based participatory research approach. *BMC Womens Health*. 2021;21:Article number: 179.

27. Holroyd-Leduc JM, Straus S, Thorpe K, Davis DA, Schmaltz H, Tannenbaum C. Translation of evidence into a self-management tool for use by women with urinary incontinence. *Journal of Age and Ageing*. 2011;40(2):227–33.

14.
15.
16.

PART VII

CONCLUSION

23

A Life Course Approach to Women's Health

Linking the Past, Present, and Future

Rebecca Hardy, Diana Kuh, and Gita D. Mishra

23.1 Introduction

There has been an enormous amount of additional relevant research since the first edition of this book was published in 2002. As with the first edition, the aim of the second edition is to review the risk factors and exposures and pathways across women's lives that contribute to health and morbidity at later ages. An understanding the trajectories in body function and structure across the life course which result in disease is given greater emphasis. Further, the last 20 years have seen an proliferation of systematic reviews, with or without meta-analysis, which provide overviews of existing evidence for many associations highlighted in the chapters.

In this concluding chapter, we pick out common themes covered in the preceding chapters, highlight new advances in women's health life course research and important methodological developments, while also looking forward to future opportunities and challenges. We finish by commenting on policy and translational implications which have the potential to improve the health of women across the life course.

23.2 Common Themes and Key Findings: Linking the Past to the Future

23.2.1 Life Course Trajectories

Since the first edition of this book, the study of functional trajectories has become increasingly prominent in life course research, demonstrating their importance in understanding ageing and disease development and their potential for identifying groups in need of intervention. Multiple chapters, including those on musculoskeletal ageing (Chapter 7), cardiovascular disease (CVD) (Chapter 5), dementia (Chapter 10), and chronic obstructive pulmonary disease (COPD) (Chapter 8), highlight how investigating a longitudinal functional phenotype complements the study of a disease endpoint, while Chapter 14, on endocrinology, outlines current knowledge of the changes in hormones across the stages of a

Rebecca Hardy, Diana Kuh, and Gita D. Mishra, *A Life Course Approach to Women's Health* In: *A Life Course Approach to Women's Health*. Second Edition. Edited by: Gita D Mishra, Rebecca Hardy, and Diana Kuh, Oxford University Press. © Oxford University Press 2023. DOI: 10.1093/oso/9780192864642.003.0023 women's life. Empirical evidence has now accumulated to demonstrate how measures such as grip strength and lung function follow the previously hypothesised life course pattern of development, peak, and age-related decline. While the mean level at any given age of muscle and bone phenotypes varies by sex, country, and ethnicity, the patterns of change over the life course remain consistent (Chapter 7).[1-3] Other measures of function, particularly those related to cardiometabolic disease, display different patterns of change with age (Chapter 5). Although more is now known about age-related trends in mean levels of many functional measures, it is not always clear what constitutes an 'optimal' or a 'healthy' trajectory. For example, the mean systolic blood pressure trajectory in the UK is likely not a healthy or natural ageing trajectory as it is influenced by high population levels of overweight and obesity (Chapter 16). Therefore, further study of heterogeneity of patterns within, as well as between populations, will likely be required to identify optimal trajectories. Multiple lung function trajectory patterns from childhood to age 50 years have been identified, although all groups demonstrated a similar pattern of change but with different peak levels and varying rates of decline (Chapter 8),[4] as have different trajectories of midlife blood pressure within UK and US samples.[5,6] The potential to use functional trajectories to identify those in need of early intervention is starting to be recognised, and guidelines highlight the importance of optimising, for example, peak bone mass[7] and lung function.[8] The value of identifying markers which can detect preclinical change, before disease onset, is further recognised in chapters considering outcomes for which there are no obvious life course phenotypes, such as cancer (Chapters 11 and 12) and osteoarthritis (Chapter 7). Potential intermediate phenotypes such as breast density for breast cancer and bone shape for osteoarthritis have been used, while there is active research to identify potential biomarkers.

While the focus has been on these long-term life course changes in function, there is also evidence of the importance of shorter-term changes and fluctuations which are less studied. For example, women's cognitive performance changes according to the phase of the menstrual cycle (Chapter 10)[9] and changes in blood pressure (BP) and other cardiometabolic measures occur during pregnancy[10,11] and may have long-term consequences. There is also evidence that variation in BP, for example between clinic visits, may predict subsequent disease risk,[12] and progress has been made on methodological approaches to examine the impact of both mean and variability.[13] To maximise understanding of change in function over different timeframes, studies need to consider the required density of repeated measures and may require a more regular measurement schedule during times of rapid change. The increased feasibility of employing wearable devices in longitudinal studies makes this more likely in future. Use of such new technology may also begin to address the persisting challenge of a lack of data in the same individuals across the whole life course. These data are needed as trajectories derived from multiple cross-sectional studies may be influenced by secular or cohort differences, although the potential and challenges of combining longitudinal data from different cohorts is an alternative approach being explored.[14] Among other methodological challenges, data harmonisation across studies is prominent. However, longitudinal data which cover large portions of the life course within a study also often require harmonisation, because the use of identical measurement procedures at every age is not always feasible.[15] Some measures of function, such as cognition, require age-appropriate measures at different developmental stages, while technological developments mean that new, improved, and more convenient instruments may be introduced, resulting in the need for measurement comparison studies.

23.2.2 Evidence on Early Life Origins of Women's Health

23.2.2.1 Advances in Understanding Prenatal Effects

As in the previous edition of this book, markers of birth size and in utero growth were re-ported to be associated with reproductive health (Chapter 2 and 4), CVD (Chapter 5), dia-betes (Chapter 6), musculoskeletal ageing (Chapter 7), lung function (Chapter 8), and breast cancer (Chapter 11), with systematic reviews and meta-analyses summarising evidence for many of these outcomes. While Barker's initial fetal origins hypothesis proposed that insults during critical periods of in utero development programmed the structure and function of body systems, birth size is only a proxy marker of such exposures. Family studies, along with recent developments in genetic methods, have started to be applied to identify whether associations between birth weight (and other measures of birth size) and health do indeed represent an intrauterine programming effect, or are a result of common genetic effects, or environmental confounding. Current evidence suggests, for example, that genetic effects appear a more likely explanation of associations between birth weight and BP[16] and type 2 diabetes mellitus (T2DM).[17,18] Understanding of the mechanisms linking maternal charac-teristics and offspring health is also accumulating. For example, maternal prepregnancy body mass index (BMI), smoking, and alcohol intake may influence daughters' age at menarche (Chapter 2); maternal occupational and pollution exposures could be related to lung function (Chapter 8); and exposure or pregnant women to intimate partner violence (IPV) has been related to a whole range of psychological and emotional outcomes in offspring (Chapter 20). The body weight chapter (Chapter 16) highlights how sibling and maternal-paternal com-parison support the hypothesised intrauterine effect of maternal diabetes on offspring BMI, but that shared environmental factors are the more likely explanation of the relationship be-tween maternal and offspring BMI. The emerging apparent variation in underlying mechan-isms means that further research is needed to understand the implication on the full range of health outcomes.

Epigenetics has been proposed as one mechanism linking intrauterine exposures and subsequent disease and a potential target for intervention.[19] While there is evidence of dif-ferential DNA methylation according to birth weight,[20] the implications remain unclear. An example of a possible epigenetic mechanism for diabetes was described in Chapter 6, whereby the loss of DNA methylation of specific genes acquired from the mother (thus pro-moting maternal gene expression), but not the father (paternal gene suppression), was asso-ciated with T2DM.[21] Epigenetic changes to the methylation of the glucocorticoid receptor gene, whose expression in the central nervous system plays a role in neuroendocrine func-tions, were highlighted in a small study of young people whose mothers were exposed to IPV during pregnancy in Chapter 20.[22] Robust evidence of transgenerational epigenetic effects and causal mechanisms mediated via epigenetics remains scarce, but accumulation of data on larger samples will likely further clarify the role of epigenetics in the intergenerational transmission of health.

23.2.2.2 Growth and the Obesity Epidemic

Given the still limited number of studies with detailed repeated measures of height and weight across life, this book does not document much additional evidence relating growth to outcomes since the last edition. More evidence has accumulated, including from Mendelian randomization (MR) studies, that short adult stature is related to CVD (Chapter 5),[23] and, conversely, that greater height is associated with increased risk of breast cancer (Chapter 11).[24] More broadly, the importance of promoting healthy early life growth is emphasised for musculoskeletal outcomes (Chapter 7). In contrast to growth, there has been a considerable accumulation of research on timing of menarche (detailed in Section 23.2.3.1), which is part of the developmental maturation process. In addition, with the rise of the obesity epidemic across much of the world, attention has perhaps turned from growth per se to the impact of childhood adiposity on subsequent health.

More recently born generations of women, at least in most high-income countries (HICs), are spending more of their life overweight or obese (Chapter 16). While high midlife BMI is associated with mortality and multiple health outcomes, the importance of life course patterns of adiposity in women is outlined in preceding chapters. For example, greater accumulation of lifetime overweight appears to be related to cardiometabolic health[25,26] (Chapter 5) and osteoarthritis (Chapter 7), while obesity in childhood is related to reproductive outcomes (Chapters 2) and the higher levels of youth-onset T2DM in women is attributed to increased rates of overweight and obesity in young girls (Chapter 6). The relationship between life course adiposity and breast cancer is more complex, with weight gain from early to later adulthood shown to be associated with increased risk of postmenopausal breast cancer, and women who were heavier in early adulthood showing reduced premenopausal cancer risk independent of later weight gain (Chapter 11). In addition, it is documented how high BMI in adolescent women, through social stigma and discrimination or through increased disease burden, results in poorer social and well-being outcomes (Chapter 16).

A key question for life course epidemiology is whether childhood overweight has a direct causal effect on health or is a result of tracking of overweight through to adulthood. A novel MR approach, using separate genetic risk scores for childhood and adult BMI, offers the potential to tease out the effect. So far, results suggest that associations between childhood body size and CVD risk are likely due to the life course tracking of high BMI (Chapter 5), although recently, childhood body size was shown to have a long-term influence on later life heart structure.[27] The possible lack of a direct causal effect of childhood BMI suggests that, among children who are overweight or obese, weight loss during transition to adulthood would be beneficial. However, considering the substantial tracking in weight from childhood to adulthood, prevention aimed in childhood is also important.

23.2.2.3 Early Life Social and Psychosocial Exposures

Stark socioeconomic inequalities both within and between countries are documented across a whole range of health outcomes in the preceding chapters. Many are demonstrated to have their origins in childhood. One obvious pathway from early life disadvantage involves a lack of social mobility across the life course (Chapter 17), with education an important key to social mobility. Life course health behaviours likely play a role in this pathway, as health-damaging behaviours in adulthood are more likely in those from disadvantaged backgrounds (Chapter 15). The role of identity and self-esteem, largely developed in adolescence is important in development of health behaviours (Chapter 15) and depression (Chapter 9), and perhaps particularly for women as girls' self-esteem decreases in adolescence, and women have lower adult levels than men.[28] Parent-child relationship quality, parenting style, and adversity may be important in the development of such characteristics, as they affect social and psychological development (Chapter 18).

In the previous edition of this book, individual childhood stressors such as parental illness and parental divorce were highlighted in relation to depression and health behaviours, but the increasing interest in a larger range of adverse childhood experiences (ACEs) including abuse and violence (Chapter 20) is evidenced in this book. Although the role of ACEs in mental health and some risky behaviours is clear (Chapters 9 and 15), there is less certainty with regards to the relationship with physical health outcomes (Chapter 5, 16). Some types of ACEs are more common in girls than in boys,[29] and there is a suggestion that experience of ACEs may be particularly detrimental for women as the stress response varies by sex. While the chapter on gender-based violence (Chapter 20) indicates that abuse has a bigger impact on women than on men, broader consistent evidence for sex and gender differences in the effect of ACEs is lacking. The variation in measurement (including retrospective versus prospective ascertainment of events and statistical approaches to modelling of the impact of multiple ACEs) may explain some of the inconsistency in the current literature.[30] It remains to be seen whether type, severity, and timing of ACEs are important for health, as these aspects are so far less studied, perhaps because of a lack of detailed data.

A key question is how these early life exposures leave a biological imprint on the body (discussed in Chapter 17). Psychological stress is the main hypothesised pathway studied to date, with the hypothalamic-pituitary-adrenal (HPA) axis being a focus of attention, although findings remain mixed.[31] Parental socioeconomic position (SEP) has been associated with alterations in the neonatal epigenome,[32] and it is suggested that early life disadvantaged SEP might speed up biological ageing[33-38]. However, there remain challenges to understand mechanisms and biomarker utility which require further research.[39-42]

23.2.3 Integrating Women's Reproductive and Social Life

23.2.3.1 Reproductive Factors Across Life and Women's Health

The links across a woman's reproductive life have been increasingly recognised, as has the link between reproductive health and other aspects of health and ageing. The chapters in the book have highlighted a myriad of such interrelationships across the life course, and while menarche, pregnancy, and menopause have been commonly studied, the impact of menstrual characteristics appears less researched and has, indeed, been highlighted as an under-researched topic during the COVID-19 pandemic.[43] Reproductive characteristics are related across life from menarche to menopause, and the potential underlying genetic commonalities and causal effects are now starting to be understood (Chapters 2 and 13).[44] Furthering understanding of the life course changes in the various hypothalamic-pituitary axes provide the possibility of linking reproductive characteristics, underlying hormonal mechanisms, and health (Chapter 14). As in the first edition of this book, it has continued to be recognised that reproductive health reflects general health, potentially marking future disease risk, and the policy implications of this are discussed in Section 23.4.

Multiple chapters detailed evidence relating to the potential effects of age at menarche and/or age at menopause on health outcomes including reproduction (Chapter 2), gynacological conditions (Chapters 3 and 4), CVD (Chapter 5), diabetes (Chapter 6), COPD (Chapter 8), cognition (Chapter 10), cancers (Chapters 11 and 12), and body size (Chapter 16). It has long been discussed as to whether observed associations between earlier menarche and poorer health are causal or attributable to the association between high childhood BMI and earlier menarche and the subsequent tracking of BMI across life. These relationships mean it is challenging to disentangle the role of menarche from that of BMI.[45] Given the availability of hundreds of genetic variants for pubertal timing, MR has been used across a range of outcomes. MR supports a causal relationship of early menarche with breast and endometrial cancer,[46] and lower levels of adult lung function;[47] and later menarche with lower bone mineral density.[48] However, for cardiometabolic health, the evidence is less clear with some suggestion that associations are due to higher life course BMI in those with early menarche.[45,49–52] Therefore, tackling childhood overweight, as well as understanding other factors that trigger early menarche (second-hand smoke and endocrine-disrupting chemicals are two exposures highlighted in the reproductive chapter) may be important to improve the health of girls in future. In contrast to the potential long-term effects on most outcomes, the effect of menarche on depression may be only short-term during the pubertal transition (Chapter 9).

The study of reproductive characteristics on women's health is a good example of integration of the biological and social processes. Associations between number of children and age at parenthood may reflect biological effects of pregnancy or be confounded by selection into parenthood or mediated by behaviour change as result of family formation and child rearing (Chapters 2 and 5). Studies have compared the relationship between number of children and CVD in men and in women in an attempt to determine the main mechanism,[53,54] and have generally found that confounding is the most likely predominant mechanism because of similar associations observed in men and women, although pregnancy may play a small role. Further, there remains a clear interrelationship between women's reproductive and socioeconomic trajectory (Chapter 17) as, for example, disadvantaged childhood SEP selects into early childbearing, and partnership and pregnancy histories influence subsequent SEP.

23.2.3.2 Cultural and Societal Change

One of the main questions for life course research, which has used studies that may have followed cohorts over decades, is the extent to which any resultant evidence is relevant to generations of women today. The rise of the obesity epidemic is a stark example of how changes in the environment, which has become increasingly obesogenic, has resulted in rapid changes in levels of overweight and obesity in childhood (Chapter 16). Therefore, studies which have provided information linking childhood BMI with adult health had much lower rates of overweight and obesity than current generations of children. As the numbers of girls categorised as obese were small in these historical cohorts, this limits the statistical power of the study to look at long-term effects. Perhaps the next edition of this book will be able to provide this information using data from longitudinal studies of those born in the 1980s or later. The weakening of traditional gender norms and socialisation processes seen in many countries over the past 40 years is highlighted in the social relationships chapter (Chapter 18), where it is hypothesised that given the importance of social relationships to women, there may be changes in the gendered patterns between social relations and health. To understand, and potentially predict, the long-term effects of early life on younger generations, it will be important to track and compare the social and biological trajectories of multiple generations of women, and to compare intermediate relationships on the pathways between early life and later health.

There are also exposures that are operating today for which there is no, or very little, equivalent in the past. For example, the impact of social media and screen use on children has generated a huge amount of research and debate. While secular increases in mental health problems have been attributed in part to high levels of screen usage, the complexity of the relationship is starting to be recognised.[55] The nearest similar societal factors, such as the role of peer pressure, even in quite recent cohorts, do not seem to provide a comparable exposure. Another example is the use of assisted reproductive technology (ART), which is likely partly explained by the secular social trend of delayed childbearing (Chapter 2). Initial studies focused on improving the live birth weight and then perinatal outcomes; however, the impact of ART is now being more comprehensively addressed through collaborations of multiple cohorts to ensure adequate statistical power. Increased risk of low birth weight, small-for-gestational age, and preterm birth were seen in offspring conceived through ART,[56,57] with differences now being shown depending on type of ART procedure.[58] Longer follow-up of children has allowed study of later growth, where, reassuringly, only small differences between ART and naturally conceived offspring were found.[59] Further follow-up of cohorts to assess longer term outcomes will be required.

23.3 New Developments and Future Opportunities and Challenges

23.3.1 Cross-Study Analysis

Chapter authors in this edition of the book were able to draw on existing summaries of evidence in the form of systematic reviews. Although there are some individual life course studies with detailed prospective information on, for example, repeated measure of growth, SEP, or ACEs, which are difficult to replicate across many studies, relevant life course research is increasingly being produced from cross-study collaborations. Genetics research led the way because of the need for very large sample sizes for genome-wide association studies (GWAS) to successfully identify genetic variants,[60] but data from multiple studies are being pooled to be able to study rare outcomes, such as premature menopause,[61] or more detailed patterns of association, such as between smoking and age at menopause.[62]

Other cross-study research in the biomedical and social sciences of relevance to a life course approach aims to study differences in prevalence, average level, or distribution of an outcome, or differences in association between exposure and outcome, by time, birth cohort, or geographical location.[63,64] The NCD Risk Factor Collaboration (NCDRisC)[65] has used data from hundreds of studies to track historic trends in cardiometabolic risk factors across the globe.[66,67] Smaller scale studies, such as those within the UK, have tracked changing life course social inequalities in health across birth cohorts,[68–70] and how outcomes of child mental health problems have changed.[71] Methodological considerations are key to this type of endeavour as differences in data selection, data processing, including harmonisation across studies, and analysis can impact conclusions.[64] Various research infrastructure initiatives and platforms have sought to aid the process of data harmonisation and to avoid replication of effort.[72–74] The potential for such collaborations to promote prospective harmonisation of data is yet to be fully realised, although some progress was made during the COVID-19 pandemic.[75] Ongoing calibration studies may be one solution to achieving the within- and between-study comparability required for longitudinal cross-study comparisons, and the creation of calibrated question banks could also enable progress.[15] One approach that is commonly used in clinical trials would be to define core outcome sets, which are a minimum set of variables that should be reported for a specific condition. This could readily be adopted by researchers for observational studies to better facilitate comparisons.

23.3.2 New Studies and New Data

The longitudinal birth cohort study remains the ideal design for life course research, but there has been a proliferation of large studies, such as UK Biobank which recruited approximately 500,000 participants aged 40–69 years between 2006 and 2010,[76] since the first edition of this book. The UK Biobank is now a longitudinal study, but it has limited and retrospective early life information, although it has been used to study life course hypotheses, such as the health consequences of age at menarche,[77] as well as for genetic analyses of relevance to a life course approach.[16] The value of linking data from longitudinal studies with administrative data is also becoming evident. For example, the ability to add to survey data the entire history of antenatal records, or of prescription usage, can completely transform the potential of a study. The Norwegian HUNT study has provided important information on drops in BP after each pregnancy through linkage to pregnancy information from the Medical Birth Registry of Norway.[78] In another example, the cumulative prevalence of endometriosis for Australian women (that was reported in Chapter 3) was determined using three data linkage sources (Medicare, pharmaceutical, and hospital data) with longitudinal survey data. Such linkages enable researchers to use a wider range of objectively collected information to enhance the questionnaire data collected from study participants. New studies are now being designed around this ability to link administrative and health records as well as the potential use of wearables—some of which are targeting precision medicine and based on huge numbers (e.g. Our Future Health, UK[79]; All of Us, US[80]), and others which are national (e.g. Early Life Cohort Feasibility Study)[81] and regional birth cohort studies (e.g. Gen V,[82] C-Gull,[83] and Queensland Family Cohort Study[84]). The benefits of linkages to other types of data, such as geographical information including air pollution,[85] are being realised, and linkage of cohorts to digital footprint information[86] is being actively pursued. Although the difficulty in obtaining historical measures of environmental exposures limits the extent to which life course questions can be addressed,[87] the health impacts of life course pollution and area deprivation have been studied.[88–90]

Many cohort studies have added genotyping information and, more recently, epigenomics and metabolomics data. The main advances in genomics to the understanding of women's health have come from GWAS, which have for the first time been able to identify large numbers of genetic loci that influence multifactorial traits (e.g. menarche and menopause timing)[91] and female-specific disease (e.g. hormone-sensitive cancer,[92,93] endometriosis,[94] and polycystic ovary syndrome[95]). Through integration with transcriptomics, epigenomics and proteomics, these studies have provided novel insights into the biological process involved in these traits (Chapter 13). Further, as larger proportions of trait variation are explained, genomic variants become invaluable for causal inference studies using MR, as highlighted above. Using genomics for precision medicine is in its infancy, but polygenic risk scores using GWAS variants are being used to predict risk of diseases such as cardiovascular disease and diabetes. Clinically useful scores for female-specific traits are not yet available, but as more of the genetic architecture is uncovered, clinical utility is likely to improve. Studies are also beginning to track more detailed subclinical phenotypes, such as those obtained through imaging, than has been previously possible, and although longitudinal data are currently limited, they will accumulate. Chapter 10, on cognition and dementia, outlines research linking women's reproductive characteristics—oral contraceptive use and menopause—to neuroimaging biomarkers of Alzheimer's Disease (AD).

There is a clear need for more research on women's health from a life course perspective in LMICs. There remains a general lack of evidence specific to LMICs. It is the case that some countries, such as China and India,[96-98] have started or will shortly commence population cohort studies on women's health. These will likely take considerable time to have collected sufficient data to be able to replicate the life course studies already conducted in HICs and to compare findings. Assuming the applicability of evidence obtained from HICs without considering the local context is likely to be problematic. For example, for women with premature ovarian insufficiency, the recommended clinical guidance is for menopausal hormone therapy use until the usual age at menopause in HICS of around 50–51 years. The suggested duration of treatment, however, may not be appropriate for women in LMICs, since in many such countries, they typically experience menopause several years earlier than in HICs.[99]

23.3.3 Methodology

Given the extended time frame between an exposure and outcome in life course epidemiology, there is considerable room for bias in traditional analysis of observational data. In the previous edition of the book, the methodological challenges were highlighted, and since then, approaches have developed considerably with more complex methods now increasingly applied in practice. In particular, approaches to identify causal relationships have come to the fore. The use of directed acyclic graphs, which provide a visual representation of the assumed causal relationships, makes clear the set of assumptions on which a model is based.[100] Advances in causal mediation analysis have resulted in more robust results relating to the understanding of pathways,[101,102] and the use of E-values to estimate the size of an unmeasured confounder required to explain away the exposure-outcome associations is being increasingly used.[103] Methods to identify the life course model that best fits the observed data have developed as highlighted in Chapter 1, although these can be challenging to implement in practice.[104-109] In addition, advances in approaches to deal with missing data[110] and selection bias,[111,112] common challenges in observational studies, have been made in the last 20 years. These new approaches have been accompanied with advances in software, but increased accessibility does not in itself ensure better analysis, highlighting the importance of building sufficient analytic capacity among researchers.[15]

Many chapters provide evidence from multiple approaches to assessing associations in order to triangulate the evidence[113] and provide a stronger causal evidence base. A common approach, much referenced in the book, is MR which uses genetic variants to instrument for an environmental exposure.[114] The effects obtained from MR studies are generally interpreted as the lifetime effect of exposure, but the interest in life course epidemiology is to study exposures at different periods of the life course. Recently, multivariable MR, an extension of MR that allows for multiple and potentially highly related exposures to be analysed, has been developed[115] and used, as described above, to disentangle the effects of childhood versus adult BMI. The development of such an approach could be of great significance to life course epidemiology. Other useful approaches, although perhaps less commonly used currently, include sibling studies,[116] negative control exposure or outcome studies,[117,118] natural experiments,[119] and, commonly used in economics, nongenetic instrumental variable analysis.[120]

23.3.4 Integrating the COVID-19 Pandemic into a Life Course Approach

As was noted in Chapter 1, the COVID-19 pandemic has cast a long shadow over preparation of this book. The pandemic provides an extreme example of a period effect which will have affected all generations, but at different stages of their life course. Yet, we argue that it is increasingly evident since the acute phase that the direct and indirect impacts of COVID-19 have become enmeshed within the wider epidemic of noncommunicable diseases (NCDs). The risk profile for adverse COVID-19 outcomes in women vary with the reproductive life stage, potentially related to the protective effects of oestrogen levels,[121] as postmenopausal women are more likely to suffer severe COVID-19 morbidity and mortality, compared with premenopausal women.[122] Consistent with the life course approach, pregnant women represent a vulnerable group, since those with severe COVID-19 during pregnancy are at possible increased risk of preterm birth[123] and stillbirth. The interaction between COVID-19 and NCDs was first apparent in the increased risk of COVID-19 morbidity and mortality for those with high BMI and preexisting conditions such as hypertension, diabetes, CVD, and respiratory diseases.[124-126] Women are more likely to experience what is commonly termed *long COVID*, and it also appears that a 10%–20% of those infected experience a variety of chronic symptoms that persist long after the viral infection has cleared.[127] In addition, and distinct from long COVID, early evidence suggests that past infection poses an increased risk of NCDs, including new onset hypertension,[128] diabetes,[129] and for dementia and AD, reflecting potential damage from COVID-19 to several organs, including the lung vasculature.[130] In addition, the pandemic has seen the prevalence of depressive and anxiety disorders increase substantially for women, and more so than for men.[131,132] The pandemic has also resulted in considerable harm in disrupting prevention and management of NCDs, such as breast and cervical cancer screening, and the existing management and treatment healthcare plans of cancer patients.[133,134] The consequences of delayed diagnosis and treatment of breast cancer will take many years to quantify in full, but one model recently estimated that the UK would see a 7.9%–9.6% increase in fatalities. These types of adverse impacts on women's health, if sustained as the hidden legacy of the pandemic, will need to be incorporated into public health policies and modelling of the future burden of NCDs.

Looking to the future, life course epidemiology needs to study how and why the long-term consequences of the pandemic vary by age and birth cohort, and how biological, psychological or socioeconomic factors earlier in life affect or modify the immediate and long-term health consequences of the pandemic.[135] Based on existing knowledge, the increased early life disadvantage, adversity, and stress and the social and economic consequences of lockdowns, educational disruption, and economic recession are likely to have long-term impacts on the current generation of children.[135] The initiation of the studies tracking the impact of the COVID-19 pandemic on children in the UK (COSMO,[136] Children of 2020s Study[137]) and United States (RECOVER),[138] as well as continued follow-up of existing cohort studies, which collected information through the pandemic, are vital to understand, and to mitigate, the longer term impacts.[139] More broadly, there needs to be greater focus on the dynamic interplay between individual life course determinants of women's health and ageing with both the global physical challenges, such as the emergence of future pandemics, climate change, antimicrobial resistance, and environmental pollution, and associated societal challenges. A focus on the long-term consequences of infectious diseases on ageing and NCDs needs to be restored and the lifetime determinants of risk and susceptibility to infectious diseases needs more emphasis.[135]

23.4 Women's Health Policy

The effects of the COVID-19 pandemic will inevitably have an impact on policy over the coming years, as highlighted in the previous section. In this section, we consider policy outside of COVID-19 and as documented in the Introduction (Chapter 1), there has been an increased national and international emphasis on the health of women and girls. In some policy documents, the use of a life course approach to tackle the challenges of improving women's health has been specifically stated. However, it remains to be seen what taking a life course approach will mean in practice as it does not necessarily coincide with what we mean by a life course approach in epidemiology. Policymakers in the UK[140] and Australia[141] are now adopting a life course approach in their women's health strategy. They aim to support new research to increase understanding of female-specific health conditions and to address data gaps to improve health care for women. Additionally, the strategies highlight the need to take a preventive approach, have broadened their view of the determinants of health, and aim to identify the critical stages, transitions, and settings where there are opportunities to promote good health or to prevent negative health outcomes, consistent with the aims of life course epidemiology. They also acknowledge that services should be centred on women's needs rather than being organised by individual condition consistent with the aspirations outlined in Chapter 21 in this book. The long-term socioeconomic implications of reproductive health across life are also starting to be realised with the recent UK policy paper on menopause and the workplace.[142] It remains to be seen whether there will remain disparate health services for women or whether a truly joined up life course approach will emerge.

23.4.1 Implications of Our Findings for Policy

23.4.1.1 Reproductive Health
Reproduction has for some years now been considered a sentinel of health and chronic disease in women, providing a window into the subclinical disease processes.[143] A life course approach pointed the way to using reproductive health service use (from menarche to menopause) to target preventive health strategies. Research highlighted in Chapters 2 and 5 indicate that adverse pregnancy outcomes, such as gestational diabetes and preeclampsia, identify women at substantial increased risk of subsequent cardiometabolic disease. Broad international and national guidelines for the postpartum follow-up of women who experienced hypertensive disorders of pregnancy and gestational diabetes do now exist,[144,145] but there remains little consensus on the ideal time to commence follow-up, and there is limited information on the efficacy of postpartum intervention clinics in reducing risk.[146] Longer term follow-up and evaluation of the effect of postpartum interventions is thus required.

While the implications of pregnancy complications for the mother herself are perhaps clear, the effects of maternal behaviour in pregnancy and intrauterine growth and pregnancy complications for her offspring are more complex. The benefit of intervention to promote maternal health and the health of women of childbearing age cannot be denied; however, care needs to be taken to ensure the results from DOHaD and life course research do not result in unnecessary maternal blame and guilt.[147,148] Society has a history of blaming mothers for poor health of their offspring, and interventions can have unintended negative consequences.[147,149] Sharp et al.[150] have argued that the implicit causal assumption of the primary importance of maternal pregnancy effects sets the agenda for DOHaD research leading to the reinforcement of the assumption. They outline useful practical strategies to maintain a critical perspective in future.[148,150] Further, work to better understand the development and communication of risk to pregnant women which respects women's autonomy and trusts them to make decisions about their own pregnancy is required.[151] As outlined in Chapter 20, on Knowledge Translation, best practice in implementation science requires engagement with women and co-design to develop appropriate interventions, especially with disadvantaged and vulnerable groups. This are some early examples where antenatal practice is being completely redeveloped with extremely vulnerable groups such as First Nation Australians.[152]

While overall health systems in LMICs may be lacking, maternal and child healthcare are typically the most well developed (as the priority areas of WHO goals). So existing antenatal and postnatal health services, perhaps delivered by a community nurse, provide a potential platform from which to add NCD prevention strategies in essentially the same concept as in HICs, even if the priorities and delivery of health interventions may differ. The development of life course approach to women's health research and translation into effective health prevention is likely to continue to be an even greater challenge for LMICs than it is for HICs.

23.4.1.2 Tackling Life Course Social Inequalities

There are wide and increasing social inequalities in health, and it is documented how many of the important early life exposures and health risk factors and behaviours are socially patterned. Therefore, addressing the underlying socioeconomic inequalities has the benefit of impacting multiple interrelated factors. For example, while life course research on the impact of ACEs on health has resulted in policy initiatives, rigorous research on their benefits and harms is currently lacking. Further, given the practical and ethical challenges related to routine enquiry about, or 'screening' for, ACEs, it is suggested that tackling the social causes of ACEs, such as poverty, may prove a promising complementary approach.[30] UK Government policies of austerity have had a damaging impact on health inequalities over the last 10 years, and the Marmot Review calls for national and local government interventions to redistribute funds.[153] It has generally been found that in countries with better welfare provision, such as Sweden and Norway, population health is better compared to countries where provision is less generous.[154,155] Initiatives aiming to provide every child the best start in life have been found to have some beneficial impacts. For example, a report from 2016 suggested that Sure Start in the UK, which is now defunded, reduced hospitalisations in children by the end of primary school, and, importantly, greatest benefits were observed among the most disadvantaged.[156] However, no benefits of Sure Start on childhood obesity were observed. Long-term follow-up of two US childhood randomised interventions found beneficial effects on health, although these were stronger in boys than in girls.[157]

Evidence in the preceding chapters overwhelmingly demonstrates the importance to women's health of life course overweight and obesity. This together with health behaviours, such as physical activity and alcohol consumption, are increasingly being demonstrated as causally related to a range of adverse health outcomes. Policies to tackle the obesity epidemic to date have had little demonstrable impact as evidenced by continued secular increases in BMI (Chapter 16) and are often assessed as ineffectual or it is suggested that they inappropriately focused on the individual or family.[158] Most educational and social marketing interventions require considerable individual agency, and it has been argued that low agency, upstream, interventions are more likely to be effective, as well as more equitable.[159] Such interventions need to be evaluated, and follow-up of longitudinal nationally representative cohorts can examine how prevalence and inequalities change in response to different policies. The reduction in consumption of sugar-sweetened beverages at a population level has been an upstream target in many countries, and the implementation of a tax on such products has been a common approach. Observational evidence from evaluations suggests that these policies can be effective in reducing the purchasing and consumption of these beverages,[160–162] as well as encouraging industry to reduce the sugar content of such products.[163] Among children, there has been much focus on school-based programs, but a systematic review of such physical activity interventions found no evidence of an effect, although the null effect was equitable across genders and SEP.[164] When translating life course evidence into intervention or policy, as for all interventions, there is a need, therefore, to assess the equity of proposed interventions and policies, as well as their overall effectiveness, if progress is to be made in reducing social inequalities in women's health.[165] Weight stigma, which may have worse socioeconomic consequences in women, also needs to be addressed, as it can result in a reluctance to seek help, which has been exacerbated during the COVID-19 pandemic.[166] Thus, implementation of policy should include consultation with women living with obesity to minimise unconscious bias, avoid stigma, and fully understand the barriers to accessing health care (see Chapter 22).

23.5 Conclusions

In the conclusions of the first edition of this book, we outlined four challenges for a life course approach to women's health. First, to identify the risk and protective factors at each stage of a woman's life that influenced independently, cumulatively, or interactively her chance of good health and the risk of disease in later life. Second, to shed light on the underlying biological, behavioural, and psychosocial pathways that operate across life and across generations. Third, to explain social, geographical, and temporal patterns of disease distribution in women, and fourth, to recommend policy interventions that are effective and sensitive to women's need at each stage of life. The first edition concluded that we had got a long way to meeting the first challenge and part way for the second and third, but that the fourth remained relatively untouched. This second edition demonstrates that progress has been made across all four challenges, including an understanding of causal mechanisms under the first and second. Life course approaches are starting to be integrated into policy, although need continued evaluation. New challenges, driven by the COVID-19 pandemic, include a greater integration of life course and infectious disease epidemiology to understand better the long-term consequences of the pandemic and other global challenges which impact on women's health. We hope that this book will, like the first, stimulate research and encourage others to take up these challenges.

Key messages and implications

- There has been a considerable amount of additional research relevant to a life course approach to women's health since the first edition of this book, although information from LMICs is still lacking.
- Important advances have been made in, for example, understanding life course trajectories of function, prenatal effects, the relevance of reproductive characteristics for health, and the biological mechanisms underlying early life exposures.
- Life course social inequalities and the obesity epidemic remain pressing public health concerns for women.
- Accumulation of new studies, new types of data, and advances in methodology have resulted in new insights and have future potential.
- A major challenge going forward is integrating impact of COVID-19 within women's life course research.
- Policy on women's health is starting to take a life course approach, but it remains to be seen what form this will take in practice.

References

1. Dodds RM, Syddall HE, Cooper R, Kuh D, Cooper C, Sayer AA. Global variation in grip strength: a systematic review and meta-analysis of normative data. *Age and Ageing*. 2016;45(2):209–16.
2. Leong DP, Teo KK, Rangarajan S, Kutty VR, Lanas F, Hui C, et al. Reference ranges of handgrip strength from 125,462 healthy adults in 21 countries: a prospective urban rural epidemiologic (PURE) study. *Journal of Cachexia, Sarcopenia and Muscle*. 2016;7(5):535–46.
3. Silva AM, Shen W, Heo M, Gallagher D, Wang Z, Sardinha LB, et al. Ethnicity-related skeletal muscle differences across the lifespan. *American Journal of Human Biology*. 2010;22(1):76–82.
4. Bui DS, Lodge CJ, Burgess JA, Lowe AJ, Perret J, Bui MQ, et al. Childhood predictors of lung function trajectories and future COPD risk: a prospective cohort study from the first to the sixth decade of life. *The Lancet Respiratory Medicine*. 2018;6(7):535–44.
5. Petruski-Ivleva N, Viera AJ, Shimbo D, Muntner P, Avery CL, Schneider ALC, et al. Longitudinal patterns of change in systolic blood pressure and incidence of cardiovascular disease. *Hypertension*. 2016;67(6):1150–6.
6. Wills AK, Lawlor DA, Muniz-Terrera G, Matthews F, Cooper R, Ghosh AK, et al. Population heterogeneity in trajectories of midlife blood pressure. *Epidemiology*. 2012;23(2):203–11.
7. Weaver CM, Gordon CM, Janz KF, Kalkwarf HJ, Lappe JM, Lewis R, et al. The National Osteoporosis Foundation's position statement on peak bone mass development and lifestyle factors: a systematic review and implementation recommendations. *Osteoporosis International*. 2016;27(4):1281–386.
8. Global Initiative for Chronic Obstructive Lung Disease. *Global strategy for prevention, diagnosis and management of chronic obstructive pulmonary disease (2020 report)*. Global Initiative for Chronic Obstructive Lung Disease; 2020.
9. Hampson E. Variations in sex-related cognitive abilities across the menstrual cycle. *Brain and Cognition*. 1990;14(1):26–43.
10. Macdonald-Wallis C, Lawlor DA, Fraser A, May M, Nelson SM, Tilling K. Blood pressure change in normotensive, gestational hypertensive, preeclamptic, and essential hypertensive pregnancies. *Hypertension*. 2012;59(6):1241–8.

11. Macdonald-Wallis C, Silverwood RJ, Fraser A, Nelson SM, Tilling K, Lawlor DA, et al. Gestational-age-specific reference ranges for blood pressure in pregnancy: findings from a prospective cohort. *Journal of Hypertension.* 2015;33(1):96–105.

12. Rothwell PM, Howard SC, Dolan E, O'Brien E, Dobson JE, Dahlöf B, et al. Prognostic significance of visit-to-visit variability, maximum systolic blood pressure, and episodic hypertension. *Lancet.* 2010;375(9718):895–905.

13. Parker RMA, Leckie G, Goldstein H, Howe LD, Heron J, Hughes AD, et al. Joint modeling of in-dividual trajectories, within-individual variability, and a later outcome: systolic blood pressure through childhood and left ventricular mass in early adulthood. *American Journal of Epidemiology.* 2020;190(4):652–62.

14. Hughes RA, Tilling K, Lawlor DA. Combining longitudinal data from different cohorts to examine the life-course trajectory. *American Journal of Epidemiology.* 2021;190(12):2680–9.

15. Hardy R, O'Neill D. Life course biological trajectories: maximising the value of longitudinal studies. *Annals of Human Biology.* 2020;47(2):227–8.

16. Warrington NM, Beaumont RN, Horikoshi M, Day FR, Helgeland Ø, Laurin C, et al. Maternal and fetal genetic effects on birth weight and their relevance to cardio-metabolic risk factors. *Nature Genetics.* 2019;51(5):804–14.

17. Stein AD, Obrutu OE, Behere RV, Yajnik CS. Developmental undernutrition, offspring obesity and type 2 diabetes. *Diabetologia.* 2019;62(10):1773–8.

18. Hughes AE, Hattersley AT, Flanagan SE, Freathy RM. Two decades since the fetal insulin hypoth-esis: what have we learned from genetics? *Diabetologia.* 2021;64(4):717–26.

19. Hanson M, Godfrey KM, Lillycrop KA, Burdge GC, Gluckman PD. Developmental plasticity and developmental origins of non-communicable disease: theoretical considerations and epigenetic mechanisms. *Progress in Biophysics and Molecular Biology.* 2011;106(1):272–80.

20. Küpers LK, Monnereau C, Sharp GC, Yousefi P, Salas LA, Ghantous A, et al. Meta-analysis of epigenome-wide association studies in neonates reveals widespread differential DNA methylation associated with birthweight. *Nature Communications.* 2019;10(1):1893.

21. Hanson RL, Guo T, Muller YL, Fleming J, Knowler WC, Kobes S, et al. Strong parent-of-origin effects in the association of KCNQ1 variants with type 2 diabetes in American Indians. *Diabetes.* 2013;62(8):2984–91.

22. Radtke KM, Ruf M, Gunter HM, Dohrmann K, Schauer M, Meyer A, et al. Transgenerational im-pact of intimate partner violence on methylation in the promoter of the glucocorticoid receptor. *Transl Psychiatry.* 2011;1:e21.

23. Lai FY, Nath M, Hamby SE, Thompson JR, Nelson CP, Samani NJ. Adult height and risk of 50 dis-eases: a combined epidemiological and genetic analysis. *BMC Medicine.* 2018;16(1):187.

24. Zhang B, Shu X-O, Delahanty RJ, Zeng C, Michailidou K, Bolla MK, et al. Height and breast cancer risk: evidence from prospective studies and Mendelian randomization. *Journal of the National Cancer Institute.* 2015;107(11):djv219.

25. Park MH, Sovio U, Viner RM, Hardy RJ, Kinra S. Overweight in childhood, adolescence and adult-hood and cardiovascular risk in later life: pooled analysis of three British birth cohorts. *PLoS One.* 2013;8(7):e70684.

26. Norris T, Cole TJ, Bann D, Hamer M, Hardy R, Li L, et al. Duration of obesity exposure between ages 10 and 40 years and its relationship with cardiometabolic disease risk factors: a cohort study. *PLoS Medicine.* 2020;17(12):e1003387.

27. O'Nunain K, Park C, Urquijo H, Leyden GM, Hughes AD, Davey Smith G, et al. A lifecourse men-delian randomization study highlights the long-term influence of childhood body size on later life heart structure. *PLoS Biology.* 2022;20(6):e3001656.

28. Kiviruusu O, Huurre T, Aro H, Marttunen M, Haukkala A. Self-esteem growth trajectory from adolescence to mid-adulthood and its predictors in adolescence. *Advances in Life Course Research.* 2015;23:29–43.

29. Jones MS, Pierce H, Shafer K. Gender differences in early adverse childhood experiences and youth psychological distress. *Journal of Criminal Justice.* 2022;83:101925.

30. Lacey RE, Minnis H. Practitioner review: twenty years of research with adverse childhood experi-ence scores—advantages, disadvantages and applications to practice. *Journal of Child Psychology and Psychiatry.* 2020;61(2):116–30.

31. Bryson HE, Price AMH, Goldfeld S, Mensah F. Associations between social adversity and young children's hair cortisol: a systematic review. *Psychoneuroendocrinology*. 2021;127:105176.

32. Simanek AM, Manansala R, Woo JMP, Meier HCS, Needham BL, Auer PL. Prenatal Socioeconomic disadvantage and epigenetic alterations at birth among children born to white British and Pakistani mothers in the Born in Bradford Study. *Epigenetics*. 2022;17(13):1976–90.

33. Raffington L, Belsky DW. Integrating DNA methylation measures of biological aging into social determinants of health research. *Current Environmental Health Reports*. 2022;9(2):196–210.

34. George A, Hardy R, Castillo Fernandez J, Kelly Y, Maddock J. Life course socioeconomic position and DNA methylation age acceleration in mid-life. *Journal of Epidemiology and Community Health*. 2021;75(11):1084–90.

35. Hughes A, Smart M, Gorrie-Stone T, Hannon E, Mill J, Bao Y, et al. Socioeconomic position and DNA methylation age acceleration across the life course. *American Journal of Epidemiology*. 2018;187(11):2346–54.

36. Ridout KK, Levandowski M, Ridout SJ, Gantz L, Goonan K, Palermo D, et al. Early life adversity and telomere length: a meta-analysis. *Molecular Psychiatry*. 2018;23(4):858–71.

37. Dowd JB, Simanek AM, Aiello AE. Socio-economic status, cortisol and allostatic load: a review of the literature. *International Journal of Epidemiology*. 2009;38(5):1297–309.

38. Belsky DW, Caspi A, Cohen HJ, Kraus WE, Ramrakha S, Poulton R, et al. Impact of early personal-history characteristics on the pace of aging: implications for clinical trials of therapies to slow aging and extend healthspan. *Aging Cell*. 2017;16(4):644–51.

39. El Khoury LY, Gorrie-Stone T, Smart M, Hughes A, Bao Y, Andrayas A, et al. Systematic under-estimation of the epigenetic clock and age acceleration in older subjects. *Genome Biology*. 2019;20(1):283.

40. Bell CG, Lowe R, Adams PD, Baccarelli AA, Beck S, Bell JT, et al. DNA methylation aging clocks: challenges and recommendations. *Genome Biology*. 2019;20(1):249.

41. Martin-Ruiz CM, Baird D, Roger L, Boukamp P, Krunic D, Cawthon R, et al. Reproducibility of telomere length assessment: an international collaborative study. *International Journal of Epidemiology*. 2014;44(5):1673–83.

42. Belsky DW, Moffitt TE, Cohen AA, Corcoran DL, Levine ME, Prinz JA, et al. Eleven telomere, epigenetic clock, and biomarker-composite quantifications of biological aging: do they measure the same thing? *American Journal of Epidemiology*. 2017;187(6):1220–30.

43. Sharp GC, Fraser A, Sawyer G, Kountourides G, Easey KE, Ford G, et al. The COVID-19 pandemic and the menstrual cycle: research gaps and opportunities. *International Journal of Epidemiology*. 2021;51(3):691–700.

44. Prince C, Sharp GC, Howe LD, Fraser A, Richmond RC. The relationships between women's reproductive factors: a Mendelian randomisation analysis. *BMC Medicine*. 2022;20(1):103.

45. Bell JA, Carslake D, Wade KH, Richmond RC, Langdon RJ, Vincent EE, et al. Influence of puberty timing on adiposity and cardiometabolic traits: a Mendelian randomisation study. *PLoS Medicine*. 2018;15(8):e1002641.

46. Day FR, Thompson DJ, Helgason H, Chasman DI, Finucane H, Sulem P, et al. Genomic analyses identify hundreds of variants associated with age at menarche and support a role for puberty timing in cancer risk. *Nature Genetics*. 2017;49(6):834–41.

47. Gill D, Sheehan NA, Wielscher M, Shrine N, Amaral AFS, Thompson JR, et al. Age at menarche and lung function: a Mendelian randomization study. *European Journal of Epidemiology*. 2017;32(8):701–10.

48. Zheng J, Frysz M, Kemp JP, Evans DM, Davey Smith G, Tobias JH. Use of Mendelian Randomization to Examine Causal Inference in Osteoporosis. *Frontiers in Endocrinology*. 2019;10:807.

49. Yuan S, Larsson SC. An atlas on risk factors for type 2 diabetes: a wide-angled Mendelian randomisation study. *Diabetologia*. 2020;63(11):2359–71.

50. Cao M, Cui B. negative effects of age at menarche on risk of cardiometabolic diseases in adulthood: a Mendelian randomization study. *Journal of Clinical Endocrinology & Metabolism*. 2019;105(2):515–22.

51. Magnus MC, Guyatt AL, Lawn RB, Wyss AB, Trajanoska K, Küpers LK, et al. Identifying potential causal effects of age at menarche: a Mendelian randomization phenome-wide association study. *BMC Medicine*. 2020;18(1):71.

52. Au Yeung SL, Jiang C, Cheng KK, Xu L, Zhang W, Lam TH, et al. Age at menarche and cardiovascular risk factors using Mendelian randomization in the Guangzhou Biobank Cohort Study. *Preventive Medicine*. 2017;101:142–8.

53. Hardy R, Lawlor D, Black S, Wadsworth M, Kuh D. Number of children and coronary heart disease risk factors in men and women from a British birth cohort. *BJOG*. 2007;114(6):721–30.

54. Kravdal Ø, Tverdal A, Grundy E. The association between parity, CVD mortality and CVD risk factors among Norwegian women and men. *European Journal of Public Health*. 2020;30(6):1133–9.

55. Orben A, Przybylski AK, Blakemore S-J, Kievit RA. Windows of developmental sensitivity to social media. *Nature Communications*. 2022;13(1):1649.

56. Goisis A, Remes H, Martikainen P, Klemetti R, Myrskylä M. Medically assisted reproduction and birth outcomes: a within-family analysis using Finnish population registers. *Lancet*. 2019;393(10177):1225–32.

57. Pinborg A, Wennerholm UB, Romundstad LB, Loft A, Aittomaki K, Söderström-Anttila V, et al. Why do singletons conceived after assisted reproduction technology have adverse perinatal outcome? Systematic review and meta-analysis. *Human Reproduction Update*. 2012;19(2):87–104.

58. Smith ADAC, Tilling K, Lawlor DA, Nelson SM. Live birth rates and perinatal outcomes when all embryos are frozen compared with conventional fresh and frozen embryo transfer: a cohort study of 337,148 in vitro fertilisation cycles. *BMC Medicine*. 2019;17(1):202.

59. Elhakeem A, Taylor AE, Inskip HM, Huang J, Tafflet M, Vinther JL, et al. Association of assisted reproductive technology with offspring growth and adiposity from infancy to early adulthood. *JAMA Network Open*. 2022;5(7):e2222106.

60. Gibson G. Population genetics and GWAS: a primer. *PLoS Biology*. 2018;16(3):e2005485.

61. Mishra GD, Pandeya N, Dobson AJ, Chung H-F, Anderson D, Kuh D, et al. Early menarche, nulliparity and the risk for premature and early natural menopause. *Human Reproduction*. 2017;32(3):679–86.

62. Zhu D, Chung H-F, Pandeya N, Dobson AJ, Cade JE, Greenwood DC, et al. Relationships between intensity, duration, cumulative dose, and timing of smoking with age at menopause: a pooled analysis of individual data from 17 observational studies. *PLoS Medicine*. 2018;15(11):e1002704.

63. O'Connor M, Spry E, Patton G, Moreno-Betancur M, Arnup S, Downes M, et al. Better together: advancing life course research through multi-cohort analytic approaches. *Advances in Life Course Research*. 2022;53:100499.

64. Bann D, Wright L, Goisis A, Hardy R, Johnson W, Maddock J, et al. Investigating change across time in prevalence or association using observational data: guidance on utility, methodology, and interpretation. *Discover Social Science and Health*. 2022;2(1):18.

65. NCD Risk Factor Collaboration. *NCD-RisC [Internet]*. NCD-RisC; 2017 [updated unknown date; cited Available from: https://ncdrisc.org.

66. Finucane MM, Stevens GA, Cowan MJ, Danaei G, Lin JK, Paciorek CJ, et al. National, regional, and global trends in body-mass index since 1980: systematic analysis of health examination surveys and epidemiological studies with 960 country-years and 9·1 million participants. *Lancet*. 2011;377(9765):557–67.

67. Danaei G, Finucane MM, Lu Y, Singh GM, Cowan MJ, Paciorek CJ, et al. National, regional, and global trends in fasting plasma glucose and diabetes prevalence since 1980: systematic analysis of health examination surveys and epidemiological studies with 370 country-years and 2·7 million participants. *Lancet*. 2011;378(9785):31–40.

68. Fluharty ME, Hardy R, Ploubidis G, Pongiglione B, Bann D. Socioeconomic inequalities across life and premature mortality from 1971 to 2016: findings from three British birth cohorts born in 1946, 1958 and 1970. *Journal of Epidemiology and Community Health*. 2021;75(2):193–6.

69. Bann D, Johnson W, Li L, Kuh D, Hardy R. Socioeconomic inequalities in childhood and adolescent body-mass index, weight, and height from 1953 to 2015: an analysis of four longitudinal, observational, British birth cohort studies. *Lancet Public Health*. 2018;3(4):e194–e203.

70. Bann D, Fluharty M, Hardy R, Scholes S. Socioeconomic inequalities in blood pressure: coordinated analysis of 147,775 participants from repeated birth cohort and cross-sectional datasets, 1989 to 2016. *BMC Medicine*. 2020;18(1):338.

71. Sellers R, Warne N, Pickles A, Maughan B, Thapar A, Collishaw S. Cross-cohort change in adolescent outcomes for children with mental health problems. *Journal of Child Psychology and Psychiatry*. 2019;60(7):813–21.

72. O'Neill D, Benzeval M, Boyd A, Calderwood L, Cooper C, Corti L, et al. data resource profile: cohort and longitudinal studies enhancement resources (CLOSER). *International Journal of Epidemiology*. 2019;48(3):675–6i.

73. Fortier I, Raina P, Van den Heuvel ER, Griffith LE, Craig C, Saliba M, et al. Maelstrom research guidelines for rigorous retrospective data harmonization. *International Journal of Epidemiology*. 2016;46(1):103–5.

74. Pinot de Moira A, Haakma S, Strandberg-Larsen K, van Enckevort E, Kooijman M, Cadman T, et al. The EU Child Cohort Network's core data: establishing a set of findable, accessible, interoperable and re-usable (FAIR) variables. *European Journal of Epidemiology*. 2021;36(5):565–80.

75. Villadsen A, Conti G, Fitzsimons E. *Parental involvement in home schooling and developmental play during lockdown—initial findings from the COVID-19 survey in five national longitudinal studies.* London: UCL Centre for Longitudinal Studies; 2020.

76. Sudlow C, Gallacher J, Allen N, Beral V, Burton P, Danesh J, et al. UK Biobank: an open access resource for identifying the causes of a wide range of complex diseases of middle and old age. *PLoS Medicine*. 2015;12(3):e1001779.

77. Day FR, Elks CE, Murray A, Ong KK, Perry JRB. Puberty timing associated with diabetes, cardiovascular disease and also diverse health outcomes in men and women: the UK Biobank study. *Scientific Reports*. 2015;5(1):11208.

78. Haug EB, Horn J, Markovitz AR, Fraser A, Vatten LJ, Macdonald-Wallis C, et al. Life course trajectories of cardiovascular risk factors in women with and without hypertensive disorders in first pregnancy: the HUNT Study in Norway. *Journal of the American Heart Association*. 2018;7(15):e009250.

79. Our Future Health. *Our Future Health [home page] [Internet].* Manchester: Our Future Health; 2022 [updated unknown date; cited 4 August 2022]. Available from: https://ourfuturehealth.org.uk/.

80. National Institutes of Health. *All of Us Research Program [Internet].* Bethesda, MD: National Institutes of Health; 2022 [updated unknown date; cited 4 August 2022]. Available from: https://allofus.nih.gov/.

81. Early Life Cohort Feasibility Study [Internet]. London: University College London; 2022 [updated unknown date; cited 4 August 2022]. Available from: https://cls.ucl.ac.uk/cls-studies/early-life-cohort-feasibility-study/.

82. Wang J, Hu YJ, Clifford S, Goldfeld S, Wake M. Selecting life course frameworks to guide and communicate large new cohort studies: Generation Victoria (GenV) case study. *Journal of Developmental Origins of Health and Disease*. 2021;12(6):829–48.

83. University of Liverpool. Children growing up in Liverpool (C-GULL) [Internet]. Liverpool: University of Liverpool; 2022 [updated unknown date; cited 4 August 2022]. Available from: https://www.liverpool.ac.uk/research/research-themes/living-well/c-gull/.

84. Borg D, Rae K, Fiveash C, Schagen J, James-McAlpine J, Friedlander F, et al. Queensland Family Cohort: a study protocol. *BMJ Open*. 2021;11(6):e044463.

85. Kuiper IN, Markevych I, Accordini S, Bertelsen RJ, Bråbäck L, Christensen JH, et al. Associations of preconception exposure to air pollution and greenness with offspring asthma and hay fever. *International Journal of Environmental Research and Public Health*. 2020;17(16):5828.

86. Shiells K, Di Cara N, Skatova A, Davis OSP, Haworth CMA, Skinner AL, et al. Participant acceptability of digital footprint data collection strategies: an exemplar approach to participant engagement and involvement in the ALSPAC birth cohort study. *Int J Popul Data Sci*. 2020;5(3):1728.

87. Murray ET, Southall H, Aucott P, Tilling K, Kuh D, Hardy R, et al. Challenges in examining area effects across the life course on physical capability in mid-life: findings from the 1946 British birth cohort. *Health & Place*. 2012;18(2):366–74.

88. Russ TC, Cherrie MPC, Dibben C, Tomlinson S, Reis S, Dragosits U, et al. Life course air pollution exposure and cognitive decline: modelled historical air pollution data and the Lothian birth cohort 1936. *Journal of Alzheimer's Disease*. 2021;79:1063–74.

89. Hansell A, Ghosh RE, Blangiardo M, Perkins C, Vienneau D, Goffe K, et al. Historic air pollution exposure and long-term mortality risks in England and Wales: prospective longitudinal cohort study. *Thorax*. 2016;71(4):330–8.

90. Jivraj S, Murray ET, Norman P, Nicholas O. The impact of life course exposures to neighbourhood deprivation on health and well-being: a review of the long-term neighbourhood effects literature. *European Journal of Public Health*. 2019;30(5):922–8.

91. He C, Murabito JM. Genome-wide association studies of age at menarche and age at natural menopause. *Molecular and Cellular Endocrinology*. 2014;382(1):767–79.

92. Zhang H, Ahearn TU, Lecarpentier J, Barnes D, Beesley J, Qi G, et al. Genome-wide association study identifies 32 novel breast cancer susceptibility loci from overall and subtype-specific analyses. *Nature Genetics*. 2020;52(6):572–81.

93. Phelan CM, Kuchenbaecker KB, Tyrer JP, Kar SP, Lawrenson K, Winham SJ, et al. Identification of 12 new susceptibility loci for different histotypes of epithelial ovarian cancer. *Nature Genetics*. 2017;49(5):680–91.

94. Nyholt DR, Low S-K, Anderson CA, Painter JN, Uno S, Morris AP, et al. Genome-wide association meta-analysis identifies new endometriosis risk loci. *Nature Genetics*. 2012;44(12):1355–9.

95. Day F, Karaderi T, Jones MR, Meun C, He C, Drong A, et al. Large-scale genome-wide meta-analysis of polycystic ovary syndrome suggests shared genetic architecture for different diagnosis criteria. *PLoS Genetics*. 2018;14(12):e1007813.

96. Kusneniwar G, Whelan RM, Betha K, Robertson JM, Ramidi PR, Balasubramanian K, et al. Cohort profile: the Longitudinal Indian Family Health (LIFE) Pilot Study, Telangana State, India. *International Journal of Epidemiology*. 2016;46(3):788–9j.

97. Zheng W, Chow W-H, Yang G, Jin F, Rothman N, Blair A, et al. The Shanghai Women's Health Study: rationale, study design, and baseline characteristics. *American Journal of Epidemiology*. 2005;162(11):1123–31.

98. Falkingham J, Evandrou M, Qin M, Vlachantoni A. Chinese women's health and wellbeing in middle life: unpacking the influence of menopause, lifestyle activities and social participation. *Maturitas*. 2021;143:145–50.

99. Golezar S, Ramezani Tehrani F, Khazaei S, Ebadi A, Keshavarz Z. The global prevalence of primary ovarian insufficiency and early menopause: a meta-analysis. *Climacteric*. 2019;22(4):403–11.

100. Tennant PWG, Murray EJ, Arnold KF, Berrie L, Fox MP, Gadd SC, et al. Use of directed acyclic graphs (DAGs) to identify confounders in applied health research: review and recommendations. *International Journal of Epidemiology*. 2020;50(2):620–32.

101. Daniel RM, De Stavola BL. Mediation analysis for life course studies. In: Ploubidis GB, Pongiglione B, De Stavola B, Daniel RM, Benova L, Grundy E, et al., eds. *Pathways to health*. Dordrecht: Springer Netherlands; 2019. pp. 1–40.

102. De Stavola BL, Daniel RM, Ploubidis GB, Micali N. Mediation analysis with intermediate confounding: structural equation modeling viewed through the causal inference lens. *American Journal of Epidemiology*. 2014;181(1):64–80.

103. Blum MR, Tan YJ, Ioannidis JPA. Use of E-values for addressing confounding in observational studies—an empirical assessment of the literature. *International Journal of Epidemiology*. 2020;49(5):1482–94.

104. Hardy R, Tilling K. Commentary: the use and misuse of life course models. *International Journal of Epidemiology*. 2016;45(4):1003–5.

105. Howe LD, Smith AD, Macdonald-Wallis C, Anderson EL, Galobardes B, Lawlor DA, et al. Relationship between mediation analysis and the structured life course approach. *International Journal of Epidemiology*. 2016;45(4):1280–94.

106. Smith AD, Hardy R, Heron J, Joinson CJ, Lawlor DA, Macdonald-Wallis C, et al. A structured approach to hypotheses involving continuous exposures over the life course. *International Journal of Epidemiology*. 2016;45(4):1271–9.

107. Mishra G, Nitsch D, Black S, De Stavola B, Kuh D, Hardy R. A structured approach to modelling the effects of binary exposure variables over the life course. *International Journal of Epidemiology*. 2008;38(2):528–37.

108. Chumbley J, Xu W, Potente C, Harris KM, Shanahan M. A Bayesian approach to comparing common models of life-course epidemiology. *International Journal of Epidemiology*. 2021;50(5):1660–70.

109. Madathil S, Joseph L, Hardy R, Rousseau M-C, Nicolau B. A Bayesian approach to investigate life course hypotheses involving continuous exposures. *International Journal of Epidemiology*. 2018;47(5):1623–35.

110. Hughes RA, Heron J, Sterne JAC, Tilling K. Accounting for missing data in statistical analyses: multiple imputation is not always the answer. *International Journal of Epidemiology*. 2019;48(4):1294–304.

111. Bradley V, Nichols TE. Addressing selection bias in the UK Biobank neurological imaging cohort. *medRxiv*. 2022:2022.01.13.22269266. https://doi.org/10.1101/2022.01.13.22269266.

112. Infante-Rivard C, Cusson A. Reflection on modern methods: selection bias—a review of recent developments. *International Journal of Epidemiology*. 2018;47(5):1714–22.

113. Lawlor DA, Tilling K, Davey Smith G. Triangulation in aetiological epidemiology. *International Journal of Epidemiology*. 2017;45(6):1866–86.

114. Davey Smith G, Ebrahim S. 'Mendelian randomization': can genetic epidemiology contribute to understanding environmental determinants of disease? *International Journal of Epidemiology*. 2003;32(1):1–22.

115. Sanderson E, Richardson TG, Morris TT, Tilling K, Davey Smith G. Estimation of causal effects of a time-varying exposure at multiple time points through multivariable mendelian randomization. *PLoS Genetics*. 2022;18(7):e1010290.

116. Strully KW, Mishra GD. Theoretical underpinning for the use of sibling studies in life course epidemiology. In: Lawlor DA, Mishra GD, eds. *Family matters. Designing, analysing and understanding family-based studies in life course epidemiology*. Oxford: Oxford University Press; 2009. pp. 35–56.

117. Dusetzina SB, Brookhart MA, Maciejewski ML. Control outcomes and exposures for improving internal validity of nonrandomized studies. *Health Services Research*. 2015;50(5):1432–51.

118. Smith GD. Negative control exposures in epidemiologic studies. *Epidemiology*. 2012;23(2):350–1; author reply 1–2.

119. Glymour MM. Natural experiments and instrumental variable analyses in social epidemiology. In: Oakes MJ, Kaufman JS, eds. *Methods in social epidemiology*. San Francisco: Jossey-Bass/Wiley; 2007. pp. 429–60.

120. Hernan MA, Robins JM. Instruments for causal inference: an epidemiologist's dream? *Epidemiology*. 2006;17(4):360–72.

121. Costeira R, Lee KA, Murray B, Christiansen C, Castillo-Fernandez J, Ni Lochlainn M, et al. Estrogen and COVID-19 symptoms: associations in women from the COVID Symptom Study. *PLoS One*. 2021;16(9):e0257051.

122. Garg R, Agrawal P, Gautam A, Pursnani N, Agarwal M, Agarwal A, et al. COVID-19 outcomes in postmenopausal and perimenopausal females: is estrogen hormone attributing to gender differences? *J Midlife Health*. 2020;11(4):250–6.

123. Ferrara A, Hedderson MM, Zhu Y, Avalos LA, Kuzniewicz MW, Myers LC, et al. Perinatal complications in individuals in California with or without SARS-CoV-2 infection during pregnancy. *JAMA Internal Medicine*. 2022;182(5):503–12.

124. Giri M, Puri A, Wang T, Guo S. Comparison of clinical manifestations, pre-existing comorbidities, complications and treatment modalities in severe and non-severe COVID-19 patients: a systemic review and meta-analysis. *Science Progress*. 2021;104(1):00368504211000906.

125. Honardoost M, Janani L, Aghili R, Emami Z, Khamseh ME. The association between presence of comorbidities and COVID-19 severity: a systematic review and meta-analysis. *Cerebrovasc Dis*. 2021;50(2):132–40.

126. Yang J, Zheng Y, Gou X, Pu K, Chen Z, Guo Q, et al. Prevalence of comorbidities and its effects in patients infected with SARS-CoV-2: a systematic review and meta-analysis. *Int J Infect Dis*. 2020;94:91–5.

127. World Health Organization. *Coronavirus disease (COVID-19): post COVID-19 condition [Internet]*. Geneva: World Health Organization; 2021 [updated 16 December 2021; cited 7 March 2022]. Available from: https://www.who.int/news-room/questions-and-answers/item/coronavirus-disease-(covid-19)-post-covid-19-condition.

128. Akpek M. Does COVID-19 cause hypertension? *Angiology*. 2022;73(7):682–7.

129. Xie Y, Al-Aly Z. Risks and burdens of incident diabetes in long COVID: a cohort study. *Lancet Diabetes & Endocrinology*. 2022;10(5):311–21.

130. Halawa S, Pullamsetti SS, Bangham CRM, Stenmark KR, Dorfmüller P, Frid MG, et al. Potential long-term effects of SARS-CoV-2 infection on the pulmonary vasculature: a global perspective. *Nature Reviews Cardiology*. 2022;19(5):314–31.

131. Santomauro DF, Mantilla Herrera AM, Shadid J, Zheng P, Ashbaugh C, Pigott DM, et al. Global prevalence and burden of depressive and anxiety disorders in 204 countries and territories in 2020 due to the COVID-19 pandemic. *Lancet*. 2021;398(10312):1700–12.

132. Alzueta E, Perrin P, Baker FC, Caffarra S, Ramos-Usuga D, Yuksel D, et al. How the COVID-19 pandemic has changed our lives: a study of psychological correlates across 59 countries. *Journal of Clinical Psychology*. 2021;77(3):556–70.

133. Alkatout I, Biebl M, Momenimovahed Z, Giovannucci E, Hadavandsiri F, Salehiniya H, et al. Has COVID-19 affected cancer screening programs? A systematic review. *Frontiers in Oncology*. 2021;11:675038.

134. Riera R, Bagattini ÂM, Pacheco RL, Pachito DV, Roitberg F, Ilbawi A. Delays and disruptions in cancer health care due to COVID-19 pandemic: systematic review. *JCO Global Oncology*. 2021;7:311–23.

135. Kuh D, Blodgett JM. Covid-19 across the life course. In: Duncan DT, Kawachi I, Morse SS, eds. *The social epidemiology of the Covid-19 pandemic*. New York: Oxford University Press; in press.

136. Centre for Education Policy and Equalising Opportunities. *COVID Social Mobility and Opportunities Study (COSMO) [Internet]*. London: University College London; 2022 [updated unknown date; cited 5 August 2022]. Available from: https://www.ucl.ac.uk/ioe/departments-and-centres/centres/centre-education-policy-and-equalising-opportunities/research-themes/schools/covid-social-mobility-and-opportunities-study-cosmo.

137. Centre For Longitudinal Studies. *Children of the 2020s Study [Internet]*. London: University College London; 2022 [updated unknown date; cited 5 August 2022]. Available from: https://cls.ucl.ac.uk/cls-studies/children-of-the-2020s-study/.

138. National Institutes of Health. *RECOVER: researching COVID to enhance recovery [Internet]*. Bethesda, MD: National Institutes of Health; 2022 [updated unknown date; cited 5 August 2022]. Available from: https://recovercovid.org/.

139. Li X, Vanderloo LM, Maguire JL, Keown-Stoneman CDG, Aglipay M, Anderson LN, et al. Public health preventive measures and child health behaviours during COVID-19: a cohort study. *Canadian Journal of Public Health*. 2021;112(5):831–42.

140. UK Government. *Women's health strategy for England [Policy paper]*. London: UK Government; 2022. CP 710.

141. Australian Government. *National women's health strategy 2020–2030*. Canberra: Australian Government; 2018.

142. Department for Work & Pensions. *Menopause and the workplace: how to enable fulfilling working lives: government response [Policy paper]*. London: UK Government; 2022.

143. Rich-Edwards JW. Reproductive health as a sentinel of chronic disease in women. *Women's Health*. 2009;5(2):101–5.

144. Lowe SA, Bowyer L, Lust K, McMahon LP, Morton M, North RA, et al. SOMANZ guidelines for the management of hypertensive disorders of pregnancy 2014. *Australian and New Zealand Journal of Obstetrics and Gynaecology*. 2015;55(5):e1–e29.

145. Government of South Australia. *South Australian perinatal practice guideline: diabetes mellitus and gestational diabetes (version 5)*. Adelaide: Government of South Australia; 2019.

146. Aldridge E, Verburg PE, Sierp S, Andraweera P, Dekker GA, Roberts CT, et al. A protocol for nurse-practitioner led cardiovascular follow-up after pregnancy complications in a socioeconomically disadvantaged population. *Frontiers in Cardiovascular Medicine*. 2020;6:184.

147. Richardson SS, Daniels CR, Gillman MW, Golden J, Kukla R, Kuzawa C, et al. Society: don't blame the mothers. *Nature*. 2014;512(7513):131–2.

148. Sharp GC, Schellhas L, Richardson SS, Lawlor DA. Time to cut the cord: recognizing and addressing the imbalance of DOHaD research towards the study of maternal pregnancy exposures. *Journal of Developmental Origins of Health and Disease*. 2019;10(5):509–12.

149. Amnesty International. *Criminalizing pregnancy: policing pregnant women who use drugs in the USA*. London: Amnesty International Ltd; 2017. AMR 51/6203/2017.

150. Sharp GC, Lawlor DA, Richardson SS. It's the mother!: how assumptions about the causal primacy of maternal effects influence research on the developmental origins of health and disease. *Social Science & Medicine*. 2018;213:20–7.

151. Blaylock R, Trickey H, Sanders J, Murphy C. WRISK voices: a mixed-methods study of women's experiences of pregnancy-related public health advice and risk messages in the UK. *Midwifery*. 2022;113:103433.

152. Kildea S, Gao Y, Hickey S, Nelson C, Kruske S, Carson A, et al. Effect of a birthing on country service redesign on maternal and neonatal health outcomes for First Nations Australians: a prospective, non-randomised, interventional trial. *Lancet Global Health*. 2021;9(5):e651–e659.

153. Marmot M, Allen J, Boyce T, Goldblatt P, Morrison J. *Health equity in England: the Marmot Review 10 years on*. London: Institute of Health Equity; 2020.

154. Bambra C. Going beyond the three worlds of welfare capitalism: regime theory and public health research. *Journal of Epidemiology and Community Health*. 2007;61(12):1098–102.

155. Álvarez-Gálvez J, Jaime-Castillo AM. The impact of social expenditure on health inequalities in Europe. *Social Science & Medicine*. 2018;200:9–18.

156. Cattan S, Conti G, Farquharson C, Ginja R. *The health effects of Sure Start*. London: Institute for Fiscal Studies; 2021.

157. Conti G, Heckman JJ, Pinto R. The effects of two influential early childhood interventions on health and healthy behaviour. *Economic Journal*. 2016;126(596):F28–F65.

158. Vallgårda S. Childhood obesity policies—mighty concerns, meek reactions. *Obesity Reviews*. 2018;19(3):295–301.

159. Adams J, Mytton O, White M, Monsivais P. Why are some population interventions for diet and obesity more equitable and effective than others? The role of individual agency. *PLoS Medicine*. 2016;13(4):e1001990.

160. Acton RB, Vanderlee L, Adams J, Kirkpatrick SI, Pedraza LS, Sacks G, et al. Tax awareness and perceived cost of sugar-sweetened beverages in four countries between 2017 and 2019: findings from the international food policy study. *International Journal of Behavioral Nutrition and Physical Activity*. 2022;19(1):38.

161. Caro JC, Corvalán C, Reyes M, Silva A, Popkin B, Taillie LS. Chile's 2014 sugar-sweetened beverage tax and changes in prices and purchases of sugar-sweetened beverages: An observational study in an urban environment. *PLoS Medicine*. 2018;15(7):e1002597.

162. Lawman HG, Bleich SN, Yan J, Hua SV, Lowery CM, Peterhans A, et al. One-year changes in sugar-sweetened beverage consumers' purchases following implementation of a beverage tax: a longitudinal quasi-experiment. *American Journal of Clinical Nutrition*. 2020;112(3):644–51.

163. Scarborough P, Adhikari V, Harrington RA, Elhussein A, Briggs A, Rayner M, et al. Impact of the announcement and implementation of the UK soft drinks industry levy on sugar content, price, product size and number of available soft drinks in the UK, 2015–19: a controlled interrupted time series analysis. *PLoS Medicine*. 2020;17(2):e1003025.

164. Love R, Adams J, van Sluijs EMF. Are school-based physical activity interventions effective and equitable? A meta-analysis of cluster randomized controlled trials with accelerometer-assessed activity. *Obesity Reviews*. 2019;20(6):859–70.

165. Jull J, Whitehead M, Petticrew M, Kristjansson E, Gough D, Petkovic J, et al. When is a randomised controlled trial health equity relevant? Development and validation of a conceptual framework. *BMJ Open*. 2017;7(9):e015815.

166. Le Brocq S, Clare K, Bryant M, Roberts K, Tahrani AA. Obesity and COVID-19: a call for action from people living with obesity. *Lancet Diabetes & Endocrinology*. 2020;8(8):652–4.

Index

For the benefit of digital users, indexed terms that span two pages (e.g., 52–53) may, on occasion, appear on only one of those pages.

Tables and figures are indicated by *t* and *f* following the page number

abdominal fat, type 2 diabetes 99
accumulation model 5
  breast cancer 196
ACE *see* adverse childhood experiences (ACE)
ACTH *see* adrenocorticotropic hormone (ACTH)
AD *see* Alzheimer's disease (AD)
ADHD (attention-deficit hyperactivity
  disorder) 302–3
adiposity
  early menopause 54
  reproductive health and 21–22
  type 2 diabetes 97
adolescence
  breast cancer 191
  depression 158, 162
  exposures during and endometriosis 39
  health behaviours 264–65
  high body mass index 278–79
  knowledge transfer and 377–78
  peer relationships 314–15
  reproductive health 23–24
  social relationships 314–15
adrenarche, hypothalamic–pituitary–adrenal axis 241
adrenocorticotropic hormone (ACTH) 240–41
  ageing 242
  pregnancy 241
adult environment
  depression 154
  health behaviours 265–66
  reproductive health 24
  social relationships 315–17
adverse childhood experiences (ACE) 335, 389
  cardiovascular disease 82–83
  childhood social inequalities in health 303–4
  cross-study analysis 391
  depression 157
  early menopause 52
  health effects 396
  obesity 281
age at menarche 19–20, 21–22
  cardiovascular disease 77
  early and endometriosis 39
  early menopause 53
  gynaecological cancers 206
  health effect 389–90
  hysterectomy 56
  type 2 diabetes 98

age at menopause
  cardiovascular disease 77–78
  disease risk factors 51–54
  health effect 389–90
ageing
  ghrelin 244–45
  hypothalamic–pituitary–adrenal axis 242
  hypothalamus–pituitary–gonadal axis 240
  leptin 246
  musculoskeletal ageing 118–20
  thyrotropic axis 243
air pollution, lung function deficits/COPD 140
airways 135
alcohol consumption 260
  binge drinking 260
  breast cancer 190
  cardiovascular disease 75
  COVID-19 pandemic 266
  endometriosis 40
  gynaecological cancers 209–10
  health behaviour effects 263, 265–66
  hysterectomy 57
  obesity and 282
  type 2 diabetes 102–3
allele frequencies, ethnicity 232
allergics 42
alveoli 135
Alzheimer's disease (AD)
  female verbal memory 171–72
  menopause 175–76
  neuroimaging biomarkers 392–93
  pathology 169–70
  protective factors 175–78
  risk factors 173–78
  sex differences 170, 172–73
AMH *see* anti-Müllerian hormone (AMH)
amyloid b (Aβ) protein 169–70
androstenedione 241
animal models, type 2 diabetes 95
antenatal care 366*t*
anti-inflammatory compounds 209
anti-Müllerian hormone (AMH) 240
  early menopause 53
antioxidants 209
anxiety 160–61
  later-life effects 328*f*
  menopausal transition 59

APOE4 174
area deprivation 301–2
ART *see* assisted reproductive treatment (ART)
aspirin 212
assisted contraception 366*t*
   see also combined oral contraceptive (COC);
     oral contraceptives; progestin-only
     contraceptive (POC)
assisted reproductive treatment (ART) 390–91
   endometriosis 40
asthma
   endometriosis 42
   lung function deficits/COPD 140
Atherosclerosis in Communities Study 102–3
attention-deficit hyperactivity disorder
     (ADHD) 302–3
attitudinal gender inequality, violence against
     women 349
Australian Longitudinal Study on Women's Health
   endometriosis 35
   obesity 278*f*
autoimmune diseases 334
   endometriosis 42
Avon Longitudinal Study of Parents and Children 75

back pain 59
Barker, David 4–5
behaviour
   change technique in urinary incontinence 379
   early menopause 53–54
   health and well-being and 318
   musculoskeletal ageing 123–25
   obesity 282
benign gynaecological conditions 208
Benn index, obesity definition 274
Better for women: Improving the Health and Wellbeing of
   Girls and Workers (Royal College of Obstetricians
   and Gynaecology) 9–10
bilateral oophorectomy 49, 50, 54
   see also surgical menopause
binge drinking 260
biology
   health and well-being and 318–19
   omic studies 228–29
birth characteristics, endometriosis 38–39
birth cohort studies 4–5
   menopause 50
birth size
   cardiovascular disease 81–82
   type 2 diabetes 95
birthweight
   Alzheimer's disease 173–74
   breast cancer 192
   cardiovascular disease 81
   early menopause 52
   endometriosis 38–39
   growth *vs.* 22–23
   gynaecological cancers in 206
   type 2 diabetes 95
blood pressure
   cardiovascular disease 75–76

high *see* hypertension
   social relationships 318–19
   systolic blood pressure 75–76, 84*f*
BMD *see* bone mineral density (BMD)
BMI *see* body mass index (BMI)
body mass index (BMI)
   age-standardised changes 275*f*
   body weight measurement 273
   breast cancer 195–96
   changes in 274–76
   genetic risk factors 388
   hysterectomy 57
   increases in 397
   limitations of 274
   musculoskeletal ageing 122–23
   older age 276
   omics 229
   prepregnancy, effects of 387
   reproductive health 24
   see also body weight
body size
   changes in 274–76
   early menopause 54
   endometriosis 40–41
   gynaecological cancers 211
body weight 273–92
   breast cancer 190, 195–96
   chronic conditions 334
   definition 273–74
   endometriosis 40
   gynaecological cancers 206, 208–9, 211
   health burden 276–79
   hysterectomy 57
   measurement 273–74
   social burden 276–79
   see also body mass index (BMI); obesity
bone mineral density (BMD)
   musculoskeletal ageing 118
   osteoporosis definition 117
brain function, sex differences 173
brain metabolism, Alzheimer's disease 173
BRCA1 223, 231
   gynaecological cancers 205
   surgical menopause 54
BRCA2 223, 231
   gynaecological cancers 205
   surgical menopause 54
breast cancer 189–202
   adolescence 191
   adult risk factors 190
   endometriosis 42
   genome-wide association studies 230*t*
   genomics and 223
   infant factors 192–93
   life course methods 193, 194*f*, 195–96
   menopausal hormone therapy 60
   pregnancy 190
   prenatal factors 192–93
   puberty 191–92
   reproductive health 25
   screening 366*t*

Breast Cancer Family Registry 191
breastfeeding
    Alzheimer's disease 173–74
    breast cancer 190, 193
    cardiovascular disease 82
    endometriosis 40
    gynaecological cancers 207
    type 2 diabetes 100–1
BRIP1 205
British Birth Cohort Study (1946) 59,
        159, 300
British Cohort Study (1970) 300
bullying 158

Canadian Institute of Health Research of Knowledge
        Translation 372
cancer, body weight 276–78
CARDIA study *see* Coronary Artery Risk
        Development in Young Adults (CARDIA) study
cardiorespiratory fitness, type 2 diabetes 101–2
cardiovascular disease (CVD) 73–92
    Alzheimer's disease risk factors 174
    body weight 276–78
    COVID-19 pandemic 394
    early life risk factors 81–83
    endometriosis 42
    experience in utero 362–63
    genetic risks 80
    later life risk factors 83
    reproductive health 25
    risk factors 75–76
    sex-specific factors 76–79
    sex-specific prevalence 74*f*
    short stature 387–88
    social inequalities 79–80, 316, 318
cardiovascular system, pregnancy in 386
caregiving
    health effects 330
    structural sexism 329–31
causal mediation analysis 393
CEE (conjugated equine oestrogen) 176–77
central metabolic regulation, endocrine
        pathways 243–46, 244*f*
    see also ghrelin; leptin
central sensitization, endometriosis 39
cerebrovascular disease 74
    endometriosis 42
cervical cancer
    hysterectomy and 210
    incidence 203
    risk factors 204*t*
    see also gynaecological cancers
cervical caner, screening 366*t*
CFB (complementary food and beverages)
        281–82
chain of risk model 5
    breast cancer 196
chain reaction, breast cancer 196
CHEK2 223, 229
    menopause timing 228
child abuse 350

childhood
    asthma 140
    body mass index and cardiovascular disease 25
    depression risk factors 157–58
    endometriosis 39
    growth and cardiovascular disease 82
    health behaviours 265
    health interventions 365, 366*t*
    intimate partner violence 344–46
    obesity and overweight 274, 276
    obesity and reproductive health 23–24
    reproductive health 23–24
    socioeconomic position 300
    trauma 334–35
    vaccinations 366*t*
Chlamydia trachomatis screening 361–62
cholesterol 75
chronic diseases
    endometriosis 41–42
    later-life effects 327, 328*f*
    see also diseases (NCDs)
chronic obstructive pulmonary disorder (COPD)
    body weight 276–78
    definition 138
    development 135–36
    life course perspective 138–39
    pathogenesis 139
    prognosis 139
    reproductive exposures 144–46
    risk factors 140–43, 142*f*
    sex differences 139–40
Cochrane Review (2014), type 2 diabetes 100
Cochrane Review (2017), menopausal hormone
        therapy 60
coding sequence variations 222
cognitive function
    decline in 318
    depression risk factors 160–61
    early menopause 52
    sex differences 170–71
cohort studies 392–93
    endometriosis 39
combined oral contraceptive (COC)
    endometriosis 39–40
    gynaecological cancers 207
    type 2 diabetes 99
community-based participatory research 378
complementary food and beverages (CFB) 281–82
computed tomography (CT), body weight 273
conjugated equine oestrogen (CEE) 176–77
Conner's conceptual model for research evaluation 373
contraception 363, 366*t*
    gynaecological cancers 207
    progestin-only contraceptive (POC) 99–100
    progestin-releasing intrauterine devices (IUDs) 207
    see also combined oral contraceptive (COC);
        oral contraceptives; progestin-only
        contraceptive (POC)
Coordinate Implementation Model 373
COPD *see* chronic obstructive pulmonary
        disorder (COPD)

Copenhagen School Health Record Registry 195
coronary artery disease 276–78
Coronary Artery Risk Development in Young Adults
　　(CARDIA) study 99–100
　cardiovascular disease 77–78
coronary heart disease 73–74
corticotropin-releasing hormone (CRH) 240–41
　pregnancy 241
cortisol 241
　ageing 242
COSMO trial 394–95
counselling, health behaviours 257–58
COVID-19 pandemic 11, 394–95, 397
　body weight 276–78
　health behaviours 266
　health care implications 367
　long-term consequences 394–95
　musculoskeletal ageing 115–16, 125
　omics studies 232–33
　reproductive health 389
　social inequalities in health 301, 302
　violence against women 350–51
COX inhibitors 212
C-reactive protein (CRP) 304
CRH see corticotropin-releasing hormone (CRH)
critical window, breast cancer 196
cross-country comparisons, social inequalities in
　　health 298
cross-study analysis 391–95
culture
　changes in 390–91
　depression 161

DCLRE1A 228
Deciphering Developmental Disorders 221
dehydroepiandrosterone (DHEA) 241, 248f
dehydroepiandrosterone sulphate (DHEAS) 241
delayed puberty 223–24
dementia 169–88
　definition 169
　see also Alzheimer's disease (AD)
DENND1A 225
depression 153–67
　across life course 153–55, 154f
　adolescence 158
　Alzheimer's disease risk factors 174
　cognitive styles 160–61
　culture 161
　evidence integration 161
　intimate partner violence 348
　later-life effects 328f
　menopause 59, 159
　older age 159
　personality 160–61
　pregnancy 159
　risk factors 155–61
　social factors 161
dermatologic characteristics,
　　endometriosis 40–41
DES see diethylstilbestrol (DES)

development
　ghrelin 244
　growth hormone 247
　hypothalamus–pituitary–gonadal axis 238
　thyrotropic axis 242–43
Developmental Origins of Health and Disease
　　(DOHaD) 4–5, 362–63, 393–94, 396
　type 2 diabetes 95
DEXA (dual-energy X-ray absorptiometry) 273
DHEA (dehydroepiandrosterone) 241, 248f
DHEAS (dehydroepiandrosterone sulphate) 241
diabetes mellitus 93–114
　cardiovascular disease 75
　COVID-19 pandemic 394
　experience in utero 362–63
　gynaecological cancers 211–12
　later-life effects 328f
　obesity 280
　see also gestational diabetes mellitus (GDM); type
　　1 diabetes mellitus (T1DM); type 2 diabetes
　　mellitus (T2DM)
diet 260–61
　COVID-19 pandemic 266
　gynaecological cancers 209
　health behaviour effects 265
　musculoskeletal ageing 124
　obesity 282
Dietary Intervention Study in Children 192
diethylstilbestrol (DES)
　breast cancer 190, 193
　cardiovascular disease 75
　endometriosis 38
directed acrylic graphs 393
disease overlap, omic studies 229
divorce 52, 59, 162, 263–64, 298–99, 317, 331, 389
　health effects 332
　social inequalities in health 298
DNA 94, 121, 156, 157, 162, 206–7, 221, 226–28, 304
　chemical modification 225
　methylation in depression 157
DOHaD see Developmental Origins of Health and
　　Disease (DOHaD)
drug discovery 229–31
drug use see illicit drug use
dual-energy X-ray absorptiometry (DEXA) 273
dynorphin 237
dysmenorrhoea 33, 39
dysthymia 154–55

early life
　Alzheimer's disease risk factors 173–74
　breast cancer 189–90
　contribution of 5–6
　depression 156–57
　origins of health 387–89
　social relationships 314–15
Early vs Late Intervention Trial with Estradiol
　　(ELITE) 176–77
ecological understanding, violence against
　　women 344, 346f, 351f

educational attainment
  Alzheimer's disease 178
  attention-deficit hyperactivity disorder 302–3
  health behaviour effects 264
  hysterectomy 56–57
  menopausal hormone therapy 61
  parents, health behaviour effects 263
  social inequalities in health 297–98, 301–2
elder abuse 350
ELITE trial 59–60
emotions
  early menopause 52
  intimate partner violence 346
endocrine-disrupting chemicals 41
endocrine pathways 237–56, 239f
  central metabolic regulation 243–46
  see also ghrelin; growth hormone/insulin-like
     growth factor (GH/IGF) axis; hypothalamic–
     pituitary–adrenal (HPA) axis; hypothalamic–
     pituitary–gonadal (HPG) axis; leptin;
     thyrotropic axis
endogenous oestrogens, breast cancer 196
endometrial cancer
  body weight 276–78
  endometriosis 42
  hysterectomy 210
  pregnancy 207
  risk factors 204t
  treatment 229–31
  tubal ligation and 210
  see also gynaecological cancers
endometriosis 33–48, 34f
  adult factors 39–41
  aetiology 37
  allergies 42
  asthma 42
  autoimmune diseases 42
  cardiovascular disease 42
  chronic diseases 41–42
  diagnostic challenges 35
  economic burden 36
  ethnicity and prevalence 34–35
  genetic factors 37–38
  genome-wide association studies 230t
  genomics and 223
  gynaecological cancers and 208
  heritability 37–38
  hysterectomy 55
  incidence rates 35
  ovarian cancer 41
  pathology 33
  prevalence and burden 34–36, 392
  quality of life and 36
  risk factors 37–41
  superficial endometriosis 35
  surgery 33
  surgical menopause 54
  in utero exposures 38–39
environment
  breast cancer 190

chemical exposure and endometriosis 41
lung function deficits/COPD 140, 144
epidemiology causal inference 231–32
epigenetics 387
  breast cancer 196
  depression 157
  musculoskeletal ageing 121
epigenomics 225
  definition 221
eQTLs 226
ethnicity, allele frequencies 232
European Community Respiratory Health Survey 145
European Institute for Gender Equality 4
exercise see physical activity

families
  history of breast cancer 190
  reconstituted families 314
  socioeconomic position (SEP) 298–99
  studies of 223
FEF$_{25\%-75\%}$ (forced expiratory flow over the middle half
     of the FVC) 136, 137t
female-to-male transsexuals 171
fertility 20
  body weight and 278
  decline pre-menopause 51
  treatment in gynaecological cancers 208
fertilization 240
FEV$_1$ (forced expiratory volume in the first
     second) 136, 137t
FEV$_1$/FVC ratio 136, 137t
  chronic obstructive pulmonary disease 138
fibroids see uterine fibroids
financial impacts, intimate partner violence 348
flour fortification 365
foetal development, early menopause 52
foetal origins of adult disease hypothesis 81
folic acid 365
follicle-stimulating hormone (FSH) 237
  development 238
  menstrual cycle 238, 239f
follicular maturation, hypothalamus–pituitary–
     gonadal axis 240
forced expiratory flow over the middle half of the FVC
     (FEF$_{25\%-75\%}$) 136, 137t
forced expiratory volume in the first second
     (FEV$_1$) 136, 137t
  see also FEV$_1$/FVC ratio
forced vital capacity (FVC) 136, 137t
  see also FEV$_1$/FVC ratio
Foundation for the National Institutes of Health
     (FNIH) 120
frailty, cardiovascular disease 83
Framework convention on Tobacco Control (2003)
     (WHO) 259
FSH see follicle-stimulating hormone (FSH)
FSHR 221
FVC (forced vital capacity) 136, 137t

gamma radiation, breast cancer 191

GDM *see* gestational diabetes mellitus (GDM)
gender
    Alzheimer's disease 178
    definition 4, 170
    social constructions 328
gender-based violence *see* violence against
        women (VAW)
gender gap
    depression 154–55, 156–57
    earnings gap 298–99
    health effects 328
gene–environment interplay, depression 156
gene expression 387
Generation R study 81–82
genetic factors
    depression 155–56, 162
    early menopause 51–52
    health behaviour effects 262–63
    hysterectomy 55–56
    lung function deficits/COPD 140
    musculoskeletal ageing 120–21
    obesity 279
    reproductive health 22
    types of differences 222
Genetics of Osteoarthritis and Lifestyle
        (GOAL) 122–23
Genome Aggregation Database (genomAD) 222
genome sequencing 223–24
    time taken 221
genome-wide association studies (GWAS) 224–25,
        230*t*, 392–93
    biological insights 228–29
    depression 155–56
    early menopause 52
    endometriosis 38
    health behaviour effects 262–63
    obesity 279
    reproductive health 22
    type 2 diabetes 93–94
genomics 222–23
    imprinting in type 2 diabetes 94
    role of 223
    technologies 223–28
Genotype-Tissue Expression (GTEx) 226
gestational age, breast cancer 193
gestational diabetes mellitus (GDM) 95, 363, 395
    obesity 280
    offspring body mass index 96
    type 2 diabetes and 100–1, 360
ghrelin 244*f*, 244–45
    ageing 244–45
    development 244
GHRH (growth hormone-releasing hormone) 246
glucocorticoids 246
GnRH *see* gonadotropin-releasing hormone (GnRH)
GOAL (Genetics of Osteoarthritis and
        Lifestyle) 122–23
gonadotropin-releasing hormone (GnRH) 237
    development 238
gray divorce economic penalty 332

Great Gatsby Curve 297–98
grip strength 385–86
    musculoskeletal ageing 119*f*
growth
    musculoskeletal ageing 122
    in utero growth *vs.* 22–23
growth hormone/insulin-like growth factor (GH/IGF)
        axis 246–48, 247*f*
    age-related changes 248
    changes across life stages 247–48, 248*f*
    development 247
    pregnancy 247–48
growth hormone-releasing hormone (GHRH) 246
growth measures, cross-study analysis 391
GWAS *see* genome-wide association studies (GWAS)
gynaecological cancers 203–18
    age at menarche 206
    alcohol consumption 209–10
    benign gynaecological conditions 208
    birthweight 206
    body size 211
    body weight 206, 208–9, 211
    breastfeeding 207
    contraception 207
    diabetes 211–12
    diet 209
    early life to menarche 203–6
    fertility treatment 208
    genetic risks 205
    height 206, 208–9
    human papilloma virus infection 206–7
    hysterectomy 210
    infertility 208
    medications 211–12
    menarche to menopause 206–11
    menopausal hormone therapy 211
    metabolic syndrome 211–12
    natural menopause, age at 210–11
    physical activity 209, 211
    pregnancy 207
    risk factors 204*t*
    sexual activity 206–7
    smoking 209–10, 211
    tubal ligation 210
    in utero exposure 206
    see also cervical cancer; uterine cancer

Haplotype Reference Consortium (HRC) 224–25
HAPO (Hyperglycaemia and Adverse Pregnancy
        Outcome) cohort 96
HbA1c levels 100–1
hCG (human chorionic hormone) 240
health behaviours 257–71
    adolescence 264–65
    adult transitions 265–66
    behavioural capital 264
    before birth 262–63
    COVID-19 pandemic 266
    current perspectives 257–58
    endometriosis 40–41

hysterectomy 57
life course framework 261–66, 262*f*
reproductive factors and 389–90
social context 258–61
socioeconomic environment 261–62, 263–64
temporal context 258–61
health care 359–70
COVID-19 pandemic 367
delivery implications 360–65, 361*f*
hysterectomy 57–58
impact of 365–67
relevant features 359–60, 360*f*
health effects
body weight 276–79
intimate partner violence 348
health inequalities, socioeconomic position
(SEP) 299–301
health policy 395–97
heart disease 328*f*
see also coronary heart disease; ischaemic heart disease
heart health, definition 10
heart rate, social relationships 318–19
height
breast cancer 195–96
gynaecological cancers 206, 208–9
weight-for-height indices 273
HICs *see* high-income countries (HICs)
high blood pressure *see* hypertension
high-income countries (HICs)
cardiovascular disease 73
childhood social inequalities in health 300
menopause 21
obesity 273, 388
social inequalities in health 296, 302
histone proteins, acetylation 225
holistic health care 361–62
hormonal contraceptives
breast cancer 190
cardiovascular disease 79
lung function deficits/COPD 144
type 2 diabetes 99–100
see also combined oral contraceptive (COC);
oral contraceptives; progestin-only
contraceptive (POC)
hormone exposure, endometriosis 38
hormone replacement therapy (HRT) *see* menopausal
hormone therapy (MHT)
hormone therapy, Alzheimer's disease 171,
175, 176–77
see menopausal hormone therapy (MHT)
hot flushes 58–59
HPA axis *see* hypothalamic–pituitary–adrenal
(HPA) axis
HPG axis *see* hypothalamic–pituitary–gonadal
(HPG) axis
HPT (hypothalamic–pituitary–thyroid) axis *see*
thyrotropic axis
HRC (Haplotype Reference Consortium) 224–25
HRT *see* menopausal hormone therapy (MHT)
human chorionic hormone (hCG) 240

Human Development Index
gynaecological cancers 203
natural menopause 50
human papillomavirus (HPV)
infection 206–7
vaccination 361–62, 366*t*
HUNT study 25, 392
3-hydroxy-3-methylglutaryl coenzyme A (HMG-CoA)
reductase 212
11-hydroxysteroid-dehydrogenase 2 241
hypercholestaemia 75
hyperglycaemia 96
type 2 diabetes 95–97
Hyperglycaemia and Adverse Pregnancy Outcome
(HAPO) cohort 96
hypertension
cardiovascular disease 76
COVID-19 pandemic 394
endometriosis 42
pregnancy 395
hypothalamic peptides 246
hypothalamic–pituitary–adrenal (HPA) axis 238–
40, 239*f*
adrenarche 241
ageing 242
changes across life course 241–42
depression 156
early menopause 52
pregnancy 241
psychological stress 389
hypothalamic–pituitary–gonadal (HPG) axis 237–
40, 239*f*
age-related changes 240
development 238
follicular maturation 240
menstrual cycle regulation 238–40
hypothalamic–pituitary–thyroid (HPT) axis *see*
thyrotropic axis
hysterectomy 55–58
gynaecological cancers 210
indications 55
risk factors for 55–58

iatrogenic menopause 49
idiopathic hypogonadotropic hypogonadism
(IHH) 223–24
IHH (idiopathic hypogonadotropic
hypogonadism) 223–24
illicit drug use 260
health behaviour effects 263
income, smoking and 260
indoor air pollution, lung function deficits/COPD 143
infants
breast cancer 192–93
obesity 281–82
infertility
endometriosis 40
gynaecological cancers 208
infiltrating endometriosis (DIE) 35
inflammation, social relationships 318–19

insufficient physical activity 261
insulin, age-related changes 246
integrated knowledge transfer 372–73
intergenerational social mobility 296–98
InterLACE (International Collaboration for a Life
    Course Approach to Reproductive Health and
    Chronic Disease Events)
    cardiovascular disease 76–77
    early menopause 53
    menopause definition 20–21
interleukin 6 (IL-6) 304
International Agency for Research on Cancer
    (IARC) 190
intimate partner violence (IPV)
    adverse health conditions 348, 349f
    childhood effects 344–46, 347f
    health effects 348
    physiological stress response 348
    social impact 348
    see also violence against women (VAW)
intracellular fibrillary tangles, Alzheimer's
    disease 169–70
in utero exposure
    growth vs. 22–23
    gynaecological cancers in 206
ionising radiation, breast cancer 191
IPV see intimate partner violence (IPV)
ischaemic heart disease 42
isolation 318
    social relationships 316–17

joint pain 59

KCNQ1 94
KEEPS (Kronos Early Estrogen Prevention Study) 59–
    60, 176–77
KLF14 94
Knowledge-to-Action (K2A) cycle 373, 374f
    menopause 375–77, 376t
knowledge translation (KT) 372–73
    across life cycle 377–79
    definition 372
    health care 375–77
    Knowledge-to-Action cycle 373, 374f
    theories, models, framework (TMFs) 373–75
Kronos Early Estrogen Prevention Study (KEEPS) 59–
    60, 176–77

Lancet Commission (2020) 169
LDL (low-density lipoprotein) cholesterol 212
leptin 245–46
    age-related changes 246
    changes across life stages 248f
    changes during development 245
    placenta-derived 246
    pregnancy 246
LGBTIQA+ population 258
LH see luteinising hormone (LH)
life course
    depression risk factors 159–60
    epidemiology 3

models 5–6
    social inequalities 396–97
    structural sexism 328–29
    trajectories 385–86
lifestyle determinants, type 2 diabetes 101–3
Lifetime Risk Pooling Project 76
LIN28B 228
LMICs see low- and middle-income studies (LMICs)
loneliness 318
    social relationships 316–17
longitudinal birth cohorts 392
longitudinal studies, wearable devices 386
low- and middle-income studies (LMICs)
    health life course perspective 393
    health systems 396
    lung function deficits/COPD 143
    obesity 273
    social inequalities in health 296
    type 2 diabetes 103, 104
low-density lipoprotein (LDL) cholesterol 212
lung anatomy 135
lung cancer, body weight 276–78
lung function 385–86
    later-life effects 328f
    life course 136–37
    lifetime trajectories 137, 138f, 141f
    reproductive exposures 144–46
    risk factors 140–43, 142f
    sex differences 139–40
    see also respiratory disease
lupus 334
luteinising hormone (LH) 237
    fertilization 240
    menstrual cycle 238, 239f

magnetic resonance imaging (MRI)
    Alzheimer's disease 176
    body weight measurement 273
major depressive disorders (MDDs) 155
MAP (mean arterial pressure) 190
Marmot Review 396
marriage status
    Alzheimer's disease 178
    depression 161
    health and 331
    social inequalities in health 298
    see also partnerships
MC3T 228
MDDs (major depressive disorders) 155
mean arterial pressure (MAP) 190
measles, mumps, rubella (MMR) vaccine 365
medical abortions, COVID-19 pandemic 367
medications, gynaecological cancers 211–12
menarche 19–20
    age at see age at menarche
    breast cancer 192
    genome-wide association studies 230t
    mean age 224–25
    menopause transition, gynaecological cancers 206–11
    timing of 223
    type 2 diabetes 97–98

Mendelian randomization (MR) studies 231–
    32, 387–88
  Alzheimer's disease 175–76
  body weight 276
  genetic variants 393–94
  musculoskeletal ageing 121
  obesity 282
  reproductive health 22
menopausal hormone therapy (MHT) 59–61
  breast cancer 190
  cardiovascular disease 77, 79
  gynaecological cancers 210, 211
  lung function deficits/COPD 144
menopause 20–21
  Alzheimer's disease 175–76
  body mass index and 283
  definition 20–21
  depression risk factors 159
  genome-wide association studies 230t
  health behaviour 265–66
  Knowledge-to-Action cycle 375–77, 376t
  lifetime risk factors 58–59
  musculoskeletal ageing 118, 121
  symptom reporting 58–59
  timing and genetics 228
  timing of 223
  type 2 diabetes 99
  see also age at menopause; natural menopause;
      surgical menopause
menstrual cycle 20
  hypothalamus–pituitary–gonadal axis 238–40, 239f
  length and endometriosis 39–40
  short and early menopause 53
  type 2 diabetes 97–98
mental health, social inequalities in health 304, 318
metabolic syndrome, gynaecological cancers 211–12
metabolomics 226–28
methodology 393–94
MHT see menopausal hormone therapy (MHT)
migraine 59
Millennium Cohort Study (2001 MCS) 280–81
mitochondrial inheritance, type 2 diabetes 94
MLH1 205
MMR (measles, mumps, rubella) vaccine 365
mortality, secular changes 300
MRC National Survey of Health and Development
    cardiovascular disease 77–78
  obesity 279
MRI see magnetic resonance imaging (MRI)
MR-pheWAS (MR phenome-wide association
    studies) 76–77
MR studies see Mendelian randomization (MR)
    studies
MSH2 205
MSH6 205
multimorbidities, musculoskeletal ageing 115–16
multiple pregnancies, early menopause 51–52
muscle mass 118
musculoskeletal ageing 115–33
  behavioural risk factors 123–25
  definitions 117–18

genetic factors 120–21
growth 122
obesity 122–23
oestrogen 121–22
phenotypic changes 118–20
publications 116f
musculoskeletal disease 328f

National Health and Nutrition Examination
    Survey (US) 75
National Health Examination and Nutrition Survey 24
National Longitudinal Study of Adolescent
    Health 102–3
National Survey of Health and Development
    (NSHD) 122–23
national vaccination programs 365
National Women's Health Strategy (Australian
    Government) 10
natural menopause 50–54
  age at 49
  biology of 51
  definition 49
  gynaecological cancers 210–11
NCDs see noncommunicable diseases (NCDs)
neural tube defects 365
neuroimaging, Alzheimer's disease 176, 392–93
neurokinin B 237
neuropeptide/Agouti-related protein (NPY/AGRP) 245
neuroticism 162
newborn screening 365, 366t
  blood spots 366t
NICE
  menopausal hormone therapy 60
  menopause guidelines 50
night sweats 58–59
Non-Communicable Disease Risk Factor Collaboration
    (NCD-RisC) 274, 391–92
noncommunicable diseases (NCDs) 6, 11
  reproductive health 25 26
North American Menopause Society 60
NPY/AGRP (neuropeptide/Agouti-related
    protein) 245
NSHD (National Survey of Health and
    Development) 122–23
nulliparity, early menopause 53
Nurses Health Study 191
nutrients
  musculoskeletal ageing 124
  sensing in omics 229
nutrition 52, 93, 95, 98, 102, 124, 140, 189–90, 192
  breast cancer 191
  cardiovascular disease 82
  overnutrition 104, 246, 280
  undernutrition 4–5, 104
  type 2 diabetes 102

obesity 397
  across life course 277f
  behavioural factors 282
  cardiovascular disease 75
  causes 279–83

obesity (*cont.*)
    childhood 389–90
    diabetes 280
    diet 282
    experience in utero 362–63
    genetics 279
    gynaecological cancers and 208
    high-income countries 388
    hyperglycaemia 96
    infant feeding 281–82
    lung function deficits/COPD 140
    musculoskeletal ageing 122–23
    physical activity 282
    policy implications 283
    prenatal body weight 280
    reproductive factors 282–83
    sarcopenia and 123
    social factors 280–81
    social relationships 318–19
    see also body weight; overweight
obesity epidemic 387–88, 390
occupational exposure, lung function deficits/
    COPD 140, 143–44
oestradiol
    development 238
    hysterectomy 56
oestrogen 204*t*, 208, 209–10, 211, 212–13, 232, 240
    cardiovascular disease 76–77
    depression 159
    endogenous, breast cancer 196
    leptin and 245
    musculoskeletal ageing 121–22
    pregnancy 241
    type 2 diabetes 97–98
oestrogen receptor (ER) negative breast
    cancer 190
older age
    body mass index (body mass index) 276
    breast cancer 190
    depression risk factors 159
    health behaviour effects 262
OMA (ovarian endometriosis) 35
omic studies 221–36
    biological insights 228–29
    drug discovery 229–31
    epidemiology causal inference 231–32
    future work 232–33
    personal risk prediction 231
    population risk prediction 231
    unmet needs 232
    see also epigenomics; genome sequencing; genome-
      wide association studies (GWAS); metabolomics;
      proteomics; transcriptomics
100,000 Genomes project 221
oral contraceptives
    Alzheimer's disease 175, 178
    hysterectomy 56
    see also combined oral contraceptive (COC);
      hormonal contraceptives; progestin-only
      contraceptive (POC)

osteoarthritis 115
    definitions 117–18
    diagnosis 120
    see also musculoskeletal ageing
Osteoarthritis Biomarkers Consortium 120
osteoporosis 115
    definition 117
    knowledge transfer and 378
    see also musculoskeletal ageing
Ottawa Model of Research Use 373
Our Vision for the Women's Health Strategy for England
    (UK Government) 9–10
ovarian cancer
    endometriosis 41
    genome-wide association studies 230*t*
    pregnancy 207
    risk factors 204*t*
    tubal ligation and 210
ovarian cysts 54
ovarian endometriosis (OMA) 35
ovarian function, hypothalamic–pituitary–adrenal
    axis 237
overweight 397
    across life course 277*f*
    see also obesity

pain disorders 39
parent-of-offspring effects, type 2 diabetes 94
parents
    conflict 314
    smoking 140
    social relationships 314
parity
    breast cancer 190
    cardiovascular disease 78
    type 2 diabetes 100–1
partnerships 331–33
    cardiovascular disease 80
    depression 161
    social relationships 317
    see also marriage status
paternal gene expression 387
PCOS *see* polycystic ovarian syndrome (PCOS)
peak expiratory flow rate (PEF) 136, 137*t*
peer relationships
    adolescence 314–15
    rejection and depression 158
PEF (peak expiratory flow rate) 136, 137*t*
pelvic infections 54
pelvic pain
    endometriosis 33
    surgical menopause 54
personality 160–61
personal risk prediction 231
perverse fluidity 297
PET (positron emission tomography), Alzheimer's
    disease 173, 176
phosphorylated tau protein 169–70
physical activity
    breast cancer 190, 191

cardiovascular disease 75
COVID-19 pandemic 266
gynaecological cancers 209, 211
health behaviour effects 265
hysterectomy 57
musculoskeletal ageing 124
obesity 282
type 2 diabetes 101–2
physical development, social inequalities in
    health 302–3
physician advice, health behaviours 257–58
physiological stress response, intimate partner
    violence 348
Pike model, breast cancer 196
placenta, leptin 246
plant-based diet, hysterectomy 57
PMS2 205
POI (premature ovarian insufficiency) 50, 223–24
policy/practice 371–81
    obesity 283
    see also knowledge translation (KT)
polycystic ovarian syndrome (PCOS) 221
    genome-wide association studies 230*t*
    genomics and 223
    gynaecological cancers and 208
    susceptibility to 225
    type 2 diabetes 98–99
polygenic risk scores (PRS) 155–56
POMC (pro-opiomelanocortin) neurons 245
populations
    patterns within and between 385–86
    risk prediction 231
positron emission tomography (PET), Alzheimer's
    disease 173, 176
postnatal life *see* early life
posttraumatic growth 351–52
posttraumatic stress disorder (PTSD), intimate partner
    violence 346, 348
preconception care 366*t*
preeclampsia 22
pregnancy 20
    Alzheimer's disease 177
    body mass index and 283
    body weight and 278
    breast cancer 190
    cardiovascular changes 386
    cardiovascular disease 25–26, 78–79
    COVID-19 pandemic 394
    depression risk factors 159
    growth hormone 247–48
    gynaecological cancers 207
    health behaviour effects 262
    hypertension 395
    hypothalamic–pituitary–adrenal axis 241
    leptin 246
    lifestyle interventions 360*f*, 363, 364*f*
    loss and cardiovascular disease 78–79
    multiple, early menopause 51–52
    outcomes of 22
    stressor effect 360, 361*f*

thyrotropic axis 243
time to *see* time to pregnancy (TTP)
premature ovarian insufficiency (POI) 50, 223–24
prenatal environment
    body weight and obesity 280
    breast cancer 192–93
    depression 156–57
    health effects 387
    reproductive health 22–23
preterm delivery, cardiovascular disease 78–79
preventative methods, knowledge transfer and 378
primary ovarian insufficiency 221
progestin-only contraceptive (POC) 99–100
progestin-releasing intrauterine devices (IUDs) 207
pro-inflammatory compounds 209
pro-opiomelanocortin (POMC) neurons 245
prostaglandins 212
proteomics 226–28
    definition 221
PRS (polygenic risk scores) 155–56
psychological distress 153–67
psychological stress 389
psychological symptoms, menopause 59
psychosocial exposures
    early life 388–89
    social inequalities in health 303–4
PTEN 205, 223
PTSD (posttraumatic stress disorder), intimate partner
    violence 346, 348
pubarche 238
puberty 19–20
    body mass index and 282–83
    breast cancer 191–92
    delayed 223–24
    depression 158
    first signs 238
    nutritional triggering 228
public health interventions 363–65
public health research 4–5

quality of life (QoL), endometriosis 36

RAD51 205
radiovascular health, reproductive health and 21–22
reconstituted families 314
record linkage studies, breast cancer 189
RECOVER trial 394–95
relational resources, social relationships 315–16
reproductive coercion 344–46
reproductive duration, type 2 diabetes 98
reproductive health 19–32
    adult environment 24
    childhood/adolescent environment 23–24
    COVID-19 pandemic 389
    endometriosis 39–40
    fertility 20
    genetic determinants 22
    health and 389–90
    indicator relationships 21–22
    interventions in 362*f*

reproductive health (*cont.*)
   lung function deficits/COPD 144–46
   menarche 19–20
   menopause 20–21
   noncommunicable diseases 25–26
   obesity 282–83
   policy implications 395–96
   pregnancy 20
   prenatal environment 22–23
   puberty 19–20
   social life and 389–91
   socioeconomic determinants 24
reproductive hormones, type 2 diabetes 97–100
resilience, violence against women 351–52
resistance exercises, type 2 diabetes 101–2
respiratory disease
   body weight 276–78
   COVID-19 pandemic 394
   experience in utero 362–63
   infections 140
   see also lung function
rheumatoid arthritis 334
RNA transcripts *see* transcriptomics
Royal College of Obstetricians and Gynaecology 9–10

sarcopenia 115
   definition 117
   obesity and 123
   see also musculoskeletal ageing
school-based activities 257–58
scRNA-seq (single-cell transcriptomics) 226
second-hand smoking 23–24
secular trends, social inequalities in health 299–300
sedentary behaviour
   type 2 diabetes 101–2
   see also physical activity
sensitive period model 5
Setler Model of Research Utilization 373
sex definition 4, 170
sex differences
   COPD 139–40
   lung disorders 136
   lung functions 139–40
   type 2 diabetes 93
sex steroids 158
sexual abuse 334
sexual activity 206–7
sexual assault 343–44
sexual health education 366*t*
SHBG 226–28
sibling studies, obesity 280
single cause-and-effect intervention models 365–67
single-cell transcriptomics (scRNA-seq) 226
single gene disorders 223–24
single nucleotide polymorphisms (SNPs) 222, 224, 225
   expression levels 228–29
   obesity 279
   personal/population risk prediction 231
   reproductive health 22
sleep disturbances, menopause 59

sleep patterns, COVID-19 pandemic 266
small-for-gestational age delivery 78–79
smoking 259*f*, 259–60
   breast cancer 190
   cardiovascular disease 75
   cessation of 265–66
   early menopause 52, 53–54
   endometriosis 38
   fibroids 57
   gynaecological cancers 209–10, 211
   health behaviour effects 262, 265
   income and 260
   lung function deficits/COPD 140, 143, 144
   obesity and 282
   second-hand smoking 23–24
   type 2 diabetes 102–3
SNPs *see* single nucleotide polymorphisms (SNPs)
social burden, body weight 276–79
social constructions, gender 328
social factors
   Alzheimer's disease 178
   cardiovascular disease 80
   depression 161
   early life 388–89
   early menopause 53–54
   health behaviours 257–61
   obesity 280–81
   reproductive life and 389–91
social impact, intimate partner violence 348
social inequalities in health
   physical development 302–3
   psychosocial exposures 303–4
social media 314–15
social relationships 313–25
   adolescence 314–15
   adult relationships 315–17
   early life 314–15
   health and well-being and 318–19
   isolation 316–17
   loneliness 316–17
   parental relationships 314
   partnerships 317
   relational resources 315–16
   social support 315–16
social support 315–16
societal gender inequality 349
society changes 390–91
socioeconomic inequalities 388
socioeconomic position (SEP) 295–312
   Alzheimer's disease 173–74
   associations 389
   breast cancer 190
   cardiovascular disease 79–80
   cross-study analysis 391
   definition 295–96
   early menopause 52
   family and work 298–99
   health behaviour effects 263–64
   health behaviours 258, 261–62, 263–64
   health inequalities 299–301

hysterectomy 56–57
intergenerational social mobility 296–98
measurement 295–96
obesity 280–81
type 2 diabetes 103–4
Socioemotional Selection Theory 316–17
solo parents 333
somatic symptoms, menopause 59
somatostatin 246
spirometry 136
chronic obstructive pulmonary disorder 140
Statistical Shape Modelling 120
STK11 205
stress
depression 156
health costs 333–34
pregnancy 360, 361*f*
type 2 diabetes 103
stroke 74
structural sexism 327–41
caregiving 329–31
life course dynamics 328–29
work history 329–31
Study of Women's Health across the Nation (SWAN) 77–78
sugar-based beverages 397
suicide
intimate partner violence 348
risk of 154–55
superficial endometriosis (SUP) 35
surgery, musculoskeletal ageing 115–16
surgical menopause 50, 54
definition 49
SVP (systolic blood pressure) 75–76, 84*f*
SWAN (Study of Women's Health across the Nation) 77–78
systolic blood pressure (SBP) 75–76, 84*f*

T1DM (type 1 diabetes mellitus) 95
T2DM *see* type 2 diabetes mellitus (T2DM)
tamoxifen 211
Tasmanian Longitudinal Health Survey 145
tau burden, sex differences 172
TCF7L2 93–94
temporal context, health behaviours 258–61
testosterone
female-to-male transsexuals 171
type 2 diabetes 97–98
thelarche 192
theories, models, framework (TMFs), knowledge
translation 373–75
thyroid disease 334
thyroid hormones 246
see also thyroxine (T4); triiodothyronine (T3)
thyroid-stimulating hormone (TSH) 242
ageing 243
birth 243
thyrotropic axis 239*f*, 242–43
ageing 243
changes across life course 242–43, 248*f*
development 242–43
pregnancy 243

thyrotropin-releasing hormone (TRH) 242
thyroxine (T4) 242
ageing 243
birth 243
time to pregnancy (TTP) 78
transcriptomics 226, 227*f*
definition 221
transgenerational epigenetic changes 346
trauma
health costs 334–35
intimate partner violence 348
TRH (thyrotropin-releasing hormone) 242
triiodothyronine (T3) 242
ageing 243
birth 243
TSH *see* thyroid-stimulating hormone (TSH)
tubal ligation, gynaecological cancers 210
twin studies 223
breast cancer 192–93
depression 162
early menopause 51–52
obesity 279
type 1 diabetes mellitus (T1DM) 95
type 2 diabetes mellitus (T2DM)
birth size 95
body weight 276–78
breastfeeding 100–1
child-onset 388
genetics 93–94
gestational diabetes and 100–1, 360
hormonal contraceptives 99–100
interuterine environment 95–97
lifestyle determinants 101–3
maternal adiposity 97
maternal hyperglycaemia 95–97
menarche 97–98
menopause 99
menstrual cycle 97–98
parent-of-offspring effects 94
parity 100–1
polycystic ovarian syndrome 98–99
prevalence 93
reproductive duration 98
reproductive hormones 97–100
socioeconomic position 103–4

UK Biobank 392
lung function deficits/COPD 145
obesity 279
omics studies 228
reproductive health 21–22
UK Labour Force Survey (2014-18) 297
UK Office of National Statistics Longitudinal
Study 297, 299
UNICEF 9–10
unmet needs, omic studies 232
urinary incontinence
behaviour change technique 379
menopausal transition 59
urinary tract infections 59

urogynaecological symptoms, menopause 59
US National Inpatient Sample 54
uterine bleeding 55
uterine cancer
   incidence 203
   see also gynaecological cancers
uterine fibroids 50, 54, 55–56, 204*t*, 208
   genome-wide association studies 230*t*
   gynaecological cancers and 208
   hysterectomy 55, 56
   smoking 57

vaccination programs 360*f*, 365
vasomotor symptoms (VMS), menopause 21,
   58–59
VAW *see* violence against women (VAW)
verbal memory
   Alzheimer's disease 171–72
   sex differences 170–71
violence against women (VAW) 343–56, 345*f*
   childhood and adult abuse 348
   contributing factors 343–44
   COVID-19 pandemic 350–51
   ecological understanding 344, 346*f*, 351*f*
   frequency and severity 350–51
   life course effect 348
   posttraumatic growth 351–52
   prevalence 343–44
   prevention 349–50
   resilience 351–52
   see also intimate partner violence (IPV)

visuospatial abilities, sex differences 170–71
vitamin D 209
VMS (vasomotor symptoms), menopause 21, 58–59
   see also vasomotor symptoms

waist circumference 274
waist-to-hip ratio 274
   endometriosis 40
weight *see* body weight
weight-for-height indices 273
Whitehall II study, type 2 diabetes 103
WHO *see* World Health Organization (WHO)
widowhood 298
Women's Health Initiative 59–60, 83, 195
Women's Health Initiative Memory Study
   (WHIMS) 176–77
Women's Health Plan (Scotland) 10
Women's Health Study 39
workplace
   health behaviours 257–58
   socioeconomic position (SEP) 298–99
   structural sexism 329–31
World Health Organization (WHO) 9–10, 117, 350,
   365–67, 372, 396
   Commission on Ending Childhood Obesity 365–67
   COVID-19 pandemic 350
   Framework convention on Tobacco Control
     (2003) 259
   obesity definition 273
   osteoporosis definition 117
   violence against women 350